DAT®

Seventh Edition

Related Kaplan Books

dent Essentials, Second Edition
Kaplan MCAT 2009–2010, Premier Program

DAT®

Seventh Edition

By the staff of Kaplan, Inc.

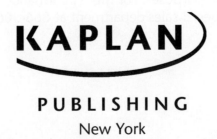

PUBLISHING
New York

© 2010 Kaplan, Inc.

Published by Kaplan Publishing, a division of Kaplan, Inc.
1 Liberty Plaza, 24th Floor
New York, NY 10006

Printed in the United States of America

10 9 8 7 6 5 4

ISBN-13: 978-1-60714-659-9

Kaplan Publishing books are available at special quantity discounts to use for sales promotions, employee premiums, or educational purposes. For more information or to purchase books, please call the Simon & Schuster special sales department at 866-506-1949.

CONTENTS

How to Use This Book

Kaplan's *DAT* is the most complete DAT preparation book available. All topics listed in the American Dental Association's Application and Preparation Materials for the DAT are included in this book. In addition to reviewing every single subject you'll need for the DAT, each chapter contains helpful notes, strategies, summaries, and pointers to help you maximize your study efforts. The margins also provide you with ample space to include your own notes. Each full-length practice DAT—one is included in the book, the other on online—will prepare you even further by simulating the complete test-taking experience. The explanations reinforce key concepts and test-taking strategies that will help you do your best on test day.

Here's how to use the various components of this book.

READ THE INTRODUCTORY SECTION

Kaplan's live DAT course has been the industry standard for decades. We've helped more people get into dental school than all the other courses combined. This section introduces you to the idiosyncrasies of the DAT and shows you how to take control of the test-taking experience on all levels.

STUDY THE TEST CONTENT

The quantity of material you need to know for the DAT is voluminous. Kaplan's *DAT* covers every subject in the Natural Sciences that you're likely to need for the test, and the Perceptual Ability chapters provide in-depth practice of each category. We also give you Reading Comprehension practice passages and a detailed review of the Quantitative Reasoning subjects.

Throughout this book, you'll see the following margin notes:

Kaplan Exclusive:
These boxes refer to material you can only find at Kaplan to give you the extra edge you need on test day.

DAT Synopsis:
These synopses are found on pages where lots of important and complex information is presented. In the days right before the DAT, make sure to review the Synopsis notes.

Real-World Analogy:
These sidebars provide "real-world" examples of important scientific principles. Being able to relate a concept to something you are familiar with from day-to-day life should help you understand and remember key information for test day.

Bridge:
We use "Bridges" to alert you to the conceptual links that occur between disciplines. Bridges contain specific chapter references for the other subjects.

Flashback:
Flashbacks refer to something you've seen earlier in the book.

TAKE KAPLAN'S FULL-LENGTH DAT PRACTICE TESTS

After you've learned valuable test-taking strategies and studied the test content, take the 2 full-length Practice Tests—timed, simulated DATs—as a test run for the real thing. The explanations for every question on the test are included in this book so you can understand your mistakes. Try not to confine your review to the explanations for the questions you've gotten wrong. Instead, read all of the explanations to reinforce key concepts and sharpen your skills.

REVIEW TO SHORE UP WEAK POINTS

If you find your performance was weak in any area, go back to the chapter in which that material was covered and review.

Different people have different learning styles. If after spending some time with this book, you feel that a live course with more individualized instruction and extensive opportunity for practice is what you need, **call us at 1-800-KAP-TEST**. We're here to help.

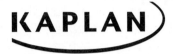

Available Online

FREE ADDITIONAL PRACTICE

kaptest.com/booksonline

As owner of this guide, you are entitled to get more DAT practice and help online. Log on to **kaptest.com/booksonline** to access a selection of DAT workshops and practice questions.

Access to this selection of online DAT practice material is free of charge to purchasers of this book. You'll be asked for a specific password derived from the text in this book, so have your book handy when you log on.

FOR ANY TEST CHANGES OR LATE-BREAKING DEVELOPMENTS

kaptest.com/publishing

The material in this book is up-to-date at the time of publication. However, the American Dental Association may have instituted changes in the test after this book was published. Be sure to read carefully the materials you receive when you register for the test. If there are any important late-breaking developments—or any changes or corrections to the Kaplan test preparation materials in this book—we will post that information online at **kaptest.com/publishing**.

FEEDBACK AND COMMENTS

kaplansurveys.com/books

We'd love to hear your comments and suggestions about this book. We invite you to fill out our online survey form at **kaplansurveys.com/books**. Your feedback is extremely helpful as we continue to develop high-quality resources to meet your needs.

Periodic Table of the Elements

Group**

Period	1 IA 1A	2 IIA 2A	3 IIIB 3B	4 IVB 4B	5 VB 5B	6 VIB 6B	7 VIIB 7B	8 ------- VIII ----- -- ------- 8 -------	9	10	11 IB 1B	12 IIB 2B	13 IIIA 3A	14 IVA 4A	15 VA 5A	16 VIA 6A	17 VIIA 7A	18 vIIIA 8A
1	1 H 1.008																	2 He 4.003
2	3 Li 6.941	4 Be 9.012											5 B 10.81	6 C 12.01	7 N 14.01	8 O 16.00	9 F 19.00	10 Ne 20.18
3	11 Na 22.99	12 Mg 24.31											13 Al 26.98	14 Si 28.09	15 P 30.97	16 S 32.07	17 Cl 35.45	18 Ar 39.95
4	19 K 39.10	20 Ca 40.08	21 Sc 44.96	22 Ti 47.88	23 V 50.94	24 Cr 52.00	25 Mn 54.94	26 Fe 55.85	27 Co 58.47	28 Ni 58.69	29 Cu 63.55	30 Zn 65.39	31 Ga 69.72	32 Ge 72.59	33 As 74.92	34 Se 78.96	35 Br 79.90	36 Kr 83.80
5	37 Rb 85.47	38 Sr 87.62	39 Y 88.91	40 Zr 91.22	41 Nb 92.91	42 Mo 95.94	43 Tc (98)	44 Ru 101.1	45 Rh 102.9	46 Pd 106.4	47 Ag 107.9	48 Cd 112.4	49 In 114.8	50 Sn 118.7	51 Sb 121.8	52 Te 127.6	53 I 126.9	54 Xe 131.3
6	55 Cs 132.9	56 Ba 137.3	57 La* 138.9	72 Hf 178.5	73 Ta 180.9	74 W 183.9	75 Re 186.2	76 Os 190.2	77 Ir 190.2	78 Pt 195.1	79 Au 197.0	80 Hg 200.5	81 Tl 204.4	82 Pb 207.2	83 Bi 209.0	84 Po (210)	85 At (210)	86 Rn (222)
7	87 Fr (223)	88 Ra (226)	89 Ac~ (227)	104 Rf (257)	105 Db (260)	106 Sg (263)	107 Bh (262)	108 Hs (265)	109 Mt (266)	110 --- ()	111 --- ()	112 --- ()		114 --- ()		116 --- ()		118 --- ()

Lanthanide Series*	58 Ce 140.1	59 Pr 140.9	60 Nd 144.2	61 Pm (147)	62 Sm 150.4	63 Eu 152.0	64 Gd 157.3	65 Tb 158.9	66 Dy 162.5	67 Ho 164.9	68 Er 167.3	69 Tm 168.9	70 Yb 173.0	71 Lu 175.0
Actinide Series~	90 Th 232.0	91 Pa (231)	92 U (238)	93 Np (237)	94 Pu (242)	95 Am (243)	96 Cm (247)	97 Bk (247)	98 Cf (249)	99 Es (254)	100 Fm (253)	101 Md (256)	102 No (254)	103 Lr (257)

ABOUT
THE DAT

INTRODUCTION TO THE DAT

The Dental Admission Test, affectionately known as the DAT, is designed to provide dental schools with common measures for comparing the qualifications of applicants. Dental schools use DAT scores to assess whether you possess the foundation upon which to build a successful dental career. In addition to evaluating your knowledge of the sciences, the test also calls for your skills in solving mathematical problems, reading comprehension, and spatial manipulation.

The DAT's power comes from its use as an indicator of your abilities. Good scores can open doors. Your power comes from preparation and mindset, because the key to DAT success is knowing what you're up against. And that's where this book comes in. We'll explain the test, review the sections one by one, share some of Kaplan's proven tips, provide you with practice questions and answers, and clue you in to what the test makers are really after. You'll get a handle on the process, find a confident new perspective, and achieve your highest possible scores.

A Fair Shake

The DAT may not be a perfect gauge of your abilities, but it's a relatively objective way to compare you with students from different backgrounds and undergraduate institutions.

REGISTRATION

The DAT is administered exclusively on computer and can be taken almost any day of the year. For the most up-to-date information regarding the exam, see the website of the American Dental Association at **ada.org** and follow the links. You'll have the opportunity to practice using the computer-based testing format at the testing center on the day of your actual DAT. The ADA also offers a computer-based tutorial on the mechanics of taking the electronic DAT at its website: **ada.org/prof/ed/testing/dat**.

To register for the DAT, pick up an Application and the DAT guide from your Pre-Med/Pre-Dental adviser, or visit ada.org to apply with credit card.

You can also write to:

ADA Department of Testing Services
211 East Chicago Avenue, Suite 600
Chicago, IL 60611
800-232-2162

After the application and fee are processed, you will receive a letter containing instructions to call an 800 number to register with the Prometric Candidate Contact Center for the DAT. By calling the 800 number, you will be able to arrange the day, time, and place to take the DAT. Prometric requires at least a 48-hour advance notice for scheduling a test. A current listing of Prometric Testing Centers can be found at www.2test.com. You are eligible to take the test for a 12-month period without reapplying. The DAT fee is $205.

For the paper (scannable form) application, fees are payable by certified check or money order. For online applications, fees are payable by credit card (Master Card or Visa).

On the day of your test, be sure to bring two forms of signed identification to the Prometric Testing Center. One of these must be a photo ID. The names on these forms of ID must match exactly the one in your application file. Don't bring study materials, cell phones, pagers, calculators, food, or drink into the testing room. You may want to bring a snack for the break (storage lockers will be provided). You will be given scratch paper to use during the test, and you will receive your score report immediately upon finishing the exam.

ANATOMY OF THE DAT

Before mastering the content and test-taking skills, you need to know exactly what you're dealing with on the DAT. It consists of four multiple-choice sections: Survey of the Natural Sciences, Perceptual Ability Test, Reading Comprehension, and Quantitative Reasoning. You will have a total of about four hours to complete the four sections. There is a 15-minute break (optional) after completing the second section.

It's a grueling experience, to say the least. If you can't approach it with confidence and stamina, you'll quickly lose your composure. That's why it's so important that you take control of the test.

In this book, we'll take an in-depth look at each DAT section, but here's a general overview.

Survey of the Natural Sciences

Time	90 minutes
Format	100 multiple-choice questions, subdivided into three science areas:
	Biology (40 questions)
	Inorganic (General) Chemistry (30 questions)
	Organic Chemistry (30 questions)
What it tests	Knowledge of university-level sciences

Perceptual Ability

Time	60 minutes
Format	90 multiple-choice questions, subdivided into six parts of 15 questions each:
	Keyholes (Apertures)
	Top-Front-End (Orthographic Projections)
	Angle Ranking
	Hole Punching
	Cube Counting
	Pattern Folding
What it tests	Ability to visualize and manipulate objects mentally in three dimensions; angle discrimination

Fill in the Blanks

There's no penalty for a wrong answer on the DAT, so never leave any question blank, even if you have time only for a wild guess.

Reading Comprehension

Time	60 minutes
Format	50 multiple-choice questions: three passages with 16–17 questions each
What it tests	ability to absorb and keep track of information in long, technical writings

Quantitative Reasoning

Time	45 minutes
Format	40 multiple-choice questions on the following topics:
	Fractions, Decimals, and Percents
	Algebra
	Word Problems
	Geometry
	Trigonometry
What it tests	Proficiency in mathematics and problem-solving skills

SCORING

You will get your score after you complete the test. Each DAT section receives its own score, based on a scale of 1–30. In addition, each Natural Sciences subsection (Biology, General Chemistry, and Organic Chemistry) also receives its own score. Finally, your scores in all sections *except* for the PAT are combined into an academic average based on the same scale.

Your score report will tell you (and dental schools) not only your scaled scores but also your percentile ranking.

Each question within a section is worth the same amount, and *there's no penalty for guessing*. That means that *you should always answer every question, whether you get to that question or not!* This is an important piece of advice, so pay it heed. Never let time run out on any section without answering every question.

Students often ask: What's a good score? Much depends on the strength of the rest of your application (if your transcript is first-rate, the pressure to strut your stuff on the DAT isn't as intense) and on where you want to go to school (different schools have different score expectations). However, recent statistics show that the average score per section is about 17.

You don't have to be perfect to do well. In the PAT section, for example, you can typically get 30 questions wrong (that's a third!) and still obtain a scaled score of 17. Even students who receive perfect scaled scores usually get a handful of questions wrong. It's important to maximize your performance on every question. Just a few questions one way or the other can make a big difference in your score.

KAPLAN'S TOP DAT TIPS

1. **Relax!**
    You don't have to get every question right to get a great score.

2. **Remember: It's primarily a thinking test.**
    Never forget the purpose of the DAT: It's designed to test your powers of analytical reasoning. You need to know the content, as each section has its own particular "language," but the underlying intention is consistent throughout the test.

3. **Avoid wrong-answer traps.**
    Try to anticipate answers before you read the answer choices. This helps boost your confidence and protects you from persuasive or tricky incorrect choices. Most wrong answer choices are logical twists on the correct choice.

4. **Think, think, think!**
    We said it before, but it's important enough to say again: Think. Don't compute.

5. **Don't look back.**
    Don't spend time worrying about questions you had to guess on. Keep moving forward. Don't let your spirit start to flag, or your attitude will slow you down. You can recheck answers within a section if you have time left, but don't worry about a section after your time has run out.

6. **Don't leave any questions unanswered.**
    There are no points taken off for wrong answers, so if you're not sure of an answer, *guess*. And guess quickly, so you'll have more time to work through other questions.

7. **Mark it up.**
    Take advantage of the "Mark" feature on the computer for questions you may want to revisit. At the end, you can review all the marked questions before submitting your answers as final. See the User's Guide to the CD-ROM at the back of this book for more information on this feature.

BIOLOGY

## 1

THE BASIS OF LIFE

ORIGIN OF LIFE
A. THE HETEROTROPH HYPOTHESIS

The first forms of life lacked the ability to synthesize their own nutrients; they required preformed molecules. These "organisms" were **heterotrophs**, which depended upon outside sources for food. The primitive seas contained **simple inorganic** and **organic** compounds such as salts, methane, ammonia, hydrogen, and water. **Energy** was present in the form of **heat, electricity, solar radiation**, including **X-rays** and **ultraviolet light, cosmic rays,** and **radioactivity**.

The presence of these building blocks and energy may have led to the synthesis of simple organic molecules such as sugars, amino acids, purines, and pyrimidines. These molecules dissolved in the "**primordial soup**," and after many years, the simple monomeric molecules combined to form a supply of macromolecules.

1. **Evidence of Organic Synthesis**
   In 1953, **Stanley L. Miller** set out to demonstrate that the application of ultraviolet radiation, heat, or a combination of these to a mixture of methane, hydrogen, ammonia, and water could result in the formation of complex organic compounds. Miller set up an apparatus in which the four gases were continuously circulated past electrical discharges from tungsten electrodes.

   After circulation of the gases for one week, Miller analyzed the liquid in the apparatus and found that an amazing variety of organic compounds, including **urea, hydrogen cyanide, acetic acid,** and **lactic acid,** had been synthesized.

2. **Formation of Primitive Cells**
   Colloidal protein molecules tend to clump together to form **coacervate droplets** (a cluster of colloidal molecules surrounded by a shell of water). These droplets tend to **absorb** and incorporate substances from the surrounding environment. In addition, the droplets tend to

possess a definite internal structure. It is highly likely that such droplets developed on the early earth. Although these coacervate droplets were not living, they did possess some properties normally associated with living organisms.

Most of these systems were **unstable**; however, a few systems may have arisen that were **stable** enough to survive. A small percentage of the droplets possessing favorable characteristics eventually developed into the first primitive cells. These first primitive cells probably possessed **nucleic acid polymers** and became capable of reproduction.

B. DEVELOPMENT OF AUTOTROPHS

The primitive heterotrophs slowly evolved complex **biochemical pathways**, which enabled them to use a wider variety of nutrients. They evolved **anaerobic respiratory processes** to convert nutrients into energy. However, these organisms required nutrients at a faster rate than they were being synthesized. Life would have ceased to exist if **autotrophic nutrition** had not developed. The pioneer autotrophs developed primitive **photosynthetic** pathways, capturing solar energy and using it to synthesize carbohydrates from carbon dioxide and water.

C. DEVELOPMENT OF AEROBIC RESPIRATION

The primitive autotrophs fixed **carbon dioxide** during the synthesis of carbohydrates and released molecular oxygen as a waste product. The addition of molecular oxygen to the atmosphere converted the atmosphere from a **reducing** to an **oxidizing** one. Some molecular oxygen was converted to ozone, which functions in the atmosphere to block high-energy radiation. In this way, living organisms **destroyed** the conditions that made their development possible. Once molecular oxygen became a major component of the earth's atmosphere, both heterotrophs and autotrophs evolved the biochemical pathways of aerobic respiration.

D. GENERAL CATEGORIES OF LIVING ORGANISMS

All living organisms can be divided into four basic categories. The **autotrophic anaerobes** include chemosynthetic bacteria. The **autotrophic aerobes** include the green plants and photoplankton. The **heterotrophic anaerobes** include yeasts. The **heterotrophic aerobes** include amoebas, earthworms, and humans.

BIOCHEMISTRY

Despite the uncertainties concerning the origin in life, it is well known that all living organisms share important characteristics. All living things are composed primarily of the elements carbon, hydrogen, oxygen, nitrogen, sulfur, and phosphorus. Traces of magnesium, iodine, iron, calcium, and other minerals are also components of **protoplasm**, the substance of life.

The unit of an element is the atom. The unit of a compound is the **molecule**. **Atoms** are joined by chemical bonds to form **compounds**. Water (H_2O), carbon dioxide (CO_2), and glucose ($C_6H_{12}O_6$) are some familiar compounds.

The chemical compounds in living matter can be divided into inorganic and organic compounds. **Inorganic compounds** are compounds that do not contain the element carbon, including salts and HCl. **Organic compounds** are made by living systems and contain carbon. They include carbohydrates, lipids, proteins, and nucleic acids.

In addition, various processes are required to maintain an organism's internal environment and regulate the basic activities of life. In this chapter and beyond, you will see how heredity, cellular organization, growth, development, reproduction, regulation, and homeostasis control the acquisition, conversion, and some of the uses of energy by a living organism.

THE CELL

The cell is the fundamental unit of all living things. Every function in biology involves a process that occurs within cells or at the interface between cells. Therefore, to understand biology, you need to appreciate the structure and function of different parts of the cell.

A. CELL THEORY

The cell was not discovered or studied in detail until the development of the microscope in the 17th century. Since then, much more has been learned, and a unifying theory known as the Cell Theory has been proposed.

The Cell Theory may be summarized as follows:

• All living things are composed of cells.

• The cell is the basic functional unit of life.

• Cells arise only from pre-existing cells.

• Cells carry genetic information in the form of **DNA**. This genetic material is passed from parent cell to daughter cell.

B. STUDYING THE CELL

Various tools are used to study the cell and its structure.

1. **Microscopy**
   Of the many tools used by scientists to study cells, the microscope is the most basic. **Magnification** is the increase in apparent size of an object. **Resolution** is the differentiation of two closely situated objects.

   a. **Compound Light Microscope**
      A compound light microscope uses two lenses or lens systems to magnify an object. The total magnification is the product of the magnification of the eyepiece and the magnification of the objective:

Total magnification = Magnification of eyepiece × Magnification of objective

      • The **diaphragm** controls the amount of light passing through the specimen.

- The **coarse adjustment** knob roughly focuses the image.
- The **fine adjustment** knob sharply focuses the image.

In general, light microscopy is used to observe nonliving specimens. Light microscopy requires contrast between cells and cell structures. Such contrast is obtained through staining techniques, which result in cell death.

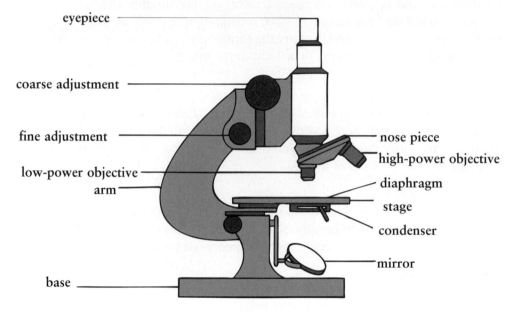

eyepiece

coarse adjustment

fine adjustment

low-power objective

arm

base

nose piece

high-power objective

diaphragm

stage

condenser

mirror

Figure 1.1

b. **Phase Contrast Microscopy**

A phase contrast microscope is a special type of light microscope that permits the study of living cells. Differences in refractive index are used to produce contrast between cellular structures. This technique does not kill the specimen.

c. **Electron Microscopy**

An electron microscope uses a beam of electrons to allow a thousandfold higher magnification than is possible with light microscopy. Unfortunately, examination of living specimens is not possible because of the preparations necessary for electron microscopy; tissues must be fixed and sectioned and, sometimes, stained with solutions of heavy metals.

2. **Centrifugation**

Differential centrifugation can be used to separate cells or mixtures of cells without destroying them in the process. Spinning fragmented cells at high speeds in the centrifuge will cause their components to sediment at different levels in the test tube on the basis of their respective densities. Denser parts, such as nuclei, endoplasmic reticulum, and mitochondria, will sink to the bottom.

CELL BIOLOGY

The components of the cell are specialized in their structure and function. These **organelles** include the nucleus, ribosomes, endoplasmic reticulum, Golgi apparatus, vesicles, vacuoles, lysosomes, mitochondria, chloroplasts, and centrioles.

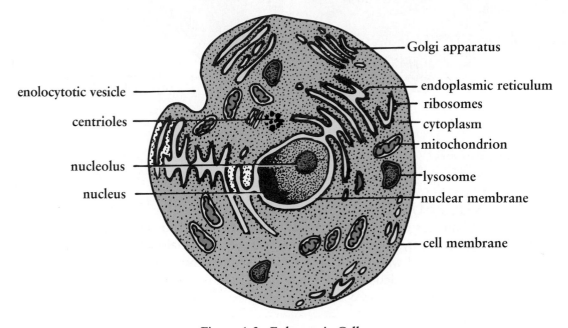

Figure 1.2. Eukaryotic Cell

A. CELL MEMBRANE

The cell membrane (plasma membrane) encloses the cell and exhibits selective permeability; it regulates the passage of materials into and out of the cell. According to the generally accepted **fluid mosaic model**, the cell membrane consists of a phospholipid bilayer with proteins embedded throughout. The lipids and many of the proteins can move freely within the membrane.

As a result of its lipid bilayer structure, a plasma membrane is readily permeable to both small, nonpolar molecules, such as oxygen, and small, polar molecules, such as water. Small charged particles are usually able to cross the membrane through protein channels. Some larger, charged molecules cross the membrane with the assistance of **carrier proteins.**

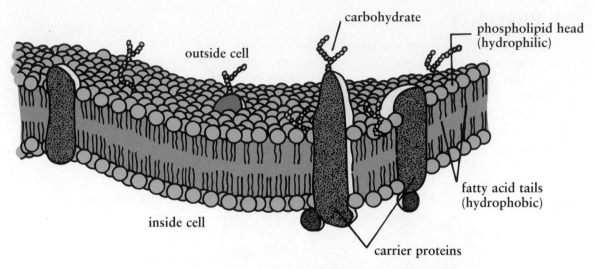

outside cell

carbohydrate

phospholipid head
(hydrophilic)

fatty acid tails
(hydrophobic)

inside cell

carrier proteins

Figure 1.3. Fluid Mosaic Model

B. NUCLEUS

The nucleus controls the activities of the cell, including cell division. It is surrounded by a nuclear membrane. The nucleus contains the DNA, which is complexed with structural proteins called **histones** to form **chromosomes**. The **nucleolus** is a dense structure in the nucleus where **ribosomal RNA** (rRNA) synthesis occurs.

C. RIBOSOME

Ribosomes are the sites of protein production and are synthesized by the nucleolus. Free ribosomes are found in the cytoplasm, while bound ribosomes line the outer membrane of the endoplasmic reticulum.

D. ENDOPLASMIC RETICULUM

The endoplasmic reticulum (ER) is a network of membrane-enclosed spaces involved in the transport of materials throughout the cell, particularly those materials destined to be secreted by the cell.

E. GOLGI APPARATUS

The Golgi apparatus receives vesicles and their contents from the smooth ER, modifies them (e.g. glycosylation), repackages them into vesicles, and distributes them to the cell surface by exocytosis.

F. MITOCHONDRIA

Mitochondria are the sites of aerobic respiration within the cell and, hence, the suppliers of energy. Each mitochondrion is bounded by an outer and inner phospholipid bilayer.

G. CYTOPLASM

Most of the cell's metabolic activity occurs in the cytoplasm. Transport within the cytoplasm occurs by **cyclosis** (streaming movement within the cell).

H. VACUOLE

Vacuoles and vesicles are membrane-bound sacs involved in the transport and storage of materials that are ingested, secreted, processed, or digested by the cell. Vacuoles are larger than vesicles and are more likely to be found in plant than in animal cells.

I. CENTRIOLES

Centrioles are a specialized **microtubule** involved in spindle organization during cell division and are not bound by a membrane. Animal cells usually have a pair of centrioles that are oriented at right angles to each other and lie in a region called the centrosome. Plant cells do not contain centrioles.

J. LYSOSOME

Lysosomes are membrane-bound vesicles that contain **hydrolytic enzymes** involved in intracellular digestion. Lysosomes break down material ingested by the cell. An injured or dying tissue may "commit suicide" by rupturing the lysosome membrane and releasing its hydrolytic enzymes; this process is called **autolysis**.

K. CYTOSKELETON

The cytoskeleton, composed of microtubules and microfilaments, gives the cell mechanical support, maintains its shape, and functions in cell motility.

TRANSPORT ACROSS THE CELL MEMBRANE

Substances can move into and out of cells in various ways. Some methods occur passively, without energy, while others are active and require energy expenditure (ATP) (see Figure 1.4).

> **KAPLAN) EXCLUSIVE**
>
> Not all cells have the same relative distribution of organelles. Form follows function: Cells that require a lot of energy for locomotion (e.g., sperm cells) have lots of mitochondria; cells involved in secretion (e.g., pancreatic islet cells) have lots of Golgi bodies; and cells such as red blood cells, which primarily serve a transport function, have no organelles at all!

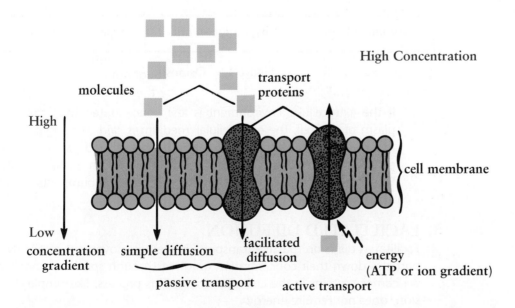

Figure 1.4. Movement Across Membranes

A. SIMPLE DIFFUSION

Simple diffusion is the net movement of dissolved particles down their concentration gradients—from a region of higher concentration to a region of lower concentration. This is a passive process that requires no external source of energy.

1. Osmosis

Osmosis is the simple diffusion of water from a region of lower solute concentration to a region of higher solute concentration. When the cytoplasm of a cell has a lower concentration of nonpenetrating solutes than the extracellular medium, the medium is said to be **hypertonic** to the cell, and water will flow out of the cell. This process, also called **plasmolysis**, will cause the cell to shrivel.

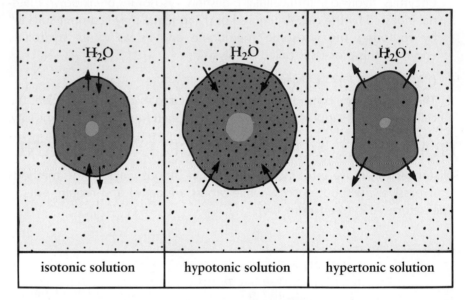

isotonic solution | hypotonic solution | hypertonic solution

Figure 1.5. Osmosis

If the extracellular environment is less concentrated than the cytoplasm of the cell, the extracellular medium is said to be **hypotonic**, and water will flow into the cell, causing it to swell and **lyse** (burst). For example, red blood cells will burst if placed in distilled water. Freshwater protozoa have contractile vacuoles to pump out excess water and prevent bursting.

B. FACILITATED DIFFUSION

Facilitated diffusion (passive transport) is the net movement of dissolved particles down their concentration gradient through special channels or via carrier proteins in the cell membrane. This process, like simple diffusion, does not require energy.

DAT Synopsis

Types of transport:

Passive diffusion
- Down gradient
- No carrier
- No energy required

Facilitated diffusion
- Down gradient
- Carrier
- No energy required

Active transport
- Against gradient
- Carrier
- Energy required

C. ACTIVE TRANSPORT

Active transport is the net movement of dissolved particles against their concentration gradient with the help of transport proteins. Unlike diffusion, active transport requires energy.

CIRCULATION

Circulation is the transportation of material within cells and throughout the body of a multicellular organism.

A. INTRACELLULAR CIRCULATION

Materials move about within a cell in a number of ways:

1. Brownian Movement
The movement of particles due to kinetic energy spreads small, suspended particles throughout the cytoplasm of the cell.

2. Cyclosis or Streaming
This is the circular motion of cytoplasm around the cell transport molecules.

3. Endoplasmic Reticulum
This provides channels throughout the cytoplasm and provides a direct continuous passageway from the plasma membrane to the nuclear membrane.

B. EXTRACELLULAR CIRCULATION

A number of systems have been devised to deal with the movement of materials on a larger scale, through the body of an organism:

1. Diffusion
If cells are in direct or close contact with the external environment, diffusion can serve as a sufficient means of transport for food and oxygen from the environment to the cells. In larger, more complex animals, diffusion is important for the transport of materials between cells and the interstitial fluid that bathes the cells.

2. Circulatory System
Complex animals, whose cells are too far from the external environment to transport materials by diffusion, require a circulatory system. This generally includes vessels to transport fluid and a pump to drive the circulation.

ENZYMES

Enzymes are organic catalysts. A catalyst is any substance that affects the rate of a chemical reaction without itself being changed. Enzymes are crucial to living things because all living systems must have **continuous, controlled** chemical activity. Enzymes regulate metabolism by speeding up or slowing down certain chemical reactions. They affect the reaction rate by decreasing the activation energy.

> ### DAT Synopsis
> Enzymes:
> - Lower activation energy of a reaction.
> - Increase the rate of the reaction.
> - Do not affect the overall ΔG of the reaction.
> - Are not changed or consumed in the course of the reaction.

Enzymes are **proteins**, and thus thousands of different enzymes can conceivably be formed. Many enzymes are conjugated proteins and have a nonprotein **coenzyme**. In these cases, both components must be present for the enzyme to function.

A. ENZYME SPECIFICITY

Enzymes are very selective; they may catalyze only one reaction or one specific class of closely related reactions. The molecule upon which an enzyme acts is called the **substrate**. There is an area on each enzyme to which the substrate binds called the **active site**. Two models describe the binding of the enzyme to the substrate:

1. **Lock and Key Theory**
   This theory holds that the spatial structure of an enzyme's active site is exactly complementary to the spatial structure of its substrate. The two fit together like a lock and key. This theory has been largely discounted.

2. **Induced Fit Theory**
   This more widely accepted theory describes the active site as having flexibility of shape. When the appropriate substrate comes in contact with the active site, the conformation of the active site changes to fit the substrate.

B. ENZYME REVERSIBILITY

Most enzyme reactions are reversible. The product synthesized by an enzyme can be decomposed by the same enzyme. An enzyme that synthesizes maltose from glucose can also hydrolyze maltose back to glucose.

C. ENZYME ACTION

Enzyme action and the reaction rate depend on several environmental factors, including temperature, pH, and the concentration of enzyme and substrate (see Figure 1.6 and 1.7).

1. **Effects of Temperature**
   In general, as the temperature increases, the rate of enzyme action increases until an optimum temperature is reached (usually around 40°C). Beyond optimal temperature, heat alters the shape of the active site of the enzyme molecule and deactivates it, leading to a rapid drop in rate.

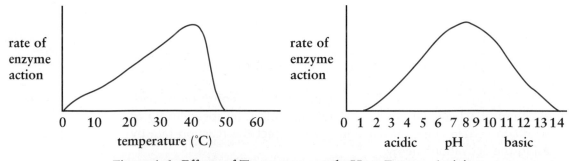

Figure 1.6. Effects of Temperature and pH on Enzyme Activity

2. **Effects of pH**

For each enzyme, there is an optimal pH above and below which enzymatic activity declines. Maximal activity of many human enzymes occurs around pH 7.2, which is the pH of most body fluids. Exceptions include **pepsin**, which works best in the highly acidic conditions of the stomach (pH = 2), and pancreatic enzymes, which work optimally in the alkaline conditions of the small intestine (pH = 8.5). In most cases, the optimal pH matches the conditions under which the enzyme operates.

3. **Effects of Concentration**

The concentrations of substrate and enzyme greatly affect the reaction rate. When the concentrations of both enzyme and substrate are low, many of the active sites on the enzyme are unoccupied,

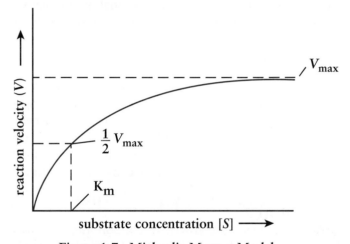

Figure 1.7. Michaelis-Menten Model

and the reaction rate is low. Increasing the substrate concentration will increase the reaction rate until all of the active sites are occupied. After this point, further increase in substrate concentration will not increase the reaction rate (the reaction has reached V_{max}).

D. EXAMPLES OF ENZYME ACTIVITY

Every reaction in the body is regulated by enzymes. Some of the basic reaction types are listed here:

1. **Hydrolysis**

Hydrolysis reactions function to digest large molecules into smaller components. **Lactase** hydrolyzes lactose to the monosaccharides glucose and galactose. **Proteases** degrade proteins to amino acids, and **lipases** break down lipids to fatty acids and glycerol.

In multicellular organisms, digestion can begin outside of the cells, in the gut. Other hydrolytic reactions occur within cells.

2. Synthesis

Synthesis reactions (including dehydrations) can be catalyzed by the same enzymes as hydrolysis reactions, but the directions of the reactions are reversed.

These reactions occurs in different parts of the cell. For example, protein synthesis occurs in the ribosomes and involves dehydration synthesis between amino acids.

Synthesis is required for growth, repair, regulation, protection, and production of food reserves, such as fat and glycogen, by the cell. The survival of an organism depends on its ability to ingest substances that it needs but cannot synthesize. Once ingested, these substances are converted into useful products.

Certain vitamin cofactors and essential amino acids cannot be synthesized by humans. If they are not available in the diet, deficiency diseases occur.

E. COFACTORS

Many enzymes require the incorporation of a nonprotein molecule to become active. These molecules, called **cofactors**, can be metal cations like Zn^{2+} or Fe^{2+} or small organic groups called coenzymes. Most coenzymes cannot be synthesized by the body and are obtained from the diet as vitamin derivatives. Cofactors that bind to the enzyme by strong covalent bonds are called **prosthetic groups**.

OVERVIEW OF CELLULAR RESPIRATION

Photosynthesis converts the energy of the sun into the chemical energy of bonds in compounds such as glucose. **Respiration** involves the conversion of the chemical energy in these bonds into the usable energy needed to drive the processes of living cells.

Carbohydrates and fats are the favored **fuel** molecules in living cells. As hydrogen is removed, bond energy is made available. The C–H bond is energy-rich; in fact, compared with other bonds, it is capable of releasing the largest amount of energy per mole. In contrast, carbon dioxide contains little usable energy. It is the stable, "energy-exhausted" end product of respiration.

During respiration, high-energy hydrogen atoms are removed from organic molecules. This is called **dehydrogenation** and is an oxidation reaction. The subsequent acceptance of hydrogen by a hydrogen acceptor (oxygen in the final step) is the reduction component of the redox reaction. Energy released by this reduction is used to form a high-energy phosphate bond in ATP. Although the initial oxidation step requires an energy input, the net result of the redox reaction is energy production. If all of this energy were released in a single step, little could be harnessed. Instead, the reductions occur in a series of steps called the **electron transport chain**.

GLUCOSE CATABOLISM

The degradative oxidation of glucose occurs in two stages, **glycolysis** and **cellular respiration**.

A. GLYCOLYSIS

The first stage of glucose catabolism is glycolysis (see Figure 1.8). Glycolysis is a series of reactions that lead to the oxidative breakdown of glucose into two molecules of **pyruvate** (the ionized form of pyruvic acid), the production of ATP, and the reduction of NAD^+ into NADH. All of these reactions occur in the **cytoplasm** and are mediated by specific enzymes.

1. Glycolytic Pathway

Note that at step 4, fructose 1,6-diphosphate is split into 2 three-carbon molecules: dihydroxyacetone phosphate and **glyceraldehyde 3-phosphate (PGAL)**. **Dihydroxyacetone phosphate** is isomerized into PGAL so that it can be used in subsequent reactions. Thus, 2 molecules of PGAL are formed per molecule of glucose, and all of the subsequent steps occur twice for each glucose molecule.

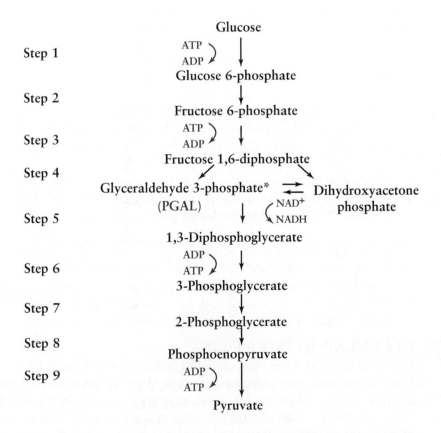

*NOTE: Steps 5–9 occur twice per molecule of glucose (see text).

Figure 1.8. Glycolysis

From 1 molecule of glucose (a six-carbon molecule), 2 molecules of pyruvate (a three-carbon molecule) are obtained. During this sequence of reactions, 2 ATP are used (in steps 1 and 3), and 4 ATP are generated (2 in step 6 and 2 in step 9). Thus, there is a net production of 2 ATP per glucose molecule. This type of phosphorylation is called **substrate-level phosphorylation**, since ATP synthesis is directly coupled with the degradation of glucose without the participation of an intermediate molecule such as NAD^+. One NADH is produced per PGAL, for a total of 2 NADH per glucose.

The net reaction for glycolysis is as follows:

$$Glucose + 2ADP + 2P_i + 2NAD^+ \rightarrow$$

$$2Pyruvate + 2ATP + 2NADH + 2H^+ + 2H_2O$$

At this stage, much of the initial energy stored in the glucose molecule has not been released and is still present in the chemical bonds of pyruvate. Depending on the capabilities of the organism, pyruvate degradation can proceed in one of two directions. Under **anaerobic** conditions (in the absence of oxygen), pyruvate is reduced during the process of fermentation. Under **aerobic** conditions (in the presence of oxygen), pyruvate is further oxidized during cell respiration in the mitochondria.

2. **Fermentation**

NAD^+ must be regenerated for glycolysis to continue in the absence of O_2. This is accomplished by reducing pyruvate into ethanol or lactic acid. Fermentation refers to all of the reactions involved in this process—glycolysis and the additional steps leading to the formation of ethanol or lactic acid. Fermentation produces only 2 ATP per glucose molecule.

Alcohol fermentation commonly occurs only in yeast and some bacteria. The pyruvate produced in glycolysis is converted to ethanol. In this way, NAD^+ is regenerated, and glycolysis can continue.

Lactic acid fermentation occurs in certain fungi and bacteria and in human muscle cells during strenuous activity. When the oxygen supply to muscle cells lags behind the rate of glucose catabolism, the pyruvate generated is reduced to lactic acid. As in alcohol fermentation, the NAD^+ used in step 5 of glycolysis is regenerated when pyruvate is reduced.

B. CELLULAR RESPIRATION

Cellular respiration is the most efficient catabolic pathway used by organisms to harvest the energy stored in **glucose**. Whereas glycolysis yields only **2 ATP** per molecule of glucose, cellular respiration can yield **36–38 ATP**. Cellular respiration is an **aerobic** process; **oxygen** acts as the final acceptor of the electrons that are passed from carrier to carrier during the final stage of glucose oxidation. The metabolic reactions of cell respiration occur in the eukaryotic mitochondrion and are catalyzed by reaction-specific enzymes.

Cellular respiration can be divided into three stages: pyruvate decarboxylation, the citric acid cycle, and the electron transport chain.

1. **Pyruvate Decarboxylation**
   The pyruvate formed during glycolysis is transported from the cytoplasm into the mitochondrial matrix where it is decarboxylated (i.e., it loses a CO_2), and the acetyl group that remains is transferred to coenzyme A to form acetyl CoA. In the process, NAD^+ is reduced to NADH.

2. **Citric Acid Cycle**
   The citric acid cycle is also known as the **Krebs cycle**. The cycle begins when the two-carbon acetyl group from acetyl CoA combines with oxaloacetate, a four-carbon molecule, to form the six-carbon citrate. Through a complicated series of reactions, 2 CO_2 are released, and oxaloacetate is regenerated for use in another turn of the cycle.

   For each turn of the citric acid cycle, 1 ATP is produced by substrate-level phosphorylation via a GTP intermediate. In addition, electrons are transferred to NAD^+ and FAD, generating NADH and $FADH_2$, respectively. These coenzymes then transport the electrons to the electron transport chain, where more ATP is produced via oxidative phosphorylation (see below). Studying the cycle, we can do some bookkeeping; keep in mind that for each molecule of glucose, 2 pyruvates are decarboxylated and channeled into the citric acid cycle.

2×3 NADH	6 NADH
2×1 FADH2	2 $FADH_2$
2×1 GTP (ATP)	2 ATP

   The net reaction of the citric acid cycle per glucose molecule is as follows:

   $$2\text{Acetyl CoA} + 6NAD^+ + 2FAD + 2GDP + 2P_i + 4H_2O \longrightarrow 4CO_2 + 6NADH + 2FADH_2 + 2ATP + 4H^+ + 2CoA$$

3. **Electron Transport Chain**
   The electron transport chain (ETC) is a complex carrier mechanism located on the inside of the **inner mitochondrial membrane**. During oxidative phosphorylation, ATP is produced when high-energy potential electrons are transferred from NADH and $FADH_2$ to oxygen by a series of carrier molecules located in the inner mitochondrial membrane. As the electrons are transferred from carrier to carrier, free energy is released, which is then used to form ATP. Most of the molecules of the ETC are **cytochromes**, electron carriers that resemble hemoglobin in the structure of their active site. The functional unit contains a central iron atom, which is capable of undergoing a reversible redox reaction; that is, it can be alternatively reduced and oxidized. Sequential redox reactions continue to occur as the electrons

are transferred from one carrier to the next; each carrier is reduced as it accepts an electron and is then oxidized when it passes it on to the next carrier. The last carrier of the ETC passes its electron to the final electron acceptor, O_2. In addition to the electrons, O_2 picks up a pair of hydrogen ions from the surrounding medium, forming water.

$$2H^+ + 2e^- + O_2 \longrightarrow H_2O$$

C. TOTAL ENERGY PRODUCTION

To calculate the net amount of ATP produced per molecule of glucose, we need to tally the number of ATP produced by substrate-level phosphorylation and the number of ATP produced by oxidative phosphorylation.

1. **Substrate-Level Phosphorylation**

   Degradation of 1 glucose molecule yields a net of 2 ATP from glycolysis and 1 ATP for each turn of the citric acid cycle. Thus, a total of 4 ATP are produced by substrate-level phosphorylation.

2. **Oxidative Phosphorylation**

   Two pyruvate decarboxylations yield 1 NADH each for a total of 2 NADH. Each turn of the citric acid cycle yields 3 NADH and 1 $FADH_2$, for a total of 6 NADH and 2 $FADH_2$ per glucose molecule. Each $FADH_2$ generates 2 ATP, as previously discussed. Each NADH generates 3 ATP except for the 2 NADH that were reduced during glycolysis; these NADH cannot cross the inner mitochondrial membrane and must transfer their electrons to an intermediate carrier molecule, which delivers the electrons to the second carrier protein complex, Q. Therefore, these NADH generate only 2 ATP per glucose. So the 2 NADH of glycolysis yield 4 ATP, the other 8 NADH yield 24 ATP, and the 2 $FADH_2$ produce 4 ATP for a total of 32 ATP by oxidative phosphorylation.

   The total amount of ATP produced during eukaryotic glucose catabolism is, therefore, 4 via substrate level phosphorylation plus 32 via oxidative phosphorylation for a total of 36 ATP. (For prokaryotes, the yield is 38 ATP, because the 2 NADH of glycolysis don't have any mitochondrial membranes to cross and therefore don't lose energy.)

Eukaryotic ATP Production per Glucose Molecule

Glycolysis

2 ATP invested (steps 1 and 3)	− 2 ATP
4 ATP generated (steps 6 and 9)	+ 4 ATP (substrate)
2 NADH × 2 ATP/NADH (step 5)	+ 4 ATP (oxidative)

Pyruvate Decarboxylation

2 NADH × 3 ATP/NADH	+ 6 ATP (oxidative)

Citric Acid Cycle

6 NADH × 3 ATP/NADH   +18 ATP (oxidative)

2 FADH$_2$ × 2 ATP/FADH$_2$ + 4 ATP (oxidative)

2 GTP × 1 ATP/GTP   + 2 ATP (substrate)

Total   **+36 ATP**

ALTERNATE ENERGY SOURCES

When glucose supplies run low, the body utilizes other energy sources. These sources are used by the body in the following preferential order: other carbohydrates, fats, and proteins. These substances are first converted to either glucose or glucose intermediates, which can then be degraded in the glycolytic pathway and the citric acid cycle.

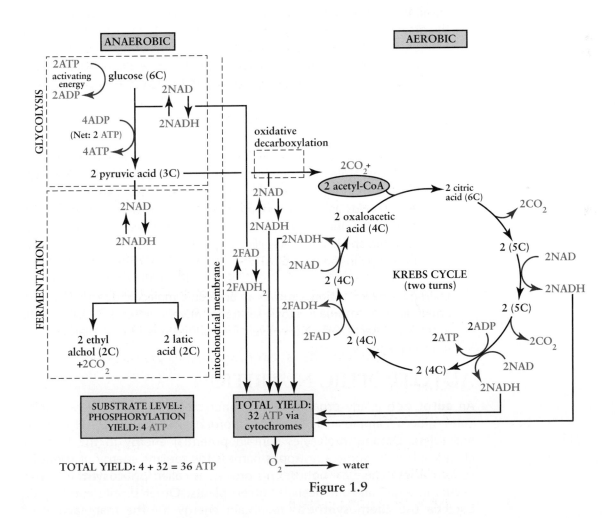

Figure 1.9

A. CARBOHYDRATES

Disaccharides are hydrolyzed into monosaccharides, most of which can be converted into glucose or glycolytic intermediates. Glycogen stored in the liver can be converted, when needed, into a glycolytic intermediate.

B. FATS

Fat molecules are stored in adipose tissue in the form of triglycerides. When needed, they are hydrolyzed by **lipases** to **fatty acids** and **glycerol** and are carried by the blood to other tissues for oxidation. Glycerol can be converted into PGAL, a glycolytic intermediate. A fatty acid must first be "activated" in the cytoplasm; this process requires 2 ATP. Once activated, the fatty acid is transported into the mitochondrion and taken through a series of beta-oxidation cycles that convert it into two-carbon fragments, which are then converted into acetyl CoA. Acetyl CoA then enters the TCA cycle. With each round of β-oxidation of a saturated fatty acid, 1 NADH and 1 $FADH_2$ are generated.

Of all the high-energy compounds used in cellular respiration, fats yield the greatest number of ATP per gram. This makes them extremely efficient energy-storage molecules. Thus, while the amount of glycogen stored in humans is enough to meet the short-term energy needs of about a day, the stored fat reserves can meet the long-term energy needs of about a month.

C. PROTEINS

The body degrades proteins only when not enough is carbohydrate or fat available. Most amino acids undergo a **transamination reaction** in which they lose an amino group to form an α-keto acid. The carbon atoms of most amino acids are converted into acetyl CoA, pyruvate, or one of the intermediates of the citric acid cycle. These intermediates enter their respective metabolic pathways, allowing cells to produce fatty acids, glucose, or energy in the form of ATP.

Oxidative deamination removes an ammonia molecule directly from the amino acid. **Ammonia** is a toxic substance in vertebrates. Fish can excrete ammonia, insects and birds convert it to uric acid, and mammals convert it into urea for excretion.

AUTOTROPHIC NUTRITION

An **autotroph** is any organism that manufactures its own organic molecules (glucose, amino acids, fats) from inorganic materials (CO_2, H_2O, mineral salts). Organic molecules contain potential energy in the form of chemical bonds. Some autotrophs harness the radiant energy of **sunlight** to form these chemical bonds. This process is called **photosynthesis** and occurs in algae and multicellular green plants. Other simple autotrophic bacteria use **chemosynthesis** to obtain energy for the manufacture of organic materials.

A. SUMMARY OF THE CALVIN CYCLE

Carbon dioxide is fixed to RBP (ribulose bisphosphate), a five-carbon sugar. The resulting unstable six-carbon molecule splits to form 2 molecules of PGA (phosphoglyceric acid). PGA is then phosphorylated and reduced (by ATP and NADPH) to form PGAL. Most of the PGAL is recycled to RBP by a complex series of reactions. In six turns of the Calvin cycle, 12 PGAL are formed from 6 carbon dioxide and 6 RBP. The 12 PGAL recombine to form 6 RBP and 1 molecule of glucose, the net product.

PGAL is generally considered the prime end product of photosynthesis, and it can be used as an immediate food nutrient; combined and rearranged to form monosaccharide sugars (e.g., glucose), which can be transported to other cells; or packaged for storage as insoluble polysaccharides, such as starch.

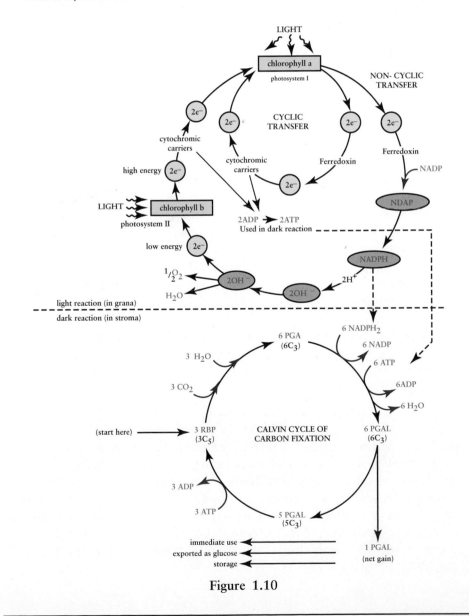

Figure 1.10

## 2

REPRODUCTION

Reproduction is the process by which an organism perpetuates itself and its species.

CELL DIVISION

Cell division is the process by which a cell doubles its organelles and cytoplasm, replicates its DNA, and then divides in two. For **unicellular organisms**, cell division is a means of reproduction, while for **multicellular organisms**, it is a method of growth, development, and replacement of worn-out cells. Cell division can follow two different courses, mitosis and meiosis.

A. MITOSIS

Mitosis is the division and distribution of the cell's DNA to its two daughter cells such that each cell receives a complete copy of the original genome. Nuclear division **(karyokinesis)** is followed by cell division **(cytokinesis)**. Prior to the initiation of mitosis, the cell undergoes a period of growth and replication of genetic material called interphase.

1. **Interphase**

   A cell normally spends at least 90 percent of its life in interphase. During this period, each chromosome is replicated so that during division, a complete copy of the genome can be distributed to both daughter cells. After replication, the chromosomes consist of two identical **sister chromatids** held together at a central region called the **centromere**. During interphase, the individual chromosomes are not visible. The DNA is uncoiled and is called **chromatin.** (Fact: Despite the number of sister chromatids, both structures are only one chromosome!)

> **DAT Synopsis**
>
> It's hard to believe but true—all the nucleated cells of your body, regardless of their structure and function, have the *exact* same chromosomes (including two sex chromosomes inside their nuclei). The only exceptions are the sex cells, which have only half the number of chromosomes as somatic cells. So the different cell types have differing structures and functions, not because their DNA is different but rather because the *expression* of what's coded in the DNA is unique to that cell type.

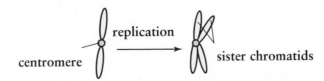

Figure 2.1. Chromosome Replication

2. **Prophase**

Centrosome

During prophase, the chromosomes condense, and the centriole pairs (in animals) separate and move towards the opposite poles of the cell. The spindle apparatus forms between them, and the nuclear membrane dissolves, allowing the spindle fibers to interact with the chromosomes.

3. **Metaphase**

The centriole pairs are now at opposite poles of the cell. The fibers of the spindle apparatus attach to each chromatid at the centromere to align the chromosomes at the center of the cell (equator), forming the **metaphase plate.**

4. **Anaphase**

The centromeres split so that each chromatid has its own distinct centromere, thus allowing sister chromatids to separate. The sister chromatids are pulled towards the opposite poles of the cell by the shortening of the spindle fibers. Spindle fibers are composed of microtubules.

5. **Telophase**

The spindle apparatus disappears. A nuclear membrane forms around each set of newly formed chromosomes. Thus, each nucleus contains the same number of chromosomes (the diploid number, 2N) as the original or parent nucleus. The chromosomes uncoil, resuming their interphase form.

6. **Cytokinesis**

Near the end of telophase, the cytoplasm divides into two daughter cells, each with a complete nucleus and its own set of organelles. In animal cells, a **cleavage furrow** forms, and the cell membrane indents along the equator of the cell and finally pinches through the cell, separating the two nuclei.

DAT Synopsis

Each chromatid is composed of a complete, double-stranded molecule of DNA. Sister chromatids are identical copies of each other. The term *chromosome* may be used to refer to either the single chromatid or the pair of chromatids attached at the centromere.

DAT Synopsis

Prophase: Chromosomes condense; spindles form.

Metaphase: Chromosomes align.

Anaphase: Sister chromatids separate.

Telophase: New nuclear membranes form.

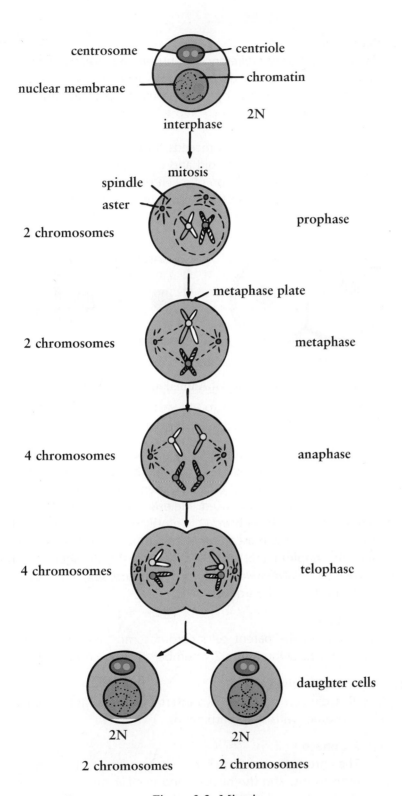

Figure 2.2. Mitosis

7. **Plant Cells**

There are two major differences between cell division in animal cells and plant cells. One is that plant cells lack centrioles. The spindle apparatus is synthesized by microtubule organizing centers, which are not visible.

Cytokinesis in animal cells proceeds through production of a cleavage furrow. Plant cells are rigid and cannot form a cleavage furrow. They divide by the formation of a **cell plate**, an expanding partition that grows outward from the interior of the cell until it reaches the cell membrane (see Figure 2.3).

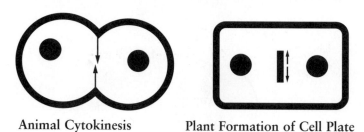

Animal Cytokinesis   Plant Formation of Cell Plate

Figure 2.3. Comparison of Animal and Plant Cell Division

B. MEIOSIS

Sexual reproduction differs from asexual reproduction in that two parents are involved. Sexual reproduction occurs via the fusion of two gametes—specialized sex cells produced by each parent. Meiosis is the process by which these sex cells are produced. Meiosis is similar to mitosis in that a cell duplicates its chromosomes before undergoing the process. However, while mitosis preserves the diploid number of the cell, meiosis produces the **haploid** (1N) number, halving the number of chromosomes. Meiosis involves two divisions of **primary sex cells**, resulting in four haploid cells called **gametes**.

1. **Interphase**

As in mitosis, the parent cell's chromosomes are replicated during interphase, resulting in the 2N number of sister chromatids.

2. **First Meiotic Division**

The first division produces two intermediate daughter cells with N chromosomes with sister chromatids.

a. **Prophase I**

The chromatin condenses into chromosomes, the spindle apparatus forms, and the nucleoli and nuclear membrane disappear. Homologous chromosomes (chromosomes that code for the same traits, one inherited from each parent), come together and intertwine in a process called **synapsis** (see Figure 2.4). Since at this stage, each chromosome consists of two sister chromatids, each synaptic pair of homologous chromosomes contains four chromatids and is, therefore, often called a **tetrad**. Sometimes chromatids of homologous chromosomes break at corresponding points and exchange equivalent pieces of DNA; this process is called **crossing over**. Note that crossing over occurs between homologous chromosomes and not between sister chromatids of the same chromosomes (the latter are identical, so crossing over would not produce any genetic variation). The chromatids involved are left with an altered but complete set of genes. Recombination among chromosomes results in increased genetic diversity within a species. Note that sister chromatids are no longer identical after recombination has occurred.

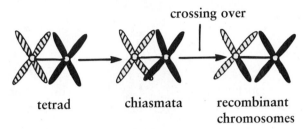

crossing over

tetrad   chiasmata   recombinant
                                   chromosomes

Figure 2.4. Synapsis

b. **Metaphase I**
Homologous pairs (tetrads) align at the equatorial plane, and each pair attaches to a separate spindle fiber by its kinetochore.

c. **Anaphase I**
The homologous pairs separate and are pulled to opposite poles of the cell. This process is called **disjunction**, and it accounts for a fundamental Mendelian law. During disjunction, each chromosome of paternal origin separates (or disjoins) from its homologue of maternal origin, and either chromosome can end up in either daughter cell. Thus, the distribution of homologous chromosomes to the two intermediate daughter cells is random with respect to parental origin. Each daughter cell will have a unique pool of genes from a random mixture of maternal and paternal origin.

d. **Telophase I**
A nuclear membrane forms around each new nucleus. At this point, each chromosome still consists of sister chromatids joined at the centromere.

3. **Second Meiotic Division**
This second division is very similar to mitosis, except that meiosis II is not preceded by chromosomal replication. The chromosomes align at the equator, separate and move to opposite poles, and are surrounded by a re-formed nuclear membrane. The new cells have the haploid number of chromosomes. Note that in human females, only one of these daughter cells becomes a functional gamete.

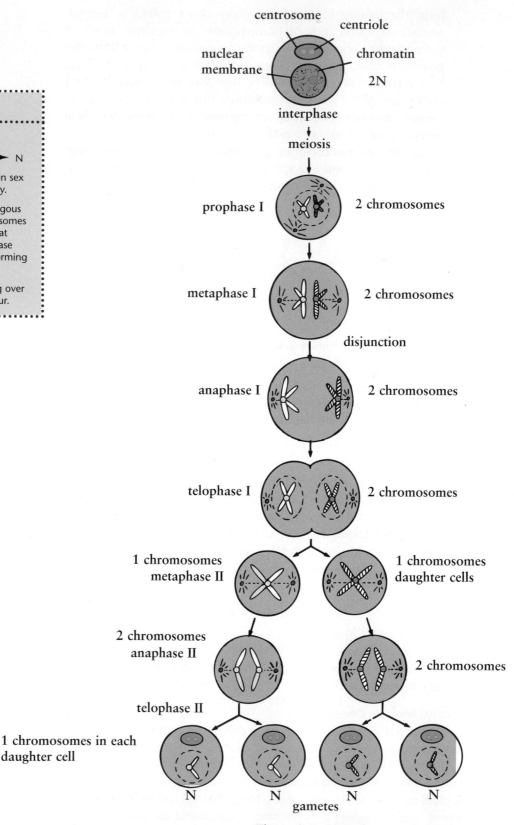

DAT Synopsis

Mitosis	Meiosis
2N → 2N	2N → N
Occurs in all dividing cells.	Occurs in sex cells only.
Homologous chromosomes don't pair up.	Homologous chromosomes pair up at metaphase plate, forming tetrads.
No crossing over.	Crossing over can occur.

centrosome
centriole
nuclear membrane
chromatin
2N
interphase
meiosis

prophase I   2 chromosomes

metaphase I   2 chromosomes

disjunction

anaphase I   2 chromosomes

telophase I   2 chromosomes

1 chromosomes metaphase II   1 chromosomes daughter cells

2 chromosomes anaphase II   2 chromosomes

telophase II

1 chromosomes in each daughter cell

N   N   N   N
gametes

Figure 2.5. Meiosis

SEXUAL REPRODUCTIVE MECHANISMS

Sexual reproduction differs from asexual reproduction in that two parents are involved and the end result is a genetically unique offspring. Sexual reproduction occurs via the fusion of two gametes—specialized sex cells produced by each parent. Sexual reproduction requires the following:

- The production of **functional sex cells** or **gametes** by adult organisms
- The union of these cells (**fertilization** or conjugation) to form a zygote
- The development of the zygote into another adult, completing the cycle

A. SEXUAL REPRODUCTION IN ANIMALS

Sexual reproduction in animals is a complex process involving the formation and fertilization of gametes and regulation of these processes by both parents.

1. Gonads

The gametes are produced in specialized organs called the gonads. The male gonads, called **testes**, produce sperm in the tightly coiled seminiferous tubules. The female gonads, called **ovaries**, produce **oocytes** (eggs). Some species are **hermaphrodites**, which have both functional male and female gonads. These include the hydra and the earthworm.

2. Spermatogenesis

Spermatogenesis, or sperm production, occurs in the seminiferous tubules. Diploid cells called spermatogonia undergo meiosis to produce four haploid sperm of equal size. The mature sperm is an elongated cell with a head, tail, neck, and body. The **head** consists almost entirely of the nucleus, which contains the paternal genome. The tail (**flagellum**) propels the sperm, while mitochondria in the neck and body provide energy for locomotion.

3. Oogenesis

Oogenesis, the production of female gametes, occurs in the ovaries. One diploid primary female sex cell undergoes meiosis in the ovaries to produce a **single mature egg**. Each meiotic division produces a **polar body**, which is a small cell that contains little more than the nucleus. The mature ovum is a large cell containing most of the cytoplasm, RNA, organelles, and nutrients needed by a developing embryo. The polar bodies rapidly degenerate.

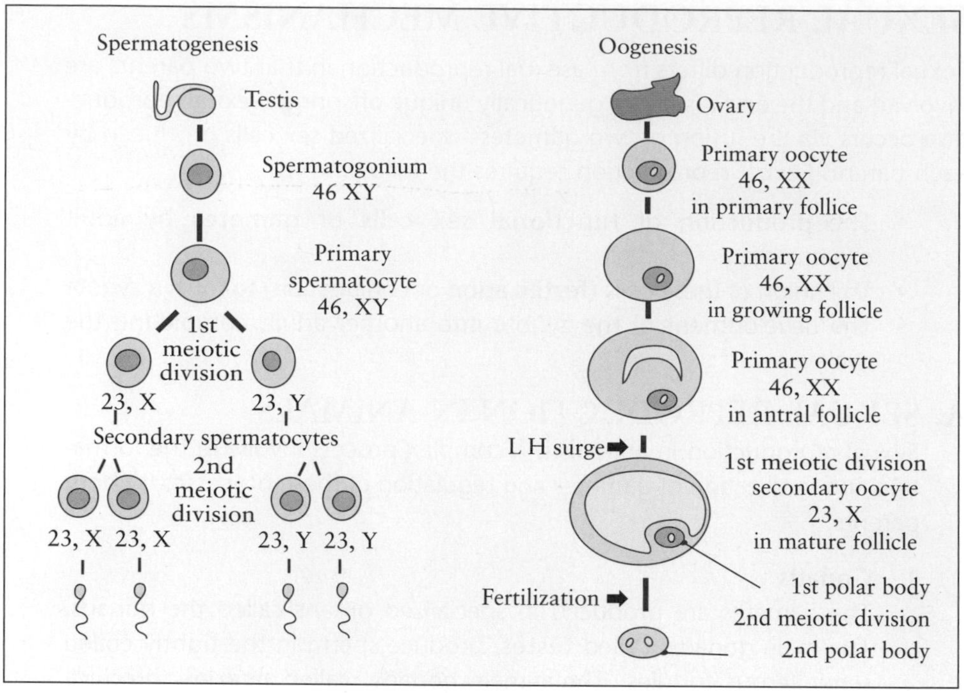

Figure 2.6. Normal Gametogenesis

4. Fertilization

Fertilization is the union of the egg and sperm nuclei to form a zygote with a diploid number of chromosomes.

a. External Fertilization

External fertilization occurs in vertebrates that reproduce in water (fish and amphibians). The female lays eggs in the water, and the male deposits sperm in the vicinity. The lack of direct passage of sperm from male to female reduces the chances of fertilization considerably. Many eggs must be laid to ensure some fertilization success. The sperm have flagella, enabling them to swim through the water to the eggs.

b. Internal Fertilization

Internal fertilization is practiced by terrestrial vertebrates and provides a direct route for sperm to reach the egg cell. This increases the chance for fertilization success, and females produce fewer eggs. The number of eggs produced is affected by other factors as well. If the early development of the offspring occurs outside of the mother's body, more eggs will be laid to increase the chances of offspring survival. The amount of parental care after birth is also related to the number of eggs produced. Species that care for their young produce fewer eggs.

B. HUMAN REPRODUCTION

1. Male Reproductive Physiology

The **testes** are located in an external pouch called the scrotum, which maintains testes temperature 2–4°C lower than body temperature, a condition essential for sperm survival. Sperm pass from the testes through the **vas deferens** to the ejaculatory duct and then to the **urethra**. The urethra passes through the penis and opens to the outside at its tip. In males, the urethra is a common passageway for both the reproductive and excretory systems. The testes are also the sites of production of **testosterone**. Testosterone regulates secondary male sex characteristics, including facial and pubic hair and voice changes.

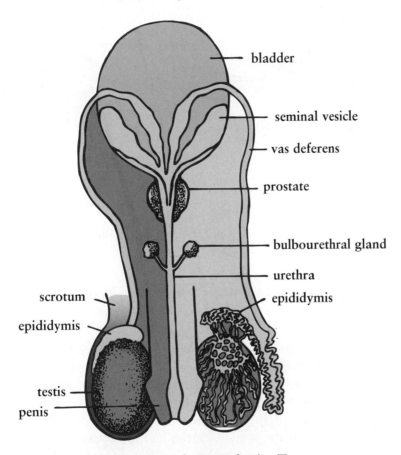

Figure 2.7. Male Reproductive Tract

DAT Synopsis

To remember the pathway of sperm, think Seven Up:

Seminiferous tubules
Epididymis
Vas Deferens
Ejaculatory Duct
(Nothing)
Urethra
Penis

2. Female Reproductive Anatomy

The **ovaries** are found in the abdominal cavity, below the digestive system. The ovaries consist of thousands of follicles; a **follicle** is a multilayered sac of cells that contains, nourishes, and protects an immature ovum. It is actually the follicle cells that produce estrogen. Once a month, an immature ovum is released from the ovary into the abdominal cavity and drawn into the nearby **oviduct**. Each fallopian tube opens into the upper end of a muscular chamber called the **uterus**, which is the site of fetal development. The lower, narrow end of the uterus is called the **cervix**. The cervix connects with the vaginal canal, which is the site of sperm deposition during intercourse and is also the passageway through which a baby is expelled during childbirth. At birth, all the eggs that a female will ovulate during her lifetime are already present in the ovaries.

3. **Female Sex Hormones**
The ovaries synthesize and secrete the female sex hormones, including estrogens and progesterone. The secretion of both estrogens and progesterone is regulated by LH and FSH, which, in turn, are regulated by GnRH.

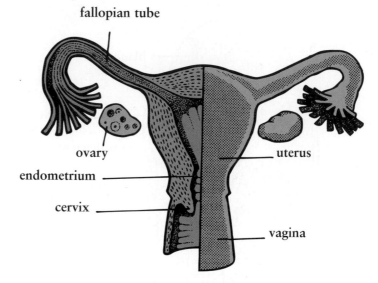

fallopian tube

ovary

endometrium

cervix

uterus

vagina

Figure 2.8. Female Reproductive Tract

a. **Estrogens**
Estrogens are steroid hormones necessary for normal female maturation. They stimulate the development of the female reproductive tract and contribute to the development of secondary sexual characteristics and sex drive. Estrogens are also responsible for the thickening of the **endometrium** (uterine wall). Estrogens are secreted by the ovarian follicles and the corpus luteum.

b. **Progesterone**
Progesterone is a steroid hormone secreted by the corpus luteum during the luteal phase of the menstrual cycle. Progesterone stimulates the development and maintenance of the endometrial walls in preparation for implantation.

4. **The Menstrual Cycle**
The hormonal secretions of the ovaries, the hypothalamus, and the anterior pituitary play important roles in the female reproductive cycle. From puberty through menopause, interactions among these hormones result in a monthly cyclical pattern known as the menstrual

cycle. The menstrual cycle may be divided into the follicular phase, ovulation, the luteal phase, and menstruation.

a. Follicular phase

The follicular phase begins with the cessation of the menstrual flow from the previous cycle. During this phase, **FSH** (follicle stimulating hormone) from the anterior pituitary promotes the development of the follicle, which grows and begins secreting estrogen.

DAT Synopsis

- Follicles mature during the follicular phase (FSH, LH).
- LH surge at midcycle triggers ovulation.
- Ruptured follicle becomes corpus luteum and secretes estrogen and progesterone to build up uterine lining in preparation for implantation; LH and FSH inhibited.
- If fertilization doesn't occur, corpus luteum atrophies, progesterone and estrogen levels decrease, menses occurs, and LH and FSH levels begin to rise again.

pituitary hormones

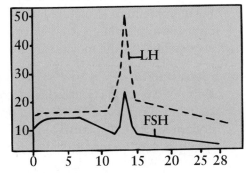

ovarian hormones

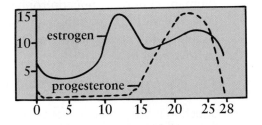

ovarian phases

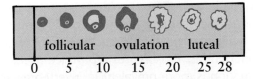

endometrial changes

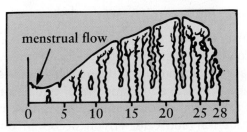

Figure 2.9

b. **Ovulation**

Midway through the cycle ovulation occurs—a mature ovarian follicle bursts and releases an ovum. Ovulation is caused by a surge in LH, which is preceded and, in part, caused by a peak in estrogen levels.

c. **Luteal phase**

Following ovulation, LH (luteinizing hormone) induces the ruptured follicle to develop into the **corpus luteum**, which secretes estrogen and progesterone. **Progesterone** causes the glands of the endometrium to mature and produce secretions that prepare it for the implantation of an embryo. Progesterone and estrogen are essential for the maintenance of the endometrium.

d. **Menstruation**

If the ovum is not fertilized, the corpus luteum atrophies. The resulting drop in progesterone and estrogen levels causes the endometrium (with its superficial blood vessels) to slough off, giving rise to the menstrual flow **(menses)**.

If fertilization occurs, the developing placenta produces **hCG** (human chorionic gonadotrophin), maintaining the corpus luteum and, thus, the supply of estrogen and progesterone that maintains the uterus, until the placenta takes over production of these hormones.

ASEXUAL REPRODUCTIVE MECHANISMS

Asexual reproduction is the production of offspring without **fertilization**. New organisms are formed by division of a single parent cell. Offspring are essentially genetic carbon copies of their parent cells. Thus, except for random mutations, the offspring are genetically identical to the parent cells. The different types of asexual reproduction are fission, budding, regeneration, and parthenogenesis. Prokaryotes reproduce asexually. Among animals, asexual reproduction is more prevalent in invertebrates than vertebrates. All **plants**, simple and complex, use asexual reproduction in some form.

A. FISSION

Binary fission is a simple form of asexual reproduction seen in prokaryotic organisms. The DNA replicates, and a new plasma membrane and cell wall grow inward along the midline of the cell, dividing it into two equally sized cells with equal amounts of cytoplasm, each containing a duplicate of the parent chromosome. A very similar process occurs in some primitive eukaryotic cells. Fission occurs in one-celled organisms, such as amoebae, paramecia, algae, bacteria.

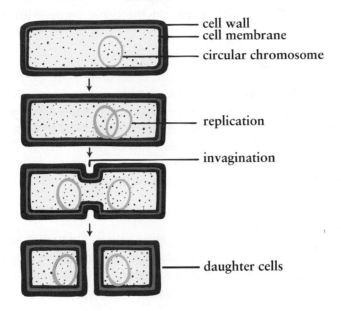

- cell wall
- cell membrane
- circular chromosome

- replication

- invagination

- daughter cells

Figure 2.10. Binary Fission

B. BUDDING

Budding is the replication of the nucleus followed by unequal cytokinesis. The cell membrane pinches inward to form a new cell, which is smaller in size but genetically identical to the parent cell and which subsequently grows to adult size. The new cell may separate immediately from the parent, or it may remain attached to it, develop as an outgrowth, and separate at a later stage. Budding occurs in hydra and yeast.

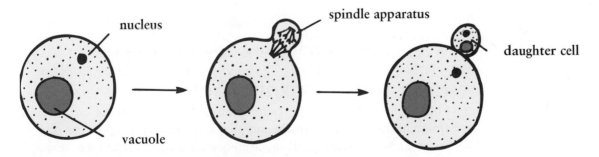

nucleus

spindle apparatus

daughter cell

vacuole

Figure 2.11. Budding

C. REGENERATION

Regeneration is the regrowth of a lost or injured body part. Replacement of cells occurs by mitosis. Some lower animals, such as hydra and starfish, have extensive regenerative capabilities. If a starfish loses an arm, it can regenerate a new one; the severed arm may even be able to regenerate an entire body, as long as the arm contains a piece of an area called the

central disk. Salamanders and tadpoles can generate new limbs (the extent of regeneration depends on the nerve damage to the severed body part).

D. PARTHENOGENESIS

Parthenogenesis is the development of an unfertilized egg into an adult organism. This process occurs naturally in certain lower organisms. For example, in most species of bees and ants, the males develop from unfertilized eggs, while the worker bees and queen bees develop from fertilized eggs. Artificial parthenogenesis can be performed in some animals. For example, the eggs of rabbits and frogs can be stimulated to develop without fertilization by electric shock or pinprick.

SEXUAL REPRODUCTION IN PLANTS

The life cycles of plants are characterized by an alternation of the diploid **sporophyte** generation and the haploid **gametophyte** generation. The relative lengths of the two stages vary with the plant type. In general, the evolutionary trend has been towards increased dominance of the sporophyte generation.

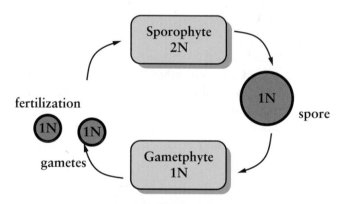

Figure 2.12. Alternating Generations of Plants

A. GAMETOPHYTE GENERATION

The haploid gametophyte generation produces **gametes** by mitosis. Union of the male and female gametes at fertilization restores the diploid sporophyte generation. Thus, the gametophytes reproduce sexually, while the sporophyte generation reproduces asexually.

GENETICS

Genetics is the study of how traits are inherited from one generation by the next. The basic unit of heredity is the **gene**. Genes are composed of **DNA** and are located on **chromosomes**. When a gene exists in more than one form, the alternative forms are called **alleles**. The genetic makeup of an individual is the individual's **genotype**; the physical manifestation of the genetic make-up is the individual's **phenotype**. Some phenotypes correspond to a single genotype, while other phenotypes correspond to several different genotypes.

MENDELIAN GENETICS

In the 1860s, Gregor Mendel developed the basic principles of genetics through his experiments with the **garden pea**. Mendel studied the inheritance of individual pea traits by performing genetic **crosses**: He took true-breeding individuals (which, if self-crossed, produce progeny only with the parental phenotype) with different traits, mated them, and statistically analyzed the inheritance of the traits in the progeny.

A. MENDEL'S FIRST LAW: LAW OF SEGREGATION

Mendel postulated four principles of inheritance:
1. Genes exist in alternative forms (now referred to as **alleles**).
2. An organism has **two alleles** for each inherited trait, one inherited from each parent.
3. The two alleles **segregate** during meiosis, resulting in gametes that carry only one allele for any given inherited trait.
4. If two alleles in an individual organism are different, only one will be fully expressed, and the other will be silent. The expressed allele is said to be **dominant**; the silent allele, **recessive**. In genetics problems, dominant alleles are typically assigned capital letters, and recessive alleles are assigned lower case letters. Organisms that contain two copies of the same allele are **homozygous** for that trait; organisms that carry two different alleles are **heterozygous**. The dominant allele appears in the phenotype. This is known as **Mendel's Law of Dominance**. In the cross shown on the following page, Yy will appear as yellow as YY.

Genes	Genotype	Phenotype
YY	Homozygous	Yellow
Yy	Heterozygous	Yellow
yy	Homozygous	Green

1. Monohybrid Cross

The principles of Mendelian inheritance can be illustrated in a cross between two true-breeding pea plants, one with purple flowers and the other with white flowers. Since only one trait is being studied in this particular mating, it is referred to as a **monohybrid cross**. The individuals being crossed are the **parental** or **P generation**; the progeny generations are the **filial** or **F generations**, with each generation numbered sequentially (e.g., F_1, F_2, etc.).

The purple flower parent has the genotype PP (i.e., it has two P alleles) and is homozygous dominant. The white flower parent has the genotype pp and is homozygous recessive. When these individuals are crossed, they produce F_1 plants that are 100 percent heterozygous (genotype = Pp). Since purple is dominant to white, all the F_1 progeny have the purple flower phenotype.

2. Punnett Square

One way of predicting the genotypes expected from a cross is by drawing a **Punnett square diagram**. The parental genotypes are arranged around a grid. Since the genotype of each progeny will be the sum of the alleles donated by the parental gametes, their genotypes can be determined by looking at the intersections on the grid. A Punnett square indicates all the potential progeny genotypes, and the relative frequencies of the different genotypes and plienotypes can be easily calculated (see Figure 3.2).

Parental: PP × pp

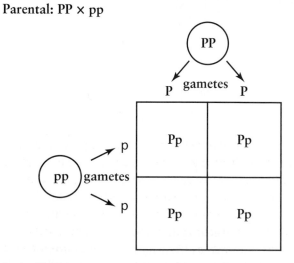

F_1 genotypes: 100% Pp (heterozygous)
F_1 phenotypes: 100% purple flowers

Figure 3.1. Monohybird Cross

When the F_1 generation from our monohybrid cross is self-crossed (i.e., Pp × Pp) the F_2 progeny are more genotypically and phenotypically diverse than their parents. Since the F_1 plants are heterozygous, they will donate a P allele to half of their descendants and a p allele to the other half. One-fourth of the F_2 plants will have the genotype PP, 50 percent will have the genotype Pp, and 25 percent will have the genotype pp. Since the homozygous dominant and heterozygous genotypes both produce the dominant phenotype, purple flowers, 75 percent of the F_2 plants will have purple flowers, and 25 percent will have white flowers (see Figure 3.2).

This is a standard pattern of Mendelian inheritance. Its hallmarks are the disappearance of the silent (recessive) phenotype in the F_1 generation and its subsequent reappearance in 25 percent of the individuals in the F_2 generation.

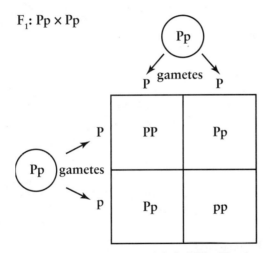

F_1: Pp × Pp

F_2 genotypes: 1:2:1; 1PP: 2Pp:1pp
F_2 phenotypes: 3:1; 3 purple:1 white

Figure 3.2. Self-Cross of F_1 Generation

3. **Testcross**

Only with a recessive phenotype can genotype be predicted with 100 percent accuracy. If the dominant phenotype is expressed, the genotype can be either homozygous dominant or heterozygous. Thus, homozygous recessive organisms always breed true. This fact can be used to determine the unknown genotype of an organism with a dominant phenotype. In a procedure known as a testcross or backcross, an organism with a dominant phenotype of unknown genotype (Ax) is crossed with a phenotypically recessive organism (genotype aa). Since the recessive parent is homozygous, it can donate only the recessive allele, a, to the progeny. If the dominant parent's genotype is AA, all of its gametes will carry an A, and thus all of the progeny will have genotype Aa. If the dominant parent's genotype is Aa, half of the progeny will be Aa and express the dominant phenotype, and half will be aa and express the recessive phenotype. In a testcross, the appearance of the recessive phenotype in the progeny indicates that the phenotypically dominant parent is genotypically heterozygous.

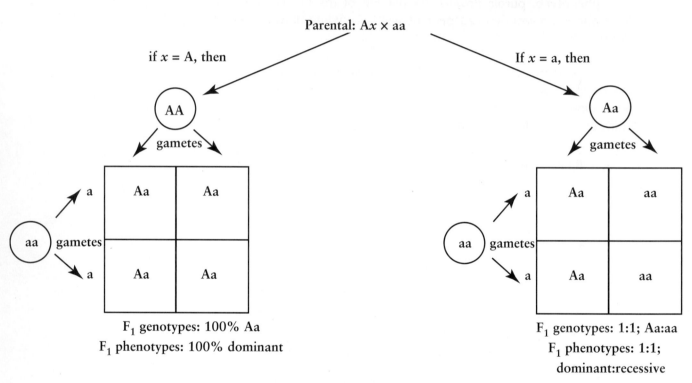

Figure 3.3. Testcross

B. MENDEL'S SECOND LAW: LAW OF INDEPENDENT ASSORTMENT

1. **Dihybrid Cross**

   The principles of the monohybrid cross can be extended to a dihybrid cross in which the parents differ in **two traits**, as long as the genes are on separate chromosomes and assort independently during meiosis. Genes on the same chromosome will stay together, unless **crossing over** occurs. Crossing over exchanges information between chromosomes and may break the linkage of certain patterns. For example, red hair is usually linked with freckles, but some blondes and brunettes have freckles as well.

   This is known as Mendel's law of independent assortment.

In the following example, a purple-flowered tall pea plant is crossed with a white-flowered dwarf pea plant; both plants are doubly homozygous (tall is dominant to dwarf, T = tall allele, t = dwarf allele; purple is dominant to white, P = purple allele, p = white allele). The purple parent's genotype is TTPP, so it produces only TP gametes; the white parent's genotype is ttpp and produces only tp gametes. The F_1, progeny will all have the genotype TtPp and will be phenotypically dominant for both traits.

When the F_1, generation is self-crossed (TtPp × TtPp), it produces four different phenotypes: tall purple, tall white, dwarf purple, and dwarf white, in the ratio 9:3:3:1, respectively. This is the typical pattern for Mendelian inheritance in a dihybrid cross between heterozygotes with independently assorting traits.

> ## DAT Synopsis
>
> Note that each trait assorts individually in a 3:1 ratio, as in a monohybrid cross. There are 9 purple tall and 3 purple dwarf, for a total of 12 purple; and there are 3 white tall and 1 white dwarf, for a total of 4 white. Hence, the purple:white ratio is 12:4 = 3:1. Likewise, the tall:dwarf ratio is 3:1.

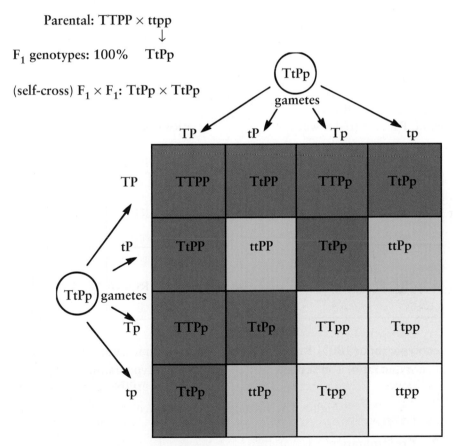

Parental: TTPP × ttpp

F_1 genotypes: 100% TtPp

(self-cross) F_1 × F_1: TtPp × TtPp

F_2 phenotypes: 9:3:3:1
9 tall purple:3 tall white:3 dwarf purple:1 dwarf white

Figure 3.4. Dihybird Cross

C. NON-MENDELIAN INHERITANCE PATTERNS

In real life, inheritance patterns are often more complicated than Mendel might have hoped. One major source of complications is in the relationship between **phenotype** and **genotype**. In theory, 100 percent of individuals with the recessive phenotype have a homozygous recessive genotype, and 100 percent of individuals with the dominant phenotype have either homozygous or heterozygous genotypes. Such clean concordance between genotype and phenotype is not always the case.

1. Incomplete Dominance

Some progeny phenotypes are apparently **blends** of the parental phenotypes. The classic example is flower color in snapdragons: Homozygous dominant red snapdragons, when crossed with homozygous recessive white snapdragons, produce 100 percent pink progeny in the F_1 generation. When F_1 progeny are self-crossed, they produce red, pink, and white progeny in the ratio of 1:2:1, respectively. The pink color is the result of the combined effects of the red and white genes in heterozygotes. An allele is incompletely dominant if the phenotype of the heterozygote is an intermediate of the phenotypes of the homozygotes.

snapdragons
R = allele for red flowers
r = allele for white flowers
Parental: RR × rr (red × white) F_1: Rr × Rr (pink × pink)

	R	R
r	Rr	Rr
r	Rr	Rr

	R	r
R	RR	Rr
r	Rr	rr

F_1 genotypic ratio: 100% Rr
F_1 phenotypic ratio: 100% pink

F_1 genotypic ratio: 1RR:2Rr:1rr
F_2 phenotypic ratio: 1 red:2 pink:1 white.

Figure 3.5. Incomplete Dominance

2. Codominance

Codominance occurs when **multiple alleles** exist for a given gene and more than one of them is **dominant**. Each dominant allele is fully dominant when combined with a recessive allele, but when two dominant alleles are present, the phenotype is the result of the expression of both dominant alleles simultaneously.

The classic example of codominance and multiple alleles is the inheritance of **ABO blood groups** in humans. Blood type is determined by three different alleles, I^A, I^B, and i. Only two alleles are present in any single individual, but the population contains all three alleles. I^A and I^B are both dominant to i. Individuals who are homozygous I^A or heterozygous I^Ai have blood type A, individuals who are homozygous I^B or heterozygous I^Bi have blood type B, and individuals who are homozygous ii have blood type O. However, I^A and I^B are codominant; individuals who are heterozygous I^AI^B have a distinct blood type, AB, which combines characteristics of both the A and B blood groups.

gametes	I^A	i
I^B	I^AI^B	I^Bi
i	I^Ai	ii

Figure 3.6. Blood Type Alleles

D. SEX DETERMINATION

Different species vary in their systems of sex determination. In sexually differentiated species, most chromosomes exist as pairs of homologues called **autosomes**, but sex is determined by a pair of **sex chromosomes**. All humans have 22 pairs of autosomes; additionally, females have a pair of homologous X chromosomes, and males have a pair of heterologous chromosomes, an X and a Y chromosome. The sex chromosomes pair during meiosis and segregate during the first meiotic division. Since females can produce only gametes containing the X chromosome, the gender of a **zygote** is determined by the genetic contribution of the **male gamete**. If the sperm carries a Y chromosome, the zygote will be male; if it carries an X chromosome, the zygote will be female. For every mating, there is a 50 percent chance that the zygote will be male and a 50 percent chance that it will be female.

Genes that are located on the X or Y chromosome are called **sex linked**. In humans, most sex-linked genes are located on the X chromosome, though some Y-linked traits have been found (e.g., hair on the outer ears).

> **DAT Synopsis**
>
> The odds of a child being a boy or a girl is 50 percent. That means that regardless of how many sons or daughters a couple might have, the odds of having a boy or girl the next time around remains 50 percent. Each fertilization is an independent event.

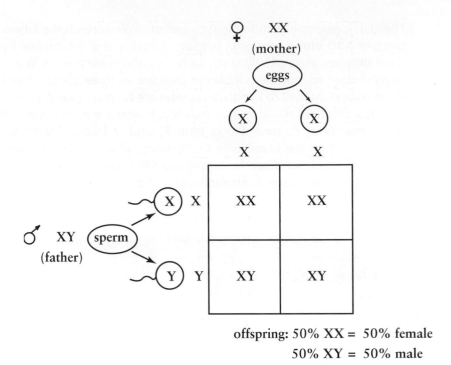

offspring: 50% XX = 50% female
50% XY = 50% male

Figure 3.7. Sex Determination in Humans

E. SEX-LINKAGE

In humans, females have two X chromosomes, and males have only one. As a result, recessive genes that are carried on the X chromosome will produce the recessive phenotypes whenever they occur in males, since no dominant allele is present to mask them. The recessive phenotype will thus be much more frequently found in males. Examples of sex-linked recessives in humans are the genes for **hemophilia** and for **color-blindness**.

The pattern of inheritance for a sex-linked recessive is somewhat complicated. Since the gene is carried on the X chromosome, and males pass the X chromosome only to their daughters, affected males cannot pass the trait to their male offspring. Affected males will pass the gene to all of their daughters. However, unless the daughter also receives the gene from her mother, she will be a phenotypically normal carrier of the trait. Since all of the daughter's male children will receive their only X chromosome from her, half of her sons will receive the recessive sex-linked allele. Thus, sex-linked recessives generally affect only males; they cannot be passed from father to son, but they can be passed from father to grandson via a daughter who is a carrier, thereby skipping a generation.

gametes	mother	
father	X^N	X^n
X^N	$X^N X^N$	$X^N X^n$
Y	$X^N Y$	$X^n Y$

Figure 3.8

F. *DROSOPHILA MELANOGASTER*

Modern work with the fruit fly (*Drosophila mefanogaster*) helped to provide explanations for Mendelian genetic patterns. The fruit fly provides several advantages for genetic research:
- It reproduces often (short life cycle).
- It reproduces in large numbers (large sample size).
- Its chromosomes (especially in the salivary gland) are large and easily recognizable in size and shape.
- Its chromosomes are few (4 pairs, 2n = 8).
- Mutations occur relatively frequently.

Through genetic and mutational analyses of *D. melanogaster*, scientists have elucidated the patterns of embryological development, discovering how genes expressed early in development can affect the adult organism.

G. ENVIRONMENTAL FACTORS

The environment can often affect the expression of a gene. Interaction between the environment and the genotype produces the phenotype. For example, *Drosophila* with a given set of genes have crooked wings at low temperature but straight wings at higher temperature.

Temperature also influences the hair color of the **Himalayan hare**. The same genes for color result in white hair on the warmer parts of the body and black hair on colder parts. If the naturally warm portions are cooled (e.g., by the application of ice), the hair will grow in black.

GENETIC PROBLEMS

Although genetic replication is very accurate, chromosome number and structure can be altered by abnormal cell division during meiosis or by mutagenic agents.

A. NONDISJUNCTION

Nondisjunction is either the failure of homologous chromosomes to separate properly during meiosis I or the failure of sister chromatids to separate properly during meiosis II. The resulting **zygote** might have either three copies of that chromosome, called **trisomy** (somatic cells will have 2N + 1 chromosomes), or a single copy of that chromosome, called **monosomy** (somatic cells will have 2N – 1 chromosomes). A classic case of trisomy is the birth defect **Down syndrome**, which is caused by trisomy of **chromosome 21**. Most monosomies and trisomies are lethal, causing the embryo to abort spontaneously early in the pregnancy.

Nondisjunction of the sex chromosomes may also occur, resulting in individuals with extra or missing copies of the X and/or Y chromosomes.

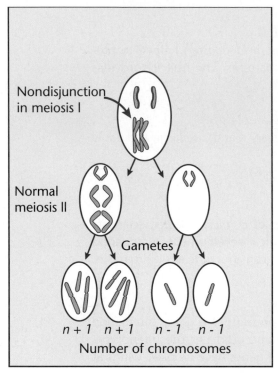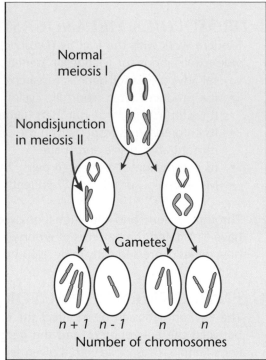

Figure 3.9

B. CHROMOSOMAL BREAKAGE

Chromosomal breakage may occur spontaneously or be induced by environmental factors, such as mutagenic agents and X-rays. The chromosome that loses a fragment is said to have a deficiency.

C. MUTATIONS

Mutations are changes in the genetic information of a cell, coded in the DNA. Mutations that occur in **somatic** cells can lead to tumors in the individual. Mutations that occur in the sex cells (**gametes**) will be transmitted to the offspring. Most mutations occur in regions of DNA that do not code for proteins and are silent (not expressed in the phenotype). Mutations that do change the sequence of amino acids in proteins are most often recessive and deleterious.

1. **Mutagenic Agents**
    Mutagenic agents induce mutations. These include cosmic rays, X-rays, ultraviolet rays, and radioactivity, as well as chemical compounds such as **colchicine** (which inhibits spindle formation, thereby causing polyploidy) or **mustard gas**. Mutagenic agents are generally also **carcinogenic**.

2. **Mutation Types**
    In a gene mutation, nitrogen bases are **added, deleted,** or **substituted,** thus creating different genes; inappropriate amino acids are inserted into polypeptide chains, and a mutated protein is produced. Therefore, a mutation is a genetic "error" with the "wrong" base or no base on the DNA at the particular position.

3. **Examples of Genetic Disorders**
    *   **Phenylketonuria** (PKU) is a molecular disease caused by the inability to produce the proper enzyme for the metabolism of **phenylalanine**. A degradation product (phenylpyruvic acid) accumulates.
    *   Sickle-cell anemia is a disease in which red blood cells become crescen shaped because they contain defective **hemoglobin**. The sickle-cell hemoglobin carries less oxygen. This disease is caused by a substitution of valine (GUA or GUG) for glutamic acid (GAA or GAG) because of a single base pair substitution in the gene coding for hemoglobin.

MOLECULAR GENETICS

Genes are composed of **DNA** (deoxyribonucleic acid), which contains information **coded** in the sequence of its base pairs, providing the cell with a blueprint for protein synthesis. These proteins regulate all life functions. Furthermore, DNA has the ability to **self-replicate**, which is crucial for cell division and, hence, for organismal reproduction. DNA is the basis of **heredity**; self-replication ensures that its coded sequence will be passed on to successive generations.

This is the central dogma of molecular genetics. DNA is **mutable** and can be altered under certain conditions, altering the corresponding characteristics in the organism. Changes in DNA are stable and can be passed from generation to generation, providing the basis for evolution.

A. STRUCTURE OF DNA
The basic unit of DNA is the **nucleotide**, which is composed of **deoxyribose** (a sugar) bonded to both a phosphate group and a nitrogenous base. There are two types of bases: **purines** and **pyrimidines**. The purines in DNA are **adenine** (A) and **guanine** (G), and the pyrimidines are **cytosine** (C) and **thymine** (T).

KAPLAN) EXCLUSIVE

If you have trouble remembering which bases are purines and which are pyrimidines, just think: CUT the PIE. Cytosine, Uracil and Thymine are PYrimidines Adenine and guanine are purines.

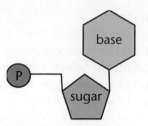

Figure 3.10. Nucleotide

The phosphate and sugar form a chain, with the bases arranged as side groups off the chain.

A DNA molecule is a **double-stranded helix** with the sugar-phosphate chains on the outside of the helix and the bases on the inside. T always forms two hydrogen bonds with A; G always forms three hydrogen bonds with C. This base-pairing forms "rungs" on the interior of the double helix that link the two polynucleotide chains together. This is known as the **Watson-Crick DNA Model**.

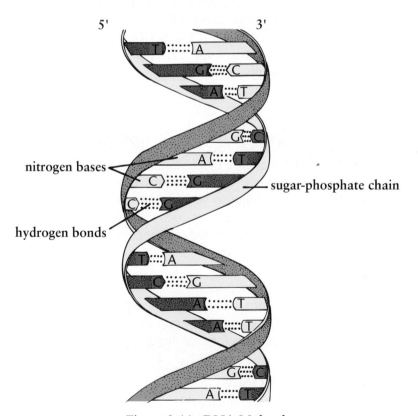

Figure 3.11. DNA Molecule

B. FUNCTION OF DNA

1. DNA Replication

The double-stranded DNA molecule unwinds and separates into two single strands. Each strand acts as a template for **complementary base-pairing** in the synthesis of two new daughter helices. Each new daughter helix contains an intact strand from the parent helix and a newly synthesized strand; thus, DNA replication is **semiconservative**. The daughter DNA helices are identical in composition to each other and to the parent DNA.

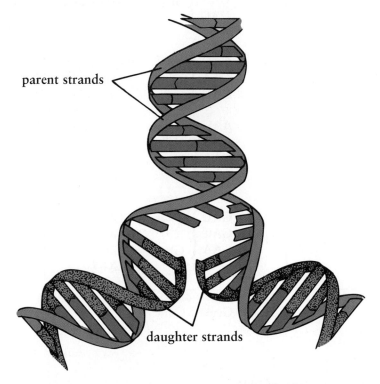

parent strands

daughter strands

Figure 3.12. Semiconservative Replication

2. The Genetic Code

The language of DNA consists of four "**letters**": A, T, C, and G. The language of **proteins** consists of 20 "words": the **20 amino acids**. The DNA language must be translated by mRNA in such a way as to produce the 20 words in the amino acid language; hence, the **triplet** code. The base sequence of mRNA is translated as a series of triplets, otherwise known as **codons**. A sequence of three consecutive bases codes for a particular amino acid (e.g., the codon GGC specifies glycine, and the codon GUG specifies valin). The genetic code is **universal** for almost all organisms.

Given that 64 different codons are possible based on the triplet code and only 20 amino acids need to be coded for, the code must

> **DAT Synopsis**
>
> Each codon represents only one amino acid, but most amino acids are represented by more than one codon.

contain **synonyms**. Most amino acids have more than one codon specifying them. This property is referred to as the **degeneracy** or **redundancy** of the genetic code.

First Base (5′)	Second Base: U	C	A	G	Third Base (3′)
U	UUU, UUC } Phe UUA, UUG } Leu	UCU, UCC, UCA, UCG } Ser	UAU, UAC } Tyr UAA, UAG } *Stop*	UGU, UGC } Cys UGA } *Stop* UGG } Trp	U C A G
C	CUU, CUC, CUA, CUG } Leu	CCU, CCC, CCA, CCG } Pro	CAU, CAC } His CAA, CAG } Gln	CGU, CGC, CGA, CGG } Arg	U C A G
A	AUU, AUC, AUA } Ile AUG } Start or Met	ACU, ACC, ACA, ACG } Thr	AAU, AAC } Asn AAA, AAG } Lys	AGU, AGC } Ser AGA, AGG } Arg	U C A G
G	GUU, GUC, GUA, GUG } Val	GGU, GGC, GGA, GGG } Ala	GAU, GAC } Asp GAA, GAG } Glu	GGU, GGC, GGA, GGG } Gly	U C A G

Figure 3.13. The Genetic Code

DAT Synopsis

DNA → DNA = replication (new DNA synthesized in 5′ → 3′ direction).
DNA → RNA = transcription (new RNA synthesized in 5′ → 3′ direction).
RNA → protein = translation (mRNA read in 5′ → 3′ direction).

C. RNA

1. The Structure of RNA

RNA, ribonucleic acid, is a polynucleotide structurally similar to DNA except that its sugar is **ribose**, it contains **uracil** (U) instead of thymine, and it is usually **single stranded**. RNA can be found in both the nucleus and the cytoplasm. There are several types of RNA, all of which are involved in some aspect of protein synthesis: mRNA, tRNA, and rRNA.

a. Messenger RNA (mRNA)

mRNA carries the complement of a DNA sequence and transports it from the **nucleus** to the **ribosomes**, where protein synthesis occurs. mRNA is assembled from ribonucleotides that are complementary to the "sense" strand of the DNA. The mRNA has the "inverted" **complementary** or negative codes of the original master on DNA. For example, since the DNA code for the amino acid valine is AAC, then the mRNA is the complementary UUG. mRNA is **monocistronic** (i.e., one mRNA strand codes for one polypeptide).

b. **Transfer RNA (tRNA)**

tRNA is a small RNA found in the cytoplasm that aids in the translation of mRNA's nucleotide code into a sequence of amino acids. tRNA brings amino acids to the ribosomes during protein synthesis. There is at least 1 type of tRNA for each amino acid; there are approximately 40 known types of tRNA.

c. **Ribosomal RNA (rRNA)**

rRNA, a structural component of ribosome, is the most abundant of all RNA types. rRNA is synthesized in the **nucleolus**.

D. PROTEIN SYNTHESIS

1. **Transcription**

Transcription is the process whereby information coded in the base sequence of DNA is transcribed into a strand of mRNA, which leaves the nucleus through nuclear pores. The remaining events of protein synthesis occur in the cytoplasm.

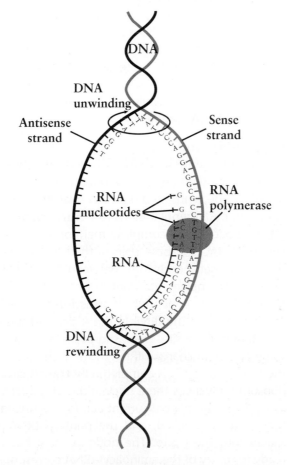

Figure 3.14.

2. Translation

Translation is the process whereby mRNA codons are translated into a sequence of amino acids. Translation occurs in the cytoplasm and involves tRNA, ribosomes, mRNA, amino acids, enzymes, and other proteins.

a. tRNA

tRNA brings amino acids to the **ribosomes** in the correct sequence for polypeptide synthesis; tRNA "recognizes" both the amino acid and the mRNA codon. This dual function is reflected in its three-dimensional structure: One end contains a three-nucleotide sequence, the **anticodon**, which is complementary to one of the mRNA codons; the other end is the site of amino acid attachment. Each amino acid has its own **aminoacyl-tRNA synthetase**, which has an active site that binds to both the amino acid and its corresponding tRNA, catalyzing their attachment to form an aminoacyl-tRNA complex.

b. Ribosomes

Ribosomes are composed of two subunits (consisting of proteins and rRNA), one large and one small, that bind together only during protein synthesis. Ribosomes have three binding sites: one for mRNA and two for tRNA. The latter are the P site (peptidyl-tRNA binding site) and the A site (aminoacyl-tRNA complex binding site). The P site binds to the tRNA attached to the growing polypeptide chain, while the A site binds to the incoming aminoacyl-tRNA complex.

c. Polypeptide synthesis

Polypeptide synthesis can be divided into three distinct stages: initiation, elongation, and termination. Synthesis begins when the ribosome binds to the mRNA near its 5′ end. The ribosome scans the mRNA until it binds to a **start codon** (AUG). The initiator aminoacyltRNA complex, methionine-tRNA (with the anticodon 3′-UAC-5′), base pairs with the start codon. In **elongation**, hydrogen bonds form between the mRNA codon in the A site and its complementary anticodon on the incoming aminoacyl-tRNA complex. A peptide bond is formed between the amino acid attached to the tRNA in the A site and the met attached to the tRNA in the P site. Following peptide bond formation, a ribosome carries uncharged tRNA in the P site and peptidyl-tRNA in the A site. The cycle is completed by **translocation**, in which the ribosome advances three nucleotides along the mRNA in the 5′ to 3′ direction. In a concurrent action, the uncharged tRNA from the P site is expelled, and the peptidyl-tRNA from the A site moves into the P site. The ribdome then has an empty A site ready for entry of the aminoacyl-tRNA corresponding to the next codon.

Polypeptide synthesis **terminates** when one of three special mRNA **termination codons** (UAA, UAG, or UGA) arrives in the A site. These codons signal the ribosome to terminate translation; they do not code for amino acids. Frequently, many ribosomes simultaneously translate a single mRNA molecule, forming a structure known as a **polyribosome**.

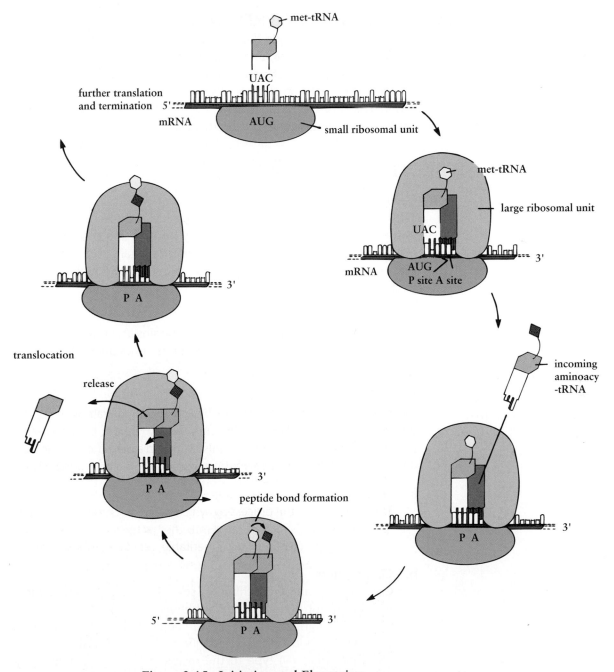

Figure 3.15. Initiation and Elongation

Following the release of the protein from the ribosome, the protein immediately assumes the characteristic native conformation. This conformation is determined by the **primary** sequence ot amino acids. Furthermore, the polypeptide chains can form intramolecular and intermolecular cross-bridges with **disulfide bonds**. The result is a complex, intertwined functional protein.

E. CYTOPLASMIC INHERITANCE

Heredity systems exist outside the nucleus. For example, **DNA** is found in **chloroplasts**, **mitochondria**, and other cytoplasmic bodies. These cytoplasmic genes may interact with nuclear genes and are important in determining the characteristics of their organelles. Drug resistance in many microorganisms is regulated by cytoplasmh rings of DNA known as **plasmids**, which contain one or more genes.

F. BACTERIAL GENETICS

1. **Bacterial Genome**

   The bacterial genome consists of a single circular chromosome located in the **nucleoid** region of the cell. Many bacteria also contain smaller circular rings of DNA called **plasmids**, which contain accessory genes. **Episomes** are plasmids that are capable of integration into the bacterial genome.

2. **Replication**

   Replication of the bacterial chromosome begins at a unique origin of replication and proceeds in both directions simultaneously. DNA is synthesized in the 5' to 3' direction.

3. **Genetic Variance**

   Bacterial cells reproduce by **binary fission** and proliferate very rapidly under favorable conditions. Although binary fission is an **asexual** process, bacteria have three mechanisms for increasing the genetic variance of a population: **transformation**, **conjugation**, and **transduction**.

   a. **Transformation**

      Transformation is the process by which a foreign chromosome fragment **(plasmid)** is incorporated into the bacterial chromosome via recombination, creating new, inheritable genetic combinations.

   b. **Conjugation**

      Conjugation can be described as **sexual mating** in bacteria; it is the transfer of genetic material between two bacteria that are temporarily joined. A cytoplasmic conjugation bridge is formed between the two cells, and genetic material is transferred from the donor male (+) type to the recipient female (−) type. Only bacteria containing plasmids called sex factors are capable of conjugating. The best studied sex factor is the **F factor** in *E. coli*.

Bacteria possessing this plasmid are termed F+ cells; those without it are called F-cells. During conjugation between an F+ and an F- cell, the F+ cell replicates its F factor and donates the copy to the recipient, converting it to an F+ cell. Genes that code for other characteristics, such as antibody resistance, may be found on the plasmids and transferred into recipient cells along with these factors.

Sometimes the sex factor becomes integrated into the bacterial genome. During conjugation, the entire bacterial chromosome replicates and begins to move from the donor cell into the recipient cell. The conjugation bridge usually breaks before the entire chromosome is transferred, but the bacterial genes that enter the recipient cell can easily recombine with the bacterial genes already present to form novel genetic combinations. These bacteria are called **Hfr** cells, meaning that they have a **high frequency of recombination**.

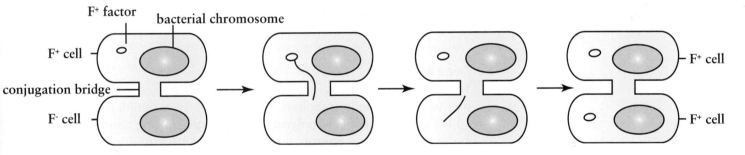

Figure 3.16. Conjugation

c. **Transduction**

   Transduction occurs when fragments of the bacterial chromosome accidentally become packaged into viral progeny produced during a viral infection. These virions may infect other bacteria and introduce new genetic arrangements through recombination with the new host cell's DNA. The closer two genes are to one another on a chromosome, the more likely they will be to transduce together. This fact allows geneticists to map genes to a high degree of precision.

d. **Recombination**

   Recombination occurs when linked genes are separated. It occurs by breakage and rearrangements of adjacent regions of DNA when organisms carrying different genes or alleles for the same traits are crossed.

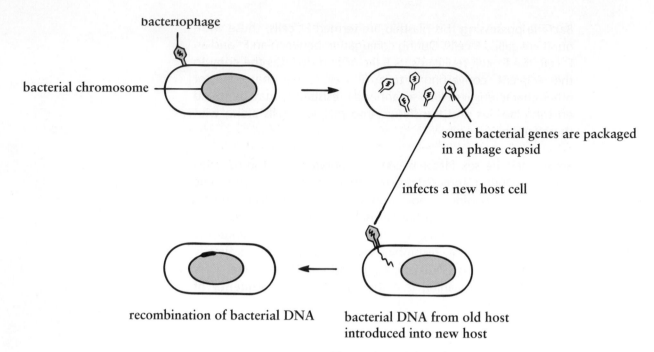

Figure 3.17. Transduction

4. **Gene Regulation**

The regulation of gene expression **(transcription)** enables prokaryotes to control their metabolism. Regulation of transcription is based on the accessibility of **RNA polymerase** to the genes being transcribed and is directed by an **operon**, which consists of **structural** genes, an **operator** gene, and a **promoter** gene. Structural genes contain sequences of DNA that code for **proteins**. The operator gene is the sequence of **nontranscribable** DNA that is the **repressor** binding site. The **promoter** gene is the noncoding sequence of DNA that serves as the initial binding site for RNA polymerase. There is also a **regulator** gene, which codes for the synthesis of a repressor molecule that binds to the operator and blocks RNA polymerase from transcribing the structural genes.

RNA polymerase must also move past the operator gene in order to transcribe the structural genes. Regulatory systems function by preventing or permitting the RNA polymerase to pass on to the structural genes. Regulation may be via **inducible systems** or **repressible systems**. Inducible systems are those that require the presence of a substance, called an **inducer**, for transcription to occur. Repressible systems are in a constant state of transcription unless a **corepressor** is present to inhibit transcription.

a. **Inducible Systems**

In an inducible system, the repressor binds to the operator, forming a barrier that prevents RNA polymerase from transcribing the structural genes. For transcription to occur, an inducer must bind to the repressor, forming an **inducer-repressor complex**. This complex cannot bind to the operator, thus permitting transcription. The proteins synthesized are thus said to be inducible. The structural genes typically code for an enzyme, and the inducer is usually the substrate, or a derivative of the substrate, upon which the enzyme normally acts. When the substrate (inducer) is present, enzymes are synthesized; when it is absent, enzyme synthesis is negligible. In this manner, enzymes are transcribed only when they are actually needed.

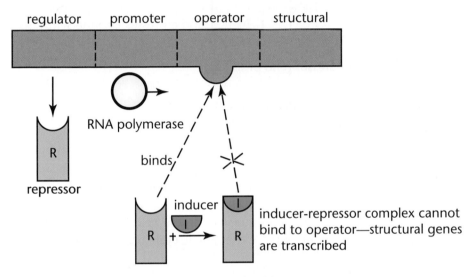

Figure 3.18. Inducible System

b. Repressible Systems

In a repressible system, the repressor is inactive until it combines with the corepressor. The repressor can bind to the operator and prevent transcription only when it has formed a repressor-corepressor complex. Corepressors are often the **end products** of the biosynthetic pathways they control. The proteins produced (usually enzymes) are said to be repressible since they are normally being synthesized; transcription and translation occur until the corepressor is synthesized. Operons containing mutations such as deletions or whose regulator genes code for defective repressors are incapable of being turned off have enzymes that are always being synthesized. These operons are referred to as **constitutive**.

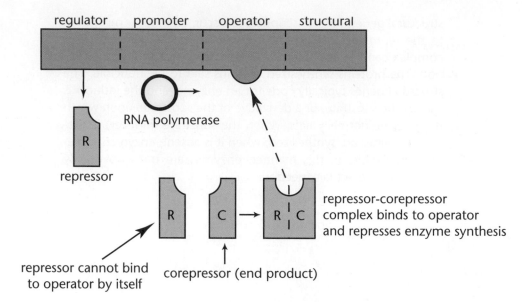

Figure 3.19. Repressible System

G. BACTERIOPHAGE

A bacteriophage is a virus that infects its host bacterium by attaching to it, boring a hole through the bacterial cell wall, and injecting its DNA while its protein coat remains attached to the cell wall. Once inside its host, the bacteriophage enters either a lytic cycle or a lysogenic cycle.

1. **Lytic Cycle**

   The phage DNA takes control of the bacterium's genetic machinery and manufactures numerous progeny. The bacterial cell then bursts **(lyses)**, releasing new virions, each capable of infecting other bacteria. Bacteriophages that replicate by the lytic cycle, killing their host cells, are called virulent. If the initial infection takes place on a bacterial **lawn** (a plated culture), then very shortly a **plaque** or clearing in the lawn occurs corresponding to the area of lysed bacteria. The physical characteristics of a plaque are useful in identifying mutant phage strains that may arise.

2. **Lysogenic Cycle**

   If the bacteriophage does not lyse its host cell, it becomes **integrated** into the bacterial genome in a harmless form (prophage), lying dormant for one or more generations. The virus may stay integrated indefinitely, replicating along with the bacterial genome. However, either spontaneously or as a result of environmental circumstances (*e.g.*, radiation, ultraviolet light, or chemicals), the prophage can re-emerge and enter a lytic cycle. Bacteria containing prophages are resistant to further infection ("superinfection") by similar phages.

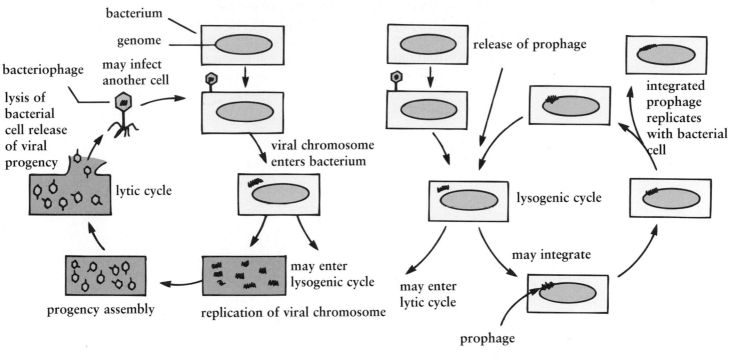

Figure 3.20. Bacteriophage Lifecycle

GENETIC TECHNOLOGY

Several techniques have proved very useful in the study of molecular genetics.

Southern blots allow for the detection of a specific DNA sequence in a specific DNA sample. In this process, DNA is cleaved into restriction fragments by restriction endonucleases that cut at specific restriction sites. Then, the fragments can be separated by gel electrophoresis. Finally, the desired sequence is detected by washing a radioactively labeled probe over a paper containing the gel's pattern.

DNA ligase joins DNA fragments by catalyzing the formation of phosphodiester bonds between DNA nucleotides.

Polymerase chain reaction (or PCR) is used for amplification of genes. PCR is composed of three steps: denaturation, primer annealing, and primer extension. First, the DNA is denatured with heat to separate the strands. A single strand acts as the template DNA, and it holds the specific sequence that needs to be amplified. In the annealing step, complementary nucleotides called primers join the single-stranded templates. Then, DNA polymerase joins deoxynucleotide triphosphates (dNTPs) to the primers, leading to the addition of nucleotides complementary to the template.

Another way to amplify genes is through **cloning DNA in bacteria**. This involves the ligation of the DNA sequence of interest with vector DNA fragments. Vector fragments are most often self-replicating phages or plasmids. Once this recombinant molecule is formed, it can be inserted into a bacteria strain, which, through transformation, will produce identical copies of the DNA.

## 4

VERTEBRATE EMBRYOLOGY

Embryology is the study of the development of a unicellular zygote into a complete multicellular organism. In the course of nine months, a unicellular human zygote undergoes cell division, cellular differentiation, and morphogenesis in preparation for life outside the uterus. Much of what is known about mammalian development stems from the study of less complex organisms, such as sea urchins and frogs.

EARLY DEVELOPMENTAL STAGES

A. FERTILIZATION

An egg can be fertilized within 12–24 hours following ovulation. Fertilization occurs in the lateral, widest portion of the oviduct when sperm traveling from the vagina encounter an egg. If more than one egg is fertilized, **fraternal twins** may be conceived.

B. CLEAVAGE

Early embryonic development is characterized by a series of rapid mitotic divisions known as cleavage. These divisions lead to an increase in cell number without a corresponding growth in cell protoplasm (i.e., the total volume of cytoplasm remains constant). Thus, cleavage results in progressively smaller cells, with an increasing ratio of nuclear to cytoplasmic material. Cleavage also increases the surface-to-volume ratio of each cell, thereby improving gas and nutrient exchange. An **indeterminate cleavage** is one that results in cells that maintain the ability to develop into a complete organism. **Identical twins** are the result of an indeterminate cleavage. A **determinate cleavage** results in cells whose future differentiation pathways are determined at an early developmental stage. Differentiation is the specialization of cells that occurs during development.

The first complete cleavage of the zygote occurs approximately 32 hours after fertilization. The second cleavage occurs after 60 hours, and the third cleavage after approximately 72 hours, at which point the eight-celled embryo reaches the uterus. As cell division continues, a solid ball of embryonic cells, known as the **morula**, is formed. **Blastulation** begins when the morula develops a fluid-filled cavity called the **blastocoel**, which by the fourth day becomes a hollow sphere of cells called the **blastula**.

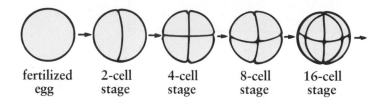

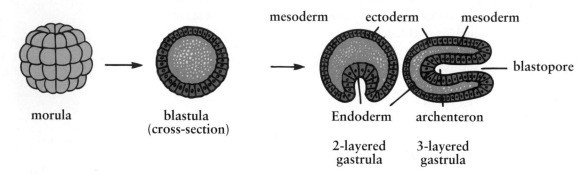

Figure 4.1. Amphibian Cleavage and Gastrulation

C. GASTRULATION

Once implanted in the uterus, cell migrations transform the single-cell layer of the blastula into a three-layered structure called a gastrula. These three primary germ layers are responsible for the differential development of the tissues, organs, and systems of the body at later stages of growth.

- **Ectoderm:** Integument (including the epidermis; hair; nails; and epithelium of the nose, mouth, and anal canal), the lens of the eye, the retina, and the nervous system
- **Endoderm:** Epithelial linings of the digestive and respiratory tracts (including die lungs) and parts of the liver, pancreas, thyroid, and bladder lining
- **Mesoderm:** Musculoskeletal system, circulatory system, excretory system, gonads, connective tissue throughout the body, and portions of digestive and respiratory organs

D. DEVELOPMENT

1. **External Development**
    The early development of many animals occurs outside of the mother's body, on land or in the water. **Fish** and **amphibians** lay eggs that are fertilized externally in the water. The embryo develops within the egg, feeding on nutrients stored in the yolk. **Reptiles, birds,** and some **mammals** (like the duck-billed platypus) develop externally on land. Fertilization occurs internally, and the fertilized egg is then laid. Eggs provide protection for the developing embryo. The eggs also include the following embryonic membranes:

    *   **Chorion**: The chorion lines the inside of the shell. It is a moist membrane that permits gas exchange.
    *   **Allantois**: This saclike structure is involved in respiration and excretion and contains numerous blood vessels to transport O_2, CO_2, water, salt, and nitrogenous wastes.
    *   **Amnion**: This membrane encloses the amniotic fluid. Amniotic fluid provides an aqueous environment that protects the developing embryo from shock.
    *   **Yolk sac**: The yolk sac encloses the yolk. Blood vessels in the yolk sac transfer food to the developing embryo.

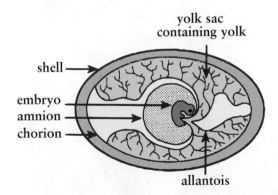

Figure 4.2.

2. **Nonplacental Internal Development**
    Early development within the body of the mother protects the young. Certain animals, including **marsupials** and some tropical fish, develop in the mother **without** a placenta. Without a placenta, exchange of food and oxygen between the young and the mother is limited. The young may be born very young.

3. **Placental Internal Development**
    The growing fetus (see Figure 4.3) receives oxygen directly from its mother through a specialized circulatory system. This system not only supplies oxygen and nutrients to the fetus but removes carbon dioxide and metabolic wastes as well. The two components of this system

are the **placenta** and the **umbilical cord**, which both develop in the first few weeks following fertilization.

The placenta and the umbilical cord are outgrowths of the four extra-embryonic membranes formed during development: the **amnion**, **chorion**, **allantois**, and **yolk sac**. The **amnion** is a thin, tough membrane containing a watery fluid called amniotic fluid. Amniotic fluid acts as a shock absorber of external pressure and localized pressure from uterine contractions during labor. Placenta formation begins with the **chorion**, a membrane that completely surrounds the amnion. A third membrane, the **allantois**, develops as an outpocketing of the gut. The blood vessels of the allantoic wall enlarge and become the umbilical vessels, which will connect the fetus to the developing placenta. The **yolk sac**, the site of early development of blood vessels, becomes associated with the umbilical vessels .

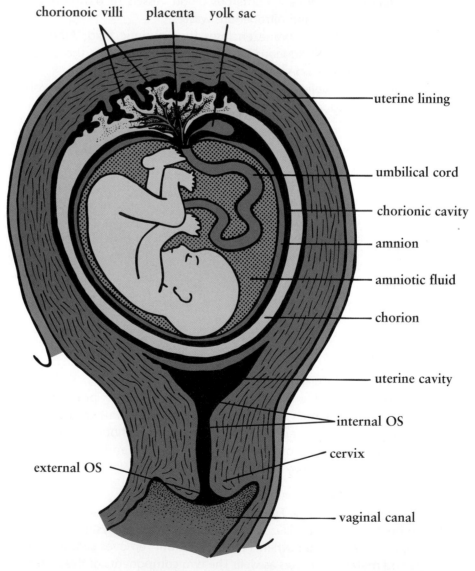

Figure 4.3. Human Fetus

E. BIRTH AND MATURATION

Childbirth is accomplished by **labor**, a series of strong uterine contractions. Labor can be divided into three distinct stages. In the first stage, the **cervix** thins and dilates, and the amniotic sac ruptures, releasing its fluids. During this time, contractions are relatively mild. The second stage is characterized by rapid contractions, resulting in the birth of the baby, followed by the cutting of the umbilical cord. During the final stage, the uterus contracts, expelling the placenta and the umbilical cord.

The embryo develops into the adult through the process of maturation, which involves cell division, growth, and differentiation. In some animals, maturation is suspended in a temporary state; for example, arthropods have a pupal stage. Mammals develop uninterrupted. Differentiation of cells is complete when all organs reach adult form.

## 5

VASCULAR SYSTEMS IN ANIMALS

CIRCULATION IN INVERTEBRATES

A. PROTOZOANS

In protozoans, movement of gases and nutrients is accomplished by simple diffusion within the cell.

B. CNIDARIANS

Hydra (see Figure 5.1) and other cnidarians have body walls that are two cells thick. All cells are in direct contact with either the internal or external environments, so there is no need for a specialized circulatory system.

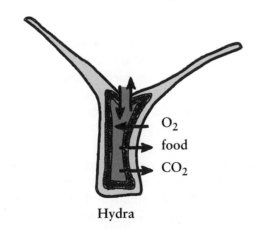

O_2
food
CO_2

Hydra

Figure 5.1

C. ARTHROPODS

Arthropods have **open circulatory systems** in which blood (interstitial fluid) is in direct contact with the body tissues. The blood is circulated primarily by body movements. Blood flows through a **dorsal vessel** and into spaces called **sinuses**, where exchange occurs.

D. ANNELIDS

The earthworm (annelida) uses a **closed circulatory system** to deliver materials to cells that are not in direct contact with the external environment. In a closed circulatory system, blood is confined to blood vessels. Blood moves towards the head in the dorsal vessel, which functions as the main heart by coordinated contractions. Five pairs of vessels called **aortic loops** connect the dorsal vessel to the ventral vessel and function as additional pumps. Earthworm blood lacks any red blood cells, but a hemoglobin-like pigment is dissolved in an aqueous solution.

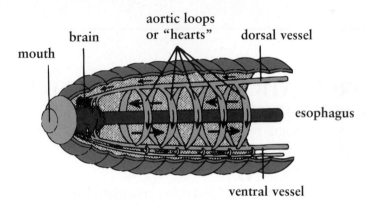

Figure 5.2. Earthworm

CIRCULATION IN HUMANS

The human cardiovascular system is composed of a muscular, four-chambered heart, a network of blood vessels, and the blood itself. Oxygenated blood is pumped from the left ventricle to the **aorta**, which branches into a series of arteries. The **arteries** branch into **arterioles** and then into microscopic **capillaries**. Exchange of gases, nutrients, and cellular waste products occurs via diffusion across capillary walls.

The capillaries then converge into venules and eventually into veins, leading deoxygenated blood through the inferior and superior vena cava back towards the heart. This blood enters the right atrium and then the right ventricle, which pumps the blood through the pulmonary arteries to the lungs so that it can pick up oxygen. Oxygenated blood returns to the heart via the pulmonary vein to enter the left atrium, which sends the blood to the left ventricle.

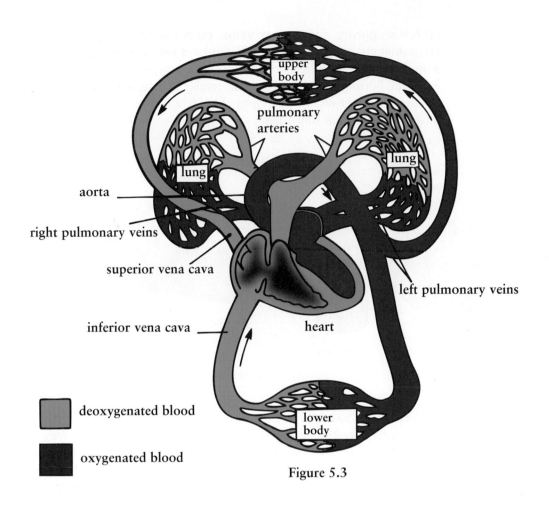

aorta

right pulmonary veins

superior vena cava

inferior vena cava

deoxygenated blood

oxygenated blood

Figure 5.3

A. THE HEART

The heart is the driving force of the circulatory system. The right and left halves can be viewed as two separate pumps: The right side of the heart pumps **deoxygenated** blood into **pulmonary** circulation (towards the lungs), while the left side pumps **oxygenated** blood into **systemic** circulation (throughout the body). The two upper chambers are called atria, and the two lower chambers are called ventricles. The atria are thin walled, while the ventricles are extremely muscular.

B. BLOOD VESSELS

The three types of blood vessels are **arteries, veins,** and **capillaries. Arteries** are thick-walled, muscular, elastic vessels that transport oxygenated blood away from the heart—except for the pulmonary arteries, which transport deoxygenated blood from the heart to the lungs. Veins are relatively thinly walled, inelastic vessels that conduct deoxygenated blood towards the heart—except for the pulmonary veins, which carry oxygenated blood from the lungs to the heart. Much of the blood flow in veins depends on their compression by skeletal muscles during movement rather than on the pumping of the heart. Venous circulation is often at odds with gravity; thus, larger **veins,** especially those in the legs, have valves that prevent backflow. Capillaries have very thin walls composed of a single layer of endothelial cells across which respiratory gases, nutrients, enzymes, hormones, and wastes can readily diffuse. **Capillaries** have the smallest diameter of all three types of vessels; red blood cells must often travel through them single file.

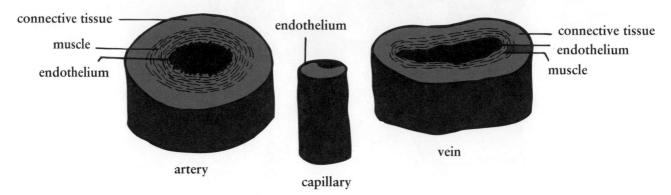

Figure 5.4

C. LYMPH VESSELS

The lymphatic system is a secondary circulatory system distinct from the cardiovascular circulation. Its vessels transport excess **interstitial fluid,** called **lymph,** to the cardiovascular system, thereby keeping fluid levels in the body constant. **Lymph** nodes are swellings along lymph vessels containing phagocytic cells **(leukocytes)** that filter the lymph, removing and destroying foreign particles and pathogens.

D. BLOOD

On the average, the human body contains four to six liters of blood. Blood has both liquid (55%) and cellular components (45%). **Plasma** is the liquid portion of the blood. It is an aqueous mixture of nutrients, salts, respiratory gases, wastes, hormones, and blood proteins (e.g., immunoglobulins, albumin, and fibrinogen). The cellular components of the blood are erythrocytes, leukocytes, and platelets.

1. **Erythrocytes (red blood cells)**

   Erythrocytes are the oxygen-carrying components of blood. An erythrocyte contains approximately 250 million molecules of hemoglobin, each of which can bind up to four molecules of oxygen. When hemoglobin binds oxygen, it is called **oxyhemoglobin.** This is the primary form of oxygen transport in the blood. Erythrocytes have a distinct biconcave, disklike shape, which gives them both increased surface area for gas exchange and greater flexibility for movement through those tiny capillaries. **Erythrocytes** are formed from stem cells in the

bone marrow, where they lose their nuclei, mitochondria, and membranous organelles. Once mature, red blood cells (RBCs) circulate in the blood for about 120 days, after which they are phagocytized by special cells in the spleen and liver.

2. **Leukocytes (white blood cells)**
Leukocytes are larger than erythrocytes and serve protective functions. Some white blood cells (WBCs) phagocytize foreign matter and organisms such as bacteria. Others migrate from the blood to tissue, where they mature into stationary cells called **macrophages**. Other WBCs, called **lymphocytes**, are involved in immune response and the production of antibodies (B cells) or cytolysis of infected cells (T cells).

3. **Platelets**
Platelets are **cell fragments** that lack nuclei and are involved in clot formation.

FUNCTIONS OF THE CIRCULATORY SYSTEM

Blood transports nutrients and O_2 to tissue and wastes and CO_2 from tissue. Platelets are involved in injury repair. Leukocytes are the main component of the immune system.

A. TRANSPORT OF GASES

Erythrocytes transport O_2 throughout the circulatory system. Actually, it is the hemoglobin molecules in erythrocytes that bind to O_2. Each hemoglobin molecule is capable of binding to four molecules of O_2. Hemoglobin also binds to CO_2.

B. TRANSPORT OF NUTRIENTS AND WASTES

Amino acids and **simple sugars** are absorbed into the bloodstream at the intestinal capillaries. After processing, they are transported throughout the body, where metabolic **waste products** (e.g., water, urea, and carbon dioxide) diffuse into capillaries from surrounding cells. These wastes are then delivered to the appropriate excretory organs.

C. CLOTTING

When platelets come into contact with the exposed collagen of a damaged vessel, they release a chemical that causes neighboring platelets to adhere to one another, forming a **platelet plug**. Subsequently, both the platelets and the damaged tissue release the clotting factor **thromboplastin**. Thromboplastin, with the aid of its cofactors calcium and vitamin K, converts the inactive plasma protein **prothrombin** to its active form, thrombin. Thrombin then converts **fibrinogen** (another plasma protein) into fibrin. Threads of **fibrin** coat the damaged area and trap blood cells to form a clot. Clots prevent extensive blood loss while the damaged vessel heals itself. The fluid left after blood clotting is called serum.

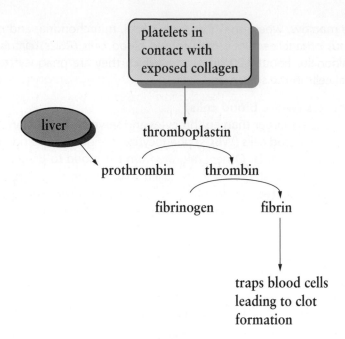

Figure 5.5

D. IMMUNOLOGICAL REACTIONS

The body has the ability to distinguish between "self" and "nonself" and to "remember" nonself entities (**antigens**) that it has previously encountered. These defense mechanisms are an integral part of the immune system. The immune system is composed of two specific defense mechanisms: **humoral** immunity, which involves the production of antibodies, and **cell-mediated** immunity, which involves cells that combat fungal and viral infection. **Lymphocytes** are responsible for both of these immune mechanisms. The body also has a number of nonspecific defense mechanisms.

1. Humoral Immunity

One of the body's defense mechanisms is the production of **antibodies**. These responses are very specific to the antigen involved. Humoral immunity is responsible for the proliferation of antibodies following exposure to antigens. Antibodies, also called **immunoglobulins** (Igs), are complex proteins that recognize and bind to specific antigens and trigger the immune system to remove them. Antibodies either attract other cells (such as leukocytes) to phagocytize the antigen or cause the antigens to clump together (**agglutinate**) and form large, insoluble complexes, facilitating their removal by phagocytic cells.

Active immunity refers to the production of antibodies during an immune response. Active immunity can be conferred by **vaccination**; an individual is injected with a weakened, inactive, or related form of a particular antigen, which stimulates the immune system to produce specific antibodies against it. Active immunity may require weeks to build up. **Passive immunity** involves the transfer of antibodies produced by another individual or organism. Passive immunity is acquired either passively or by injection. For example, during pregnancy, some maternal antibodies cross the placenta and enter fetal circulation, conferring passive immunity upon the fetus. Although passive immunity is acquired immediately, it is very short-lived, lasting only as long as the antibodies circulate in the blood system. Passive immunity is usually not very specific. **Gamma globulin**, the fraction of the blood containing a wide variety of antibodies, can be used to confer temporary protection against hepatitis and other diseases by passive immunity.

2. **Nonspecific Defense Mechanisms**
   The body employs a number of nonspecific defenses against foreign material:
   - **Skin** is a physical barrier against bacterial invasion. In addition, pores on the skin's surface secrete sweat, which contains an enzyme that attacks bacterial cell walls.
   - Passages (e.g., the respiratory tract) are lined with ciliated, **mucous-coated epithelia**, which filter and trap foreign particles.
   - **Macrophages** engulf and destroy foreign particles.
   - The **inflammatory** response is initiated by the body in response to physical damage. Injured cells release **histamine**, which causes blood vessels to dilate, thereby increasing blood flow to the damaged region. **Granulocytes** attracted to the injury site phagocytize antigenic **material**. An inflammatory response is often accompanied by a **fever**.
   - Proteins called **interferons** are produced by cells under viral attack. Interferons diffuse to other cells, where they help prevent the spread of the virus.

   Inappropriate response to certain foods and pollen can cause the body to form antibodies and release histamine. These responses are called **allergic** reactions.

3. **Rejection of Transplants**
   Transplanted tissues or organs are detected as foreign bodies by the recipient's immune system. Resulting immune response can cause the transplant to be **rejected**. Immuno-suppressing drugs can be used to lower the immune response to transplants and decrease the likelihood of rejection.

4. **ABO Blood Types**
   Erythrocytes have characteristic cell-surface proteins **(antigens)**. Antigens are macromolecules that are foreign to the host organism and trigger an immune response. The two major groups of red blood cell antigens are the **ABO group** and the **Rh factor**.

Blood Type	Antigen on Red Blood Cell	Antibodies Produced
A	A	anti-B
B	B	anti-A
AB (universal recipient)	A and B	none
O (universal donor)	none	anti-A and anti-B

Type A blood has the A antigen present. A type A individual will recognize type A antigen as self and will not respond to it. It is extremely important during blood transfusions that **donor** and **recipient** blood types be appropriately matched. The aim is to avoid transfusion of red blood cells that will be clumped ("rejected") by antibodies present in the recipient's plasma. The rule of blood matching is as follows: If the donor's antigens are already in the recipient's blood, no clumping occurs. **Type AB** blood is termed the "**universal recipient**," as it has neither anti-A nor anti-B antibodies. **Type O** blood is considered to be the "**universal donor**"; it will not elicit a response from the recipient's immune system since it does not possess any surface antigens.

5. **Rh Factor**

    The Rh factor is another antigen that may be present on the surface of red blood cells. Individuals may be Rh+, possessing the Rh antigen, or Rh–, lacking the Rh antigen. Consideration of the Rh factor is particularly important during **pregnancy**. An Rh– woman can be sensitized by an **Rh+ fetus** if fetal red blood cells (which will have the Rh factor) enter maternal circulation during birth. If this woman subsequently carries another Rh+ fetus, the anti-Rh antibodies she produced when sensitized by the first birth may cross the placenta and destroy fetal red blood cells. This results in a severe anemia for the fetus, known as **erythroblastosis fetalis**. Erythroblastosis is not caused by ABO blood type mismatches between mother and fetus, since anti-A and anti-B antibodies cannot cross the placenta.

## 6

ENDOCRINOLOGY

CHEMICAL REGULATION IN ANIMALS

The endocrine system acts as a means of internal communication, coordinating the activities of the organ systems. Endocrine glands synthesize and secrete chemical substances called **hormones** directly into the circulatory system. (In contrast, **exocrine glands**, such as the gall bladder, secrete substances that are transported by ducts.)

Glands that synthesize and/or secrete hormones include the pituitary, hypothalamus, thyroid, parathyroids, adrenals, pancreas, testes, ovaries, pineal, kidneys, gastrointestinal glands, heart, and thymus (see Figure 6.1). Some hormones regulate a single type of cell or organ, while others have more widespread actions. The **specificity** of hormonal action is usually determined by the presence of specific receptors on or in the target cells.

A. ADRENAL GLANDS

The adrenal glands are situated on top of the **kidneys** and consist of the **adrenal cortex** and the **adrenal medulla**.

1. **Adrenal Cortex**
   In response to stress, **ACTH** (produced by the anterior pituitary) stimulates the adrenal cortex to synthesize and secrete the steroid hormones, which are collectively known as **corticosteroids.** The corticosteroids, derived from cholesterol, include glucocorticoids, mineralocorticoids, and cortical sex hormones.

   a. **Glucocorticoids**
      Glucocorticoids, such as **cortisol** and **cortisone**, are involved in glucose regulation and protein metabolism. Glucocorticoids raise blood glucose levels by promoting protein breakdown and **gluconeogenesis** and decreasing protein synthesis. Glucocorticoids raise the plasma glucose levels and are antagonistic to the effects of insulin.

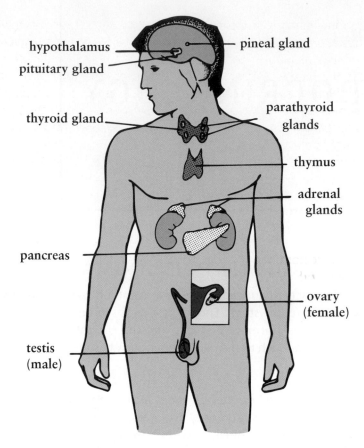

Figure 6.1. Human Endocrine System

b. **Mineralocorticoids**

Mineralocorticoids, particularly **aldosterone**, regulate plasma levels of sodium and potassium and, consequently, the total extracellular water volume. Aldosterone causes active reabsorption of sodium and passive reabsorption of water in the **nephron.** This results in a rise in both blood volume and blood pressure. Excess production of aldosterone results in excess retention of water with resulting hypertension (high blood pressure).

c. **Cortical sex hormones**

The adrenal cortex secretes small quantities of **androgens** (male sex hormones) like androstenedione and dehydroepiandrosterone in both males and females. Since, in males, most of the androgens are produced by the **testes,** the physiologic effect of the adrenal androgens is quite small. In females, however, overproduction of the adrenal androgens may have masculinizing effects, such as excessive facial hair.

2. **Adrenal Medulla**

The adrenal medulla produces **epinephrine** (adrenaline) and **norepinephrine** (noradrenaline), both of which belong to a class of amino acid-derived compounds called **catecholamines.**

Epinephrine increases the conversion of glycogen to glucose in liver and muscle tissue, causing a rise in blood glucose levels and an increase in the basal metabolic rate. Both epinephrine and norepinephrine increase the rate and strength of the heartbeat, and they dilate and constrict blood vessels in such a way as to increase the blood supply to skeletal muscle, the heart, and the brain, while decreasing the blood supply to the kidneys, skin, and digestive tract. These effects are known as the "fight or flight response" and are elicited by sympathetic nervous stimulation in response to stress. Epinephrine will inhibit certain "vegetative" functions, like digestion, which are not immediately important for survival. Both of these hormones are also **neurotransmitters.**

3. **Control of Adrenal Hormones**

Release of adrenal cortical hormones is under the control of adrenocorticotrophic hormone (ACTH), a hormone secreted by the **anterior pituitary gland.** ACTH stimulates the production of glucocorticoids and sex steroids; aldosterone production is controlled by a different mechanism.

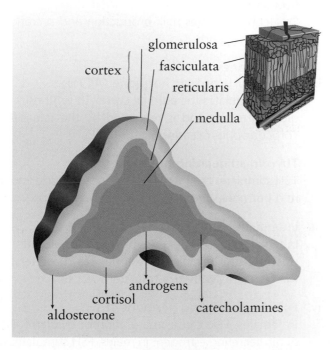

Figure 6.2

B. PITUITARY GLAND

The pituitary (**hypophysis**) is a small, trilobed gland lying at the base of the brain. The two main lobes, anterior and posterior, are functionally distinct. (In humans, the third lobe, the intermediate lobe, is rudimentary.)

1. Anterior Pituitary

The anterior pituitary synthesizes both direct hormones, which directly stimulate their target organs, and tropic hormones, which stimulate other endocrine glands to release hormones. The hormonal secretions of the anterior pituitary are regulated by hypothalamic secretions called releasing/inhibiting hormones or factors.

a. Direct hormones

i. Growth hormone (GH, somatotropin)

GH promotes bone and muscle growth. In children, a GH deficiency can lead to stunted growth (**dwarfism**), while overproduction of GH results in **gigantism.** Overproduction of GH in adults causes **acromegaly,** a disorder characterized by a disproportionate overgrowth of bone, localized especially in the skull, jaw, feet, and hands.

ii. Prolactin

Prolactin stimulates milk production and secretion in female mammary glands.

b. Tropic hormones

i. Adrenocorticotropic hormone (ACTH)

ACTH stimulates the adrenal cortex to synthesize and secrete glucocorticoids and is regulated by the releasing hormone corticotrophin-releasing factor (CRF).

ii. Thyroid-stimulating hormone (TSH)

TSH stimulates the thyroid gland to synthesize and release thyroid hormones, including thyroxin.

iii. Luteinizing hormone (LH)

In females, LH stimulates ovulation and formation of the **corpus luteum**. In males, LH stimulates the interstitial cells of the testes to synthesize testosterone.

iv. Follicle-stimulating hormone (FSH)

In females, FSH causes maturation of ovarian follicles, which begin secreting estrogen; in males, FSH stimulates maturation of the seminiferous tubules and sperm production.

v. Melanocyte-stimulating hormone (MSH)

MSH is secreted by the intermediate lobe of the pituitary. In mammals, the function of MSH is unclear, but in frogs, MSH causes darkening of the skin via induced dispersion of molecules of pigment in melanophore cells.

2. Posterior Pituitary

The posterior pituitary (**neurohypophysis**) does not synthesize hormones; it stores and releases the peptide hormones **oxytocin** and **ADH**, which are produced by the neurosecretory cells of the hypothalamus. Hormone secretion is stimulated by action potentials descending from the hypothalamus.

a. Oxytocin

Oxytocin, which is secreted during childbirth, increases the strength and frequency of uterine muscle contractions. Oxytocin secretion is also induced by suckling; oxytocin stimulates milk secretion in the mammary glands.

b. Antidiuretic hormone (ADH, vasopressin)

ADH increases the permeability of the nephron's **collecting duct** to water, thereby promoting water reabsorption and increasing blood volume. ADH is secreted when plasma osmolarity increases, as sensed by osmoreceptors in the hypothalamus, or when blood volume decreases, as sensed by baroreceptors in the circulatory system.

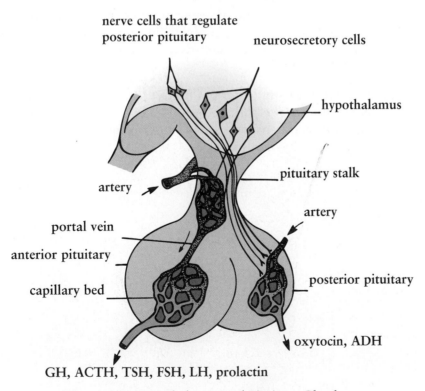

Figure 6.3. Hypothalamus and Pituitary Gland

C. HYPOTHALAMUS

The hypothalamus is part of the forebrain and is located directly above the pituitary gland. The hypothalamus receives neural transmissions from other parts of the brain and from peripheral nerves, which trigger specific responses from its neurosecretory cells. The neurosecretory cells regulate pituitary gland secretions via negative feedback mechanisms and through the actions of inhibiting and releasing hormones.

1. **Interactions with Anterior Pituitary**

   Hypothalamic-releasing hormones stimulate or inhibit the secretions of the anterior pituitary. For example, **GnRH** stimulates the anterior pituitary to secrete **FSH** and **LH.** Releasing hormones are secreted into the hypothalamic-hypophyseal portal system. In this circulatory pathway, blood from the capillary bed in the hypothalamus flows through a **portal vein** into the anterior pituitary, where it diverges into a second capillary network. In this way, releasing hormones can immediately reach the anterior pituitary.

   A complicated feedback system regulates the secretions of the endocrine system. For example, when the plasma levels of adrenal cortical hormones drop, hypothalamic cells (via a negative feedback mechanism) release ACTH-releasing factor (ACTH-RF) into the portal system. When the plasma concentration of corticosteroids exceeds the normal plasma level, the steroids themselves exert an inhibitory effect on the hypothalamus.

2. **Interactions with Posterior Pituitary**

   Neurosecretory cells in the hypothalamus synthesize both **oxytocin** and **ADH** and transport them via their axons into the posterior pituitary for storage and secretion.

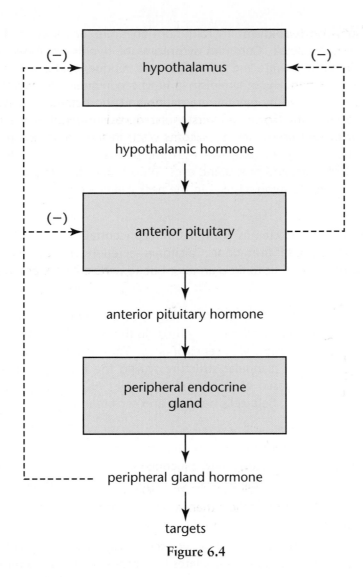

Figure 6.4

D. THYROID

The thyroid gland is a bilobed structure located on the ventral surface of the trachea. It produces and secretes thyroxin and triiodothyronine (the thyroid hormones) and calcitonin.

1. **Thyroid Hormones (Thyroxine and Triiodothyronine)**

Thyroxine (T_4) and triiodothyronine (T_3) are derived from the iodination of the amino acid **tyrosine**. Thyroid hormones are necessary for growth and neurological development in children. They increase the rate of metabolism throughout the body.

In **hypothyroidism,** thyroid hormones are undersecreted or not secreted at all. Common symptoms of hypothyroidism include a slowed heart rate and respiratory rate, fatigue, cold intolerance, and weight gain. Hypothyroidism in newborn infants, called **cretinism,** is characterized by mental retardation and short stature. In **hyperthyroidism,** the thyroid is overstimulated, resulting in the oversecretion of thyroid hormones. Symptoms often include increased metabolic rate, feelings of excessive warmth, profuse sweating, palpitations, weight loss, and protruding eyes. In both disorders, the thyroid often enlarges, forming a bulge in the neck called a goiter.

2. Calcitonin

Calcitonin decreases plasma Ca^{2+} concentration by inhibiting the release of Ca^{2+} from bone. Calcitonin secretion is regulated by plasma Ca^{2+} levels. Calcitonin is antagonistic to parathyroid hormone.

E. PANCREAS

The pancreas is both an **exocrine** organ and an **endocrine** organ. The exocrine function is performed by the cells that secrete digestive enzymes into the small intestine via a series of ducts. The endocrine function is performed by small glandular structures called the **islets of Langerhans,** which are composed of alpha and beta cells. Alpha cells produce and secrete glucagon; beta cells produce and secrete insulin.

1. Glucagon

Glucagon stimulates protein and fat degradation, the conversion of glycogen to glucose, and gluconeogenesis, all of which serve to increase blood glucose levels. Glucagon's action are largely antagonistic to those of insulin.

2. Insulin

Insulin is a protein hormone secreted in response to a high blood glucose concentration. It stimulates the uptake of glucose by muscle and adipose cells and the storage of glucose as glycogen in muscle and liver cells, thus lowering blood glucose levels. It also stimulates the synthesis of fats from glucose and the uptake of amino acids. Insulin's actions are antagonistic to those of **glucagon** and the **glucocorticoids.** Underproduction of insulin, or an insensitivity to insulin, leads to **diabetes mellitus,** which is characterized by hyperglycemia (high blood glucose levels).

F. PARATHYROID GLANDS

The parathyroid glands are four small, pea-shaped structures embedded in the posterior surface of the thyroid. These glands synthesize and secrete parathyroid hormone (PTH), which regulates plasma Ca^{2+} concentration. PTH raises the Ca^{2+} concentration in the blood by increasing bone resorption and decreasing Ca^{2+} excretion in the kidneys. Calcium in bone is bonded to phosphate, and breakdown of the bone releases phosphate as well as calcium. Parathyroid hormone compensates for this by stimulating excretion of phosphate by the kidneys.

DAT Synopsis

Insulin decreases plasma glucose.

Glucagon increases plasma glucose.

Don't forget that growth hormone, the glucocorticoids, and epinephrine are also capable of increasing plasma glucose.

DAT Synopsis

PTH increases Ca^{2+}.
CalciTONIN decreases Ca^{2+}.
(CalciTONIN tones down Ca^{2+}.)

If you remember this simple principle, you'll be able to *predict* their respective effects on bone, intestinal absorption of calcium, and urinary excretion/reabsorption of calcium. You don't need to memorize anything, just *think.*

G. KIDNEYS

When blood volume falls, the kidneys produce **renin**—an enzyme that converts the plasma protein angiotensinogen to angiotensin I. Angiotensin I is converted to angiotensin II, which stimulates the adrenal cortex to secrete **aldosterone.** Aldosterone helps to restore blood volume by increasing sodium reabsorption at the kidney, leading to an increase in water. This removes the initial stimulus for renin production.

H. GASTROINTESTINAL HORMONES

Ingested food stimulates the stomach to release the hormone gastrin. **Gastrin** is carried to the gastric glands and stimulates the glands to secrete HCl in response to food in the stomach. Secretion of pancreatic juice, the exocrine secretion of the pancreas, is also under hormone control: The hormone **secretin** is released by the small intestine when acidic food material enters from the stomach. Secretin stimulates the secretion of an alkaline bicarbonate solution from the pancreas, which neutralizes the acidity of the chyme (partially digested food coming from the stomach). The hormone **cholecystokinin** is released from the small intestine in response to the presence of fats and causes the contraction of the gallbladder and release of bile into the small intestine. **Bile** is involved in the digestion of fats.

I. PINEAL GLAND

The pineal gland is a tiny structure at the base of the brain that secretes the hormone **melatonin.** The role of melatonin in humans is unclear, but it is believed to play a role in the regulation of circadian rhythms—physiological cycles lasting 24 hours. Melatonin secretion is regulated by light and dark cycles in the environment. In primitive vertebrates, melatonin lightens the skin by concentrating pigment granules in melanophores. (Melatonin is an antagonist to MSH.)

MECHANISM OF HORMONE ACTION

Hormones are classified on the basis of their chemical structure into two major groups: peptide hormones and steroid hormones. There are two ways in which hormones affect the activities of their target cells: via extracellular receptors or intracellular receptors.

A. PEPTIDES

Peptide hormones range from simple, short peptides (amino acid chains) such as ADH, to complex polypeptides, such as insulin. Peptide hormones act as first messengers. Their binding to **specific receptors** on the surface of their target cells triggers a series of enzymatic reactions within each cell, the first of which may be the conversion of ATP to cyclic adenosine monophosphate (cAMP); this reaction is catalyzed by the membrane-bound enzyme adenylate cyclase. **Cyclic AMP** acts as a **second messenger,** relaying messages from the extracellular peptide hormone to cytoplasmic enzymes and initiating a series of successive reactions in the cell. This is an example of a cascade effect; with each step, the hormone's effects are amplified. Cyclic AMP activity is inactivated by the cytoplasmic enzyme phosphodiesterase.

B. STEROIDS

Steroid hormones, such as estrogen and aldosterone, belong to a class of lipid-derived molecules with a characteristic ring structure. They are produced by the testes, ovaries, placenta, and adrenal cortex. Because they are lipid soluble, steroid hormones enter their target cells directly and bind to specific receptor proteins in the cytoplasm. This receptor-hormone complex enters the nucleus and directly activates the expression of specific genes by binding to receptors on the chromatin. This induces a change in mRNA transcription and protein synthesis.

## 7

NERVOUS SYSTEM

The **nervous system** enables organisms to receive and respond to **stimuli** from their external and internal environments. **Neurons** are the functional units of the nervous system. A neuron converts stimuli into **electrochemical signals,** which are conducted through the nervous system. The nervous system responds to stimuli more rapidly than the endocrine system.

NEURON
A. STRUCTURE

The neuron is an elongated cell consisting of several dendrites, a cell body, and a single axon. **Dendrites** are cytoplasmic extensions that receive information and transmit it towards the cell body. The **cell body (soma)** contains the nucleus and controls the metabolic activity of the neuron. The **axon** is a long cellular process that transmits impulses away from the cell body. Most mammalian axons are sheathed by an insulating substance known as **myelin,** which allows axons to conduct impulses faster. Myelin is produced by cells known as glial cells. (**Oligodendrocytes** produce myelin in the central nervous system, and **Schwann cells** produce myelin in the peripheral nervous system.) The gaps between segments of myelin are called **nodes of Ranvier.** The axons end as swellings known as **synaptic terminals** (sometimes also called synaptic boutons or knobs). **Neurotransmitters** are released from these terminals into the **synapse**

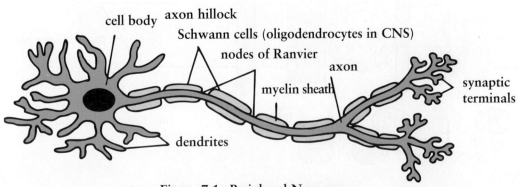

Figure 7.1. Peripheral Nerve

(or synaptic cleft), which is the gap between the axon terminals of one cell and the dendrites of the next cell. Axons traveling from the spine to the tip of the foot may be very long.

B. FUNCTION

Neurons are specialized to receive signals from sensory receptors or from other neurons in the body and transfer this information along the length of the axon. Impulses, known as **action potentials**, travel the length of the axon and invade the nerve terminal, thereby causing the release of neurotransmitter into the synapse. When a neuron is at rest, the potential difference between the extracellular space and the intracellular space is called the **resting potential**.

1. Resting Potential

Even at rest, a neuron is **polarized**. This potential difference is the result of an unequal distribution of ions between the inside and outside of the cell. A typical resting membrane potential is **–70 millivolts** (mV), which means that the inside of the neuron is more negative than the outside. This difference is due to selective ionic permeability of the neuronal cell membrane and is maintained by the **active transport** by the **Na^+/K^+ pump** (also called the Na^+/K^+ ATPase).

The concentration of K^+ is higher inside the neuron than outside; the concentration of Na^+ is higher outside than inside. Additionally, negatively charged proteins are trapped inside of the cell. The resting potential is created because the neuron is **selectively permeable** to K^+, so K^+ diffuses down its concentration gradient, leaving a net negative charge inside. (Neurons are **impermeable** to Na^+, so the cell remains polarized.)

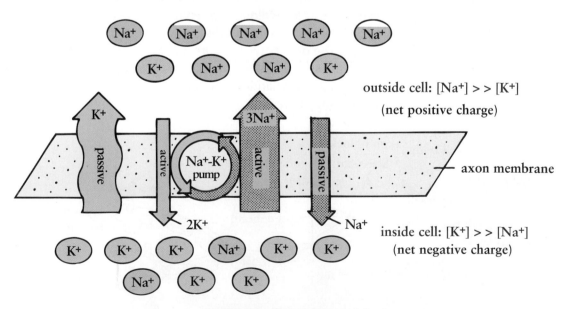

Figure 7.2. Resting Potential of a Neuron

Because the transmission of action potentials lead, to the disruption of the ionic gradients, the gradients must be restored by the Na^+/K^+ pump. This pump, using ATP energy, transports 3 Na^+ out for every 2 K^+ it transports into the cell.

2. **Action Potential**
The nerve cell body receives both excitatory and inhibitory impulses from other cells. If the cell becomes sufficiently excited or depolarized (i.e., the inside of the cell becomes less negative), an **action potential** is generated. The minimum **threshold** membrane potential (usually around –50 mV) is the level at which an action potential is initiated.

Ion channels located in the nerve cell membrane open in response to these changes in voltage and are, therefore, called voltage-gated ion channels. An action potential begins when **voltage-gated Na^+ channels** open in response to **depolarization**, allowing Na^+ to rush down its electrochemical gradient into the cell, causing a rapid further depolarization of that segment of the cell. The voltage-gated Na^+ channels then close, and **voltage-gated K^+ channels** open, allowing K^+ to rush out down its electrochemical gradient. This returns the cell to a more negative potential, a process known as **repolarization**. In fact, the neuron may shoot past the resting potential and become even more negative inside than normal; this is called **hyperpolarization**. Immediately following an action potential, it may be very difficult or impossible to initiate another action potential; this period of time is called the **refractory period**.

The action potential is often described as an **all-or-none response**. This means that whenever the threshold membrane potential is reached, an action potential with a consistent size and duration is produced. The nerve fires either maximally or not at all. Stimulus intensity is coded by the **frequency** of action potentials.

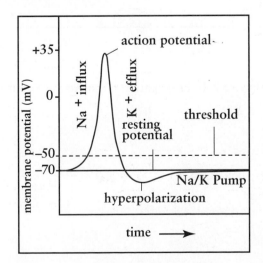

Figure 7.3. Action Potential

3. Impulse Propagation

Although axons can theoretically propagate action potentials bidirectionally, information transfer will occur only in one direction: from dendrite to synaptic terminal. (This is because synapses operate only in one direction and because refractory periods make the backward travel of action potentials impossible.) Different axons can propagate action potentials at **different speeds**. The greater the **diameter** of the axon and the more heavily it is **myelinated**, the faster the impulses will travel. Myelin increases the conduction velocity by insulating segments of the axon, so the membrane is permeable to ions only in the nodes of Ranvier. In this way, the action potential "jumps" from node to node.

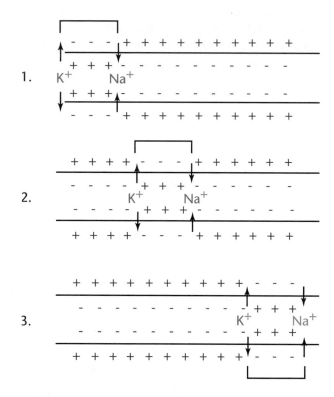

Figure 7.4. Propagation of an Action Potential

SYNAPSE

The synapse is the gap between the **axon terminal** of one neuron (called the **presynaptic neuron** because it is before the synapse) and the **dendrites** of another neuron **(postsynaptic neuron)**. Neurons may also communicate with postsynaptic cells other than neurons, such as cells in muscles or glands; these are called effector cells. The nerve terminal contains thousands of membrane-bound vesicles full of chemical messengers known as **neurotransmitters**. When the action potential arrives at the nerve terminal and depolarizes it, the synaptic vesicles fuse with the presynaptic membrane and release neurotransmitter into the synapse. The neurotransmitter **diffuses** across the synapse and acts on receptor proteins embedded in the postsynaptic membrane. The neurotransmitter can lead to depolarization of the postsynaptic cell and consequent firing of an action potential. Neurotransmitter is removed from the synapse in a variety of ways: It may be taken back up into the nerve terminal (via a protein known as an uptake carrier), where it may be reused or degraded; it may be degraded by enzymes located in the synapse (e.g., **acetylcholinesterase** inactivates the neurotransmitter **acetylcholine**); or it may simply diffuse out of the synapse.

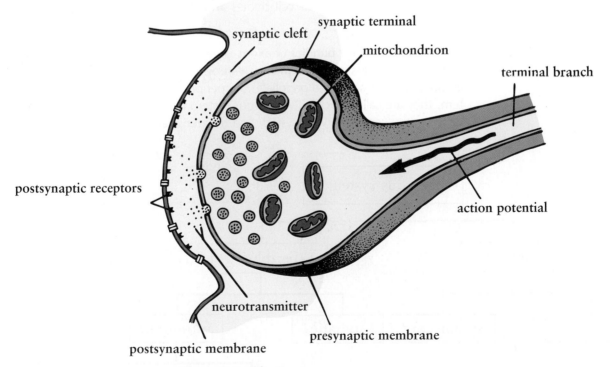

Figure 7.5. The Synapse

A. EFFECTS OF DRUGS

- **Curare** blocks the postsynaptic acetylcholine receptors so that acetylcholine is unable to interact with the receptor. This leads to paralysis by blocking nerve impulses to muscles.
- **Botulism toxin** prevents the release of acetylcholine from the presynaptic membrane and also results in paralysis.
- **Anticholinesterases** are used as nerve gases and in the insecticide parathion. As the name implies, these substances inhibit the activity of the **acetylcholinesterase** enzyme. As a result, the acetylcholine is not degraded in the synapse and continues to affect the postsynaptic membrane. Therefore, no coordinated muscular contractions can take place.

VERTEBRATE NERVOUS SYSTEM

> **DAT Synopsis**
>
> Afferent neurons are sensory neurons, and efferent neurons are motor neurons.

There are many different kinds of neurons in the vertebrate nervous system. Neurons that carry **sensory** information about the external or internal environment to the brain or spinal cord are called **afferent neurons**. Neurons that carry **motor** commands from the brain or spinal cord to various parts of the body (e.g., muscles or glands) are called **efferent neurons**. Some neurons (**interneurons**) participate only in local circuits, linking sensory and motor neurons in the brain and spinal cord; their cell bodies and their nerve terminals are in the same location.

Nerves are essentially **bundles of axons** covered with connective tissue. A network of nerve fibers is called a **plexus**. Neuronal cell bodies often cluster together: Such clusters are called **ganglia** in the periphery; in the central nervous system, they are called **nuclei**. The nervous system itself is divided into two major systems, the **central** nervous system and the **peripheral** nervous system.

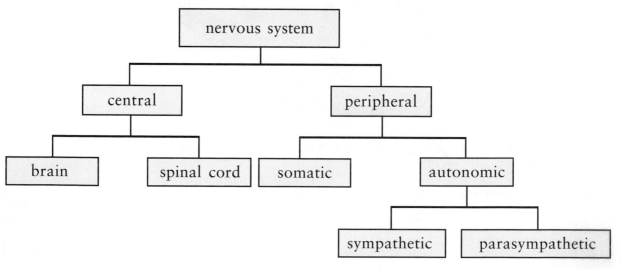

Figure 7.6. Organization of Vertebrate Nervous System

A. CENTRAL NERVOUS SYSTEM

The central nervous system (CNS) consists of the brain and spinal cord.

1. **Brain**

   The brain is a mass of neurons that resides in the skull. Its functions include interpreting sensory information, forming motor plans, and cognitive function (thinking). The brain consists of an outer portion called the gray matter (cell bodies) and an inner white matter (myelinated axons). The brain can be divided into the forebrain, midbrain, and hindbrain.

   a. **Forebrain**

      The forebrain consists of the **telencephalon** and the **diencephalon**. A major component of the telencephalon is the **cerebral cortex**, which is the highly convoluted gray matter that can be seen on the surface of the brain. The cortex processes and integrates sensory input and motor responses and is important for memory and creative thought. The **olfactory bulb** is the center for reception and integration of olfactory input.

      The **diencephalon** contains the thalamus and hypothalamus. The **thalamus** is a relay and integration center for the spinal cord and cerebral cortex. The **hypothalamus** controls visceral functions, such as hunger, thirst, sex drive, water balance, blood pressure, and temperature regulation. It also plays an important role in the control of the endocrine system.

   b. **Midbrain (Mesencephalon)**

      The midbrain is a relay center for visual and auditory impulses. It also plays an important role in motor control.

   c. **Hindbrain**

      The hindbrain is the **posterior** part of the brain and consists of the cerebellum, the pons, and the medulla. The **cerebellum** helps to modulate motor impulses initiated by the cerebral cortex and is important in the maintenance of balance, hand-eye coordination, and the timing of rapid movements. One function of the **pons** is to act as a relay center to allow the cortex to communicate with the cerebellum. The **medulla** (also called the medulla oblongata) controls many vital functions, such as breathing, heart rate, and gastrointestinal activity. Together, the midbrain, pons, and medulla constitute the **brainstem**.

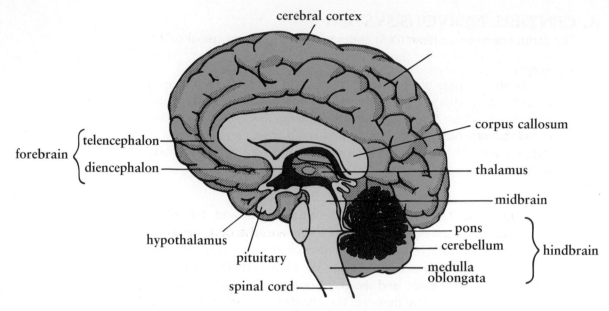

Figure 7.7. Human Brain

2. Spinal Cord

The spinal cord is an elongated extension of the brain that acts as the conduit for sensory information to the brain and motor information from the brain. The spinal cord can also integrate simple motor responses (e.g., **reflexes**) by itself. A cross section of the spinal cord reveals an outer white matter area containing motor and sensory axons and an inner gray matter area containing nerve cell bodies. Sensory information enters the spinal cord through the **dorsal horn**; the cell bodies of these sensory neurons are located in the dorsal root ganglia. All motor information exits the spinal cord through the **ventral horn**. For simple reflexes, like the knee-jerk reflex, sensory fibers (entering through the dorsal root ganglion) synapse directly on ventral horn motor fibers. Other reflexes include interneurons between the sensory and motor fibers, which allow for some processing in the spinal cord.

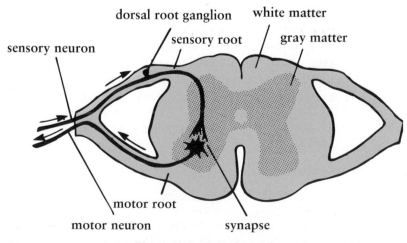

Figure 7.8. Spinal Cord

B. PERIPHERAL NERVOUS SYSTEM

The peripheral nervous system (PNS) consists of nerves and ganglia. The sensory nerves, which enter the CNS, and the motor nerves, which leave the CNS, are part of the peripheral nervous system. The PNS has two primary divisions, the **somatic** and the **autonomic** nervous systems, each of which has both motor and sensory components.

1. **Somatic Nervous System**

   The somatic nervous system (SNS) innervates skeletal muscles and is responsible for voluntary movement.

2. **Autonomic Nervous System**

   The autonomic nervous system (ANS) is sometimes also called the **involuntary nervous system** because it regulates the body's internal environment without the aid of conscious control. The autonomic innervation of the body includes both sensory and motor fibers. The ANS innervates **cardiac** and **smooth muscle**. Smooth muscle is located in areas such as blood vessels, the digestive tract, the bladder, and bronchi, so it isn't surprising that the ANS is important in blood pressure control, gastrointestinal motility, excretory processes, respiration, and reproductive processes. The ANS is comprised of two subdivisions, the **sympathetic** and the **parasympathetic** nervous systems, which generally act in opposition to one another.

   a. **Sympathetic nervous system**

      The sympathetic division is responsible for the "**flight or fight**" responses that ready the body for action in an emergency situation. It increases blood pressure and heart rate, it increases blood flow to skeletal muscles, and it decreases gut motility. It also dilates the bronchioles to increase gas exchange. The sympathetic nervous system uses **norepinephrine** as its primary neurotransmitter.

   b. **Parasympathetic nervous system**

      The parasympathetic division acts to conserve energy and restore the body to resting activity levels following exertion ("**rest and digest**"). It acts to lower heart rate and to increase gut motility. One very important parasympathetic nerve that innervates many of the thoracic and abdominal viscera is called the **vagus nerve**. It uses **acetylcholine** as its primary neurotransmitter.

SPECIAL SENSES

The body has a number of organs that are specialized receptors, designed to detect stimuli.

A. THE EYE

The eye detects light energy (as **photons**) and transmits information about intensity, color, and shape to the brain. The eyeball is covered by a thick, opaque layer known as the **sclera**, which is also known as the white of the eye. Beneath the sclera is the **choroid** layer, which helps to supply the retina with blood. The choroid is a dark, pigmented area that reduces reflection in the eye. The innermost layer of the eye is the **retina**, which contains the **photoreceptors** that sense light.

The transparent **cornea** at the front of the eye bends and focuses light rays. The rays then travel through an opening called the **pupil**, whose diameter is controlled by the pigmented, muscular **iris**. The iris responds to the intensity of light in the surroundings (light makes the pupil constrict). The light continues through the lens, which is suspended behind the pupil. The **lens**, the shape and **focal length** of which is controlled by the **ciliary muscles**, focuses the image onto the retina.

In the retina are **photoreceptors**, which transduce light into action potentials. There are two main types of photoreceptors: cones and rods. **Cones** respond to high-intensity illumination and are sensitive to color, while **rods** detect low-intensity illumination and are important in night vision. The cones and rods contain various pigments that absorb specific wavelengths of light. The cones contain three different pigments that absorb red, green, and blue wavelengths; the rod pigment, **rhodopsin**, absorbs a single wavelength. The photoreceptor cells synapse onto **bipolar cells**, which in turn synapse onto **ganglion cells**. Axons of the ganglion cells bundle to form the optic nerves, which conduct visual information to the brain. The point at which the optic nerve exits the eye is called the **blind spot** because photoreceptors are not present there. A small area of the retina, called the **fovea**, is densely packed with cones and is important for high-acuity vision.

The eye contains a **jellylike material**, called **vitreous humor**, which helps maintain its shape and optical properties. **Aqueous humor** is formed by the eye and exits through ducts to join the venous blood.

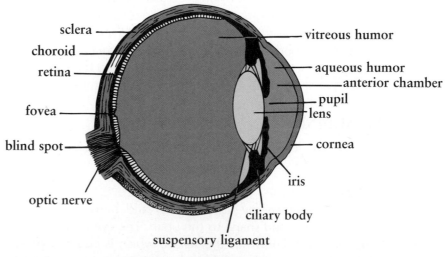

Figure 7.9. Human Eye

1. Disorders of the Eye
- **Myopia (nearsightedness)** occurs when the image is focused in front of the retina.
- **Hyperopia (farsightedness)** occurs when the image is focused behind the retina.
- **Astigmatism** is caused by an irregularly shaped cornea.
- **Cataracts** cause the lens to become opaque; light cannot enter the eye, and blindness results.
- **Glaucoma** is an increase of **pressure** in the eye due to the blocking of the outflow of the aqueous humor.

B. THE EAR

The ear transduces **sound** energy **(pressure waves)** into impulses perceived by the brain as sound. Sound waves pass through three regions as they enter the ear. First, they enter the **outer ear**, which consists of the auricle (external ear) and the **auditory canal**. At the end of the auditory canal is the **tympanic membrane** (eardrum) of the middle ear, which vibrates at the same frequency as the incoming sound. Next, the three bones, or **ossicles** (malleus, incus, and stapes), amplify the stimulus and transmit it through the oval window, which leads to the fluid-filled inner ear. The inner ear consists of the **cochlea** and the **vestibular apparatus**, which is involved in maintaining equilibrium. Vibration of the ossicles exerts pressure on the fluid in the cochlea, stimulating **hair cells** in the **basilar membrane** to transduce the pressure into action potentials, which travel via the auditory (cochlear) nerve to the brain for processing.

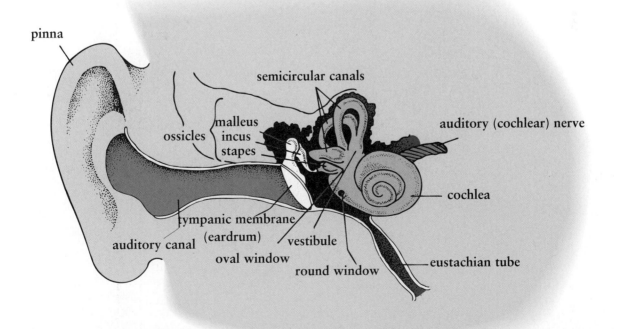

Figure 7.10. Human Ear

INVERTEBRATE NERVOUS SYSTEMS

A. PROTOZOA

Unicellular organisms possess no organized nervous system. The single-celled organisms may respond to stimuli such as touch, heat, light, and chemicals.

B. CNIDARIA

Cnidarians have a simple nervous system called a **nerve net**. This network of nerve cells may have limited centralization. Some jellyfish have clusters of cells and pathways that coordinate the relatively complex movements required for swimming.

C. ANNELIDA

Earthworms possesses a primitive **central nervous system**, consisting of a defined ventral nerve cord, and an anterior "brain" of fused ganglia (i.e., clusters of nerve cell bodies). Definite nerve pathways lead from receptors to effectors.

D. ARTHROPODA

Arthropod brains are similar to those of annelids, but more specialized sense organs are present (e.g., **compound** or **simple eyes**, **tympanum** for detecting sound).

## 8

RESPIRATION

Respiration refers to the utilization of **oxygen** by an organism. This process includes the intake of oxygen from the environment, the transport of oxygen in the blood, and the ultimate oxidation of fuel molecules in the cell. **External respiration** refers to the entrance of air into the lungs and the gas exchange between the alveoli and the blood. **Internal respiration** includes the exchange of gas between the blood and the cells and the intracellular processes of respiration.

RESPIRATION IN INVERTEBRATES

A. UNICELLULAR AND SIMPLE MULTICELLULAR ORGANISMS

  1. **Protozoa and Hydra (Phylum: Cnidaria)**
      In these organisms, every cell is in contact with the external environment (water), and respiratory gases can be exchanged between the cell and the environment by simple diffusion through the cell membrane.

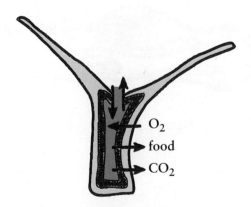

Figure 8.1. Hydra

B. ANNELIDS

Mucus secreted by cells on the external surface of the earthworm's body provides a moist surface for gaseous exchange by diffusion. The circulatory system brings O_2 to the cells and waste products, such as CO_2, back to the skin for excretion.

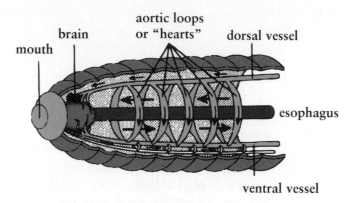

Figure 8.2

C. ARTHROPOD PHYLUM

The respiratory system of a grasshopper consists of a series of respiratory tubules, called **tracheae**, whose branches reach to almost every cell. These tubes access the surface in openings called **spiracles**. This system thus permits the intake, distribution, and removal of respiratory gases directly between the air and the body cells by diffusion. No carrier of oxygen is needed in this respiratory system, and the efficiency of this system allows insects to have a relatively effortless open circulatory system.

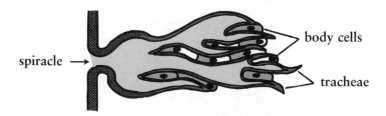

Figure 8.3

RESPIRATION IN HUMANS

In the human respiratory system, air enters the **lungs** after traveling through a series of respiratory **airways**. The air passages consists of the nose, pharynx (throat), larynx, trachea, bronchi, bronchioles, and the alveoli. Gas exchange between the lungs and the circulatory system occurs across the very thin walls of the **alveoli**, which are air-filled sacs at the terminals of the airway branches. Three hundred million alveoli provide approximately 100 m^2 of moist respiratory surface for gas exchange. Following gas exchange, air rushes back through the respiratory pathway and is exhaled.

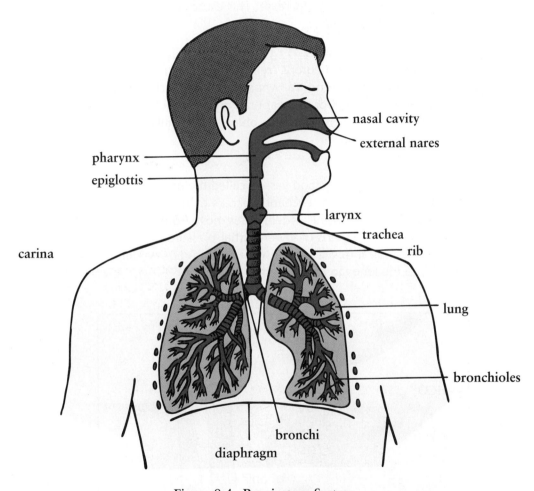

Figure 8.4. Respiratory System

A. VENTILATION

Ventilation of the lungs (breathing) is the process by which air is **inhaled** and **exhaled**. The purpose of ventilation is to take in oxygen from the atmosphere and eliminate carbon dioxide from the body.

During **inhalation**, the diaphragm contracts and flattens, and the external intercostal muscles contract, pushing the rib cage and chest wall up and out. This causes the thoracic cavity to increase in **volume**. This volume increase, in turn, reduces the pressure, causing the lungs to expand and fill with air.

Exhalation is generally a passive process. The lungs and chest wall are highly elastic and tend to recoil to their original positions following inhalation. The diaphragm and external intercostal muscles relax, and the chest wall pushes inward. The consequent decrease in thoracic cavity volume causes the air pressure to increase. This causes the lungs to deflate, forcing air out of the alveoli.

B. CONTROL OF VENTILATION

Ventilation is regulated by neurons (referred to as **respiratory centers**) located in the **medulla oblongata**, whose rhythmic discharges stimulate the intercostal muscles and/or the diaphragm to contract. When the partial pressure of CO_2 rises, the medulla oblongata stimulates an increase in the rate of ventilation.

C. GAS EXCHANGE

A dense network of minute blood vessels called the **pulmonary capillaries** surrounds the alveoli. Gas exchange occurs by diffusion across these capillary walls and those of the alveoli; gases move from regions of higher partial pressure to regions of lower partial pressure. Oxygen diffuses from the alveolar air into the blood, while carbon dioxide diffuses from the blood into the lungs to be exhaled.

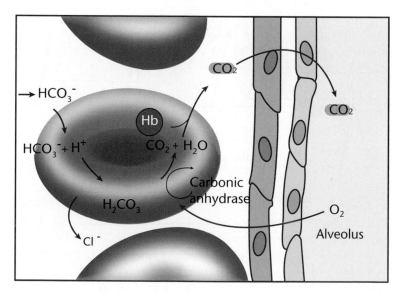

Figure 8.5

## 9

MUSCLES AND LOCOMOTION

The musculoskeletal system forms the basic internal framework of the vertebrate body. Muscles and bones work in close coordination to produce voluntary movement. In addition, bone and muscle perform a number of other independent functions. Unicellular organisms may rely on specialized organelles for locomotion. Invertebrates have developed a number of systems for locomotion. Physical support and locomotion are the functions of animal skeletal systems. The muscular system generates force.

UNICELLULAR LOCOMOTION

Protozoans and primitive algae may move by beating **cilia** or **flagella**. The cilia and flagella of all eukaryotic cells possess the same basic structure. Each contains a cylindrical stalk of 11 microtubules—9 paired microtubules arranged in a circle with 2 single microtubules in the center. Flagella achieve movement by means of the **power stroke**, a thrusting movement generated by the sliding action of microtubules. Return of the cilium or flagellum to its original position is termed the **recovery stroke**. Amoeba extend **pseudopodia** for locomotion; the advancing cell membrane extends forward, allowing the cell to move.

INVERTEBRATE LOCOMOTION

A. HYDROSTATIC SKELETONS

1. **Flatworms**

    The muscles within the body wall of advanced **flatworms**, such as **planaria**, are arranged in two antagonistic layers, **longitudinal** and **circular**. The muscles contract against the resistance of the **incompressible fluid** within the animal's tissues (this fluid is termed the **hydrostatic skeleton**). Contraction of the circular layer of muscles causes the incompressible interstitial fluid to flow longitudinally, lengthening the animal. Conversely, contraction of the longitudinal layer of muscles shortens the animal. The same type of hydrostatic skeleton assists in the locomotion of annelids, in which each segment of the animal can expand or contract independently.

2. **Segmented Worms (annelids)**

Earthworms advance principally by the action of muscles on a hydrostatic skeleton. Bristles in the lower part of each segment, called **setae**, anchor the earthworm temporarily in the earth while muscles push it ahead.

B. EXOSKELETON

An exoskeleton is a **hard skeleton** that covers all muscles and organs of some invertebrates. Exoskeletons are found principally in **arthropods** (e.g., insects). Insect exoskeletons are composed of **chitin**. All exoskeletons are composed of noncellular material secreted by the epidermis. While offering the animal some protection, exoskeletons impose limitations on growth. Thus, periodic **molting** and deposition of a new skeleton are necessary to permit body growth.

VERTEBRATE SKELETON

An **endoskeleton** serves as the framework within all vertebrate organisms. Muscles are attached to the bones, permitting movement. The endoskeleton also provides protection by surrounding delicate vital organs in bone. The rib cage protects the thoracic organs (heart and lungs), while the skull and vertebral column protect the brain and spinal cord. The two major components of the skeleton are cartilage and bone.

A. STRUCTURE OF THE SKELETON

1. **Cartilage**

Cartilage is a type of **connective tissue** that is softer and more flexible than bone. Cartilage is retained in adults in places where firmness and flexibility are needed—for example, in humans, the external ear, the nose, the walls of the larynx and trachea, and the skeletal joints contain cartilage.

2. **Bone**

Bone is a specialized type of mineralized **connective** that has the ability to withstand physical stress. Ideally designed for body support, bone tissue is hard and strong while, at the same time, somewhat elastic and lightweight. There are two basic types of bone: **compact bone** and **spongy bone**.

- **Compact bone** is dense bone that does not appear to have any cavities when observed with the naked eye. The bony matrix is deposited in structural units called **osteons (Haversian systems)**. Each osteon consists of a central microscopic channel, called a **Haversian canal**, surrounded by a number of concentric circles of bony matrix (calcium phosphate), called lamellae.
- **Spongy bone** is much less dense and consists of an interconnecting lattice of bony **spicules** (trabeculae); the cavities between the spicules are filled with yellow and/or red bone marrow. Yellow marrow is inactive and infiltrated by adipose tissue; red marrow is involved in blood cell formation.

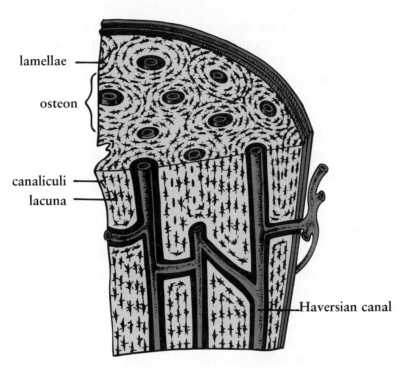

lamellae

osteon

canaliculi

lacuna

Haversian canal

Figure 9.1. Microscopic Bone Structure

3. **Osteocytes**

Two other types of cells found in bone tissue are osteoblasts and osteoclasts. **Osteoblasts** synthesize and secrete the organic constituents of the bone matrix; once they have become surrounded by their matrix, they mature into osteocytes. **Osteoclasts** are large, multinucleated cells involved in bone resorption.

4. **Bone Formation**

Bone formation occurs by either **endochondral ossification** or by **intramembranous ossification**. In endochondral ossification, existing **cartilage** is replaced by bone. Long bones arise primarily through endochondral ossification. In intramembranous ossification, mesenchymal (embryonic, undifferentiated) connective tissue is transformed into, and replaced by, bone.

DAT Synopsis

OsteoBLASTS: Build bone.

OsteoCLASTS: Destroy bone (also called bone resorption).

B. ORGANIZATION OF VERTEBRATE SKELETON

The **axial skeleton** is the basic framework of the body, consisting of the skull, vertebral column, and the rib cage. It is the point of attachment of the **appendicular** skeleton, which includes the bones of the appendages and the pectoral and pelvic girdles.

Bones are held together in a number of ways. Sutures or immovable joints hold the bones of the skull together. Bones that do move relative to one another are held together by **movable joints** and are additionally supported and strengthened by **ligaments**. Ligaments serve as bone-to-bone connectors. Tendons attach skeletal muscle to bones and bend the skeleton at the movable joints.

The point of attachment of a muscle to a stationary bone (the proximal end in limb muscles) is called the **origin**. The point of attachment of a muscle to the bone that moves (distal end in limb muscles) is called the **insertion**. **Extension** indicates a straightening of a joint, while **flexion** refers to a bending of a joint.

MUSCULAR SYSTEM

Muscle tissue consists of bundles of specialized **contractile fibers** held together by connective tissue. There are three morphologically and functionally distinct types of muscle in mammals: **skeletal muscle**, **smooth muscle**, and **cardiac muscle**.

A. SKELETAL MUSCLE

Skeletal muscle is responsible for **voluntary** movements and is innervated by the somatic nervous system. Each fiber is a **multinucleated** cell created by the fusion of several mononucleated embryonic cells. Embedded in the fibers are filaments called **myofibrils**, which are further divided into contractile units called **sarcomeres**. The myofibrils are enveloped by a modified endoplasmic reticulum that stores calcium ions and is called the **sarcoplasmic reticulum**. The cytoplasm of a muscle fiber is called sarcoplasm, and the cell membrane is called the sarcolemma. The sarcolemma is capable of propagating an **action potential**, and is connected to a system of transverse tubules (T system) oriented perpendicularly to the myofibrils. The T system provides channels for ion flow throughout the muscle fibers and can also propagate an action potential. Because of the high energy requirements of contraction, **mitochondria** are very abundant in muscle cells, distributed along the myofibrils. Skeletal muscle has **striations** of light and dark bands and is, therefore, also referred to as **striated muscle**.

B. THE SARCOMERE

1. Structure

The sarcomere is composed of **thin** and **thick** filaments. The thin filaments are chains of **actin** molecules. The thick filaments are composed of organized bundles of **myosin** molecules.

Electron microscopy reveals that the sarcomere is organized as follows: **Z lines** define the boundaries of a single sarcomere and anchor the thin filaments. The **M line** runs down the center of the sarcomere. The **I band** is the region containing thin filaments only. The **H zone** is the region containing thick filaments only. The **A band** spans the entire length of the thick filaments and any overlapping portions of the thin filaments. Note that during contraction, the A band is not reduced in size, while the H zone and I band are.

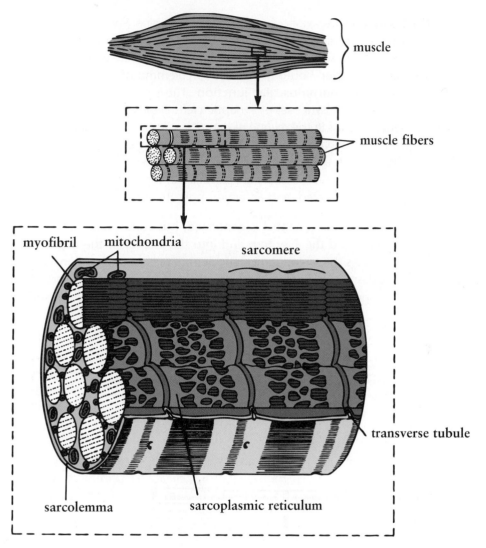

myofibril   mitochondria   sarcomere

transverse tubule

sarcolemma   sarcoplasmic reticulum

Figure 9.2. Skeletal Muscle

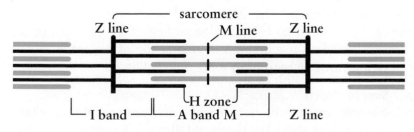

sarcomere

Z line   M line   Z line

H zone

I band   A band M   Z line

Figure 9.3. Sarcomere

2. Contraction

Muscle contraction is stimulated by a message from the somatic nervous system sent via a motor neuron. The link between the nerve terminal (synaptic bouton) and the sarcolemma of the muscle fiber is called the **neuromuscular junction**. The space between the two is known as the synapse, or synaptic cleft. Depolarization of the motor neuron results in the release of neurotransmitters (e.g., **acetylcholine**) from the nerve terminal. The neurotransmitter diffuses across the synaptic cleft and binds to special receptor sites on the sarcolemma. If enough of these receptors are stimulated, the permeability of the sarcolemma is altered, and an action potential is generated.

Once an action potential is generated, it is conducted along the sarcolemma and the T system and into the interior of the muscle fiber. This causes the sarcoplasmic reticulum to release **calcium ions** into the sarcoplasm. Calcium ions initiate the contraction of the sarcomere. Actin and myosin slide past each other, and the sarcomere contracts.

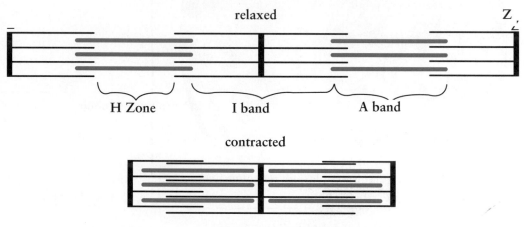

relaxed

Z

H Zone   I band   A band

contracted

Figure 9.4. Contraction

3. Stimulus and Muscle Response

Individual muscle fibers generally exhibit an **all-or-none response**; only a stimulus above a minimal value, called the **threshold value**, can elicit contraction. The strength of the contraction of a single muscle fiber cannot be increased, regardless of the strength of the stimulus. However, the strength of contraction of the entire muscle can be increased by **recruiting** more muscle fibers.

a. Simple twitch

A simple twitch is the response of a single muscle fiber to a brief stimulus at or above the **threshold** stimulus. It consists of a latent period, a contraction period, and a relaxation period. The **latent period** is the time between stimulation and the onset of contraction. During this time lag, the action potential spreads along the sarcolemma, and Ca^{2+} ions are released. Following the **contraction period**, there is a brief **relaxation period** in which the muscle is unresponsive to a stimulus; this period is known as the **absolute refractory period**.

b. **Summation and tetanus**

When the fibers of a muscle are exposed to very frequent stimuli, the muscle cannot fully relax. The contractions begin to combine, becoming stronger and more prolonged. This is known as temporal **summation**. The contractions become continuous when the stimuli are so frequent that the muscle cannot relax. This type of contraction is known as **tetanus** and is stronger than a simple twitch of a single fiber. If tetanus is maintained, the muscle will fatigue, and the contraction will weaken.

simple twitch (single fiber)

summation and tetanus (whole muscle)

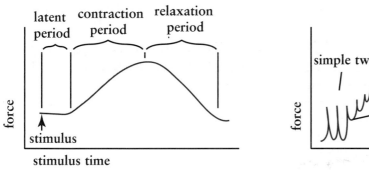
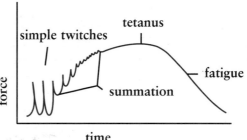

Figure 9.5. Simple Twitch and Summation/Tetanus

c. **Tonus**

Tonus is a state of partial contraction. Muscles are never completely relaxed and maintain a partially contracted state at all times.

C. SMOOTH MUSCLE

Smooth muscle is responsible for involuntary actions and is innervated by the **autonomic** nervous system. Smooth muscle is found in the digestive tract, bladder, uterus, and blood vessel walls, among other places. Smooth muscle cells possess **one** centrally located nucleus. Smooth muscles lack the striations of skeletal muscle.

D. CARDIAC MUSCLE

The muscle tissue of the heart is composed of cardiac muscle fibers. These fibers possess characteristics of both skeletal and smooth muscle fibers. As in skeletal muscle, actin and myosin filaments are arranged in sarcomeres, giving cardiac muscle a striated appearance. However, cardiac muscle cells generally have only one or two centrally located nuclei.

ENERGY RESERVES

ATP is the primary source of energy for muscle contraction. Very little ATP is actually stored in the muscles, and other forms of energy must be stored and rapidly converted to ATP.

A. CREATINE PHOSPHATE AND ARGININE PHOSPHATE

In vertebrates and some invertebrates, particularly echinoderms, energy can be temporarily stored in a high-energy compound called **creatine phosphate**. Many invertebrates utilize a similar compound called arginine phosphate.

B. MYOGLOBIN

Myoglobin is a hemoglobin-like protein found in muscle tissue. Myoglobin has a high oxygen affinity and maintains the oxygen supply in muscles by binding oxygen tightly.

## 10

DIGESTION

Animals are **heterotrophic** and thus unable to synthesize their own nutrients. Food provides the raw material for energy, repair, and growth of tissues. The food must first be **ingested**. **Digestion** consists of the degradation of large molecules into smaller molecules, which can be **absorbed** into the bloodstream and used directly by cells. **Intracellular** digestion occurs within the cell, usually in membrane-bound vesicles. **Extracellular** digestion refers to a digestive process that occurs outside of the cell, within a lumen or tract.

DIGESTION IN UNICELLULAR ORGANISMS

In unicellular organisms, food capture is effected primarily by **phagocytosis**. Food vacuoles form immediately following ingestion. In the **amoeba**, pseudopods surround and engulf food (phagocytosis) and enclose it in food vacuoles. **Lysosomes** (containing digestive enzymes) fuse with the food vacuole and release their digestive enzymes, which act upon the nutrients. The resulting simpler molecules diffuse into the cytoplasm. The unusable end products are eliminated from the vacuole.

In the paramecium (see Figure 10.1), cilia sweep food into the oral groove and **cytopharynx**. A food vacuole forms around food at the lower end of the cytopharynx. Eventually, the vacuole breaks off into the cytoplasm and progresses towards the anterior end of the cell. Enzymes are secreted into the vacuole, and the products diffuse into the cytoplasm. Solid wastes are expelled at the anal pore.

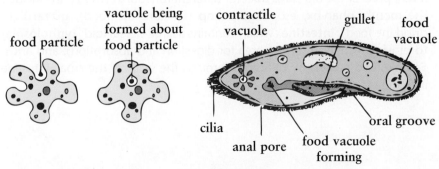

Figure 10.1

DIGESTION IN INVERTEBRATES

Multicellular organisms have developed numerous adaptations for food capture and ingestion, digestion, and absorption. In many animals, the **physical breakdown** of large particles of food into small particles begins by cutting and grinding in the mouth and churning in the digestive tract. The molecular composition is unchanged, but the surface area of the substrates on which the enzymes act is increased. **Chemical breakdown** of molecules is accomplished by enzymatic hydrolysis. The smaller digested nutrients (glucose, amino acids, fatty acids, and glycerol) pass through the semipermeable plasma membrane of the gut cells to be further metabolized or transported.

A. CNIDARIANS

The hydra (see Figure 10.2) uses intracellular and extracellular digestion. **Tentacles** bring food to the mouth (ingestion) and release the particles into a cup likesac. The endodermal cells lining this gastrovascular cavity secrete enzymes into the cavity. Thus, digestion principally occurs outside the cells (extracellular). However, once the food is reduced to small fragments, the gastrodermal cells engulf the nutrients, and digestion is completed intracellularly. Undigested food is expelled through the **mouth**. Every cell is exposed to the external environment, thereby facilitating intracellular digestion.

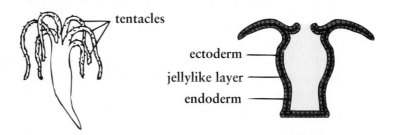

Figure 10.2

B. ANNELIDS

Like higher animals, **earthworms** (see Figure 10.3) have a one-way digestive tract with both a mouth and an anus. This allows **specialization** of different parts of the digestive tract for different functions. These parts include the mouth, pharynx, esophagus, **crop** (to store the food), **gizzard** (to grind the food), **intestine** (which contains a large dorsal fold [**typholosole**] to provide increased surface area for digestion and absorption), and **anus**. Soluble food passes, by diffusion, through the walls of the small intestine into the blood.

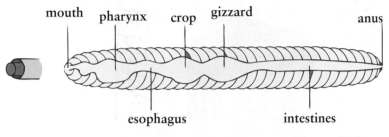

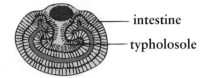

Figure 10.3

C. ARTHROPODS

Insects (see Figure 10.4) have a digestive system similar to that of the earthworm. They also have jaws for chewing and **salivary glands**, which improve food digestion.

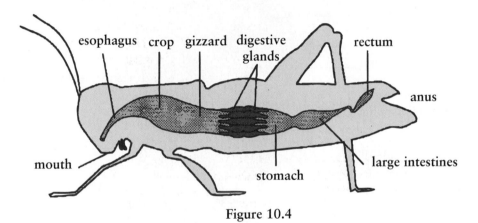

Figure 10.4

DIGESTION IN HUMANS

The human digestive tract (see Figure 10.5) begins with the **oral cavity** and continues with the **pharynx**, the **esophagus**, the **stomach**, the **small intestine**, the **large intestine**, and the anus. Accessory organs, such as the salivary glands, the pancreas, the liver, and the gall bladder, also play essential roles in digestion.

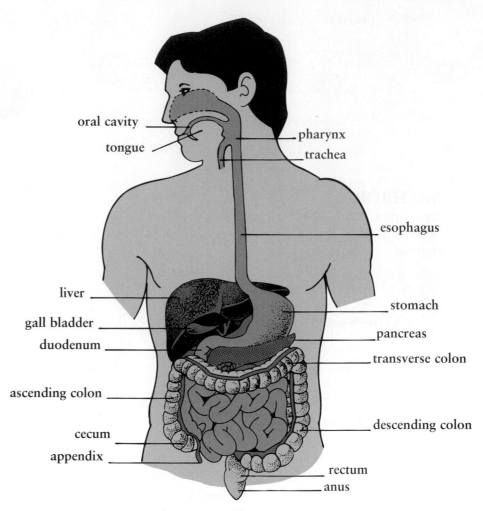

Figure 10.5. Human Digestive Tract

A. THE ORAL CAVITY

The oral cavity (the mouth) is where the **mechanical** and **chemical** digestion of food begins. Mechanical digestion is the breakdown of large food particles into smaller particles through the biting and chewing action of teeth **(mastication)**. Chemical digestion refers to the enzymatic breakdown of macromolecules into smaller molecules. It begins in the mouth when the salivary glands secrete **saliva**. Saliva **lubricates** food to facilitate swallowing and provides a solvent for food particles. Saliva is secreted in response to a nervous reflex triggered by the presence of food in the oral cavity. Saliva contains the enzyme **salivary amylase (ptyalin)**, which hydrolyzes starch to maltose (a disaccharide).

B. THE ESOPHAGUS

The esophagus is the muscular tube leading from the mouth to the stomach. Food is moved down the esophagus by rhythmic waves of involuntary muscular contractions called **peristalsis**.

C. THE STOMACH

The stomach, a large, muscular organ located in the upper abdomen, stores and partially digests food. The walls of the stomach are lined by the thick gastric mucosa, which contains the glands. These glands secrete **mucus**, which protects the stomach lining from the harshly acidic juices (pH = 2) present in the stomach. They also secrete **pepsin**, which is a protein-hydrolyzing enzyme, and hydrochloric acid (HCl), which kills bacteria, dissolves the intercellular "glue" holding food tissues together, and activates certain proteins. The churning of the stomach produces an acidic, semi-fluid mixture of partially digested food known as **chyme**. The chyme passes into the first segment of the small intestine, the **duodenum**, through the pyloric sphincter.

D. THE SMALL INTESTINE

Chemical digestion is completed in the small intestine. The small intestine is divided into three sections: the duodenum, the jejunum, and the ileum. The small intestine is highly **adapted** to **absorption**. To maximize the surface area available for digestion and absorption, the intestine is extremely long (greater than six meters in length) and highly coiled. In addition, numerous fingerlike projections, called **villi**, extend out of the intestinal wall (see Figure 10.6). Villi contain capillaries and lacteals (vessels of the lymphatic system). Amino acids and monosaccharides pass through the villi walls into the capillary system. Large fatty acids and glycerol pass into the lacteals and are then reconverted into fats (fatty acid + glycerol). Note that some nutrients are actively absorbed (i.e., requiring energy), such as glucose and amino acids, while others are passively absorbed.

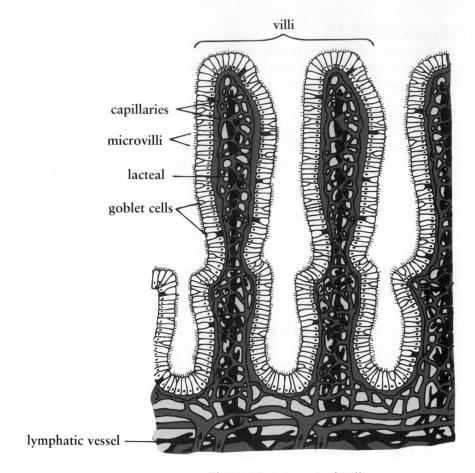

villi

capillaries

microvilli

lacteal

goblet cells

lymphatic vessel

Figure 10.6. Intestinal Villi

Most digestion in the small intestine occurs in the duodenum, where the secretions of the intestinal glands, pancreas, liver, and gall bladder mix with the acidic chyme entering from the stomach. The intestinal mucosa secretes **lipases** (for fat digestion), **aminopeptidases** (for polypeptide digestion) and **disaccharidases** (for the digestion of maltose, lactose, and sucrose). The disaccharidase **lactase** breaks down lactose (milk sugar). This enzyme is present in infants, but many adults lack the enzyme and are **lactose-intolerant**. Lactose in the small intestine cannot be digested and is metabolized by bacteria, producing intestinal discomfort.

E. THE LIVER

The liver produces **bile**, which is stored in the **gall bladder** prior to release into the small intestine. Bile contains no enzymes; it **emulsifies** fats, breaking down large globules into small droplets. Emulsification of fats exposes a greater surface area of the fat to the action of pancreatic lipase. In the absence of bile, fats cannot be digested.

F. THE PANCREAS

The pancreas produces enzymes such as **amylase** for carbohydrate digestion, **trypsin** for protein digestion, and **lipase** for fat digestion. The pancreas secretes a bicarbonate-rich juice that neutralizes the acidic chyme
arriving form the stomach. The pancreatic enzymes operate optimally at
this higher pH.

G. THE LARGE INTESTINE

The large intestine is approximately 1.5 meters long and functions in the
absorption of salts and the absorption of any water not already absorbed
by the small intestine. The **rectum** provides for transient storage of feces
prior to elimination through the anus.

DIGESTION IN PLANTS AND FUNGI

Plants have no digestive system, but intracellular digestive processes similar to
those of animals do occur, coordinating the utilization of nutrients with their
production.

A. INTRACELLULAR DIGESTION

Plants store insoluble polymers, starches, lipids, and proteins in the cells.
The principle storage food is starch (a glucose polysaccharide), found in
large quantities in seeds, stems, and roots. When nutrients are required,
the storage polymers are broken down to simpler molecules (glucose, fatty
acids, glycerol, and amino acids) by enzyme **hydrolysis**. The simple products can be used in the storage cell itself or transported by diffusion to
other cells.

B. EXTRACELLULAR DIGESTION

Some heterotrophic organisms, such as fungi, must obtain preformed
organic molecules (nutrients) from the environment. Enzymes are secreted, hydrolyzing complex nutrients into simpler molecules, which are then
absorbed. Once inside, the simpler molecules can be used for energy or to
synthesize larger molecules.

For example, the **rhizoids** of bread mold, a typical saprophyte that lives on
dead organic material, secrete enzymes into the external environment (the
bread). Digestion produces simple soluble end products (glucose, amino
acids, fatty acids, and glycerol), which are absorbed by diffusion into the
rhizoid and transported throughout the mold.

In the plant kingdom, the **Venus flytrap** comes the closest to actual ingestion. When a fly arrives, certain sensitive tissues entrap the insect.
Enzymes are secreted to digest the fly and absorb the soluble end products. This is, of course, extracellular digestion. Note that the Venus flytrap
is still an autotroph—it photosynthesizes to produce glucose. It uses the
insect as a **nitrate** source, because the flytrap grows in nitrogen-poor soils.

## 11

EXCRETION

Excretion refers to the removal of **metabolic wastes** produced in the body. It is distinguished from **elimination**, the removal of indigestible material. Most of the body's activities produce metabolic wastes that must be removed. **Aerobic respiration** leads to the production of **carbon dioxide** and water. **Deamination** of amino acids in the liver leads to the production of **nitrogenous wastes** like urea and ammonia. All metabolic processes lead to the production of mineral salts, which must be excreted by the kidneys.

EXCRETION IN INVERTEBRATES
A. EXCRETION IN PROTOZOANS AND CNIDARIANS
In these phyla, all cells are in contact with the external, aqueous environment. Water soluble wastes, such as **ammonia** and **carbon dioxide**, can exit the cells by simple diffusion through the cell membrane. This type of excretion is **passive**. Some freshwater **protozoa**, such as the paramecium, possess a contractile **vacuole**—an organelle specialized for water excretion by active transport. Excess water, which continually diffuses into the cell from the hypotonic environment (freshwater), is collected and periodically pumped out of the cell. This permits the cell to maintain its volume and pressure.

B. EXCRETION IN ANNELIDS
In earthworms, carbon dioxide excretion occurs directly through the moist skin. Two pairs of **nephridia** in each body segment excrete water, mineral salts, and nitrogenous wastes in the form of urea (see Figure 11.1).

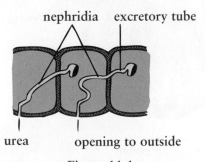

Figure 11.1

C. EXCRETION IN ARTHROPODS

In insects, carbon dioxide is released from the tissues into adjacent tube-like **tracheae**, which are continuous with the external air through openings called **spiracles**. Nitrogenous wastes are excreted in the form of solid **uric acid** crystals. The use of solid nitrogenous wastes is an adaptation for the conservation of water. Mineral salts and uric acid accumulate in the **Malphigian tubules** and are then transported to the intestine to be expelled with the solid wastes of digestion.

EXCRETION IN HUMANS

The principal organs of excretion in humans are the lungs, liver, skin, and kidneys. In the **lungs,** carbon dioxide and water vapor diffuse from the blood and are continually exhaled. Sweat glands in the **skin** excrete water and dissolved salts (and a small quantity of urea). Perspiration serves to regulate body temperature, since the evaporation of sweat produces cooling. The **liver** processes nitrogenous wastes, blood pigment wastes, and other chemicals for excretion. Urea is produced by the deamination of amino acids in the liver and diffuses into the blood for ultimate excretion in the **kidneys.** Bile salts and red blood pigments are excreted as bile and pass out with the feces. The kidneys function to maintain the osmolarity of the blood; excrete numerous waste products and toxic chemicals; and conserve glucose, salt, and water.

A. THE KIDNEYS

The kidneys regulate the concentration of salt and water in the blood through the formation and **excretion** of urine. The kidneys are bean shaped and are located behind the stomach and liver. Each kidney is composed of approximately 1 million units, called **nephrons.**

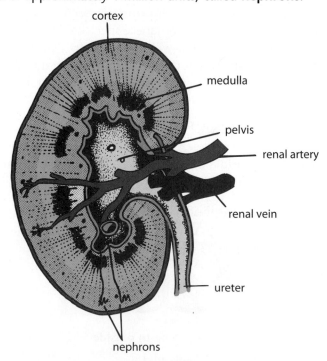

Figure 11.2

1. **Structure**

The kidney is divided into three regions: the outer **cortex**, the inner **medulla**, and the renal **pelvis**. A **nephron** consists of a bulb called **Bowman's capsule**, which embraces a special capillary bed called a **glomerulus**. Bowman's capsule leads into a long, coiled tubule, which is divided into functionally distinct units: the **proximal convoluted tubule**, the **loop of Henle**, the **distal convoluted tubule**, and the **collecting duct**. The nephron is positioned such that the loop of Henle runs through the medulla, while the convoluted tubules and Bowman's capsule are in the cortex. Concentrated urine in the collecting tubules flows into the pelvis of the kidney, a funnel-like region that opens directly into the **ureter**. The ureters from each kidney empty into the **urinary bladder**, where urine collects until expelled via the **urethra**. Most of the nephron is surrounded by a complex **peritubular capillary** network to facilitate reabsorption of amino acids, glucose, salts, and water.

> **DAT Synopsis**
>
> Imagine that the glomerulus is like a sieve or collander. Small molecules dissolved in the fluid will pass through the glomerulus (e.g., glucose that is later reabsorbed), while large molecules, such as proteins and blood cells, will not. If blood cells or protein are found in the urine, this indicates a problem at the level of the glomerulus.

2. **Urine Formation**

Filtration, secretion, and reabsorption are the three processes that lead to urine formation.

  a. **Filtration**

  Blood pressure forces 20 percent of the blood plasma entering the **glomerulus** through the capillary walls and into the surrounding **Bowman's capsule**. The fluid and small solutes entering the nephron are called the **filtrate**. The filtrate is isotonic with blood plasma. Particles too large to filter through the glomerulus, such as blood cells and albumin, remain in the circulatory system. Filtration is a passive process driven by the hydrostatic pressure of the blood.

  b. **Secretion**

  The nephron secretes substances such as acids, bases, and ions like potassium and phosphate from the interstitial fluid into the filtrate by both **passive** and **active** transport. Materials are secreted from the peritubular capillaries into the nephron tubule.

  c. **Reabsorption**

  Essential substances (**glucose**, salts, and amino acids) and water are **reabsorbed** from the filtrate and returned to the blood. Reabsorption occurs primarily in the proximal convoluted tubule and is an active process. Movement of these molecules is accompanied by the passive movement of water. This results in the formation of concentrated urine, which is **hypertonic** to the blood.

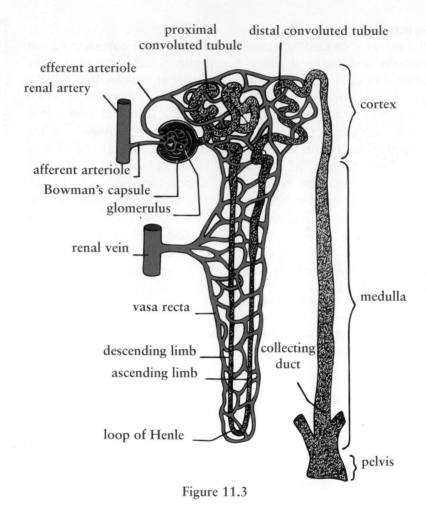

Figure 11.3

3. Nephron Function

Through the selective permeability of its walls and the maintenance of an osmolarity gradient, the nephron reabsorbs nutrients, salts, and water from the filtrate and returns them to the body, thus maintaining the bloodstream's solute concentration.

a. Osmolarity gradient

The selective permeability of the tubules establishes an osmolarity gradient in the surrounding interstitial fluid. By exiting and then re-entering at different segments of the nephron, solutes create an osmolarity gradient, with tissue osmolarity increasing from **cortex** to **inner medulla**. The solutes that contribute to the maintenance of the gradient are urea and salt (Na^+ and Cl^-). The osmolarity of urine (determined by the concentration of dissolved particles) is established in the collecting tubule by means of this **countercurrent-multiplier system**: The anatomic arrangement of the loop of Henle within the kidney permits the establishment of the concentration gradient that permits the reabsorption of 99 percent of the filtrate in the collecting tubules. Thus, the production of concentrated urine is possible.

b. **Concentration of urine**

The countercurrent system causes the medium in the medulla of the kidney to be **hyperosmolar** with respect to the dilute filtrate flowing in the collecting tubule. As the filtrate flowing in the collecting tubules passes through this region of the kidney, on its way to the pelvis and ureter, water flows out of the collecting tubules by **osmosis**. This water is removed by capillaries flowing in the medulla. The reabsorption of water in this zone of the kidney, which permits the concentration of urine, depends on the permeability of the collecting tubules to water. Regulation of the permeability of the collecting tubule to water is accomplished by the hormone **ADH (vasopressin)**. ADH increases the permeability of the collecting duct to water, allowing more water to be absorbed and more concentrated urine to be formed.

## 12

ANIMAL BEHAVIOR

PATTERNS OF ANIMAL BEHAVIOR
A. SIMPLE REFLEXES

Reflexes are simple, automatic responses to simple stimuli. Reflexes can be defined as reliable occurrences of particular behavioral responses following a given environmental stimulus. A simple reflex is controlled at the **spinal cord**, connecting a two-neuron pathway from the **receptor** (afferent neuron) to the **motor** (efferent neuron). The efferent nerve innervates the effector (e.g., a muscle or gland). Reflex behavior is important in the behavioral response of lower animals. It is less important in the behavioral repertoire of higher forms of life, such as the vertebrates.

sensory neuron ⟶ interneuron ⟶ motor neuron
(contained in the spinal cord)

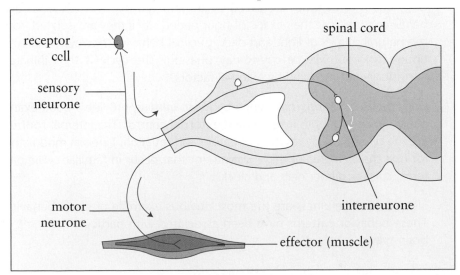

Figure 12.1

B. COMPLEX REFLEXES

More complex reflex patterns involve neural integration at a higher level—the **brainstem** or even the **cerebrum**. For example, the "**startle response**" alerts an animal to a significant stimulus. It can occur in response to potential danger or to hearing one's name called. The startle response involves the interaction of many neurons, a system termed the **reticular activating system**.

C. FIXED-ACTION PATTERNS

Fixed-action patterns are complex, coordinated, **innate** behavioral responses to specific patterns of stimulation in the environment. The stimulus that elicits the behavior is referred to as the **releaser**. Because fixed-action patterns are innate, they are relatively unlikely to be modified by learning. An animal has a repertoire of fixed-action patterns and only a limited ability to develop new ones. The particular stimuli that trigger a fixed-action pattern are more readily modified, provided certain cues or elements of the stimuli are maintained.

An example of a fixed-action pattern is the retrieval and maintenance response of many female birds to an egg of their species. Certain kinds of stimuli are more effective than others in triggering a fixed-action pattern. For example, an egg with the characteristics of that species will be more effective than one that only crudely resembles the natural egg. Another type of fixed-action pattern is the characteristic movements made by animals that herd or flock together, such as the swimming actions of fish and the flying actions of locusts.

D. BEHAVIOR CYCLES

Daily cycles of behavior are called **circadian rhythms**. Animals with such behavior cycles lose their exact 24-hour periodicity if they are isolated from the natural phases of light and dark. Cyclical behavior, however, will continue with approximate day-to-day phasing. The cycle is thus initiated intrinsically but modified by external factors.

Daily cycles of eating, maintained by most animals, provide a good example of cycles with both **internal** and **external** control. The internal controls are the natural bodily rhythms of eating and satiation. External modulators include the elements of the environment that occur in familiar cyclic patterns, such as dinner bells and clocks.

Sleep and wakefulness are the most obvious example of cyclic behavior. These behavior patterns have been associated with particular patterns of brain waves.

E. ENVIRONMENTAL RHYTHMS

In many situations, patterns of behavior are established and maintained mainly by periodic **environmental stimuli**. (A human example of this is the response to traffic light signals.) Just as environmental stimuli influence many naturally occurring biological rhythms, biological factors influence behavior governed by periodic environmental stimuli.

LEARNING

Learned behavior involves **adaptive responses** to the environment. Learning is a complex phenomenon that occurs to some extent in all animals. In lower animals, instinctual or innate behaviors are the predominant determinants of behavior patterns, and learning plays a relatively minor role in the modification of these predetermined behaviors. In higher animals, the major share of the response to the environment is learned. The capacity for learning adaptive responses is closely correlated with the degree of **neurologic development** (i.e., the capacity of the nervous system, particularly the cerebral cortex, for flexibility).

A. HABITUATION

Habituation is one of the simplest learning patterns, involving the suppression of the normal startle responses to stimuli. Repeated stimulation will result in decreased responsiveness to that stimulus. The normal autonomic response to that stimulus would serve no useful purpose when the stimulus becomes a part of the background environment, so the response to the stimulus is suppressed. If the stimulus is no longer regularly applied, the response tends to recover over time. This is referred to as **spontaneous recovery**. Recovery of the response can also occur with a modification of the stimulus.

B. CLASSICAL CONDITIONING

Classical or **Pavlovian** conditioning involves the association of a normally **autonomic** or visceral response with an environment stimulus. For this reason, the response learned through Pavlovian conditioning is sometimes called a **conditioned reflex**. In Pavlovian conditioning, the normal, innate stimulus for a reflex is replaced by one chosen by the experimenter.

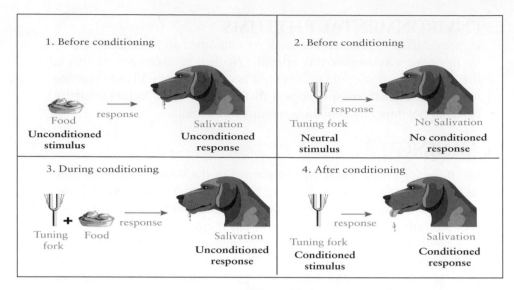

Figure 12.2

1. **Pavlov's Experiments**

   Pavlov, who won a Nobel prize for his work on digestive physiology, studied the **salivation reflex** in dogs. In 1927, he discovered that if a dog was presented with an **arbitrary stimulus** (e.g., a bell) and then presented with food, it would eventually salivate on hearing the bell alone. The food elicited the unconditioned response of salivation. After repeated association of the bell with the food, the bell alone could elicit the salivation reflex. Thus, the innate or unconditioned response would occur with the selected stimulus. Pavlov's terminology, still used today, is described below:

   - An established (innate) reflex consists of an **unconditioned stimulus** (US) (e.g., food for salivation), and the response that is naturally elicited is termed the **unconditioned response** (UR) (e.g., salivation).
   - A neutral stimulus is a stimulus that will not by itself elicit the response (prior to conditioning). During conditioning, the neutral stimulus (the bell) and the unconditioned stimulus (the food) are presented together. Eventually, the neutral stimulus is able to elicit the response in the absence of the unconditioned stimulus, and it is then called the conditioned stimulus (CS). Pavlov's example of a conditioned stimulus is the sound of a bell for salivation.
   - The product of the conditioning experience is termed the **conditioned reflex**. The conditioned reflex in Pavlov's experiment was salivation (the conditioned response) following a previously neutral stimulus (now the conditioned stimulus) such as the sound tone.

- Pavlov defined **conditioning** as the establishment of a new reflex (association of stimulus with response) by the addition of a new, previously neutral stimulus to the set of stimuli that are already capable of triggering the response. Thus, Pavlov added a bell tone to the set of stimuli, originally including food, that trigger salivation in the dogs.

2. **Pseudoconditioning**

Pseudoconditioning is a phenomenon that can be confused with true classical conditioning. A critical test of conditioning is the determination of whether the conditioning process is actually necessary for the production of a response by a previously "neutral stimulus." In many cases, the so-called "neutral" stimulus is able to elicit the response even before conditioning and, hence, is not really a neutral stimulus. Pseudoconditioning can be avoided by carefully evaluating all prospective stimuli before conditioning begins.

C. OPERANT OR INSTRUMENTAL CONDITIONING

Operant or instrumental conditioning involves conditioning responses to stimuli with the use of **reward** or **reinforcement**. When the organism exhibits a specific behavioral pattern that the experimenter would like to see repeated, the animal is rewarded. The reinforcement or reward increases the likelihood that the behavior will appear—it has been "reinforced." Although this instrumental conditioning was originally applied to conditioning responses under the voluntary control of the organism, it has been successfully applied more recently to the conditioning of visceral responses, such as changes in heartbeat.

1. **Experiments of B. F. Skinner**

B. F. Skinner first demonstrated the principles of operant conditioning and reinforcement. In the original operant conditioning experiments, he used the well-known "Skinner box," consisting of a cage with a lever or key and a food dispenser. A food pellet was delivered whenever the animal pressed the lever. Thus, depression of the lever was the operant response under study. In later experiments, Skinner varied the type of reinforcement. Reinforcers fell into two categories:

a. **Positive reinforcement**

Positive reinforcement or **reward** includes providing food, light, or electrical stimulation of the animal's brain "pleasure centers." Following positive reinforcement, the animal was much **more likely** to repeat the desired behavioral response (i.e., to press the bar). In a sense, the animal has developed a positive connection between the action (response) and the reward (stimulus that followed). This type of conditioning is likely to be involved in normal habit formation.

b. Negative reinforcement
Negative reinforcement also involves stimulating the brain's pleasure centers. However, in contrast to positive reinforcement, negative reinforcement links the **lack** of certain behavior with a reward (i.e., a bird may learn that it will receive a food pellet if it does *not* peck on a yellow circle in its cage).

In this case, the animal has developed a negative connection between action (response) and reward (stimulus that followed). Thus, the animal has developed a *positive* connection between the *lack* of the action and the reward, and the animal is **less likely** to repeat the behavioral response.

c. Punishment
Punishment involves conditioning an organism so that it will **stop** exhibiting a given behavior pattern. Punishment may involve painfully shocking the organism each time the chosen behavior appears. After punishment, the organism is **less likely** to repeat the behavioral response. The animal develops a negative connection between the stimulus and the response.

d. Habit family hierarchy
A stimulus is usually associated with several possible responses, each response having a different probability of occurrence. These stimulus-behavioral associations are believed to be ordered in a **habit family hierarchy**. For example a chicken may respond to a light in many ways, but if one particular response is rewarded, it will occur with higher probability in the future. Reward strengthens a specific behavioral response and raises its order in the hierarchy. Punishment weakens a specific behavioral response and lowers its order in the hierarchy.

D. MODIFICATIONS OF CONDITIONED BEHAVIOR
1. Extinction
Extinction is the gradual **elimination** of conditioned responses in the absence of reinforcement (i.e., the "unlearning" of the response pattern). In **instrumental and operant conditioning**, the response is diminished and finally eliminated in the absence of reinforcement. The response is not completely unlearned—rather, it is inhibited in the absence of reinforcement. It will rapidly reappear if the reinforcement is returned. In **classical conditioning**, extinction occurs when the unconditioned stimulus is removed or was never sufficiently paired with the conditioned stimulus. The conditioned stimulus must be paired with the unconditioned stimulus, at least part of the time, for the maintenance of the conditioned response. After sufficient time elapses following extinction, the conditioned response may again be elicited by the conditioned stimulus. The recovery of the conditioned response after extinction is called **spontaneous recovery**.

2. Generalization and Discrimination

Stimulus generalization is the ability of a conditioned organism to respond to stimuli that are similar, but not identical, to the original conditioned stimulus. The less similar the stimulus is to the original conditioned stimulus, the less the response will be. For example, an organism may be conditioned to respond to a stimulus of 1,000 Hz tone, but it may respond to stimuli somewhat higher or lower in pitch as well. **Stimulus discrimination** involves the ability of the learning organism to respond differentially to slightly different stimuli. For example, if rewards are given to only a very narrow range of sound (such as a tone of 990 to 1,010 Hz) but not to stimuli outside this range, the organism will also learn not to respond to stimuli that are very different in tone. A **stimulus generalization gradient** is established after the organism has been conditioned, whereby stimuli further and further away from the original conditioned stimulus elicit responses with decreasing magnitude.

LIMITS OF BEHAVIORAL CHANGE

A. IMPRINTING

Imprinting is a process in which environmental patterns or objects presented to a developing organism during a brief **"critical period"** in early life become accepted permanently as an element of its behavioral environment (i.e., "stamped in" and included in an animal's behavioral response). A duckling passes through a critical period in which it learns that the first large moving object it sees is its mother. In the natural environment, this is usually the case. However, other objects can be substituted during this period, and the duckling will follow anything that is substituted for its mother. This phenomenon was first identified by the ethologist **Konrad Lorenz**, who swam in a pond amongst newly hatched ducklings separated from their mother and found that they eventually followed him as if he were their mother.

B. CRITICAL PERIOD

Critical periods are specific time periods during an animal's early development when it is physiologically able to develop specific behavioral patterns. If the proper environmental pattern is not present during the critical period, the behavioral pattern will not develop properly. In addition to the critical period described above, some animals have a **visual critical period**. If light is not present during this period, visual effectors will not develop properly.

INTRASPECIFIC INTERACTIONS

Intraspecific interactions occur as a means of communication between members of a species.

A. BEHAVIORAL DISPLAYS

A display may be defined as an **innate behavior** that has evolved as a signal for **communication** between members of the same species. According to this definition, a song, call, or an intentional change in an animal's physical characteristics are considered displays. Categories of displays include the following:

- **Reproductive displays** are specific behaviors found in all animals, including humans. Many animals have evolved a variety of complex actions that function as signals in preparation for mating.
- **Agonistic displays** are such things as a dog's display of appeasement when it wags its tail or the dog's **antagonistic** behavior when it directs its face straight and raises its body.
- Other displays include various **dancing** procedures exhibited by **honeybees**, especially the scout honeybee, to convey information concerning the quality and location of food sources. Displays utilizing auditory, visual, chemical, and tactile elements are often used as means of communication.

B. PECKING ORDER

The relationships among members of the same species living as a contained social group frequently become stable for a period of time. When food, mates, or territory are disputed, a **dominant** member of the species will prevail over a **subordinate** one. The social hierarchy is frequently referred to as the **pecking order**. It minimizes violent intra specific aggressions by defining stable relationships among members of the group.

C. TERRITORIALITY

Members of most land-dwelling species **defend** a limited area or territory from intrusion by other members of the species. These territories are typically occupied by a male or a male-female pair and are frequently used for mating, nesting, and feeding. Territoriality serves the adaptive function of **distributing** members of the species so that the environmental resources are not depleted in a small region; furthermore, intraspecific competition is reduced. Although there is frequently a minimum size for any species' territory, the territory size varies with the population size and density. The larger the population, the smaller the territories are likely to be.

D. RESPONSE TO CHEMICALS

The **olfactory sense** is immensely important as a means of communication in many animals. Many animals secrete substances, called **pheromones**, that influence the behavior of other members of the same species. Pheromones can be classified as one of two types:

1. **Releaser pheromones** trigger a reversible behavioral change in the recipient. For example, female silkworms secrete a very powerful attracting pheromone, so powerful that a male responds to 1 ten-millionth of a gram from a distance of two miles or more. **Sex-attractant** pheromones are secreted by many animals, including cockroaches, queen honeybees, and gypsy moths. In addition to sex-attracting purposes, releaser pheromones are secreted as **alarm** and **toxic defensive** substances.

2. **Primer pheromones** produce long-term behavioral and physiological alterations in recipient animals. For example, pheromones from male **mice** may affect the **estrous cycles** of females. Pheromones have also been shown to limit sexual reproduction in areas of high animal density. Primer pheromones are important in social insects such as ants, bees, and termites, where they regulate role determination and reproductive capacities.

ECOLOGY

Ecology is the study of the **interactions** between organisms and their environment. The **environment** encompasses all that is external to the organism and is necessary for its existence. An organism's environment contains two components—the physical **(abiotic)** environment and the living **(biotic)** environment. The physical environment includes climate, temperature, availability of light and water, and the local topology. The biotic environment includes all living things that directly or indirectly influence the life of the organism, including the relationships that exist between organisms.

LEVELS OF BIOLOGICAL ORGANIZATION
A. ORGANISM

The organism is the individual unit of an ecological system, but the organism itself is composed of smaller units. The organism contains many organ systems, which are made up of **organs**. Organs are formed from **tissues**, tissues from **cells**, cells from many different **molecules**, molecules from **atoms**, and atoms from subatomic particles.

B. POPULATION

A population is a group of organisms of the same species **living together** in a given location. Examples of populations include dandelions on a lawn, flies in a barn, minnows of a certain species in a pond, and lions in a grassland. A **species** is any group of similar organisms that are capable of reproducing fertile offspring. Environmental factors, such as nutrients, water, and sunlight limitations, aid in maintaining populations at relatively constant levels.

C. COMMUNITIES

A community consists of populations of different plants and animal species interacting with each other in a given environment. The term **biotic community** is used to include only the populations and not their physical environment. An **ecosystem** includes the community and the environment. Generally, a community contains populations from all five kingdoms, monerans, protists, plants, fungi, and animals, all depending upon each other for survival. The following are examples of communities:

- A **lawn** contains dandelions, grasses, mushrooms, earthworms, nematodes, and bacteria.
- A **pond** contains dragonflies, algae, minnows, insect larvae, etc.
- A **forest** contains moss, pine, bacteria, lichens, ferns, deer, chipmunks, spiders, foxes, etc.
- The **sea** contains fish, whales, plankton, etc.

D. ECOSYSTEM

An ecosystem or ecological community encompasses the interaction between living **biotic communities** and the **nonliving environment.** In studying the ecosystem, the biologist emphasizes the effects of the biotic community on the environment and the environment on the community. The examples listed above for communities are also examples of ecosystems.

E. BIOSPHERE

The biosphere includes all portions of the planet that support life—the **atmosphere**, the **lithosphere** (rock and soil surface), and the **hydrosphere** (the oceans). It is a relatively thin zone extending a few feet beneath the earth's surface, several miles into the deepest sea, and several miles into the atmosphere.

THE ENVIRONMENT
A. PHYSICAL ENVIRONMENT

1. Water

Water is the major component of the internal environment of all living things. Water may be readily available, or the organism may possess adaptations for storage and conservation of water.

2. Temperature

Temperature must be maintained at an optimal level. Protoplasm is destroyed at temperatures below 0°C and at high temperatures. Organisms have adaptations necessary for protection against these extremes. The temperature of a geographic location depends upon its latitude and altitude. The same changes in habitat that occur as one approaches the colder polar regions occur as one ascends towards the colder regions of a mountain top.

3. **Sunlight**

   Sunlight is the ultimate source of energy for all organisms. Green plants must compete for sunlight in forests. They have adapted to capture as much sunlight as possible by growing broad leaves, branching, growing to greater height, or producing vine growths. The **photic zone** in water, the top layer through which light can penetrate, is where all aquatic photosynthetic activity takes place. In the **aphotic zone**, only animal life and other heterotrophic life exist.

4. **Oxygen Supply**

   This poses no problem for **terrestrial** life since the air contains approximately 20 percent oxygen. Aquatic plants and animals utilize the small amount of oxygen **dissolved** in water. Pollution can significantly lower oxygen content in water and threaten aquatic life.

5. **Substratum (soil or rock)**

   The substratum determines the nature of plant and animal life in the soil. Soil is affected by a number of factors:

   - **Acidity (pH):** Rhododendrons and pines are more suited for growth in acid soil. Acid rain may make soil pH too low for most plant growth.
   - The **texture** of soil and its clay content determine the water-holding capacity of the soil. Willows require moist soil. Most plants grow well in **loams,** which contain high percentages of each type of soil.
   - **Minerals,** including **nitrates** and **phosphates,** affect the type of vegetation that can be supported. Beach sand has been leached of all minerals and is generally unable to support plant life.
   - **Humus** quantity is determined by the amount of decaying plant and animal life in the soil.

B. BIOTIC FACTORS IN THE ENVIRONMENT

Organisms belonging to the same or different species influence each other's development. Living things interact with other living organisms and with their physical environment.

INTERACTIONS WITHIN THE ECOSYSTEM

Complex interactions exist among the constituents of an ecosystem. These interactions involve a cyclic flow of energy and materials.

A. THE NICHE

The niche defines the functional role of an organism in its ecosystem. The niche is distinct from the **habitat**—the latter is the physical place where an organism lives. The characteristics of the habitat aid in defining the niche, but additional factors must also be considered. The niche describes what the organism eats, where and how it obtains its food, what climactic factors it can tolerate and which are optimal, the nature of its parasites and predators, where and how it reproduces, etc. The concept of niche embodies every aspect of an organism's existence.

It is implicit in the definition of *niche* that no two species can ever occupy the same niche. Organisms occupying the same niche compete for the same limited resources: food, water, light, oxygen, space, minerals, and reproductive sites. There may be many organisms in this niche, but they are all of the same species and thus have the same requirements. The niche is so specific that a species can be identified by the niche it occupies.

Species occupying similar niches utilize at least one resource in common. Therefore, they will compete for that resource. This competition can have a number of outcomes:

- One species may be competitively superior to the other and drive the second to **extinction**.
- One species may be competitively superior in some regions, and the other may be superior in other regions under different environmental conditions. This would result in the elimination of one species in some places and the other in other places.
- The two species may rapidly evolve in **divergent** directions under the strong selection pressure resulting from intense competition. Thus, the two species would rapidly evolve greater differences in their niches.

B. NUTRITIONAL INTERACTIONS WITHIN THE ECOSYSTEM

1. Autotrophs

Autotrophs are organisms that manufacture their own food. The green plants utilize the energy of the sun to manufacture food. Chemosynthetic bacteria obtain energy from the oxidation of inorganic sulfur, iron, and nitrogen compounds.

2. Heterotrophs

Heterotrophs cannot synthesize their own food and must depend upon autotrophs or other heterotrophs in the ecosystem to obtain food and energy.

a. **Herbivores**

These animals consume only **plants** or plant foods. The toughness of **cellulose-containing** plant tissues has led to the development of structures for crushing and grinding that can extract plant fluids. Herbivores have long digestive tracts that provide greater surface area and time for digestion. However, they cannot digest much of the food they consume. **Symbiotic bacteria** capable of digesting cellulose inhabit the digestive tracts of herbivores and allow the breakdown and utilization of cellulose.

Herbivores are more adept in **defense** than carnivores because they are often prey. Many herbivores, such as cows and horses, have hoofs instead of toes for faster movement on the grasslands. They have incisors adapted for cutting and molars adapted for grinding their food. Insects or other invertebrates can also be herbivores.

b. **Carnivores**

Carnivores are animals that eat only other **animals**. In general, carnivores possess pointed teeth and fanglike canine teeth for tearing flesh. They have shorter digestive tracts due to the easier digestibility of animal food.

c. **Omnivores**

Omnivores are animals that eat both **plants** and **animals**.

C. INTERSPECIFIC INTERACTIONS

A community is not simply a collection of different species living within the same area. It is an **integrated system** of species that are dependent upon one another for survival. The major types of interspecific interactions are symbiosis, predation, saprophytism, and scavenging.

1. **Symbiosis**

Symbionts live together in an intimate, often permanent association, which may or may not be beneficial to both participants. Some symbiotic relationships are **obligatory**; that is, one or both organisms cannot survive without the other. Symbiotic relationships are classified according to the benefits the symbionts receive. The types of symbiotic relationships include commensalism, mutualism and parasitism.

a. **Commensalism**

One organism is benefited by the association, and the other is not affected. The host neither discourages nor fosters the relationship. Some examples include the following:

- **Remora and shark:** The remora (sharksucker) attaches itself by a holdfast device to the underside of a shark. Through this association, the remora obtains the food the shark discards, wide geographic dispersal, and protection from enemies. The shark is totally indifferent to the association.
- **Barnacle and whale:** The barnacle is a sessile crustacean that attaches to the whale and obtains wider feeding opportunities through the migrations of the whale.

b. **Mutualism**

A symbiotic relationship from which both organisms derive some benefit. Some examples are the following:

- **Tick bird and rhinoceros:** The bird receives food in the form of ticks on the skin of the rhinoceros. The rhinoceros has its ticks removed and is warned of danger by the rapid departure of the bird.
- **Lichen:** Lichen is a very intimate association between a fungus and an algae. Lichens are found on rocks and tree barks. The green algae produces food for itself and the fungus by **photosynthesis**. The meshes of fungal threads support the algae and conserve rainwater. The fungus also provides carbon dioxide and nitrogenous wastes for the algae, all of which are needed for photosynthesis and protein synthesis. Lichens are significant in that they are pioneer organisms in the order of ecological succession on bare rock.
- **Nitrogen-fixing bacteria and legumes:** Nitrogen-fixing bacteria invade the roots of legumes, and infected cells grow to form root nodules. In the nodule, the legume provides nutrients for the bacteria, and the bacteria fixes nitrogen (by changing it to a soluble nitrate, a mineral essential for protein synthesis by the plant). These bacteria are a major source of usable nitrogen, which is needed by all plants and animals.
- **Protozoa and termites:** Termites chew and ingest wood but are unable to digest the **cellulose**. Protozoa in the digestive tract of the termite secrete an enzyme that digests the cellulose. Both organisms share the carbohydrates. Thus, the protozoan is guaranteed protection and a steady food supply, while the termite is able to obtain nourishment from the ingested wood.
- **Intestinal bacteria and humans:** Bacteria utilize some of the food material not fully digested by humans and manufacture vitamin K.

c. **Parasitism**

A parasite benefits at the expense of the host. Parasitism exists when competition for food is most intense. Few autotrophs (green plants) exist as parasites (mistletoe is an exception). Parasitism flourishes among organisms such as bacteria, fungi, and animals. Some parasites cling to the exterior surface of the host (**ectoparasites**) using suckers or clamps. They may bore through the skin and suck out blood and nutrients. Leeches, ticks, and sea lampreys employ these techniques. Other parasites (**endoparasites**) live within the host. To gain entry, they must pass through defenses such as skin, digestive juices, antibodies, and white blood cells. Parasites possess special adaptations to overcome these defenses.

Parasitism is advantageous and efficient. The parasite lives with a minimum expenditure of energy. Parasites may even have parasites of their own. Thus, a mammal may have parasitic worms, which in turn are parasitized by bacteria, which in turn are victims of bacteriophages.

i. **Virus and host cell**

All viruses are parasites. They contain nucleic acids surrounded by a protein coat and are nonfunctional outside the host. Upon entry of the viral nucleic acid into the host, the virus takes over the host cell functions and redirects them into replication of itself. The life functions of the bacterial cell slow down or cease.

ii. **Disease bacteria and animals**

Most bacteria are either chemosynthetic or **saprophytic** (bacteria of decay). Diphtheria is parasitic upon man, anthrax on sheep, tuberculosis on cows or on man.

iii. **Disease fungi and animals**

Most fungi are saprophytic. **Ringworm** is parasitic on man.

iv. **Worms and animals**

Parasitic relationships exist between the tapeworm and man. It is interesting to note that successful parasites do not kill their hosts; this would lead to the death of the parasite. The more dangerous the parasite, the less the chance it will survive.

2. **Predation**

Predators are free-living organisms that feed on other living organisms. This definition of predation includes both **carnivores** and **herbivores**. The effects of predators on their prey vary. The predator may severely limit the numbers or distribution of the prey, and the prey, may become extinct. On the other hand, the predator may only slightly affect the prey, because the predator is scarce or commonly utilizes another food source. In many cases, the predator aids in controlling the numbers of the prey but not so much as to endanger the existence of the prey population. Predator-prey relationships evolve towards a balance in which the predator is a regulatory influence on the prey but not a threat to its survival. Examples of predators include the hawk, lion, humans, and Venus flytrap.

3. **Saprophytism**

Saprophytes include those protists and fungi that **decompose** (digest) dead organic matter externally and absorb the nutrients; they constitute a vital link in the cycling of material within the ecosystem. Examples of saprophytes include mold, mushrooms, bacteria of decay, and slime molds.

4. **Scavengers**

Scavengers are animals that consume dead animals. They therefore require no adaptations for hunting and killing their prey. Decomposers, such as the bacteria of decay may be considered scavengers. Examples of scavengers include the vulture and hyena. The snapping turtle is an organism that may be considered both a scavenger and a predator.

D. INTRASPECIFIC INTERACTIONS

Competition is not restricted to **interspecific** interactions (relations between species). Individuals belonging to the same species utilize the same resources; if a particular resource is limited, then these organisms must compete with one another. Members of the same species compete, but they must also **cooperate**. Intraspecific cooperation may be extensive (formation of societies in animal species) or may be nearly nonexistent. Relationships between individuals within a species are influenced by both disruptive and cohesive forces. Competition is the chief disruptive force. Cohesive forces include reproduction and protection from predators and destructive weather.

E. INTERACTIONS BETWEEN ORGANISMS AND THEIR ENVIRONMENT

1. **Osmoregulation**

Animals have developed many adaptations for maintaining their internal osmolarity and conserving water.

- **Saltwater fish** live in a **hyperosmotic** environment, which causes them to lose water and take in salt. They are constantly in danger of dehydration and must compensate by constant drinking and active excretion of salt across their gills.
- **Freshwater fish** live in a **hypo-osmotic** environment, which causes intake of excess water and excessive salt loss. These fish correct this condition by seldom drinking, absorbing salts through the gills, and excreting dilute urine.
- **Insects** excrete solid uric acid crystals to conserve water.
- Desert animals possess adaptations for avoiding desiccation (drying up). The **camel** can tolerate a wide range of body temperatures and possesses fat layers in regions that are exposed to solar radiation. The **horned toad** has thick, scaly skin, which prevents water loss. Other desert animals burrow in the sand during the day and search for food at night, thereby avoiding the intense heat that causes water loss.
- Plants possess adaptations for conservation of water. Nondesert plants possess waxy **cuticles** on leaf surfaces and stomata on the lower leaf surfaces only. They shed leaves in winter to avoid water loss. Desert plants have extensive root systems, **fleshy stems** to store water, **spiny leaves** to limit water loss, extra thick cuticles, and few stomata.

2. **Thermoregulation**

Cellular respiration only transfers a fraction of the energy derived from the oxidation of carbohydrates into the high-energy bonds of ATP. Roughly **60 percent** of the total energy is given off as heat. The vast majority of animals and plants are cold-blooded or **poikilothermic**, and most of their heat energy escapes to the environment. The body temperature of poikilotherms is very close to that of their surroundings. Since an organism's metabolism is closely tied to its body temperature, the activity of poikilothermic animals is radically affected by environmental temperature changes. As the temperature rises, these organisms become more active. As temperatures fall, they become sluggish and lethargic.

Some animals, notably **mammals** and **birds**, are warm-blooded or **homeothermic**. They have evolved physical mechanisms that allow them to make use of the heat produced as a consequence of respiration. Physical adaptations like fat, hair, and feathers retard heat loss. Homeotherms maintain constant body temperatures that are higher than the temperature of environment. They are less dependent upon environmental temperature than poikilothermic animals and are able to inhabit a comparatively wider range of environments.

RELATIONSHIPS WITHIN THE ECOSYSTEM
A. ENERGY FLOW

All living things require energy to carry on their life functions. The complex pathways involved in the transfer of energy through the living components of the ecosystem (biotic community) may be mapped in the form of a **food chain** or **food web**.

1. **Food Chain**

   Energy from the sun enters living systems through the **photosynthetic** production of glucose by green plants. Within the food chain, energy is transferred from the original sources in green plants through a series of organisms with repeated stages of consumption and finally decomposition. Thus, there are producers, primary consumers, secondary consumers, and decomposers.

   a. **Producers**

   The **autotrophic** green plants and **chemosynthetic** bacteria are the producers. They utilize the energy of the sun and simple raw materials (carbon dioxide, water, minerals) to manufacture carbohydrates, proteins, and lipids. The radiant energy of the sun is captured and stored in the C–H bond. Producers always form the initial step in any food chain. The wheat plant is a typical producer.

   b. **Primary consumers**

   Primary consumers are animals that consume green plants (**herbivores**). Examples include the cow, grasshopper, and elephant.

   c. **Secondary consumers**

   Secondary consumers are animals that consume the primary consumers (**carnivores**). These include frogs, tigers, and dragonflies.

   d. **Tertiary consumers**

   These are animals that feed on secondary consumers.

   e. **Decomposers**

   Decomposers include **saprophytic** organisms and organisms of decay, which include bacteria and fungi. The producers and consumers concentrate and organize materials of the environment into complex living substances. Living things give off wastes during their lifetime and eventually die. Bacteria and fungi decompose the organic wastes and dead tissues to simpler compounds, such as nitrates and phosphates, which are returned to the environment to be used again by living organisms. These processes are demonstrated in **food webs** and **material cycles** (nitrogen, carbon, and water).

2. Food Web

The food chain is not a simple linear chain but an intricate web. Almost every species is consumed by one or more other species, some of which are on different food chain levels. The result is a series of branches and cross-branches among all the food chains of a community to form a web. The greater the number of pathways in a community food web, the more stable the community. For example, owls eat rabbits. If rabbits died off because of disease, there would be more vegetation available to mice. Mice would thrive and provide substitute food for owls. Meanwhile, the decimated rabbit population would have a better chance of recovering while owls concentrated their predation on mice.

3. Food Pyramids

Without a constant input of **energy** from the sun, an ecosystem would soon run down. As food is transferred from one level of the food chain to the next, a transfer of energy occurs. According to the second law of thermodynamics, every energy transfer involves a loss of energy. In addition to the energy lost in the transfer, each level of the food chain utilizes some of the energy it obtains from the food for its own metabolism (i.e., to support life functions) and loses some additional energy in the form of heat. A pyramid of energy is thus a fundamental property of all ecosystems at all levels.

a. Pyramid of energy

Each member of a food chain utilizes some of the energy it obtains from its food for its own metabolism (life functions) and loses some additional energy in the form of heat. Since this means a loss of energy at each feeding level, the producer organism at the base of the pyramid contains the greatest amount of energy. Less energy is available for the primary consumer and still less for secondary and tertiary consumers. The smallest amount of available energy is thus at the top of the pyramid.

b. Pyramid of mass

Since organisms at the upper levels of the food chain derive their food energy from organisms at lower levels, and since energy is lost from one level to the next, each level can support a successively smaller biomass. Three hundred pounds of foliage (producer) may support 125 lb. of insects. This may support 50 lb. of insectivorous hens, who in turn will be just the right amount to sustain 25 lb. of hawks.

c. **Pyramid of numbers**

Consumer organisms that are higher in the food chain are usually larger and heavier than those further down. Since the lower organisms have a greater total mass, there must be a greater number of lower-level organisms. (A large bass eats tiny minnows but eats many of them.) With the greatest number of organisms at the base (producer level) and the smallest number at the top (final consumer level), we have a pyramid of numbers.

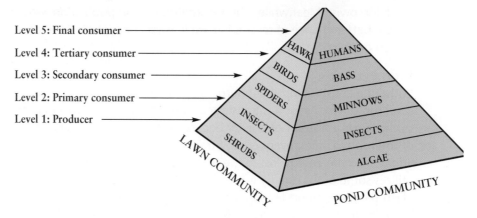

Level 5: Final consumer

Level 4: Tertiary consumer

Level 3: Secondary consumer

Level 2: Primary consumer

Level 1: Producer

HAWK HUMANS

BIRDS BASS

SPIDERS MINNOWS

INSECTS INSECTS

SHRUBS ALGAE

LAWN COMMUNITY

POND COMMUNITY

Figure 13.1

Note: Since other factors, such as the generation time and the size of the organisms, must be considered, the pyramids of numbers and biomass do not apply to all levels at all times (unlike the pyramid of energy). In general, as the pyramid is ascended, there is (1) less energy content, (2) less mass, and (3) fewer organisms.

B. MATERIAL CYCLES

Material is cycled and recycled between organisms and their environments, passing from inorganic forms to organic forms and then back to the inorganic forms. Many of these cycles are accomplished largely through the action of scavengers (such as hyenas and vultures) and decomposers (saprophytes such as bacteria and fungi).

1. **Nitrogen Cycle**

Nitrogen is an essential component of amino acids and nucleic acids, which are the building blocks for all living things. Since there is a finite amount of nitrogen on the earth, it is important that it be recovered and reused.

- Elemental nitrogen is chemically inert and cannot be used by most organisms. Lightning and nitrogen-fixing bacteria in the roots of legumes change the nitrogen to the usable, soluble nitrates.
- The nitrates are absorbed by plants and are used to synthesize nucleic acids and plant proteins.

- Animals eat the plants and synthesize specific animal proteins from the plant proteins. Both plants and animals give off wastes and eventually die.
- The nitrogen locked up in the wastes and dead tissues is released by the action of the bacteria of decay, which convert the proteins into ammonia.
- Two fates await the ammonia (NH_3). Some is nitrified to nitrites by chemosynthetic bacteria and then to usable nitrates by nitrifying bacteria. The rest is denitrified. This means the ammonia (NH_3) is broken down to release free nitrogen, which returns to the beginning of the cycle. Note that four kinds of bacteria are involved in this cycle: **decay, nitrifying, denitrifying,** and **nitrogen fixing.** The bacteria have no use for the excretory ammonia, nitrites, nitrates, and nitrogen they produce. These materials are essential, however, for the existence of other living organisms.

P1232-33

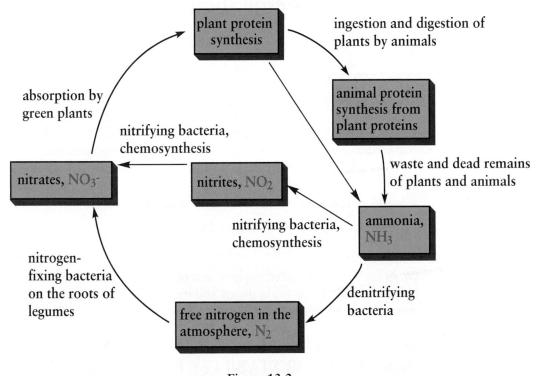

Figure 13.2

2. **Carbon Cycle**
   - **Gaseous CO_2** enters the living world when plants use it to produce glucose via photosynthesis. The carbon atoms in CO_2 are bonded to hydrogen and other carbon atoms. The plant uses the glucose to make starch, proteins, and fat.
   - Animals eat plants and use the digested nutrients to form carbohydrates, fats, and proteins characteristic of the species. A part of these organic compounds is used as fuel in respiration in plants and animals.

- The metabolically produced CO_2 is released to the air. The rest of the organic carbon remains locked within an organism until its death (except for wastes given off), at which time decay processes by bacteria return the CO_2 to the air.

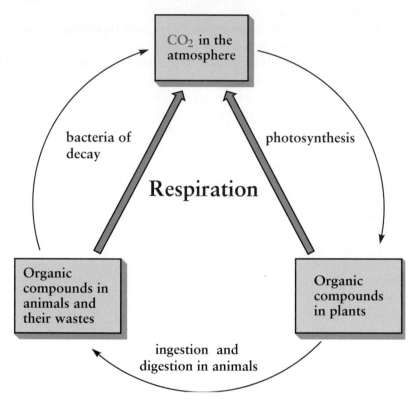

Figure 13.3

3. **Other Cycles**

Other cycles recycle water, oxygen, and phosphorus. These substances are used by almost all living things and must be returned by the biotic community to the environment so they can be reused.

STABILITY IN THE ECOSYSTEM
A. CONDITIONS FOR STABILITY IN AN ECOSYSTEM

An ecosystem is self-sustaining and, therefore, will be stable if there is a relatively stable physical environment (abiotic factors) and a relatively stable biotic community. A stable ecosystem requires a constant **energy source** and a living system incorporating this energy into organic compounds. **Cycling** of materials between the living system and its environment is critical.

B. THE CLIMAX COMMUNITY

A climax community is the **stable**, living (**biotic**) part of the ecosystem described above in which populations exist in balance with each other and with the environment. The type of climax community depends upon all the abiotic factors: rainfall, soil conditions, temperature, shade, etc. A climax community persists until a major climactic or geological change disturbs the abiotic factors or a major biotic change (such as disease, mutations, etc.) affects the populations. Once the equilibrium is upset, new climax conditions are produced, and new communities will be established in the ecosystem.

C. ECOLOGICAL SUCCESSION

Ecological succession is the orderly process by which one biotic community replaces or succeeds another until a climax community is established. Each community stage, or **sere**, in an ecological succession is identified by a **dominant** species—the one that exerts control over the other species that are present. Thus, in a grassland community, grass is the dominant species.

Changes occur because each community that establishes itself changes the **environment**, making it more unfavorable for itself and more favorable for the community that is to succeed it. Successive communities are composed of populations that are able to exist under the new conditions. Finally, a stage arises in which a population alters the environment in such a way that the original conditions giving rise to that population are re-created. Replacement stops, and we have our **climax community**, an ecological steady-state. This climax community is permanent in the ecosystem, unless the abiotic factors are drastically altered by climactic or geologic upheavals. If this happens, a new series of successions is initiated.

- **Example 1**—Consider a barren rocky area in the northeastern United States, barren perhaps as a result of a severe forest fire. **Lichen** may be the first or **pioneer organism** to resettle this virgin area. Recall that a lichen is an association between an alga and a fungus that can live on a rocky surface. Acids produced by the lichen attack the rocks and help to form bits of soil. Since lichens thrive only a solid surface, conditions are now worse for the lichen but better for mosses. Airborne spores of mosses land on the soil and germinate. The result is a new **sere** with the moss as the dominant species in the community. As the remains of the moss build up the soil still more, annual grasses and then perennial grasses with deeper roots become the dominant species. As time marches on, we find shrubs and then trees. The first trees are the sun-loving gray birch and poplar. As more and more trees compete for the sun, these trees are replaced by white pine and finally **maples** and **beeches**, which grow in deep shade—the climax community.

The growth of maples and beeches produces the same conditions that originally favored their appearance. And so this community remains for thousands of years. In the final maple-beech community, you would find foxes, deer, chipmunks, and plant-eating insects. These are animals that would not have been found in the original barren rock terrain. However, one forest fire can kill the entire community. Ecological succession then starts all over again, commencing with the lichen and the bare rock.

It is important to note again that the dominant species of the climax community depends on such **physical factors** as temperature, nature of the soil, rainfall, etc. Thus, the climax community in New York State at higher elevations is hemlock-beech-maple, while at lower elevations, the climax plant is more often oak-hickory. In cold Maine, the climax community is dominated by the pine; in the wet areas of Wisconsin, by cypress; in sandy New Jersey, by pine; on a cold, windy mountain top, by scrub oak.

- **Example 2**—Ecological succession in a pond. A quick summary:
  - **Step 1:** Pond: Plants such as algae, pondweed. Animals such as protozoa, water insects, small fish.
  - **Step 2:** Shallow water pond fills in: Reeds, cattails, water lilies.
  - **Step 3:** Moist land: Grass, herbs, shrubs, willow trees; frogs, snakes.
  - **Step 4:** Woodland: Climax tree—perhaps pine or oak.

WORLD BIOMES (MAJOR COMMUNITIES)
A. TERRESTRIAL BIOMES

The evolutionary **origin** of plants and animals can be traced to the seas. To survive on land, these organisms had to develop adaptations to face an environment with a (1) relative lack of water, (2) relative lack of food and supporting medium, (3) varying temperature (as compared to the oceans, which have a relatively constant temperature), and (4) varying composition of the soil as compared to the definite salt composition in the oceans. The conditions in different terrestrial and climate regions selected for plants and animals possessing suitable adaptations. Each **geographic region** is inhabited by a distinct community, called a **biome**, existing in the major climate areas.

Land biomes are characterized and named according to the **climax vegetation** of the region. The climax vegetation is the vegetation that becomes dominant and stable after years of evolutionary development. Since plants are important as food producers, they determine the nature of the inhabiting animal population, and thus the climax vegetation determines the **climax animal population**. Some types of terrestrial biomes are these:

1. **Desert Biome**
   Deserts receive fewer than 10 inches of rain each year; the rain is concentrated within a few heavy cloudbursts. The growing season in the desert is restricted to those days after rainfalls. Generally, small plants and animals inhabit the desert. Most desert plants conserve water actively (cactus, sagebrush, mesquite). Desert animals live in burrows (insects and lizards). Few birds and mammals are found in the deserts except those that have developed adaptations for maintaining constant body temperatures. Examples of deserts include the Sahara in Africa and the Gobi in Asia.

2. **Grassland Biome**
   Grasslands are characterized by a low rainfall (usually 10–30 inches per year), although considerably more than the desert biomes receive. Grasslands provide no shelter for **herbivorous mammals** (bison, antelope, cattle, zebra) from carnivorous predators. Animals that do inhabit the grasslands have developed long legs, and many are hoofed. Examples of grasslands include the prairies east of the Rockies, the steppes of the Ukraine, and the pampas of Argentina.

3. **Tropical Rain Forest Biome**
   Rain forests are "**jungles**" characterized by **high temperatures** and **torrential rains**. The climax community includes a dense growth of vegetation that does not shed its leaves. Vegetation such as vines and **epiphytes** (plants growing on other plants) and animals such as monkeys, lizards, snakes, and birds inhabit the typical rain forests. Trees grow closely together; sunlight hardly reaches the forest floor. The floor is inhabited by **saprophytes**, living off dead organic matter. Tropical rain forests are found in Central Africa, Central America, the Amazon basin, and Southeast Asia.

4. **Temperate Deciduous Forest Biome**
   Temperate deciduous forests have cold winters, warm summers, and a moderate rainfall. Trees such as **beech, maple, oaks** and **willows** shed their leaves during the cold winter months. Animals in temperate deciduous forests include the deer, fox, woodchuck, and squirrel. These biomes are found in the northeast and central-eastern United States and in Central Europe.

5. **Temperate Coniferous Forest Biome**
   These forests are cold, dry, and inhabited by **fir, pine,** and **spruce** trees. Much of the vegetation has evolved adaptations for water conservation, such as needle-shaped leaves. These forests are found in the extreme northern part of the United States and in southern Canada.

6. **Taiga Biome**

Taigas receive less rainfall than the temperate forests; have long, cold winters; and are inhabited by a single coniferous tree: the **spruce**. The forest floors in the taiga contain moss and lichens. The chief animal inhabitant is the moose; however, the black bear, wolf, and some birds are found there. Taigas exist in the extreme northern parts of Canada and Russia.

7. **Tundra Biome**

The tundra is a treeless, frozen plain found between the taiga lands and the northern ice sheets. There is only a very short summer and, thus, a very short growing season when the ground becomes wet and marshy. Lichens, moss, polar bears, musk oxen, and arctic hens are found in the tundra.

8. **Polar Region**

The polar region is a frozen area with no vegetation or terrestrial animals. Animals that do inhabit polar regions generally live near the polar oceans.

B. TERRESTRIAL BIOME AND ALTITUDE

The sequence of biome between the equator and the poles is comparable to the sequence of regions on mountains. The nature of those regions are determined by the same decisive factors—temperatures and rainfall. For example, the base of the mountain would resemble the biome of a temperate deciduous area. As one ascends the mountain, one would pass a coniferous-like biome, then taiga like, tundra like, and polar like biomes.

C. AQUATIC BIOMES

More than 70 percent of the earth's surface is covered by water. Most of the earth's plant and animal life is found in water. As much as 90 percent of the earth's food and oxygen production (**photosynthesis**) takes place in the water. Aquatic biomes are classified according to criteria quite different from the criteria used to classify terrestrial biomes. Plants have little controlling influence in communities of aquatic biomes compared to their role in terrestrial biomes. Aquatic areas are the most stable ecosystems; the conditions affecting temperature, amount of available oxygen and carbon dioxide, and amount of suspended or dissolved materials are stable over very large areas and show little tendency to change. Therefore, aquatic food webs and aquatic communities are balanced. There are two types of major aquatic biomes: **marine** and **freshwater**.

1. **Marine Biomes**

The oceans connect to form one continuous body of water, which controls the earth's temperature by absorbing solar heat. Water has the distinctive property of being able to absorb or utilize large amounts of heat without undergoing a great temperature change. Marine biomes contain a relatively constant amount of nutrient materials and dissolved salts.

Although ocean conditions are more uniform than those on land, distinct zones in the marine biomes exist.

- **Intertidal zone:** The region exposed at low tides that undergoes variations in temperature and periods of dryness. Populations in the intertidal zones include algae, sponges, clams, snails, sea urchins, starfish, and crabs.
- **Littoral zone:** The region on the continental shelf that contains ocean area with depths up to 600 feet and extends several hundred miles from the shores. Populations in littoral zone regions include algae, crabs, crustacea, and many different species of fish.
- **Pelagic zone:** Typical of the open seas, this can be divided into photic and aphotic zones (see Figure 13.4).
  - **Photic zone:** The **sunlit layer** of the open sea extending to a depth of 250–600 feet. It contains **plankton**, passively drifting masses of microscopic photosynthetic and heterotrophic organisms, and **nekton**, active swimmers such as fish, sharks, or whales that feed on plankton and smaller fish. The chief autotroph is the **diatom**, an algae.
  - **Aphotic zone:** The region beneath the photic zone that receives **no sunlight**. There is no photosynthesis in the aphotic zone, and only heterotrophs exist here. **Deep-sea organisms** in this zone have adaptations enabling them to survive in very cold water with high pressures and in complete darkness. The zone contains **nekton** and **benthos** (the crawling and sessile organisms). Some are scavengers, and some are predators. The habitat of the aphotic zone is fiercely competitive.

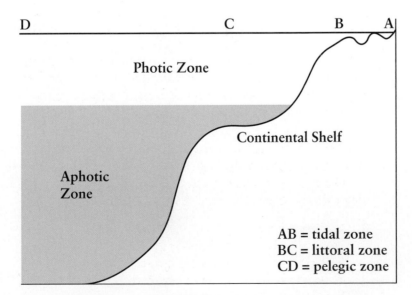

Figure 13.4

2. Freshwater Biomes

Rivers, lakes, ponds, marshes—the links between the oceans and land—contain freshwater. Rivers are the routes by which ancient marine organisms reached land and evolved terrestrial adaptations. Many forms failed to adapt to land and developed adaptations for freshwater. Others developed special adaptations suitable for both land and freshwater. As in **marine biomes**, factors affecting life in freshwater include **temperature**, **transparency** (illumination due to suspended mud particles), **depth** of water, available carbon dioxide and **oxygen**, and most important, the **salt concentration**. Freshwater biomes differ from saltwater biomes in three basic ways:

1. Freshwater is **hypotonic,** creating a diffusion gradient that results in the passage of water into the cell. Freshwater organisms have homeostatic mechanisms to maintain water balance by the regular **removal** of **excess water**. These include the contractile vacuoles of protozoa and excretory systems of fish. Plant cells have rigid cell walls and thus build up cell pressure (cell **turgor**) as water flows in. This pressure counteracts the gradient pressure, stops the influx of water, and establishes a water balance.
2. In rivers and streams, strong, swift **currents** exist, and thus fish that have developed strong muscles and plants with rootlike **holdfasts** have survived and were selected for.
3. Freshwater biomes, except very large lakes, are affected by variations in climate and weather. **Temperature** of freshwater bodies varies considerably; they may freeze or dry up, and mud from their floors may be stirred up by storms.

CLASSIFICATION

TAXONOMIC CLASSIFICATION
A. TAXONOMY

Billions of years of evolution have led to the great diversity of living organisms we see today. Scientists have tried to categorize relationships among the vast number of different organisms. The science of classification and the nomenclature used are known as **taxonomy**. The modern classification system seeks to group organisms on the basis of **evolutionary relationships**. In this system, the bat, whale, horse, and humans are placed in the same class of animals because they have all descended from a common ancestor. Since much of early evolutionary history is not known, there is some disagreement among biologists as to the best classification system to employ, particularly with regard to groups of unicellular organisms. Taxonomy takes into account anatomical and structural characteristics; modes of excretion, movement, and digestion; genetic makeup; and biochemical capabilities. Taxonomic organization proceeds from the largest, broadest group to the smaller, more specific subgroups.

B. CLASSIFICATION AND SUBDIVISIONS

The modern scheme of taxonomy has **five kingdoms** for all living organisms. Each kingdom is divided into several major **phyla** (in the animal kingdom) or **divisions** (in other kingdoms). A phylum or division has several **subphyla** or **subdivisions**, which are further divided into **classes**. Each class includes multiple **orders**. Orders are subdivided into **families**, and each family is made up of many **genera** (singular *genus*). The **species** is the final, smallest subdivision. Organisms of the same species can mate with one another to produce fertile offspring.

Kingdom
     Phylum (Division)
          Subphylum (Subdivision)
               Class
                    Order
                         Family
                              Genus
                                   Species

For example, the full classification of humans is **Kingdom**: Animal, **Phylum**: Chordata, **Subphylum**: Vertebrata, **Class**: Mammalia, **Order**: Primates, **Family**: Hominidae, **Genus**: *Homo,* **Species**: *sapiens.*

C. ASSIGNMENT OF SCIENTIFIC NAMES

All organisms are assigned a scientific name consisting of the **genus** and **species** name of that organism. Thus, humans are *Homo sapiens,* and the common housecat is *Felis domestica*. This follows a scheme originated by the biologist Carl Linn (Carolus Linnaeus).

CLASSIFICATION INTO KINGDOMS (A MODERN APPROACH)

Biologists originally divided all living things into two categories: plants and animals. This division ignored a number of different organisms. One type of modern classification system recognizes five kingdoms: Monera, Protista, Plantae, Fungi, and Animalia. Another classification system utilizes three kingdoms: Monera, Plantae (including Fungi), and Animalia (including Protista).

A. VIRUSES

Viruses are generally not considered to be living organisms. They cannot function outside of a host cell and are dependent upon the host's reproductive machinery to replicate. Therefore, they have not been placed in any of the five kingdoms.

B. MONERA

Monerans are **prokaryotes**. They lack a nucleus or any membrane-bound organelles. All monerans are single-celled organisms that reproduce asexually.

C. PROTISTA

The protist kingdom contains primitive **eukaryotic** organisms with both plant-like and animal-like characteristics. These organisms are either single cells or colonies of similar cells with no differentiation of specialized tissues. Each protist cell possesses the capability to carry out all of the life processes. The protist kingdom contains all simple eukaryotes that cannot be clas-sified as plants or animals. For example, the protists of the genus *Euglena* demonstrate the motility of animals and the photosynthetic capabilities of plants.

D. FUNGI

Fungi may be considered nonphotosynthetic plants (i.e., they resemble plants in that they are **multicellular, differentiated,** and **nonmotile**). Fungi are **not photosynthetic**. They are either **saprophytic** (i.e., bread mold) or **parasitic** (i.e., athlete's foot fungus). Their modes of reproduction are varied and unique. In addition, their cell walls are composed of chitin, not cellulose (as in plants).

E. PLANTAE

The plant kingdom includes multicellular organisms that exhibit differentiation of tissues and are **nonmotile** and **photosynthetic**. Many plants exhibit an alternation of generations and a distinct embryonic phase.

F. ANIMALIA

The animal kingdom contains the **multicellular,** generally **motile, heterotrophic** organisms that have **differentiated** tissues (and organs in higher forms).

VIRUSES

Viruses do not carry out physiological or biochemical processes outside of a host. They may be considered **nonliving**, although they are highly advanced parasites. Viruses are capable of taking over their host's cellular machinery and directing the replication of the viral genome and protein coat. Viruses have **lytic** and **lysogenic** life cycles. They contain either **DNA** or **RNA** and some essential enzymes surrounded by a protein coat. Viruses that exclusively infect bacteria are called **bacteriophages**.

KINGDOM MONERA

Monerans, also called **bacteria**, are prokaryotic cells. They may exist as single cells or as aggregates of cells that stick together after division.

A. CYANOBACTERIA

Cyanobacteria, also called blue-green algae, live primarily in fresh water but also exist in marine environments. They possess a cell wall and **photosynthetic pigments**, but they have no flagella, true nucleus, chloroplasts, or mitochondria. They can withstand extreme temperatures and are believed to be directly descended from the first organisms that developed photosynthetic capabilities.

B. OTHER BACTERIA

Bacteria are single-celled prokaryotes with a single double-stranded circular loop of DNA that is not enclosed by a nuclear membrane. Almost all forms have **cell walls**. They play active roles in **biogeochemical cycles**, the recycling of various chemicals such as carbon, nitrogen, phosphorous, and sulfur. Bacteria may be classified by their **morphological** appearances; **cocci** (round), **bacilli** (rods), and **spirilla** (spiral). Some forms are **duplexes** (diplococci), **clusters** (staphylococci), and **chains** (streptococci). Bacteria are ubiquitous, and many possess a wide variety of complex biochemical pathways.

NOTE: Much of the information that follows concerning eukaryotic classification is presented to improve your background in the features of living things. The general trends should be understood, but the specific details need not be memorized, with the exception of the classification of higher vertebrates.

KINGDOM PROTISTA

Most protists are unicellular, but there exist some colonial forms as well as some simple multicellular organisms that are neither plants nor animals. Protists are **eukaryotes** and possess a membrane-bound nucleus and organelles. The kingdom protista includes two major categories—**protozoa** and **algae**. The kingdom is divided into many phyla, which fall primarily into these two categories.

A. PROTOZOA

Traditionally, protozoans are considered those single-celled organisms that are **heterotrophic**, like little animals. This category of protists includes a number of phyla. The **rhizopods**, including amoebas, move with cellular extensions called pseudopods. The **ciliophors** have cilia that are used for feeding and locomotion.

B. ALGAE

Algae are primarily **photosynthetic** organisms. They include the **phyto-plankton**, which are important sources of food for many marine organisms. *Euglena* may be considered an algal protist because they photosynthesize. *Euglena* can also act as heterotrophs and move about with flagellum. The blue, green, and red algae can be multicellular and are sometimes placed in the animal kingdom.

C. PROTISTS RESEMBLING FUNGI

The slime molds are often placed in kingdom fungi. However, they appear to be more directly related to the protists. They are arranged in a **coenocytic** (many nuclei) mass of **protoplasm**. The slime mold undergoes a unique life cycle containing animal-like and plantlike stages. These stages include fruiting bodies and unicellular flagellated spores. Slime molds reproduce asexually by sporulation.

KINGDOM FUNGI

Fungi are eukaryotes and primarily multicellular. All fungi are **heterotrophs**. This differentiates them from the plant kingdom. They may be **saprophytic**, decomposing dead organic material, or parasitic. In either case, fungi **absorb** their food from their environment. Fungi reproduce by asexual **sporulation** or by intricate sexual processes. Some varieties of *Eumycophyta* utilize extracellular digestion. Notable types are mushrooms, yeast, and lichens.

KINGDOM ANIMALIA

A. GENERAL CHARACTERISTICS OF ALL ANIMALS (METAZOA)

1. **Differentiation of Tissues, Organs, and Organ Systems**
   Simple multicellular animals, such as sponges, coelenterates, and flatworms, have minimal differentiation. Most of their cells are in direct contact with the outside environment. In these organisms, few systems (such as the digestive systems and the reproductive systems) are required to support the life processes. In more advanced animals, specialized tissues and systems facilitate digestion, locomotion, circulation, message conduction (nervous system), and support.

2. **Alimentation**
   All animals, except some parasites like the tapeworm, ingest bulk foods (holotrophic), digest them, and then eliminate the remains.

3. **Locomotion**
   All animals employ some form of locomotion to acquire nutrients. Some are sessile (stationary) and create currents to trap food. Locomotion is also important for protection, mate selection, and reproduction.

4. **Bilateral Symmetry**
   Most animals have right and left sides that are mirror images. The head is directed **anteriorly**. However, some animals, such as the echinoderms and cnidarians, are radially symmetrical.

5. **Nervous System**
   Animals possess a system enabling them to receive stimuli and control their actions. They have sense organs, specialized conductors, and higher brain centers for coordination and learning.

6. **Chemical-Coordinating System**
   Animals secrete chemicals (hormones) that operate in conjunction with the nervous system to maintain a steady state or **homeostasis**.

B. PORIFERA (SPONGES)

The sponges have two layers of cells, have pores, are sessile, and have a low degree of cellular specialization.

C. CNIDARIANS

Cnidarians, also called coelenterates, contain a digestive sac that is sealed at one end (gastrovascular cavity). Two layers of cells are present—the **ectoderm** and the **endoderm**. Cnidarians have many specialized features, including tentacles, stinging cells, and net nerves (e.g., hydra, jellyfish, sea anemone, coral).

D. PLATYHELMINTHES (FLATWORMS)

Flatworms are ribbonlike, are **bilaterally symmetrical**, and possess three layers of cells, including a solid mesoderm. They do not have circulatory systems, and their nervous system consists of eyes, an anterior brain ganglion, and a pair of longitudinal nerve cords.

E. NEMATODA (ROUND WORMS)

Round worms possess long digestive tubes and an anus. A solid mesoderm is present. Nematodes lack circulatory systems. They possess nerve cords and an anterior nerve ring (e.g., hookworm, trichina, free-living soil nematodes).

F. ANNELIDA (SEGMENTED WORMS)

Segmented worms possess a **coelom** (a true body cavity) contained in the mesoderm. Annelids have well-defined systems, including nervous, circulatory, and excretory systems (e.g., earthworms, leeches).

G. MOLLUSCA

Mollusks are soft bodied and possess mantles that often secrete calcareous (**calcium carbonate**) exoskeletons. They breathe by gills and contain chambered hearts, blood sinuses, and a pair of ventral nerve cords (e.g., clams, snails, and squid).

H. ARTHROPODA

Arthropods have jointed appendages, chitinous exoskeletons, and open circulatory systems (sinuses). The three most important classes of arthropods are insects, arachnids, and crustaceans.

- **Insects** possess three pairs of legs, spiracles, and tracheal tubes designed for breathing outside of an aquatic environment.
- **Arachnids** have four pairs of legs and "book lungs" (e.g., scorpion, spider).
- **Crustaceans** have a segmented body with a variable number of appendages and possess gills (e.g., lobster, crayfish, shrimp).

I. ECHINODERMS

Echinoderms are spiny, are **radially** symmetrical, contain a water-vascular system, and possess the capacity for regeneration of parts. There is evolutionary evidence suggesting a link between echinoderms and chordates (e.g., starfish, sea urchin).

J. CHORDATES

Chordates are characterized by a stiff dorsal rod, called the **notochord**, present at some stage of embryologic development. They have paired gill slits and a tail extending beyond the anus at some point during development. The **lancelets** and **tunicates** (like **amphioxus**) are chordates but not **vertebrates**.

> **DAT Synopsis**
>
> Amphioxus is an example of a chordate that is not a vertebrate. It has a notochord but no backbone.

Vertebrates are the most advanced subphylum of the chordates. Vertebrates include **amphibians, reptiles, birds, fish**, and **mammals**. In addition to the chordate characteristics described above, vertebrates also possess bones, called vertebrae, which form the **backbone**. Bony vertebrae replace the notochord of the embryo and protect the nerve cord; a bony case protects the brain (i.e., the skull). Vertebrates can be divided into the following **classes**:

1. **Fish**

   All fish possess a two-chambered heart and gills and utilize external fertilization for reproduction.

   - **Jawless fish** are eel-like; retain the notochord throughout life; and have a cartilaginous internal skeleton, no jaws, and a sucking mouth. Jawless fish include the class Agnatha. Examples include the lamprey and hagfish.
   - **Cartilaginous fish** possess jaws and teeth. A reduced notochord exists as segments between cartilaginous vertebrae. An example is the shark.
   - **Bony fish** are the most prevalent type of fish. They have scales and lack a notochord in the adult form. During development, cartilage is replaced by a bony skeleton. Examples include the sturgeon, trout, and tuna.

2. **Amphibia**

   The larval stage, known as the **tadpole**, is found in water, possesses gills and a tail and has no legs. The adult amphibian lives on land; has **lungs**, two pairs of legs, no tail, a three-chambered heart, and no scales; and utilizes external fertilization. Eggs are laid in water with a jellylike secretion. Examples include the frog, salamander, toad, and newt.

3. **Reptiles**

   Reptiles are **terrestrial** animals. They breathe air by means of **lungs**, lay leathery eggs, and utilize **internal fertilization**. Reptiles are cold-blooded (**poikilothermic**) and have scales and a three-chambered heart. Examples include the turtle, lizard, snake, and crocodile.

4. **Birds**

Birds possess a four-chambered heart. They are **warm-blooded** (homeothermic), and their eggs are surrounded by shells. Examples include the hen and eagle.

5. **Mammals**

Mammals are warm-blooded animals that feed their offspring with milk produced in mammary glands.

- **Monetremes** lay leathery eggs, have horny bills, and have milk (mammary) glands with numerous openings but no nipples. Examples include the duckbill platypus and spiny anteater.
- **Marsupials** are **pouched** mammals. The embryo begins development in the uterus and completes development while attached to nipples in the abdominal pouch. Examples include the kangaroo and opossum.
- **Placental mammals** have embryos that develop fully in the uterus. The placenta attaches the embryo to the uterine wall and provides for the exchange of food, oxygen, and waste material. Examples include the bat, whale, mouse, and man.

EVOLUTION

The change in the genetic makeup of a population over time is termed **evolution**. Evolution is explained by the constant propagation of new variations in the genes of a species, some of which impart an **adaptive advantage**.

EVIDENCE OF EVOLUTION
A. FOSSIL RECORD

Fossils are the most direct evidence of evolutionary change. They represent the remains of an extinct ancestor. Fossils are generally found in sedimentary rocks.

1. **Types of Fossils**

   Many types of fossils can provide information. Paleontologists can find **actual remains**, including teeth, bones, etc., found in rock, tar pits, ice, and amber (the fossil resin of trees). **Petrification** is the process in which minerals replace the cells of an organism. **Imprints** are impressions left by an organism (i.e., footprints). **Molds** form in hollow spaces of rocks, as the organisms within decay. **Casts** are formed by minerals deposited in molds.

B. COMPARATIVE ANATOMY

1. Homologous Structures

Homologous structures have the same basic anatomical features and **evolutionary origins**. They demonstrate similar evolutionary patterns with late divergence of form due to differences in exposure to evolutionary forces. Examples of homologous structures include the wings of a bat, the flippers of a whale, the forelegs of horses, and the arms of man.

2. Analogous Structures

Analogous structures have **similar functions** but may have different evolutionary origins and entirely different patterns of development. The wings of a fly (membranous) and the wings of a bird (bony and covered with feathers) are analogous structures. Analogous organs demonstrate superficial resemblance that cannot be used as a basis for classification.

C. COMPARATIVE EMBRYOLOGY

The **stages of development** of the embryo resemble the stages in an organism's evolutionary history. The human embryo passes through the stages that demonstrate common ancestry. The **two-layer gastrula** is similar to the structure of the **hydra**, a cnidarian. The three-layer gastrula is similar in structure to the flatworm. Gill slits, which are present in the embryo, indicate a common ancestry with fish.

The similarity of stages suggests a common ancestry and development history rather than an identical early development to that of the hydra, flatworm, and fish. The earlier the stage at which the development begins to diverge, the more dissimilar the adult organisms will be. Thus, it is difficult to differentiate between the embryo of a human and that of a gorilla until relatively late in the development of each embryo.

Embryological development suggests other evidence of evolution. The avian embryo has teeth, suggesting a reptile stage. The larvae of some mollusks resemble annelids. Human embryos possess a tail.

D. COMPARATIVE BIOCHEMISTRY (PHYSIOLOGY)

Most organisms demonstrate the same basic needs and **metabolic processes**. They require the same nutrients and contain similar cellular organelles and energy storage forms (ATP). For example, **respiratory processes** are very similar in most organisms. The similarity of the enzymes involved in these processes suggests that all organisms must contain some DNA sequences in common. The closer the organisms in the evolutionary scheme, the greater the similarity of their chemical constituents (enzymes, hormones, antibodies, blood) and **genetic information**. Thus, we can conclude that all organisms are descended from a common, primitive ancestral form. The chemical similarity of the blood of different organisms very closely parallels the evolutionary pattern. A chimpanzee's blood shows close similarity to that of a human but is quite different from that of a rabbit or fish. Thus, the more time that has elapsed since the **divergence** of two species, the more different their biochemical characteristics.

E. VESTIGIAL STRUCTURES

Vestigial structures appear to be useless but apparently had some ancestral function. There are many examples of vestigial structures in humans, other animals, and plants.

- In humans, the **appendix** is small and useless. In herbivores, it assists in the digestion of cellulose.
- In humans, the **tail** is reduced to a few useless bones (coccyx) at the base of the spine.
- **Splints** on legs of horse are the vestigial remains of the two side toes of *Eohippus*.
- The **python** has legs that are reduced to useless bones embedded in the sides of the adult. The whale has similar hind-limb bones.

F. GEOGRAPHIC BARRIERS

Species multiplication is generally accompanied by **migration** to lessen **intraspecific competition**. Separation of a widely distributed population by emerging geographic barriers increases the likelihood of genetic adaptations on either side of the barrier. Each population may evolve specific adaptations to the environment in which it lives, in addition to the accumulation of neutral (random, nonadaptive) changes. These adaptations will remain unique to the population in which they evolve—provided that interbreeding is prevented by the barrier. In time, genetic differences will reach the point where successful interbreeding becomes impossible within the population, and **reproductive isolation** would be maintained if the barrier were removed.

- **Example: Marsupials**—A line of pouched mammals paralleling the development of placental mammals developed on the **Australian** side of a large water barrier. The geographic barrier protected the more primitive pouched mammals from competition with modern placental mammals. This barrier resulted in the development of uniquely Australian plants and animals (e.g., the kangaroo, duckbill platypus, pouched wolves, and eucalyptus tree).

Systematics is a field of study that constructs and studies evolutionary relationships. A **phylogeny** is the evolutionary history of a group of organisms. In phylogenetic relationships, species should be somewhat similar to their ancestors, keeping in mind that because of genetic divergence, those similarities will fade with time since separation increases.

Cladistics is used to classify organisms based on their phylogenetic relationships. Cladograms are constructed to predict how an ancestor has evolved into its proposed descendents. Each subtree of the cladogram is called a **clade**; members of a clade possess some kind of derived characteristic that distinguishes them from other clades. In constructing these clades, scientists utilize the principal of parsimony; that is, the least complex explanation. So if one cladogram assumes five evolutionary events and another assumes only two, then the latter will be more accepted.

THEORIES OF EVOLUTION
A. LAMARCKIAN EVOLUTION

This discredited theory held that new organs or changes in existing ones arose because of the needs of the organism. The amount of change was thought to be based on the **use or disuse** of the organ. The theory of use and disuse was based upon a **fallacious** understanding of genetics. Any useful characteristic acquired in one generation was thought to be transmitted to the next. An example was that of early giraffes, who were though to have stretched their necks to reach for leaves on higher branches of trees. The offspring were believed to have inherited the valuable trait of longer necks as a result of this excessive use.

Modern genetics has disproved theories of acquired characteristics. **Only changes in the DNA of the sex cells can be inherited**. Changes acquired during an individual's life are changes in the characteristics and organization of somatic cells. Weissman showed that these changes are not inherited in an experiment in which he cut off the tails of mice for 20 generations (somatic change) only to find that the 21st generation was born with tails.

DAT Synopsis

If you see any hint of the buzz phrases "use and disuse" or "inheritance of acquired characteristics," think Lamarck. And don't forget—Lamarck was wrong!

B. DARWIN'S THEORY OF NATURAL SELECTION

In Darwin's theory, pressures in the environment select for the organism most fit to survive and reproduce. Darwin outlined a number of basic agents leading to evolutionary change:

1. **Overpopulation**

   More offspring are produced than can survive, so there is insufficient food, air, light, and space to support the entire population.

2. **Variations**

   Offspring naturally show differences (variations) in their characteristics compared to their parents. Darwin did not know the source of these differences. De Vries later suggested **mutations** as the cause of variations. Some mutations are beneficial, although most are harmful.

3. **Competition (Struggle for Survival)**

   The developing population must compete for the necessities of life. Many young must die, and the number of adults in the population generally remains constant from generation to generation.

4. **Natural Selection**

   Some organisms in a species have variations that give them an advantage over other members of the species. For example, a giraffe with a variation of a longer neck would be able to get more food from higher branches of a tree and would be more fit for survival. This principle is encapsulated in the phrase "survival of the fittest."

5. **Inheritance of the Variations**

   The individuals that survive (those with the favorable variations) live to adulthood, reproduce their own kind, and thus **transmit** these favorable variations or adaptations to their offspring. These favored genes gradually dominate the gene pool.

6. **Evolution of New Species**

   Over many generations of natural selection, the favorable changes (adaptations) are perpetuated in the species. The accumulation of these favorable changes eventually results in such significant changes of the gene pool that we can say a new species has evolved. These physical changes in the gene pool were perpetuated or selected for by environmental conditions.

   - **Example**—The rapid evolution of **DDT-resistant** insects illustrates the theory of natural selection. A change in the environment, such as the introduction of DDT, constitutes a favorable change for the DDT-resistant mutant flies. These mutants existed before the environmental change. Now, conditions select for survival of DDT-resistant mutants.

DAT Synopsis

Natural Selection:

- Chance variations occur thanks to mutation and recombination.
- If the variation is "selected for" by the environment, that individual will be more "fit" and more likely to survive to reproductive age.
- Survival of the fittest leads to an increase of those favorable genes in the gene pool.

FORCES OF EVOLUTION

A. POPULATION GENETICS

A **population** includes all members of a particular species inhabiting a given location. The **gene pool** of a population is the sum total of all the alleles for any given trait in the population. **Gene frequency** is the decimal fraction representing the presence of an allele for all members of a population that have this particular gene locus. The letter *p* is used for the frequency of the **dominant allele** of a particular gene locus. The letter *q* represents the frequency of the **recessive allele**. For a given gene locus, $p + q = 1$.

1. **The Hardy-Weinberg Principle**

   Evolution can be viewed as a result of changing gene frequencies within a population. Gene frequency is the relative frequency of a particular allele. When the gene frequencies of a population are not changing, the gene pool is stable, and the population is not evolving. However, this is true only in ideal situations in which the following five conditions are met:

   1) The population is very large.
   2) There are no mutations that affect the gene pool.
   3) Mating between individuals in the population is random.
   4) There is no net migration of individuals into or out of the population.
   5) The genes in the population are all equally successful at reproducing.

   Under these idealized conditions, a certain equilibrium will exist among all of the genes in a gene pool, which is described by the **Hardy-Weinberg equation**.

   For a gene locus with only two alleles, T and t, p = the frequency of allele T and q = the frequency of allele t. By definition, for a given gene locus, $p + q = 1$, since the combined frequencies of the alleles must total 100%. Thus $(p + q)^2 = (1)^2$ and

$$p^2 + 2pq + q^2 = 1$$

   where p^2 = frequency of TT (dominant homozygotes)

   $2pq$ = frequency of Tt (heterozygotes)

   q^2 = frequency of tt (recessive homozygotes)

The Hardy-Weinberg equation may be used to determine gene frequencies in a large population in the absence of microevolutionary change (defined by the five conditions given above). For example, individuals from a nonevolving population can be randomly crossed to demonstrate that the gene frequencies remain constant from generation to generation. Assume that in the original gene pool the gene frequency of the dominant gene for tallness, T, is .80, and the gene frequency of the recessive gene for shortness, t, is .20. Thus, $p = .80$ and $q = .20$. In a cross between two heterozygotes, the resulting F_1 genotype frequencies are 64% TT, 16% + 16% = 32% Tt, and 4% tt (see the Punnett square below).

	$p = .80$ (T)	$q = .20$ (t)
$p = .80$ (T)	($p^2 = .64$) TT = 64%	($pq = .16$) Tt = 16%
$q = .20$ (t)	($pq = .16$) Tt = 16%	($q^2 = .04$) tt = 4%

The gene frequencies of the F_1 generation can be calculated as follows:

64% TT = 64% T allele + 0% t allele.
32% Tt = 16% T allele + 16% t allele.
4% tt = 0% T allele + 4% t allele.

Gene frequencies = 80% T allele + 20% t allele.

Thus, $p = .80$ and $q = .20$. These frequencies are the same as those in the parent generation, demonstrating Hardy-Weinberg equilibrium in a nonevolving population.

B. MICROEVOLUTION
No population can be represented indefinitely by the Hardy-Weinberg equilibrium, because such idealized conditions do not exist in nature. Real populations have **unstable** gene pools and **migrating** populations. The agents of microevolutionary change—natural selection, mutation, assortive mating, genetic drift, and gene flow—are all deviations from the five conditions of a Hardy-Weinberg population.

1. **Natural Selection**
   Genotypes with favorable variations are selected through natural selection, and the frequency of favorable genes increases within the gene pool. Genotypes with low adaptive values tend to disappear.

2. **Mutation**
   Gene mutations change allele frequencies in a population, shifting gene equilibria.

3. **Assortive Mating**
   If mates are not randomly chosen, but rather selected according to criteria such as phenotype and proximity, the relative genotype ratios will be affected and will depart from the predictions of the Hardy-Weinberg equilibrium. On the average, the allele frequencies in the gene pool remain unchanged.

4. **Genetic Drift**
Genetic drift refers to changes in the composition of the gene pool due to chance. Genetic drift tends to be more pronounced in small populations, where it is sometimes called the founder effect.

5. **Gene Flow**
Migration of individuals between populations will result in a loss or gain of genes and thus change the composition of a population's gene pool.

C. SPECIATION

Speciation is the evolution of new species, which are groups of individuals who can interbreed freely with each other but not with members of other species. Different selection pressures act upon the gene pools of each group, causing them to evolve independently. Changes in the environment change the survival value of certain traits, and the gene frequencies for these traits change accordingly. Eventually, the populations will become sufficiently different from each other as to become reproductively isolated. They are then considered to be distinct **species**.

1. **Demes**
A deme is a **small local population**. For example, all the beavers along a specific portion of a river form a deme. Many demes may belong to a specific species. Members of a deme resemble one another more closely than they resemble the members of other demes. They are closely related genetically, since mating between members of the same deme occurs more frequently. Also they are influenced by similar environmental factors and thus are subject to the same selection processes.

2. **Development of New Species**
If the gene pools within a species become sufficiently different so that two individuals cannot mate and produce fertile offspring, two different species have developed. Gene flow is impossible between two species. Genetic **variation**, changes in the **environment**, **migration** to new environments, **adaptation** to new environments, **natural selection**, and **isolation** are all factors that lead to speciation.

3. **Adaptive Radiation**
Adaptive radiation is the emergence of a number of lineages from a **single ancestral species**. A single species may **diverge** into a number of distinct species; the differences between them are those adaptive to a distinct lifestyle, or **niche**. A classic example is Darwin's finches of the Galapagos island chain. Over a comparatively short period of time, a single species of finch underwent adaptive radiation, resulting in 13 species of finches, some of them on the same island. Such adaptations minimized the competition among the birds, enabling each emerging species to become firmly established in its own environmental niche.

4. **Evolutionary History**

Dissimilar species have been found to have evolved from a common ancestor. Biologists seek to understand the evolutionary relationships among the species alive today. This evolutionary history is termed **phylogeny**. Evolutionary history may be visualized as a branching tree, where the common ancestor is found at the trunk and the modern species at the tips of the branches. It is interesting to note that groups in different branches develop in similar ways when exposed to similar environments. This is known as **convergent evolution**. For example, fish and dolphins have come to resemble one another physically, although they belong to different classes of vertebrates. They evolved certain similar features in adapting to the conditions of aquatic life.

Descendants of an ancestral **pouched mammal** include the pouched wolf, anteater, mouse, and mole. They have developed **parallel** to the placental wolf, anteater, mouse, and mole. These pouched mammals and their placental counterparts faced similar, though geographically separate environments; thus, they developed similar adaptations.

The concepts of **adaptive radiation** and **phylogeny** form the basis for the methods employed in developing a system for the classification of living things.

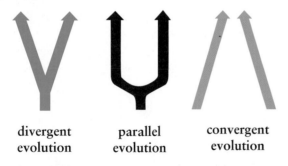

divergent   parallel   convergent
evolution   evolution   evolution

Figure 15.1 Evolutionary Patterns

5. **Isolation**

Genetic isolation often results from the **geographic isolation** of a population into two groups. When groups are isolated from each other, no gene flow occurs between them. Any difference arising from mutations or new combinations of genes will be maintained in the isolated population. Over time, these genetic differences may become significant enough to make mating impossible. In this way, a new species is formed.

GENERAL CHEMISTRY

## 1

ATOMIC STRUCTURE

Chemistry is the study of the nature and behavior of matter. The **atom** is the basic building block of matter, representing the smallest unit of a chemical element. An atom in turn is composed of subatomic particles called **protons**, **neutrons**, and **electrons**. The protons and neutrons in an atom form the **nucleus**, the core of the atom. The electrons exist outside the nucleus in characteristic regions of space called **orbitals**. All atoms of an **element** show similar chemical properties and cannot be further broken down by chemical means.

SUBATOMIC PARTICLES

A. PROTONS

Protons carry a single positive charge and have a mass of approximately one **atomic mass unit** or amu (see below). The **atomic number** (Z) of an element is equal to the number of protons found in an atom of that element. All atoms of a given element have the same atomic number.

B. NEUTRONS

Neutrons carry no charge and have a mass only slightly larger than that of protons. Different isotopes of one element have different numbers of neutrons but the same number of protons. The **mass number** of an atom is equal to the total number of protons and neutrons. The convention $^{A}_{Z}X$ is used to show both the atomic number and mass number of an X atom, where Z is the atomic number and A is the mass number.

C. ELECTRONS

Electrons carry a charge equal in magnitude but opposite in sign to that of protons. An electron has a very small mass—approximately 1/1,837th the mass of a proton or neutron—which is negligible for most purposes. The electrons farthest from the nucleus are known as **valence electrons.** The farther the valence electrons are from the nucleus, the weaker the attractive force of the positively charged nucleus, and the more likely the valence electrons are to be influenced by other atoms. Generally, the valence electrons and their activity determine the reactivity of an atom. In a neutral atom, the number of electrons is equal to the number of protons.

A positive or negative charge on an atom is due to a loss or gain of electrons; the result is called an **ion**.

Some basic features of the three subatomic particles are shown in Table 1.1.

Table 1.1

Subatomic Particle	Symbol	Relative Mass	Charge	Location
Proton	$_1^1 H$	1	+1	Nucleus
Neutron	$_0^1 n$	1	0	Nucleus
Electron	e^-	0	−1	Electron orbitals

Example: Determine the number of protons, neutrons, and electrons in a Nickel-58 atom and in a Nickel-60 2+ cation.

Solution: ^{58}Ni has an atomic number of 28 and a mass number of 58. Therefore, ^{58}Ni has 28 protons, 28 electrons, and 58 − 28, or 30, neutrons.

In the $^{60}Ni^{2+}$ species, the number of protons is the same as in the neutral ^{58}Ni atom. However, $^{60}Ni^{2+}$ has a positive charge because it has lost two electrons; thus, Ni^{2+} 26 electrons. Also, the mass number is two units higher than for the ^{58}Ni atom, and this difference in mass must be due to two extra neutrons; thus, it has a total of 32 neutrons.

ATOMIC WEIGHTS AND ISOTOPES
A. ATOMIC WEIGHTS

The atomic mass of an atom is the relative mass of that atom compared to the mass of a carbon-12 atom, which is used as a standard with an assigned mass of 12.000. Atomic masses are expressed in terms of atomic mass units (amu), with one amu being defined as exactly one-twelfth the mass of the carbon-12 atom, approximately 1.66×10^{-24} grams (g). A more common convention used to define the mass of an atom is **atomic weight**. The atomic weight is the weight in grams of one mole (mol) of a given element and is expressed in terms of g/mol. A mole is a unit used to count particles and is represented by **Avogadro's number**, 6.022×10^{23} particles. For example, the atomic weight of carbon is 12.0 g/mol, which means that 6.022×10^{23} carbon atoms weigh 12.0 g (see "Molecules and Moles" in chapter 4).

B. ISOTOPES

For a given element, multiple species of atoms with the same number of protons (same atomic number) but different numbers of neutrons (different mass numbers) exist; these are called **isotopes** of the element. Isotopes are referred to either by the convention described above or, more commonly, by the name of the element followed by the mass number. For example, carbon-12 ($^{12}_{6}C$) is a carbon atom with 6 protons and 6 neutrons, while carbon-14 ($^{14}_{6}C$) is a carbon atom with 6 protons and 8 neutrons. Since isotopes have the same number of protons and electrons, they generally exhibit the same chemical properties.

In nature, almost all elements exist as a collection of two or more isotopes, and these isotopes are usually present in the same proportions in any sample of a naturally occurring element. The presence of these isotopes accounts for the fact that the accepted atomic weight for most elements is not a whole number. The masses listed in the periodic table are weighted averages that account for the relative abundance of various isotopes.

> Example: Element Q consists of three different isotopes: A, B, and C. Isotope A has an atomic mass of 40.00 amu and accounts for 60.00% of naturally occurring Q. The atomic mass of isotope B is 44.00 amu and accounts for 25.00% of Q. Finally, isotope C has an atomic mass of 41.00 amu and a natural abundance of 15.00%. What is the atomic weight of element Q?
>
> Solution: 0.60(40 amu) + 0.25(44 amu) + 0.15(41 amu)
>
> = 24.00 amu + 11.00 amu + 6.15 amu = 41.15 amu
>
> The atomic weight of element Q is 41.15 g/mol.

BOHR'S MODEL OF THE HYDROGEN ATOM

In 1911, Ernest Rutherford provided experimental evidence that an atom has a dense, positively charged nucleus that accounts for only a small portion of the volume of the atom. In 1900, Max Planck developed the first **quantum theory,** proposing that energy emitted as electromagnetic radiation from matter comes in discrete bundles called **quanta.** The energy value of a quantum is given by the equation $E = hf$ where h is a proportionality constant known as **Planck's constant,** equal to 6.626×10^{-34} J•s, and f (sometimes designated v) is the **frequency** of the radiation.

A. THE BOHR MODEL

In 1913, Niels Bohr used the work of Rutherford and Planck to develop his model of the electronic structure of the hydrogen atom. Starting from Rutherford's findings, Bohr assumed that the hydrogen atom consisted of a central proton around which an electron travelled in a circular orbit and that the centripetal force acting on the electron as it revolved around the nucleus was the electrical force between the positively charged proton and the negatively charged electron.

Bohr's model used the quantum theory of Planck in conjunction with concepts from classical physics. In classical mechanics, an object, such as an electron, revolving in a circle may assume an infinite number of values for its radius and velocity. Therefore, the angular momentum ($L = mvr$) and kinetic energy ($KE = mv^2/2$) can take on any value. However, by incorporating Planck's quantum theory into his model, Bohr placed conditions on the value of the angular momentum. Like Planck's energy, the angular momentum of an electron is quantized according to the following equation:

$$\text{angular momentum} = nh/2\pi$$

where h is Planck's constant and n is a quantum number that can be any positive integer. Since h, 2, and π are constants, the angular momentum changes only in discrete amounts with respect to the quantum number, n.

Bohr then equated the allowed values of the angular momentum to the energy of the electron. He obtained the following equation:

$$E = -R_H/n^2$$

where R_H is an experimentally determined constant (known as the Rydberg constant) equal to 2.18×10^{-18} J/electron. Therefore, like angular momentum, the energy of the electron changes in discrete amounts with respect to the quantum number.

A value of zero energy was assigned to the state in which the proton and electron were separated completely, meaning that there was no attractive force between them. Therefore, the electron in any of its quantized states in the atom would have a negative energy as a result of the attractive forces between the electron and proton. This explains the negative sign in the above equation for energy.

B. APPLICATIONS OF THE BOHR MODEL

In his model of the structure of hydrogen, Bohr postulated that an electron can exist only in certain fixed energy states. In terms of quantum theory, the energy of an electron is **quantized.** Using this model, certain generalizations concerning the characteristics of electrons can be made. The energy of the electron is related to its orbital radius: The smaller the radius, the lower the energy state of the electron. The smallest orbit (radius) an electron can have corresponds to $n = 1$, which is the ground state of the hydrogen electron. At the **ground state** level, the electron is in its lowest energy state. The Bohr model is also used to explain the atomic emission spectrum and atomic absorption spectrum of hydrogen, and it is helpful in interpretation of the spectra of other atoms.

1. **Atomic Emission Spectra**

   At room temperature, the majority of atoms in a sample are in the ground state. However, electrons can be excited to higher energy levels, by heat or other energy, to yield the excited state of the atom. Because the lifetime of the excited state is brief, the electrons will return rapidly to the ground state, emitting energy in the form of photons. The electromagnetic energy of these photons may be determined using the following equation:

   $$E = hc/\lambda$$

   where h is Planck's constant, c is the velocity of light (3.00×10^8 m/s), and λ is the wavelength of the radiation.

   The different electrons in an atom will be excited to different energy levels. When these electrons return to their ground states, each will emit a photon with a wavelength characteristic of the specific transition it undergoes. The quantized energies of light emitted under these conditions do not produce a continuous spectrum (as expected from classical physics). Rather, the spectrum is composed of light at specific frequencies and is thus known as a line spectrum, where each line on the emission spectrum corresponds to a specific electronic transition. Because each element can have its electrons excited to different distinct energy levels, each possesses a unique **atomic emission spectrum,** which can be used as a fingerprint for the element. One application of atomic emissions spectroscopy is in the analysis of stars; while a physical sample can not be taken, the light from a star can be resolved into its component wavelengths, which are then matched to the known line spectra of the elements.

   The Bohr model of the hydrogen atom explained the atomic emission spectrum of hydrogen, which is the simplest emission spectrum among all the elements. The group of hydrogen emission lines corresponding to transitions from upper levels $n > 2$ to $n = 2$ is known as the **Balmer series** (four wavelengths in the visible region), while the group corresponding to transitions between upper levels $n > 1$ to $n = 1$ is known as the **Lyman series** (higher energy transitions, occur in the UV region).

   When the energy of each frequency of light observed in the emission spectrum of hydrogen was calculated according to Planck's quantum theory, the values obtained closely matched those expected from energy level transitions in the Bohr model. That is, the energy associated with a change in the quantum number from an initial value n_i to a final value n_f is equal to the energy of Planck's emitted photon. Thus,

   $$E = hc/\lambda = -R_H[1/(n_i)^2 - 1/(n_f)^2]$$

> **DAT Synopsis**
>
> Note that all systems tend towards minimal energy. Thus, atoms of any element will generally exist in the ground state unless subjected to extremely high temperatures or irradiation.

and the energy of the emitted photon corresponds to the precise difference in energy between the higher-energy initial state and the lower-energy final state.

2. **Atomic Absorption Spectra**

When an electron is excited to a higher energy level, it must absorb energy. The energy absorbed as an electron jumps from an orbital of low energy to one of higher energy is characteristic of that transition. This means that the excitation of electrons in a particular element results in energy absorptions at specific wavelengths. Thus, in addition to an emission spectrum, every element possesses a characteristic **absorption spectrum.** Not surprisingly, the wavelengths of absorption correspond directly to the wavelengths of emission since the energy difference between levels remains unchanged. Absorption spectra can thus be used in the identification of elements present in a gas phase sample.

QUANTUM MECHANICAL MODEL OF ATOMS

While the concepts put forth by Bohr offered a reasonable explanation for the structure of the hydrogen atom and ions containing only one electron (such as He^{1+} and Li^{2+}), they did not explain the structures of atoms containing more than one electron. This is because Bohr's model does not take into consideration the repulsion between multiple electrons surrounding one nucleus. Modern quantum mechanics has led to a more rigorous and generalized study of the electronic structure of atoms. The most important difference between the Bohr model and modern quantum mechanical models is that Bohr's assumption that electrons follow a circular orbit at a fixed distance from the nucleus is no longer considered valid. Rather, electrons are described as being in a state of rapid motion within regions of space around the nucleus called **orbitals.** An orbital is a representation of the probability of finding an electron within a given region. In the current quantum mechanical description of electrons, pinpointing the exact location of an electron at any given point in time is impossible. This idea is best described by the **Heisenberg uncertainty principle,** which states that it is impossible to determine, with perfect accuracy, the momentum and the position of an electron simultaneously. This means that if the momentum of the electron is being measured accurately, its position will change, and vice versa.

DAT Synopsis

Note that the magnitude of ΔE is the same for absorption or emission between any two energy levels. The sign of ΔE indicates whether the energy goes in or out.

A. QUANTUM NUMBERS

Modern atomic theory states that any electron in an atom can be completely described by four **quantum numbers:** n, ℓ, m_ℓ, and m_s. Furthermore, according to the **Pauli exclusion principle,** no two electrons in a given atom can possess the same set of four quantum numbers. The position and energy of an electron described by its quantum numbers is known as its **energy state.** The value of n limits the values of ℓ, which in turn limits the values of m_ℓ. The values of the quantum numbers qualitatively give information about the orbitals: n about the size, ℓ about the shape, and m_ℓ about the orientation of the orbital. All four quantum numbers are discussed below.

1. **Principal Quantum Number**

    The first quantum number is commonly known as the **principal quantum number** and is denoted by the letter n. This is the quantum number used in Bohr's model that can theoretically take on any positive integer value. The larger the integer value of n, the higher the energy level and radius of the electron's orbit. The maximum number of electrons in energy level n (electron shell n) is $2n^2$. The difference in energy between adjacent shells decreases as the distance from the nucleus increases, since it is related to the expression $(1/n_2{}^2 - 1/n_1{}^2)$. For example, the energy difference between the third and fourth shells ($n = 3$ to $n = 4$) is less than that between the second and third shells ($n = 2$ to $n = 3$).

    > **DAT Synopsis**
    >
    > For any principal quantum number n, there will be n possible values for ℓ.

2. **Azimuthal Quantum Number**

    The second quantum number is called the **azimuthal (angular momentum) quantum number** and is designated by the letter ℓ. The second quantum number refers to the **subshells** or **sublevels** that occur within each principal energy level. For any given n, the value of ℓ can be any integer in the range of 0 to $n - 1$. The four subshells corresponding to $\ell = 0$, 1, 2, and 3 are known as the s, p, d, and f subshells, respectively. The maximum number of electrons that can exist within a subshell is given by the equation $4\ell + 2$. The greater the value of ℓ, the greater the energy of the subshell. However, the energies of subshells from different principal energy levels may overlap. For example, the $4s$ subshell will have a lower energy than the $3d$ subshell because its average distance from the nucleus is smaller.

3. **Magnetic Quantum Number**

    The third quantum number is the **magnetic quantum number** and is designated m_ℓ. An orbital is a specific region within a subshell that may contain no more than two electrons. The magnetic quantum number specifies the particular orbital within a subshell where an electron is highly likely to be found at a given point in time. The possible values of m_ℓ are all integers from ℓ to $-\ell$, including 0. Therefore, the

s subshell, where there is one possible value of m_ℓ (0), will contain 1 orbital; likewise, the p subshell will contain 3 orbitals, the d subshell will contain 5 orbitals, and the f subshell will contain 7 orbitals. The shape and energy of each orbital are dependent upon the subshell in which the orbital is found. For example, a p subshell has three possible m_ℓ values (–1, 0, +1). The three dumbbell-shaped orbitals are oriented in space around the nucleus along the x, y, and z axes and are often referred to as p_x, p_y, and p_z.

4. **Spin Quantum Number**

The fourth quantum number, also called the **spin quantum number**, is denoted by m_s. The spin of a particle is its intrinsic angular momentum and is a characteristic of a particle, like its charge. In classical mechanics, an object spinning about its axis has an angular momentum; however, this does not apply to the electron. Classical analogies often are inapplicable in the quantum world.

In any case, the two spin orientations are designated: $+\frac{1}{2}$ and $-\frac{1}{2}$.

Whenever two electrons are in the same orbital, they must have opposite spins. Electrons in different orbitals with the same m_s values are said to have **parallel** spins.

The quantum numbers for the orbitals in the second principal energy level, with their maximum number of electrons noted in parentheses, are shown in Table 1.2. Electrons with opposite spins in the same orbital are often referred to as **paired**.

Table 1.2

n	2(8)			
ℓ	0(2)		1(6)	
$m\ell$	0(2)	+1(2)	0(2)	−1(2)
m_s	$+\frac{1}{2}, -\frac{1}{2}$	$+\frac{1}{2}, -\frac{1}{2}$	$+\frac{1}{2}, -\frac{1}{2}$	$+\frac{1}{2}, -\frac{1}{2}$

B. ELECTRON CONFIGURATION AND ORBITAL FILLING

For a given atom or ion, the pattern by which subshells are filled and the number of electrons within each principal level and subshell are designated by an **electron configuration**. In electron configuration notation, the first number denotes the principal energy level, the letter designates the subshell, and the superscript gives the number of electrons in that subshell. For example, $2p^4$ indicates that there are four electrons in the second (p) subshell of the second principal energy level.

When writing the electron configuration of an atom, it is necessary to remember the order in which subshells are filled. Subshells are filled from lowest to highest energy, and each subshell will fill completely before electrons begin to enter the next one. The $(n + \ell)$ rule is used to rank subshells by increasing energy. This rule states that the lower the values of the first and second quantum numbers, the lower the energy of the subshell. If two subshells possess the same $(n + \ell)$ value, the subshell with the lower n value has a lower energy and will fill first. The order in which the subshells fill is shown in the following chart.

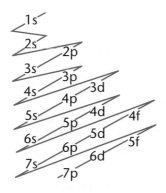

Figure 1.1

Example: Which will fill first, the 3d subshell or the 4s subshell?

Solution: For 3d, $n = 3$ and $\ell = 2$, so $(n + \ell) = 5$. For 4s, $n = 4$ and $\ell = 0$, so $(n + \ell) = 4$. Therefore, the 4s subshell has lower energy and will fill first. This can also be determined from the chart by examination.

To determine which subshells are filled, you must know the number of electrons in the atom. In the case of uncharged atoms, the number of electrons equals the atomic number. If the atom is charged, the number of electrons is equal to the atomic number plus the extra electrons if the atom is negative, or the atomic number minus the electrons if the atom is positive.

In subshells that contain more than one orbital, such as the 2p subshell with its three orbitals, the orbitals will fill according to **Hund's rule.** Hund's rule states that within a given subshell, orbitals are filled such that there are a maximum number of half-filled orbitals with parallel spins. Electrons "prefer" empty orbitals to half-filled ones, because a pairing energy must be overcome for two electrons carrying repulsive negative charges to exist in the same orbital.

Example: What are the written electron configurations for nitrogen (N) and iron (Fe) according to Hund's rule?

Solution: Nitrogen has an atomic number of 7. Thus, its electron configuration is $1s^2\,2s^2\,2p^3$. According to Hund's rule, the two s-orbitals will fill completely, while the three p-orbitals will each contain one electron, all with parallel spins.

$$\underline{\uparrow\downarrow} \qquad \underline{\uparrow\downarrow} \qquad \underline{\uparrow}\;\underline{\uparrow}\;\underline{\uparrow}$$
$$1s^2 \qquad\quad 2s^2 \qquad\quad 2p^3$$

Iron has an atomic number of 26, and its 4s subshell fills before the 3d. Using Hund's rule, the electron configuration will be

$$\underline{\uparrow\downarrow}\quad\underline{\uparrow\downarrow}\quad\underline{\uparrow\downarrow}\,\underline{\uparrow\downarrow}\,\underline{\uparrow\downarrow}\quad\underline{\uparrow\downarrow}\quad\underline{\uparrow\downarrow}\,\underline{\uparrow\downarrow}\,\underline{\uparrow\downarrow}\quad\underline{\uparrow\downarrow}\,\underline{\uparrow}\,\underline{\uparrow}\,\underline{\uparrow}\,\underline{\uparrow}\quad\underline{\uparrow\downarrow}$$
$$1s^2\quad 2s^2\qquad 2p^6\qquad 3s^2\qquad 3p^6\qquad\quad 3d^6\qquad 4s^2$$

Iron's electron configuration is written as $1s^2\,2s^2\,2p^6\,3s^2\,3p^6\,3d^6\,4s^2$. Subshells may be listed either in the order in which they fill (e.g., 4s before 3d) or with subshells of the same principal quantum number grouped together, as shown here. Both methods are correct.

The presence of paired or unpaired electrons affects the chemical and magnetic properties of an atom or molecule. If the material has unpaired electrons, a magnetic field will align the spins of these electrons and weakly attract the atom. These materials are said to be **paramagnetic.** Materials that have no unpaired electrons and are slightly repelled by a magnetic field are said to be **diamagnetic.**

C. VALENCE ELECTRONS

The valence electrons of an atom are those electrons that are in its outer energy shell *or* that are available for bonding. For elements in Groups IA and IIA, only the outermost s electrons are valence electrons. For elements in Groups IIIA through VIIIA, the outermost s and p electrons in the highest energy shell are valence electrons. For transition elements, the valence electrons are those in the outermost s subshell and in the d subshell of the next-to-outermost energy shell. For the inner transition elements, the valence electrons are those in the s subshell of the outermost energy shell, the d subshell of the next-to-outermost energy shell, and the f subshell of the energy shell two levels below the outermost shell.

IIIA–VIIA elements beyond Period II might, under some circumstances, accept electrons into their empty d subshell, which gives them more than eight valence electrons (see exceptions to the octet rule in "Bonding" in chapter 3).

> **DAT Synopsis**
>
> Period II elements cannot expand their octets, since the energy gap between the 2p and the 3s sublevels is too large.

Example: Which are the valence electrons of elemental iron, elemental selenium, and the sulfur atom in a sulfate ion?

Solution: Iron has 8 valence electrons: 2 in its 4s subshell and 6 in its 3d subshell.

Selenium has 6 valence electrons: 2 in its 4s subshell and 4 in its 4p subshell. Selenium's 3d electrons are not part of its valence shell.

Sulfur in a sulfate ion has 12 valence electrons: its original 6 plus 6 more from the oxygens to which it is bonded. Sulfur's 3s and 3p subshells can only contain 8 of these 12 electrons; the other 4 electrons have entered the sulfur atom's 3d subshell, which in elemental sulfur is empty (see chapter 3, Figure 3.1).

Periodic Table of the Elements

Group

Period

Period	1 IA 1A	2 IIA 2A	3 IIIB 3B	4 IVB 4B	5 VB 5B	6 VIB 6B	7 VIIB 7B	8 -------	9 VIII -- ------- 8 -------	10 -----	11 IB 1B	12 IIB 2B	13 IIIA 3A	14 IVA 4A	15 VA 5A	16 VIA 6A	17 VIIA 7A	18 vIIIA 8A
1	1 H 1.008																	2 He 4.003
2	3 Li 6.941	4 Be 9.012											5 B 10.81	6 C 12.01	7 N 14.01	8 O 16.00	9 F 19.00	10 Ne 20.18
3	11 Na 22.99	12 Mg 24.31											13 Al 26.98	14 Si 28.09	15 P 30.97	16 S 32.07	17 Cl 35.45	18 Ar 39.95
4	19 K 39.10	20 Ca 40.08	21 Sc 44.96	22 Ti 47.88	23 V 50.94	24 Cr 52.00	25 Mn 54.94	26 Fe 55.85	27 Co 58.47	28 Ni 58.69	29 Cu 63.55	30 Zn 65.39	31 Ga 69.72	32 Ge 72.59	33 As 74.92	34 Se 78.96	35 Br 79.90	36 Kr 83.80
5	37 Rb 85.47	38 Sr 87.62	39 Y 88.91	40 Zr 91.22	41 Nb 92.91	42 Mo 95.94	43 Tc (98)	44 Ru 101.1	45 Rh 102.9	46 Pd 106.4	47 Ag 107.9	48 Cd 112.4	49 In 114.8	50 Sn 118.7	51 Sb 121.8	52 Te 127.6	53 I 126.9	54 Xe 131.3
6	55 Cs 132.9	56 Ba 137.3	57 La* 138.9	72 Hf 178.5	73 Ta 180.9	74 W 183.9	75 Re 186.2	76 Os 190.2	77 Ir 190.2	78 Pt 195.1	79 Au 197.0	80 Hg 200.5	81 Tl 204.4	82 Pb 207.2	83 Bi 209.0	84 Po (210)	85 At (210)	86 Rn (222)
7	87 Fr (223)	88 Ra (226)	89 Ac~ (227)	104 Rf (257)	105 Db (260)	106 Sg (263)	107 Bh (262)	108 Hs (265)	109 Mt (266)	110 --- ()	111 --- ()	112 --- ()		114 --- ()		116 --- ()		118 --- ()

Lanthanide Series*	58 Ce 140.1	59 Pr 140.9	60 Nd 144.2	61 Pm (147)	62 Sm 150.4	63 Eu 152.0	64 Gd 157.3	65 Tb 158.9	66 Dy 162.5	67 Ho 164.9	68 Er 167.3	69 Tm 168.9	70 Yb 173.0	71 Lu 175.0
Actinide Series~	90 Th 232.0	91 Pa (231)	92 U (238)	93 Np (237)	94 Pu (242)	95 Am (243)	96 Cm (247)	97 Bk (247)	98 Cf (249)	99 Es (254)	100 Fm (253)	101 Md (256)	102 No (254)	103 Lr (257)

## 2

THE PERIODIC TABLE

In 1869, the Russian chemist Dmitri Mendeleev published the first version of his periodic table, in which he showed that ordering the elements according to atomic weight produced a pattern where similar properties periodically recurred. This table was later revised, using the work of the physicist Henry Moseley, to organize the elements on the basis of increasing atomic number. Using this revised table, the properties of certain elements that had not yet been discovered were predicted: A number of these predictions were later borne out by experimentation. The substance of this work is summarized in the **periodic law,** which states that the chemical properties of the elements are dependent, in a systematic way, upon their atomic numbers.

In the periodic table used today, the elements are arranged in **periods** (rows) and **groups** (columns). There are seven periods, representing the principal quantum numbers $n = 1$ to $n = 7$, and each period is filled sequentially. Groups represent elements that have the same electronic configuration in their **valence,** or outermost shell, and share similar chemical properties. The electrons in the outermost shell are called **valence electrons.** They are involved in chemical bonding and determine the chemical reactivity and properties of the element. The Roman numeral above each group represents the number of valence electrons. There are two sets of groups, designated A and B. The A elements are the **representative elements,** which have either s or p sublevels as their outermost orbitals. The B elements are the **nonrepresentative elements**, including the **transition elements,** which have partly filled d sublevels, and the **lanthanide** and **actinide series,** which have partly filled f sublevels. The electron configuration for the valence electrons is given by the Roman numeral and letter designations. For example, an element in Group VA will have a valence electron configuration of s^2p^3 ($2 + 3 = 5$ valence electrons).

PERIODIC PROPERTIES OF THE ELEMENTS

The properties of the elements exhibit certain trends, which can be explained in terms of the position of the element in the periodic table or in terms of the electron configuration of the element. All elements seek to gain or lose valence electrons so as to achieve the stable octet formation possessed by the **inert** or noble gases of Group VIII. Two other important trends exist within the periodic table. First, as one goes from left to right across a period, electrons are added one at a time; the electrons of the outermost shell experience an increasing amount of nuclear attraction, becoming closer and more tightly bound to the nucleus. Second, as one goes down a given column, the outermost electrons become less tightly bound to the nucleus. This is because the number of filled principal energy levels (which shield the outermost electrons from attraction by the nucleus) increases downward within each group. These trends help explain elemental properties such as atomic radius, ionization potential, electron affinity, and electronegativity.

A. ATOMIC RADII

The **atomic radius** of an element is equal to one-half the distance between the centers of two atoms of that element that are just touching each other. In general, the atomic radius decreases across a period from left to right and increases down a given group; the atoms with the largest atomic radii will be located at the bottom of groups and in Group I.

As one moves from left to right across a period, electrons are added one at a time to the outer energy shell. Electrons within a shell cannot shield one another from the attractive pull of protons. Therefore, since the number of protons is also increasing, producing a greater positive charge attracting the valence electrons, the effective nuclear charge increases steadily across a period. This causes the atomic radius to decrease.

As one moves down a group of the periodic table, the number of electrons and filled electron shells will increase, but the number of valence electrons will remain the same. Thus, the outermost electrons in a given group will feel the same amount of effective nuclear charge, but electrons will be found farther from the nucleus as the number of filled energy shells increases. Thus, the atomic radii will increase.

B. IONIZATION ENERGY

The **ionization energy** (IE), or **ionization potential,** is the energy required to remove an electron completely from a gaseous atom or ion. Removing an electron from an atom always requires an input of energy (is **endothermic**; see "States and State Functions" in chapter 6). The closer and more tightly bound an electron is to the nucleus, the more difficult it will be to remove, and the higher the ionization energy will be. The **first ionization energy** is the energy required to remove one valence electron from the parent atom, the **second ionization energy** is the energy needed to remove a second valence electron from the univalent ion to form the divalent ion, and so on. Successive ionization energies grow increasingly large (i.e., the second ionization energy is always greater than the first ionization energy). For example:

$$\text{Mg } (g) \longrightarrow \text{Mg}^+ (g) + e^- \quad \text{First Ionization Energy} \quad = \quad 7.646 \text{ eV}$$

$$\text{Mg}^+ (g) \longrightarrow \text{Mg}^{2+} (g) + e^- \quad \text{Second Ionization Energy} \quad = \quad 15.035 \text{ eV}$$

Ionization energy increases from left to right across a period as the atomic radius decreases. Moving down a group, the ionization energy decreases as the atomic radius increases. Group I elements have low ionization energies because the loss of an electron results in the formation of a stable octet.

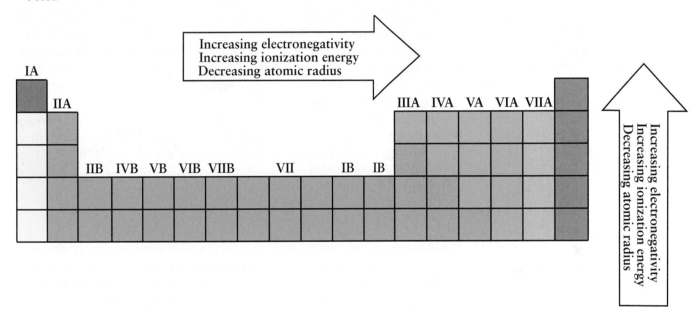

Figure 2.1

C. ELECTRON AFFINITY

Electron affinity is the energy change that occurs when an electron is added to a gaseous atom, and it represents the ease with which the atom can accept an electron. The stronger the attractive pull of the nucleus for electrons (**effective nuclear charge**, or Z_{eff}), the greater the electron affinity will be. In discussing electron affinities, two sign conventions are used. The more common one states that a positive electron affinity value represents energy release when an electron is added to an atom; the other states that a negative electron affinity represents a release of energy. In this discussion, the first convention will be used.

Generalizations can be made about the electron affinities of particular groups in the periodic table. For example, the Group IIA elements, or **alkaline earths**, have low electron affinity values. These elements are relatively stable because their s subshell is filled. Group VIIA elements, or **halogens**, have high electron affinities because the addition of an electron to the atom results in a completely filled shell, which represents a stable electron configuration. Achieving the stable octet involves a release of energy, and the strong attraction of the nucleus for the electron leads to a high energy change. The Group VIII elements, or **noble gases**, have electron affinities on the order of zero, since they already possess a stable octet and cannot readily accept an electron. Elements of other groups generally have low values of electron affinity.

DAT Synopsis

L → R	Atomic Radius ↓
	Ionization Energy ↑
	Electronegativity ↑
Top → Bottom	
	Atomic Radius ↑
	Ionization Energy ↓
	Electronegativity ↓

DAT Synopsis

To recall the various trends, remember this: Cesium, Cs, is the largest, most metallic, and least electronegative of all naturally occurring elements. It also has the smallest ionization energy and the least exothermic electron affinity.

D. ELECTRONEGATIVITY

Electronegativity is a measure of the attraction an atom has for electrons in a chemical bond. The greater the electronegativity of an atom, the greater its attraction for bonding electrons. Electronegativity values are not determined directly. The most common electronegativity scale is the Pauling electronegativity scale, where the values range from 0.7 for the most electropositive elements, like cesium, to 4.0 for the most electronegative element, fluorine. Electronegativities are related to ionization energies: Elements with low ionization energies have low electronegativities because their nuclei do not attract electrons strongly, while elements with high ionization energies have high electronegativities because of the strong pull the nucleus has on electrons. Therefore, electronegativity increases from left to right across periods. In any group, the electronegativity decreases as the atomic number increases as a result of the increased distance between the valence electrons and the nucleus (i.e., greater atomic radius).

TYPES OF ELEMENTS

The elements of the periodic table may be classified into three categories: **metals,** located on the left side and in the middle of the periodic table; **nonmetals,** located on the right side of the table; and **metalloids (semimetals),** found along a diagonal line between the other two.

A. METALS

Metals are shiny solids (except for mercury) at room temperature and generally have high melting points and densities. Metals have the characteristic ability to be deformed without breaking. The ability of a metal to be hammered into shapes is called **malleability,** and the ability to be drawn into wires is called **ductility.** Many of the characteristic properties of metals, such as large atomic radius, low ionization energy, and low electronegativity, are due to the fact that the few electrons in the valence shell of a metal atom can easily be removed. Because the valence electrons can move freely, metals are good conductors of heat and electricity. Groups IA and IIA represent the most reactive metals and will be discussed below. The transition elements, also discussed later, are metals that have partially filled *d*-orbitals.

B. NONMETALS

Nonmetals are generally brittle in the solid state and show little or no metallic luster. They have high ionization energies and electronegativities and are usually poor conductors of heat and electricity. Most nonmetals share the ability to gain electrons easily, but otherwise they display a wide range of chemical behaviors and reactivities. The nonmetals are located on the upper right side of the periodic table; they are separated from the metals by a line cutting diagonally through the region of the periodic table containing elements with partially filled *p*-orbitals.

C. METALLOIDS

The metalloids or semimetals are found along the line between the metals and nonmetals in the periodic table, and their properties vary considerably. Their densities, boiling points, and melting points fluctuate widely. The electronegativities and ionization energies of metalloids lie between those of metals and nonmetals; therefore, these elements possess characteristics of both those classes. For example, silicon has a metallic luster, yet it is brittle and is not an efficient conductor. The reactivity of metalloids is dependent upon the element with which they are reacting. For example, boron (B) behaves as a nonmetal when reacting with sodium (Na) and as a metal when reacting with fluorine (F). The elements classified as metalloids are boron, silicon, germanium, arsenic, antimony, and tellurium.

DAT Synopsis

Metalloids are intermediate in properties between metals and nonmetals. Such properties include electrical conductivity; thus, semimetals tend to make good semiconductors.

THE CHEMISTRY OF GROUPS

A. ALKALI METALS

The **alkali metals** are the elements of Group IA. They possess most of the physical properties common to metals, yet their densities are lower than those of other metals. The alkali metals have only one loosely bound electron in their outermost shell, giving them the largest atomic radii of all the elements in their respective periods. Their metallic properties and high reactivity are determined by the fact that they have low ionization energies; thus, they easily lose their valence electron to form univalent cations. Alkali metals have low electronegativities and react very readily with nonmetals, especially halogens.

B. ALKALINE EARTHS

The **alkaline earths** are the elements of Group IIA, which also possess many characteristically metallic properties. Like the alkali metals, these properties are dependent upon the ease with which they lose electrons. The alkaline earths have two electrons in their outer shell and thus have smaller atomic radii than the alkali metals. However, the two valence electrons are not held very tightly by the nucleus, so they can be removed to form divalent cations. Alkaline earths have low electronegativities and positive electron affinities.

C. HALOGENS

The **halogens**, Group VIIA, are highly reactive nonmetals with seven valence electrons (one short of the favored octet configuration). Halogens are highly variable in their physical properties. For instance, the halogens range from gaseous (F_2 and Cl_2) to liquid (Br_2) to solid (I_2) at room temperature. Their chemical properties are more uniform: The electronegativities of halogens are very high, and they are particularly reactive towards alkali metals and alkaline earths, which "want" to donate electrons to the halogens to form stable ionic crystals. Fluorine (F) has the highest electronegativity of all the elements.

D. NOBLE GASES

The **noble gases**, also called the **inert gases**, are found in Group VIII (also called Group O). They are fairly nonreactive because they have a complete valence shell, which is an energetically favored arrangement. This gives them little or no tendency to gain or lose electrons, high ionization energies, and no real electronegativities. They possess low boiling points and are all gases at room temperature.

E. TRANSITION ELEMENTS

The **transition elements**, Groups IB to VIIIB, are all considered metals; hence, they are also called the **transition metals**. These elements are very hard and have high melting points and boiling points. As one moves across a period, the five *d*-orbitals become progressively more filled. The *d* electrons are held only loosely by the nucleus and are relatively mobile, contributing to the malleability and high electrical conductivity of these elements. Chemically, transition elements have low ionization energies and may exist in a variety of positively charged forms or **oxidation states.** This is because transition elements are capable of losing various numbers of electrons from the *s*- and *d*-orbitals of their valence shell. Theoretically, the transition metals in Group VIIIB could have eight different oxidation states, from +1 to +8; however, they typically do not exhibit so many. For instance, copper (Cu), in Group IB, can exist in either the +1 or the +2 oxidation state, and manganese (Mn), in Group VIIB, occurs in the +2, +3, +4, +6, or +7 state. Because of this ability to attain positive oxidation states, transition metals form many different ionic and partially ionic compounds. The dissolved ions can form **complex ions** with either molecules of water **(hydration complexes)** or with nonmetals, forming highly colored solutions and compounds (e.g., $CuSO_4 \cdot 5H_2O$), and this complexation may enhance the relatively low solubility of certain compounds (e.g., AgCl is insoluble in water but quite soluble in aqueous ammonia due to the formation of the complex ion $[Ag(NH_3)_2]^+$). The formation of complexes causes the *d*-orbitals to be split into two energy sublevels. This enables many of the complexes to absorb certain frequencies of light—those containing the precise amount of energy required to raise electrons from the lower to the higher *d* sublevel. The frequencies not absorbed—known as the **subtraction frequencies**—give the complexes their characteristic colors.

## 3

BONDING AND CHEMICAL INTERACTIONS

The atoms of many elements can combine to form **molecules.** The atoms in most molecules are held together by strong attractive forces called **chemical bonds.** These bonds are formed via the interaction of the valence electrons of the combining atoms. The chemical and physical properties of the resulting molecules are often very different than their constituent elements. In addition to the very strong forces within a molecule, there are weaker intermolecular forces between molecules. These **intermolecular forces,** although weaker than the intramolecular chemical bonds, are of considerable importance in understanding the physical properties of many substances.

DAT Synopsis

When elements combine to form a compound, a whole new set of physical and chemical properties arises.

BONDING

Many molecules contain atoms bonded according to the **octet rule,** which states that an atom tends to bond with other atoms until it has eight electrons in its outermost shell, thereby forming a stable electron configuration similar to that of the Group VIII (noble gas) elements. **Exceptions** to this rule are as follows: **hydrogen,** which can have only two valence electrons (the configuration of He); lithium and beryllium, which bond to attain two and four valence electrons, respectively; boron, which bonds to attain six; and elements beyond the second row, such as phosphorus and sulfur, which can expand their octets to include more than eight electrons by incorporating d-orbitals.

When classifying chemical bonds, it is helpful to introduce two distinct types: ionic bonds and covalent bonds. In **ionic bonding,** an electron(s) from an atom with a smaller ionization energy is transferred to an atom with a greater electron affinity, and the resulting ions are held together by electrostatic forces. In **covalent bonding,** an electron pair is shared between two atoms. In many cases, the bond is partially covalent and partially ionic; we call such bonds **polar covalent bonds.**

IONIC BONDS

When two atoms with large differences in electronegativity react, there is a complete transfer of electrons from the less electronegative atom to the more electronegative atom. The atom that loses electrons becomes a positively charged ion, or **cation,** and the atom that gains electrons becomes a negatively charged ion, or **anion.** For this transfer to occur, the difference in electronegativity must be greater than 1.7. In general, the elements of Groups I and II (low electronegativities) bond ionically to elements of Group VII (high electronegativities). Elements of Groups I and II give up their electrons to achieve a noble gas configuration, while Group VII elements gain an electron to achieve the noble gas configuration. For example, Na + Cl $\longrightarrow$ Na$^+$ Cl$^-$ (sodium chloride). The electrostatic force of attraction between the charged ions is called an **ionic** or **electrovalent bond.**

Ionic compounds have characteristic physical properties. They have high melting and boiling points due to the strong electrostatic forces between the ions. They can conduct electricity in the liquid and aqueous states, though not in the solid state. Ionic solids form crystal lattices consisting of infinite arrays of positive and negative ions in which the attractive forces between ions of opposite charge are maximized, while the repulsive forces between ions of like charge are minimized.

COVALENT BONDS

When two or more atoms with similar electronegativities interact, the energy required to form ions is greater than the energy that would be released upon the formation of an ionic bond (i.e., the process is not energetically favorable). However, since a complete transfer of electrons cannot occur, such atoms achieve a noble gas electron configuration by **sharing** electrons in a covalent bond. The binding force between the two atoms results from the attraction that each electron of the shared pair has for the two positive nuclei.

Covalent compounds contain discrete molecular units with weak intermolecular forces. Consequently, they are low-melting solids and do not conduct electricity in the liquid or aqueous states.

A. PROPERTIES OF COVALENT BONDS

Atoms can share more than one pair of electrons. Two atoms sharing one, two, or three electron pairs are said to be joined by a **single, double,** or **triple covalent bond,** respectively. The number of shared electron pairs between two atoms is called the **bond order;** hence, a single bond has a bond order of one, a double bond has a bond order of two, and a triple bond has a bond order of three.

A covalent bond can be characterized by two features: **bond length** and **bond energy.**

1. **Bond Length**
   Bond length is the average distance between the two nuclei of the atoms involved in the bond. As the number of shared electron pairs increases, the two atoms are pulled closer together, leading to a decrease in bond length. Thus, for a given pair of atoms, a triple bond is shorter than a double bond, which is shorter than a single bond.

2. **Bond Energy**
   Bond energy is the energy required to separate two bonded atoms. For a given pair of atoms, the strength of a bond (and therefore the bond energy) increases as the number of shared electron pairs increases. (Bond energy is further discussed in "States and State Functions" in chapter 6.)

B. COVALENT BOND NOTATION

The shared valence electrons of a covalent bond are called the **bonding electrons**. The valence electrons not involved in the covalent bond are called **nonbonding electrons**. The unshared electron pairs can also be called **lone electron pairs**. A convenient notation, called a **Lewis structure**, is used to represent the bonding and nonbonding electrons in a molecule, facilitating chemical "bookkeeping." The number of valence electrons attributed to a particular atom in the Lewis structure of a molecule is not necessarily the same as the number would be in the isolated atom, and the difference accounts for what is referred to as the **formal charge** of that atom. Often, more than one Lewis structure can be drawn for a molecule; this phenomenon is called **resonance**. Lewis structures, formal charge, and resonance are discussed in detail below.

1. **Lewis Structures**
   A Lewis structure, or **Lewis dot symbol,** is the chemical symbol of an element surrounded by dots, each representing one of the *s* and/or *p* valence electrons of the atom. The Lewis symbols of the elements found in the second period of the periodic table are shown in Table 3.1.

Table 3.1

·Li	Lithium	·N̈·	Nitrogen
·Be·	Beryllium	·Ö:	Oxygen
·Ḃ·	Boron	·F̈:	Fluorine
·C̈·	Carbon	:N̈e:	Neon

Just as a Lewis symbol is used to represent the distribution of valence electrons in an atom, it can also be used to represent the distribution of valence electrons in a molecule. For example, the Lewis symbol of an F ion is $:\overset{..}{\underset{.}{F}}:^-$; the Lewis structure of an F_2 molecule is $:\overset{..}{\underset{.}{F}}\!\!-\!\!\overset{..}{\underset{.}{F}}:$.

Certain steps must be followed in assigning a Lewis structure to a molecule. These steps are outlined below, using HCN as an example.

- Write the skeletal structure of the compound (i.e., the arrangement of atoms). In general, the least electronegative atom is the central atom. Hydrogen (always) and the halogens F, Cl, Br, and I (usually) occupy the end position.

    In HCN, H must occupy an end position. Of the remaining two atoms, C is the least electronegative and, therefore, occupies the central position. The skeletal structure is as follows:

    $$H - C - N$$

- Count all the valence electrons of the atoms. The number of valence electrons of the molecule is the sum of the valence electrons of all atoms present:

    > H has 1 valence electron;
    > C has 4 valence electrons;
    > N has 5 valence electrons; therefore,
    > HCN has a total of 10 valence electrons.

- Draw single bonds between the central atom and the atoms surrounding it. Place an electron pair in each bond (bonding electron pair).

    $$H : C : N$$

    Each bond has 2 electrons, so $10 - 4 = 6$ valence electrons remain.

- Complete the octets (8 valence electrons) of all atoms bonded to the central atom, using the remaining valence electrons still to be assigned. (Recall that H is an exception to the octet rule since it can have only 2 valence electrons.) In this example, H already has 2 valence electrons in its bond with C.

    $$:H : C : \overset{..}{\underset{..}{N}}:$$

- Place any extra electrons on the central atom. If the central atom has less than an octet, try to write double or triple bonds between the central and surrounding atoms using the nonbonding, unshared lone electron pairs.

The HCN structure above does not satisfy the octet rule for C because C possesses only 4 valence electrons. Therefore, 2 lone electron pairs from the N atom must be moved to form two more bonds with C, creating a triple bond between C and N. Finally, bonds are drawn as lines rather than pairs of dots.

$$H - C \equiv N:$$

Now the octet rule is satisfied for all three atoms, since C and N have 8 valence electrons and H has 2 valence electrons.

2. Formal Charges

The number of electrons officially assigned to an atom in a Lewis structure does not always equal the number of valence electrons of the free atom. The difference between these two numbers is the **formal charge** of the atom. Formal charge can be calculated using the following formula:

$$\text{Formal charge} = V - \frac{1}{2}N_{bonding} - N_{nonbonding}$$

where V is the number of valence electrons in the free atom, $N_{bonding}$ is the number of bonding electrons, and $N_{nonbonding}$ is the number of nonbonding electrons.

The formal charge of an ion or molecule is equal to the sum of the formal charges of the individual atoms comprising the ion or molecule.

Example: Calculate the formal charge on the central N atom of $[NH_4]^+$.

Solution: The Lewis structure of $[NH_4]^+$ is

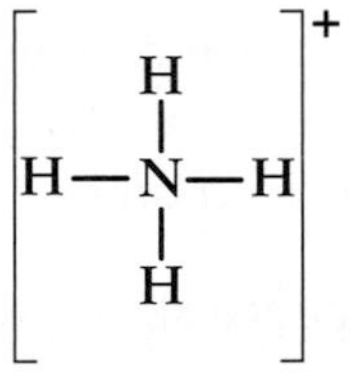

$$\left[\begin{array}{c} H \\ | \\ H - N - H \\ | \\ H \end{array} \right]^+$$

Nitrogen is in Group VA ; thus, it has 5 valence electrons.

In $[NH_4]^+$, N has 4 bonds (i.e., 8 bonding electrons and no nonbonding electrons).

So $V = 5$; $N_{bonding} = 8$; $N_{nonbonding} = 0$.

Formal charge $= 5 - \frac{1}{2}(8) - 0 = +1$.

Thus, the formal charge on te N atom in $[NH_4]^+$ is +1.

3. Resonance

For some molecules, two or more nonidentical Lewis structures can be drawn; these are called **resonance structures.** The molecule doesn't actually exist as either one of the resonance structures but is rather a composite, or hybrid, of the two. For example, SO_2 has three resonance structures, two of which are minor: $O = S - O$ and $O - S = O$. The actual molecule is a hybrid of these three structures (spectral data indicate that the two S–O bonds are identically equivalent). This phenomenon is known as resonance, and the actual structure of the molecule is called the **resonance hybrid.** Resonance structures are expressed with a double-headed arrow between them; thus,

$$\ddot{O}=\ddot{S}=\ddot{O} \longleftrightarrow \ddot{O}=\ddot{S}-\ddot{O}: \longleftrightarrow :\ddot{O}-\ddot{S}=\ddot{O}$$

represents the resonance structures of SO_2.

The last two resonance structures of sulfur dioxide shown above have equivalent energy or stability. Often, nonequivalent resonance structures may be written for a molecule. In these cases, the more stable the structure, the more that structure contributes to the character of the resonance hybrid. Conversely, the less stable the resonance structure, the less that structure contributes to the resonance hybrid. The structure on the left of the diagram above is the most stable. Formal charges are often useful for qualitatively assessing the stability of a particular resonance structure. The following guidelines are used:

- A Lewis structure with small or no formal charges is preferred over a Lewis structure with large formal charges.

- A Lewis structure in which negative formal charges are placed on more electronegative atoms is more stable than one in which the formal charges are placed on less electronegative atoms.

Example: Write the resonance structures for [NCO]⁻.

Solution: 1. C is the least electronegative of the three given atoms, N, C, and O. Therefore, the C atom occupies the central position in the skeletal structure of [NCO]⁻.

N C O

2. N has 5 valence electrons;

C has 4 valence electrons;

O has 6 valence electrons;

and the species itself has one negative charge.

Total valence electrons = 5 + 4 + 6 + 1 = 16.

3. Draw single bonds between the central C atom and the surrounding atoms, N and O. Place a pair of electrons in each bond.

$$N : C : O$$

4. Complete the octets of N and O with the remaining $16 - 4 = 12$ electrons.

$$:\ddot{N}:C:\ddot{O}:$$

5. The C octet is incomplete. There are three ways in which double and triple bonds can be formed to complete the C octet. Two lone pairs from the O atom can be used to form a triple bond between the C and O atoms:

$$:\ddot{N}-C\equiv O:$$

Or 1 lone electron pair can be taken from both the O and the N atoms to form two double bonds, one between N and C and the other between O and C:

$$:\ddot{N}=C=\ddot{O}:$$

Or 2 lone electron pairs can be taken from the N atom to form a triple bond between the C and N atoms:

$$:N\equiv C-\ddot{O}:$$

These three are all resonance structures of $[NCO]^-$.

6. Assign formal charges to each atom of each resonance structure.

The most stable structure is

$$:N\equiv C-\ddot{O}:$$

since the negative formal charge is on the most electronegative atom, O.

4. **Exceptions to the Octet Rule**
Atoms found in or beyond the third period can have more than eight valence electrons, since some of the valence electrons may occupy *d*-orbitals. These atoms can be assigned more than four bonds in Lewis structures. When drawing the Lewis structure of the sulfate ion, giving the sulfur 12 valence electrons permits three of the five atoms to be assigned a formal charge of zero. The sulfate ion can be drawn in six resonance forms, each with the two double bonds attached to a different combination of oxygen atoms.

DAT Synopsis

The octet "rule" is really not much of a rule. It always applies to neutral atoms and anions of C, N, O, and F only. It often (not always!) applies to the halogens and other representative elements, but it never applies to H, He, Li, Be, or to neutral B and Al.

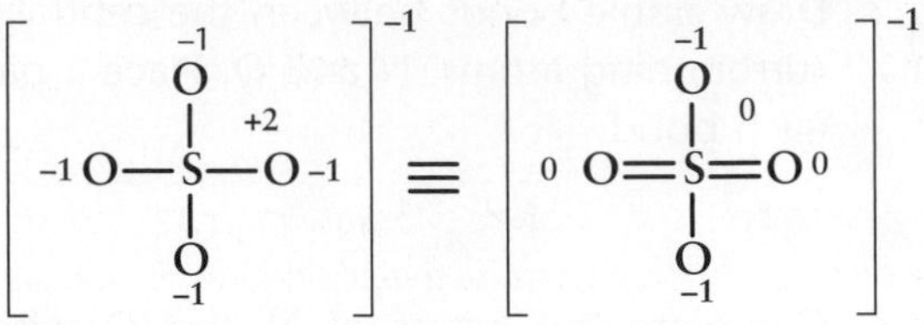

$$\left[\begin{array}{c} \overset{-1}{O} \\ | \\ _{-1}O-\overset{+2}{S}-O_{-1} \\ | \\ \underset{-1}{O} \end{array} \right]^{-1} \equiv \left[\begin{array}{c} \overset{-1}{O} \\ \| \ ^{0} \\ _{0}O=\overset{}{S}=O_{0} \\ \| \\ \underset{-1}{O} \end{array} \right]^{-1}$$

Figure 3.1

C. TYPES OF COVALENT BONDING

The nature of a covalent bond depends on the relative electronegativities of the atoms sharing the electron pairs. Covalent bonds are considered to be **polar** or **nonpolar** depending on the difference in electronegativities between the atoms.

1. **Polar Covalent Bond**

   Polar covalent bonding occurs between atoms with small differences in electronegativity, generally in the range of 0.4 to 1.7 Pauling units. The bonding electron pair is not shared equally but is pulled more towards the element with the higher electronegativity. As a result, the more electronegative atom acquires a partial negative charge, δ^-, and the less electronegative atom acquires a partial positive charge, δ^+, giving the molecule partially ionic character. For instance, the covalent bond in HCl is polar because the two atoms have a small difference in electronegativity (approx. 0.9). Chlorine, the more electronegative atom, attains a partial negative charge, and hydrogen attains a partial positive charge. This difference in charge between the atoms is indicated by an arrow crossed (like a plus sign) at the positive end pointing to the negative end, as shown in Figure 3.2.

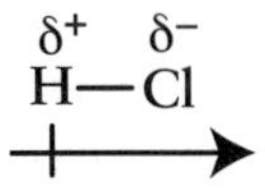

$$\overset{\delta^+ \quad \delta^-}{H-Cl}$$
$$\longmapsto$$

Figure 3.2

A molecule that has such a separation of positive and negative charges is called a polar molecule. The **dipole moment** itself is a vector quantity, μ, defined as the product of the charge magnitude (q) and the distance between the two partial charges (r):

$$\mu = qr$$

The dipole moment is denoted by an arrow pointing from the positive to the negative charge and is measured in Debye units (coulomb-meters).

2. **Nonpolar Covalent Bond**

   Nonpolar covalent bonding occurs between atoms that have the same electronegativities. The bonding electron pair is shared equally, with no separation of charge across the bond. Not surprisingly, nonpolar covalent bonds occur in diatomic molecules, such as H_2, Cl_2, O_2, and N_2.

3. **Coordinate Covalent Bond**

In a coordinate covalent bond, the shared electron pair comes from the lone pair of one of the atoms in the molecule. Once such a bond forms, it is indistinguishable from any other covalent bond. Distinguishing such a bond is useful only in keeping track of the valence electrons and formal charges. Coordinate bonds are typically found in Lewis acid-base compounds (see chapter 10, Acids and Bases). A **Lewis acid** is a compound that can accept an electron pair to form a covalent bond; a **Lewis base** is a compound that can donate an electron pair to form a covalent bond. For example, Figure 3.3 shows the reaction between borontrifluoride (BF_3) and ammonia (NH_3).

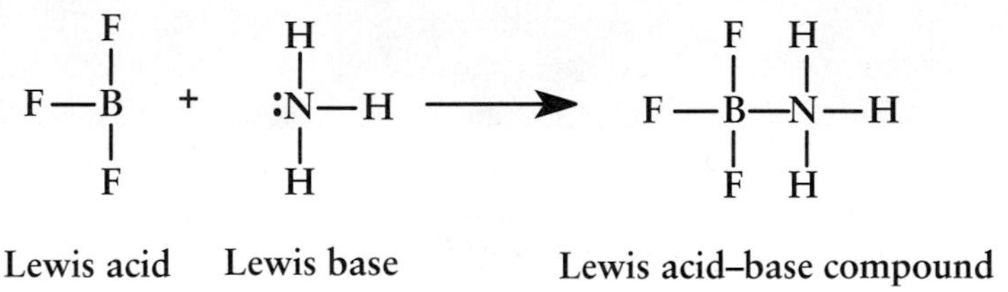

Lewis acid   Lewis base   Lewis acid–base compound

Figure 3.3

NH_3 donates a pair of electrons to form a coordinate covalent bond; thus, it acts as a Lewis base. BF_3 accepts this pair of electrons to form the coordinate covalent bond; thus, it acts as a Lewis acid.

D. GEOMETRY AND POLARITY OF COVALENT MOLECULES

1. The Valence Shell Electron-Pair Repulsion Theory

The valence shell electron-pair repulsion (VSEPR) theory uses Lewis structures to predict the molecular geometry of covalently bonded molecules. It states that the three-dimensional arrangement of atoms surrounding a central atom is determined by the repulsions between the bonding and the nonbonding electron pairs in the valence shell of the central atom. These electron pairs arrange themselves as far apart as possible, thereby minimizing repulsion.

The following steps are used to predict the geometrical structure of a molecule using the VSEPR theory.

1. Draw the Lewis structure of the molecule.

2. Count the total number of bonding and nonbonding electron pairs in the valence shell of the central atom.

3. Arrange the electron pairs around the central atom so that they are as far apart from each other as possible. For example, the compound AX_2 has the Lewis structure X : A : X. A has two bonding electron pairs in its valence shell. To make these electron pairs as far apart as possible, their geometric structure should be linear:

$$X - A - X$$

Valence electron arrangements are summarized in Table 3.2.

Table 3.2

Regions of Electron Density	Example	Geometric Arrangement of Electron Pairs Around the Central Atom	Shape	Angle between Electron Pairs
2	$BeCl_2$	X—A—X	linear	180.0°
3	BH_3	AX₃ triangular planar BeF₃	trigonal planar	120.0°
4	CH_4	AX₄ tetrahedral CH₄	tetrahedral	109.05°
5	PCl_5	AX₅ triangular bipyramidal PCl₅	trigonal bipyramidal	90.0°, 120°, 180°
6	SF_6	AX₆ octahedral SF₆	octahedral	90.0°, 180.0°

Example: Predict the geometry of NH_3.

Solution: 1. The Lewis structure of NH_3 is

$$\overset{\displaystyle H}{\underset{\displaystyle \bullet\bullet}{H-N-H}}$$

2. The central atom, N, has 3 bonding electron pairs and 1 nonbonding electron pair for a total of 4 electron pairs.

3. The 4 electron pairs will be farthest apart when they occupy the corners of a tetrahedron. Since 1 of the 4 electron pairs is a lone pair, the observed geometry is trigonal pyramidal (see Figure 3.4).

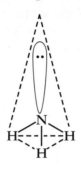

Figure 3.4

In describing the shape of a molecule, only the arrangement of atoms (not electrons) is considered. Even though the electron pairs are arranged tetrahedrally, the shape of NH_3 is pyramidal. It is not trigonal planar because the lone pair repels the 3 bonding electron pairs, causing them to move as far away as possible.

Example: Predict the geometry of CO_2.

Solution: The Lewis structure of CO_2 is $\ddot{\text{O}}\text{::}\text{C}\text{::}\ddot{\text{O}}\text{:}$.

The double bond behaves just like a single bond for purposes of predicting molecular shape. This compound has two groups of electrons around the carbon. According to the VSEPR theory, the two sets of electrons will orient themselves 180° apart, on opposite sides of the carbon atom, minimizing electron repulsion. Therefore, the molecular structure of CO_2 is linear: $\ddot{\text{O}}\text{=}\text{C}\text{=}\ddot{\text{O}}\text{:}$.

2. **Polarity of Molecules**

A molecule with a net dipole moment is called polar, as previously mentioned, because it has positive and negative poles. The polarity of a molecule depends on the polarity of the constituent bonds and on the shape of the molecule. A molecule with nonpolar bonds is always nonpolar; a molecule with polar bonds may be polar or nonpolar depending on the orientation of the bond dipoles.

A molecule of two atoms bound by a polar bond must have a net dipole moment and, therefore, be polar. The two equal and opposite partial charges are localized at the ends of the molecule on the two atoms. A molecule consisting of more than two atoms bound with polar bonds may be either polar or nonpolar, since the overall dipole moment of a molecule is the vector sum of the individual bond dipole moments. If the molecule has a particular shape such that the bond dipole moments cancel each other (i.e., if the vector sum is zero), then the result is a nonpolar molecule. For instance, CCl_4 has four polar C–Cl bonds. According to the VSEPR theory, the shape of CCl_4 is tetrahedral. The four bond dipoles point to the vertices of the tetrahedron and cancel each other, resulting in a nonpolar molecule (see Figure 3.5).

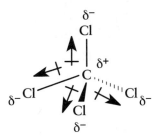

Figure 3.5. No Net Dipole Moment

However, if the orientation of the bond dipoles are such that they do not cancel out, the molecules will have a net dipole moment and, therefore, be polar. For instance, H_2O has two polar O–H bonds. According to the VSEPR model, its shape is angular. The two dipoles add together to give a net dipole moment to the molecule, making the H_2O molecule polar (see Figure 3.6).

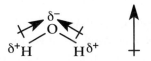

Figure 3.6. Net Dipole Moment

E. ATOMIC AND MOLECULAR ORBITALS

A description of the quantum numbers has already been given in chapter 1 (see "Quantum Mechanical Model of Atoms"). The azimuthal quantum number ℓ describes the orbitals of each n shell. The shapes of these orbitals represent the probability of finding an electron at any given instant. When $\ell = 0$, the orbital is an *s*-orbital. *s*-orbitals are spherically symmetric. The 1*s*-orbital ($n = 1$, $\ell = 0$) is plotted in Figure 3.7.

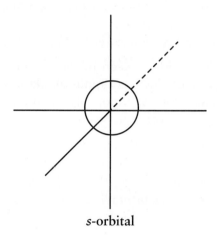

s-orbital

Figure 3.7

When $\ell = 1$, there are three possible orbitals (since the magnetic quantum number, m_ℓ, may equal –1, 0, or 1). These are called *p*-orbitals and have a dumbbell shape. The three *p*-orbitals, designated p_x, p_y, and p_z, are oriented at right angles to each other; the p_x-orbital is plotted in Figure 3.8.

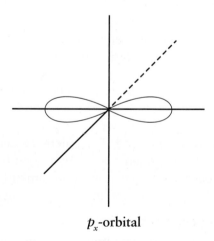

p_x-orbital

Figure 3.8

Plus and minus signs, determined from the mathematics of the wave function, are assigned to each lobe of the *p*-orbitals. The shapes of the five *d*-orbitals ($\ell = 2$, $m_\ell = -2, -1, 0, 1, 2$) and the seven *f*-orbitals ($\ell = 3$, $m_\ell = -3, -2, -1, 0, 1, 2, 3$) are more complex and need not be memorized. When two atoms bond to form a molecule, the atomic orbitals interact to form a **molecular orbital,** which describes the probability of finding the bonding electrons. Molecular orbitals are obtained by adding the wave functions of the atomic orbitals. Qualitatively, this is described by the **overlap** of two atomic orbitals. If the signs of the two atomic orbitals are the

Flashback to Chapter 1

Quantum numbers revisited:

- For any value of *n*, there are *n* values of ℓ ($0 \rightarrow n - 1$).

- $\ell = 0 \rightarrow s$.

  $\ell = 1 \rightarrow p$.

  $\ell = 2 \rightarrow d$.

- For any value of ℓ, there are $2\ell + 1$ values of m_ℓ (number of orbitals); values themselves will range from $-\ell$ to ℓ.

Bridge to Organic Chemistry

It is the pi bonds of alkenes, alkynes, aromatic compounds, and carboxylic acid derivates that lend the functionality so important in organic chemistry. Molecular orbitals are discussed further in Organic Chemistry, chapter 3.

same, a **bonding orbital** is formed. If the signs are different, an **antibonding orbital** is formed. In addition, two different types of overlap are possible. When orbitals overlap head-to-head, the resulting bond is called a **sigma** (σ) bond. When the orbitals are parallel, a **pi** (π) bond is formed.

THE INTERMOLECULAR FORCES

The attractive forces that exist between molecules are collectively known as **intermolecular forces**. These include **dipole-dipole interactions, hydrogen bonding,** and **dispersion forces**. Dipole-dipole interactions and dispersion forces are often referred to as **van der Waals forces.**

A. DIPOLE-DIPOLE INTERACTIONS

Polar molecules tend to orient themselves such that the positive region of one molecule is close to the negative region of another molecule. This arrangement is energetically favorable because an attractive dipole force is formed between the two molecules.

Dipole-dipole interactions are present in the solid and liquid phases but become negligible in the gas phase because the molecules are generally much farther apart. Polar species tend to have higher boiling points than nonpolar species of comparable molecular weight.

B. HYDROGEN BONDING

Hydrogen bonding is a specific, unusually strong form of dipole-dipole interaction, which may be either intra- or intermolecular. When hydrogen is bound to a highly electronegative atom, such as fluorine, oxygen, or nitrogen, the hydrogen atom carries little of the electron density of the covalent bond. This positively charged hydrogen atom interacts with the partial negative charge located on the electronegative atoms of nearby molecules. Substances that display hydrogen bonding tend to have unusually high boiling points compared with compounds of similar molecular formula that do not hydrogen bond. The difference derives from the energy required to break the hydrogen bonds. Hydrogen bonding is particularly important in the behavior of water, alcohols, amines, and carboxylic acids (see the Organic Chemistry section for further discussion).

C. DISPERSION FORCES

The bonding electrons in covalent bonds may appear to be equally shared between two atoms, but at any particular point in time, they will be located randomly throughout the orbital. This permits unequal sharing of electrons, causing rapid polarization and counterpolarization of the electron cloud and formation of short-lived dipoles. These dipoles interact with the electron clouds of neighboring molecules, inducing the formation of more dipoles. The attractive interactions of these short-lived dipoles are called dispersion or **London forces.**

Dispersion forces are generally weaker than other intermolecular forces. They do not extend over long distances and are, therefore, most important when molecules are close together. The strength of these interactions within a given substance depends directly on how easily the electrons in the molecules can move (i.e., be polarized). Large molecules in which the electrons are far from the nucleus are relatively easy to polarize and, therefore, possess greater dispersion forces. If not for dispersion forces, the noble gases would not liquefy at any temperature, since no other intermolecular forces exist between the noble gas atoms. The low temperature at which the noble gases liquefy is to some extent indicative of the magnitude of dispersion forces between the atoms.

DAT Synopsis

These intermolecular forces are the binding forces that keep a substance together in its solid or liquid state (see chapter 8). These same forces determine whether two substances are miscible or immiscible in the solution phase (see chapter 9).

## 4

COMPOUNDS AND STOICHIOMETRY

A **compound** is a pure substance that is composed of two or more elements in a fixed proportion. Compounds can be broken down chemically to produce their constituent elements or other compounds. All elements, except for some of the noble gases, can react with other elements or compounds to form new compounds. These new compounds can react further to form yet different compounds.

MOLECULES AND MOLES

A **molecule** is a combination of two or more atoms held together by covalent bonds. It is the smallest unit of a compound displaying the properties of that compound. Molecules may contain two atoms of the same element, as in N_2 and O_2, or may be comprised of two or more different atoms, as in CO_2 and $SOCl_2$. Molecules are usually discussed in terms of molecular weights and moles.

Ionic compounds do not form true molecules. In the solid state, they can be considered to be a nearly infinite, three-dimensional array of the charged particles of which the compound is composed. Since no actual molecule exists, molecular weight becomes meaningless, and the term **formula weight** is used in its place.

A. MOLECULAR WEIGHT

Like atoms, molecules can be characterized by their weight. The molecular weight is the sum of the atomic weights (in amu) of the atoms in the molecule. Similarly, the formula weight of an ionic compound is found by adding up the atomic weights according to the empirical formula of the substance.

Example: What is the molecular weight of $SOCl_2$?

Solution: To find the molecular weight of SOCl2, add together the atomic weights of each of the atoms.

$$1S = 1 \times 32 \text{ amu} = 32 \text{ amu}$$
$$1O = 1 \times 16 \text{ amu} = 16 \text{ amu}$$
$$2Cl = 2 \times 35.5 \text{ amu} = 71 \text{ amu}$$
$$\text{molecular weight} = 119 \text{ amu}$$

B. MOLE

A mole is defined as the amount of a substance that contains the same number of particles that are found in a 12.000 g sample of carbon-12. This quantity, **Avogadro's number,** is equal to 6.022×10^{23}. One mole of a compound has a mass in grams equal to the molecular weight of that compound in amu and contains 6.022×10^{23} molecules of the compound. For example, 62 g of H_2CO_3 represents one mole of carbonic acid and contains 6.022×10^{23} H_2CO_3 molecules. The mass of 1 mole of a compound is called its **molar weight** or **molar mass** and is usually expressed as g/mol. Therefore, the molar mass of H_2CO_3 is 62 g/mol.

The following formula is used to determine the number of moles present:

$$\text{mol} = \frac{\text{Weight of Sample (g)}}{\text{Molar Weight (g / mol)}}$$

Example: How many moles are in 9.52 g of $MgCl_2$?

Solution: First, find the molar mass of $MgCl_2$.

$$1(24.31 \text{ g/mol}) + 2(35.45 \text{ g/mol}) = 95.21 \text{ g/mol}$$

Now, solve for the number of moles.

$$\frac{9.52}{95.21 \text{ g/mol}} = 0.10 \text{ mol of } MgCl_2$$

C. EQUIVALENT WEIGHT

For some substances, it is useful to define a measure of reactive capacity. This expresses the fact that some molecules are more potent than others in performing certain reactions. An example of this is the ability of different acids to donate protons (H^+ ions) in solution (see chapter 10, Acids and Bases). For instance, 1 mole of HCl can donate 1 mol of hydrogen ions, while 1 mol of H_2SO_4 can donate 2 moles of hydrogen ions. This difference is expressed using the term **equivalent:** 1 mole of HCl contains 1 equivalent of hydrogen ions, while 1 mol of H_2SO_4 contains 2 equivalents of hydrogen ions. To determine the number of equivalents a compound contains, a new measure of weight called **gram-equivalent weight (GEW)** was developed.

$$\text{Equivalents} = \frac{\text{Weight of Compound}}{\text{Gram Equivalent Weight}}$$

and

$$\text{Gram Equivalent Weight} = \frac{\text{Molar Mass}}{n}$$

where n is usually either the number of hydrogens used per molecule of acid in a reaction or the number of hydroxyl groups used per molecule of base in a reaction. This value is strictly dependent on reaction conditions. By using equivalents, it is possible to say that one equivalent of acid will neutralize one equivalent of base, a statement that may not necessarily be true when dealing with moles.

REPRESENTATION OF COMPOUNDS
A. LAW OF CONSTANT COMPOSITION

The **law of constant composition** states that any sample of a given compound will contain the same elements in the identical mass ratio. For instance, every sample of H_2O will contain two atoms of hydrogen for every atom of oxygen, or, in other words, one gram of hydrogen for every eight grams of oxygen.

B. EMPIRICAL AND MOLECULAR FORMULAS

There are two ways to express a formula for a compound. The **empirical formula** gives the simplest whole number ratio of the elements in the compound. The **molecular formula** gives the exact number of atoms of each element in the compound and is usually a multiple of the empirical formula. For example, the empirical formula for benzene is CH, while the molecular formula is C_6H_6. For some compounds, the empirical and molecular formulas are the same, as in the case of H_2O. An ionic compound, such as NaCl or $CaCO_3$, will have only an empirical formula.

C. PERCENT COMPOSITION

The percent composition by mass of an element is the weight percent of the element in a specific compound. To determine the percent composition of an element X in a compound, the following formula is used:

$$\% \text{ Composition} = \frac{\text{Mass of X in Formula}}{\text{Formula Weight of Compound}} \times 100\%$$

The percent composition of an element may be determined using either the empirical or molecular formula. If the percent compositions are known, the empirical formula can be derived. It is possible to determine the molecular formula if both the percent compositions and molecular weight of the compound are known.

Example: What is the percent composition of chromium in $K_2Cr_2O_7$?

Solution: The formula weight of $K_2Cr_2O_7$ is calculated as follows:

2(39 g/mol) + 2(52 g/mol) + 7(16 g/mol) = 294 g/mol

$$\% \text{ composition of Cr} = \frac{2(52 g/mol)}{294 g/mol} = \times 100\%$$

$$= 0.354 \times 100\%$$

$$= 35.4\%$$

Example: What are the empirical and molecular formulas of a compound that contains 40.9% carbon, 4.58% hydrogen, and 54.52% oxygen and has a molecular weight of 264 g/mol?

Method One: First, determine the number of moles of each element in the compound by assuming a 100 gram sample; this converts the percentage of each element present directly into grams of that element. Then convert grams to moles:

$$\#\text{mol of C} = \frac{40.9 \text{ g}}{12 \text{ g/mol}} = 3.41 \text{ mol}$$

$$\#\text{mol of H} = \frac{4.58g}{1g/mol} = 4.58 \text{ mol}$$

$$\#\text{mol of O} = \frac{54.52g}{16g/mol} = 3.41 \text{ mol}$$

Next, find the simplest whole number ratio of the elements by dividing the number of moles by the smallest number obtained in the previous step.

$$\text{C:} \frac{3.41}{3.41} = 1.00 \qquad \text{H:} \frac{4.58}{3.41} = 1.33 \qquad \text{O:} = \frac{3.41}{3.41} = 1.00$$

Finally, the empirical formula is obtained by converting the numbers obtained into whole numbers (multiplying them by an integer value).

$$C_1H_{1.33}O_1 \times 3 = C_3H_4O_3$$

$C_3H_4O_3$ is the empirical formula. To determine the molecular formula, divide the molecular weight by the weight represented by the empirical formula. The resultant value is the number of empirical formula units in the molecular formula.

The empirical formula weight of $C_3H_4O_3$ is calculated as follows:

$$3(12 \text{ g/mol}) + 4(1 \text{ g/mol}) + 3(16 \text{ g/mol}) = 88 \text{ g/mol}$$

$$\frac{264 \text{ g/mol}}{88 \text{g/mol}} = 3$$

$C_3H_4O_3 \times 3 = C_9H_{12}O_9$ is the molecular formula.

Method Two: When the molecular weight is given, it is generally easier to find the molecular formula first. This is accomplished by multiplying the molecular weight by the given percentages to find the grams of each element present in one mole of compound, then dividing by the respective atomic weights to find the mole ratio of the elements:

$$\text{\#mol of C} = \frac{(0.409)(264) \text{ g}}{12 \text{ g/mol}} = 9 \text{ mol}$$

$$\text{\#mol of H} = \frac{(0.0458)(264) \text{ g}}{1 \text{ g/mol}} = 12 \text{ mol}$$

$$\text{\#mol of O} = \frac{(0.5452)(264) \text{ g}}{16 \text{ g/mol}} = 9 \text{ mol}$$

Thus, the molecular formula, $C_9H_{12}O_9$, is the direct result.

The empirical formula can now be found by reducing the subscript ratio to the simplest integral values.

TYPES OF CHEMICAL REACTIONS

There are many ways in which elements and compounds can react to form other species; memorizing every reaction would be impossible, as well as unnecessary. However, nearly every inorganic reaction can be classified into at least one of four general categories.

A. COMBINATION REACTIONS

Combination reactions are reactions in which two or more **reactants** form one **product**. The formation of sulfur dioxide by burning sulfur in air is an example of a combination reaction.

$$S (s) + O_2 (g) \rightarrow SO_2 (g)$$

B. DECOMPOSITION REACTIONS

A **decomposition reaction** is defined as one in which a compound breaks down into two or more substances, usually as a result of heating or electrolysis. An example of a decomposition reaction is the breakdown of mercury (II) oxide (the sign Δ represents the addition of heat).

$$2 \text{ HgO } (s) \xrightarrow{\Delta} 2 \text{ Hg } (\ell) + O_2 (g)$$

C. SINGLE-DISPLACEMENT REACTIONS

Single-displacement reactions occur when an atom (or ion) of one compound is replaced by an atom of another element. For example, zinc metal will displace copper ions in a copper sulfate solution to form zinc sulfate.

$$Zn\ (s) + CuSO_4\ (aq) \rightarrow Cu\ (s) + ZnSO_4\ (aq)$$

Single-displacement reactions are often further classified as **redox** reactions. (These will be discussed in more detail in chapter 11, Redox Reactions and Electrochemistry.)

D. DOUBLE-DISPLACEMENT REACTIONS

In **double-displacement reactions**, also called **metathesis reactions**, elements from two different compounds displace each other to form two new compounds. This type of reaction occurs when one of the products is removed from the solution as a precipitate or gas or when two of the original species combine to form a weak electrolyte that remains undissociated in solution. For example, when solutions of calcium chloride and silver nitrate are combined, insoluble silver chloride forms in a solution of calcium nitrate.

$$CaCl_2\ (aq) + 2\ AgNO_3\ (aq) \rightarrow Ca(NO_3)_2\ (aq) + 2\ AgCl\ (s)$$

NET IONIC EQUATIONS

Because reactions such as displacements often involve ions in solution, they can be written in ionic form. In the example where zinc is reacted with copper sulfate, the **ionic equation** would be

$$Zn\ (s) + Cu^{2+}\ (aq) + SO_4^{2-}\ (aq) \rightarrow Cu\ (s) + Zn^{2+}\ (aq) + SO_4^{2-}\ (aq)$$

When displacement reactions occur, there are usually **spectator ions** that do not take part in the overall reaction but simply remain in solution throughout. The spectator ion in the equation above is sulfate, which does not undergo any transformation during the reaction. A **net ionic reaction** can be written showing only the species that actually participate in the reaction:

$$Zn\ (s) + Cu^{2+}\ (aq) \rightarrow Cu\ (s) + Zn^{2+}\ (aq)$$

Net ionic equations are important for demonstrating the actual reaction that occurs during a displacement reaction.

NEUTRALIZATION REACTIONS

Neutralization reactions are a specific type of double displacements that occur when an acid reacts with a base to produce a solution of a salt and water. For example, hydrochloric acid and sodium hydroxide will react to form sodium chloride and water:

$$HCl\ (aq) + NaOH\ (aq) \rightarrow NaCl\ (aq) + H_2O\ (\ell)$$

(This type of reaction will be discussed further in "Salt Formation" in chapter 10.)

A. BALANCING EQUATIONS

Chemical equations express how much and what type of reactants must be used to obtain a given quantity of product. From the law of conservation of mass, the mass of the reactants in a reaction must be equal to the mass of the products. More specifically, chemical equations must be balanced so that there are the same number of atoms of each element in the products as there are in the reactants. **Stoichiometric coefficients** are used to indicate the number of moles of a given species involved in the reaction. For example, the reaction for the formation of water is:

$$2\ H_2\ (g) + O_2\ (g) \rightarrow 2\ H_2O\ (g)$$

The coefficients indicate that two moles of H_2 gas must be reacted with one mole of O_2 gas to produce two moles of water. In general, stoichiometric coefficients are given as whole numbers.

Example: Balance the following reaction.

$$C_4H_{10}\ (\ell) + O_2\ (g) \rightarrow CO_2\ (g) + H_2O\ (\ell)$$

Solution: First, balance the carbons in reactants and products.

$$C_4H_{10} + O_2 \rightarrow 4\ CO_2 + H_2O$$

Second, balance the hydrogens in reactant and products.

$$C_4H_{10} + O_2 \rightarrow 4\ CO_2 + 5\ H_2O$$

Third, balance the oxygens in the reactants and products.

$$2\ C_4H_{10} + 13\ O_2 \rightarrow 8\ CO_2 + 10\ H_2O$$

Finally, check that all of the elements, and the total charges, are balanced correctly. If there is a difference in total charge between the reactants and products, then the charge will also have to be balanced. Instructions for balancing charge are found in "Oxidation-Reduction Reaction" in chapter 11.

> **DAT Synopsis**
>
> When balancing equations, focus on the least represented elements first and work your way to the most represented element of the reaction (usually oxygen or hydrogen).

B. APPLICATIONS OF STOICHIOMETRY

Once an equation has been balanced, the ratio of moles of reactant to moles of products is known, and that information can be used to solve many types of stoichiometry problems. It is important to use proper units when solving such problems. If and when you are faced with doing the calculations, the units should cancel out so that the units obtained in the answer represent those asked for in the problem.

Example: How many grams of calcium chloride are needed to prepare 72 g of silver chloride according to the following equation?

$$CaCl_2 \ (aq) + 2AgNO_3 \ (aq) \rightarrow Ca(NO_3)_2 \ (aq) + 2AgCl \ (s)$$

Solution: Noting first that the equation is balanced, 1 mole of $CaCl_2$ yields 2 moles of AgCl when it is reacted with 2 moles of $AgNO_3$. The molar mass of $CaCl_2$ is 110 g, and the molar mass of AgCl is 144 g.

$$72g \ AgCl \times \frac{1 \ mol \ AgCl}{144 \ g \ AgCl} \times \frac{1 \ mol \ CaCl_2}{2 \ mol \ AgCl} \times \frac{110 \ g \ CaCl_2}{1 \ mol \ CaCl_2} = 27.5 \ g \ CaCl_2$$

Thus, 27.5 g of $CaCl_2$ are needed to produce 72 g of AgCl.

1. **Limiting Reactant**

When reactants are mixed, they are seldom added in the exact stoichiometric proportions as shown in the balanced equation. Therefore, in most reactions, one of the reactants will be consumed first. This reactant is known as the **limiting reactant** because it limits the amount of product that can be formed in the reaction. The reactant that remains after all of the limiting reactant is used up is called the **excess reactant.**

Example: If 28 g of Fe react with 24 g of S to produce FeS, what would be the limiting reactant? How many grams of excess reactant would be present in the vessel at the end of the reaction?

The balanced equation is Fe + S $\xrightarrow{\Delta}$ FeS.

Solution: First, the number of moles for each reactant must be determined.

$$28 \ g \ Fe \times \frac{1 \ mol \ Fe}{56 \ g} = 0.5 \ mol \ Fe$$

$$24 \ g \ S \times \frac{1 \ mol \ S}{32 \ g} = 0.75 \ mol \ S$$

Since 1 mole of Fe is needed to react with 1 mole of S, and there are 0.5 moles Fe for every 0.75 moles S, the limiting reagent is Fe. Thus, 0.5 moles of Fe will react with 0.5 moles of S, leaving an excess of 0.25 moles of S in the vessel. The mass of the excess reactant will be

$$mass \ of \ S = 0.25 \ mol \ S \times \frac{32 \ g}{1 \ mol \ S}$$
$$= 8 \ g \ of \ S$$

> **DAT Synopsis**
>
> When the quantities of two reactants are given, you are dealing with a limiting reactant problem.

2. Yields

The **yield** of a reaction, which is the amount of product predicted or obtained when the reaction is carried out, can be determined or predicted from the balanced equation. There are three distinct ways of reporting yields. The **theoretical yield** is the amount of product that can be predicted from a balanced equation, assuming that all of the limiting reagent has been used, that no competing side reactions have occurred, and all of the product has been collected. The theoretical yield is seldom obtained; therefore, chemists speak of the **actual yield,** which is the amount of product that is isolated from the reaction experimentally.

The term **percent yield** is used to express the relationship between the actual yield and the theoretical yield and is given by the following equation:

$$\text{Percent Yield} = \frac{\text{Actual Yield}}{\text{Theoretical Yield}} \times 100\%$$

Example: What is the percent yield for a reaction in which 27 g of Cu is produced by reacting 32.5 g of Zn in excess $CuSO_4$ solution?

Solution: The balanced equation is as follows:

$$Zn\ (s) + CuSO_4\ (aq) \rightarrow Cu\ (s) + ZnSO_4\ (aq)$$

Calculate the theoretical yield for Cu.

$$32.5 \text{ g Zn} \times \frac{1 \text{ mol Zn}}{65 \text{ g}} = 0.5 \text{ mol Zn}$$

$$0.5 \text{ mol Zn} \times \frac{1 \text{ mol Cu}}{1 \text{ mol Zn}} = 0.5 \text{ mol Cu}$$

$$0.5 \text{ mol Cu} \times \frac{64 \text{ g}}{1 \text{ mol Cu}} = \text{theoretical yield}$$

Finally, determine the percent yield.

$$\frac{27 \text{ g}}{32 \text{ g}} \times 100\% = 84\%$$

DAT Synopsis

Since we are given "excess" copper(II) sulfate, we know that zinc is the limiting reactant.

## 5

CHEMICAL KINETICS AND EQUILIBRIUM

When studying a chemical reaction, it is important to consider not only the chemical properties of the reactants but also the **conditions** under which the reaction occurs, the **mechanism** by which it takes place, the rate at which it occurs, and the **equilibrium** (or steady state) towards which it proceeds.

CHEMICAL KINETICS

Chemical kinetics is the study of the rates of reactions, the effect of reaction conditions on these rates, and the mechanisms implied by such observations.

A. REACTION MECHANISMS

The **mechanism** of a reaction is the actual series of steps through which a chemical reaction occurs. Knowing the accepted mechanism of a reaction often helps to explain the reaction's rate, position of equilibrium, and thermodynamic characteristics (see chapter 6). Consider the reaction below:

$$\text{Overall reaction: } A_2 + 2\,B \rightarrow 2\,AB$$

This equation seems to imply a mechanism in which two molecules of B collide with one molecule of A_2 to form two molecules of AB. But suppose instead that the reaction actually takes place in two steps.

Step 1:	$A_2 + B \rightarrow A_2B$	(Slow)
Step 2:	$A_2B + B \rightarrow 2\,AB$	(Fast)

Note that these two steps add up to the overall (net) reaction. A_2B, which does not appear in the overall reaction because it is neither a reactant nor a product, is called an **intermediate.** Reaction intermediates are often difficult to detect, but a proposed mechanism can be supported through kinetic experiments.

> **DAT Synopsis**
>
> Mechanisms as they are usually written are actually hypothetical; it is most appropriate to refer to them as "proposed mechanisms."

The slowest step in a proposed mechanism is called the **rate-determining step**, because the overall reaction cannot proceed faster than that step.

B. REACTION RATES

1. Definition of Rate

Consider a reaction $2A + B \rightarrow C$ in which 1 mole of C is produced from every 2 moles of A and 1 mole of B. The rate of this reaction may be described in terms of either the disappearance of reactants over time or the appearance of products over time.

$$\text{rate} = \frac{\text{decrease in concentration of reactants}}{\text{time}} = \frac{\text{increase in concentration of products}}{\text{time}}$$

Because the concentration of a reactant decreases during the reaction, a minus sign is placed before a rate that is expressed in terms of reactants. For the reaction above, the rate of reaction with respect to A is $-\Delta[A]/\Delta t$, with respect to B is $-\Delta[B]/\Delta t$, and with respect to C is $\Delta[C]/\Delta t$. In this particular reaction, the three rates are not equal. According to the stoichiometry of the reaction, A is used up twice as fast as B ($-\frac{1}{2}\Delta[A]/\Delta t = -\Delta[B]/\Delta t$), and A is consumed twice as fast as C is produced ($-\frac{1}{2}\Delta[A]/\Delta t = \Delta[C]/\Delta t$). To show a standard rate of reaction in which the rates with respect to all substances are equal, the rate for each substance should be divided by its stoichiometric coefficient.

$$\text{rate} = -\frac{1}{2}\frac{\Delta[A]}{\Delta t} = -\frac{\Delta[B]}{\Delta t} = \frac{\Delta[C]}{\Delta t}$$

In general, for the reaction

$$a\,A + b\,B \rightarrow c\,C + d\,D,$$

$$\text{rate} = -\frac{1}{a}\frac{\Delta[A]}{\Delta t} = -\frac{1}{b}\frac{\Delta[B]}{\Delta t} = \frac{1}{c}\frac{\Delta[C]}{\Delta t} = \frac{1}{d}\frac{\Delta[D]}{\Delta t}$$

Rate is expressed in the units of moles per liter per second (mol/L × s) or molarity per second (molarity/s).

2. **Rate Law**
For nearly all forward, irreversible reactions, the rate is proportional to the product of the concentrations of the reactants, each raised to some power. For the general reaction

$$a\,A + b\,B \rightarrow c\,C + d\,D$$

the rate is proportional to $[A]^x\,[B]^y$; that is,

$$\text{rate} = k\,[A]^x\,[B]^y$$

This expression is the **rate law** for the general reaction above, where k is the **rate constant.** Multiplying the units of k by the concentration factors raised to the appropriate powers gives the rate in units of concentration/time. The exponents *x* and *y* are called the **orders of reaction;** *x* is the order with respect to A, and *y* is the order with respect to B. These exponents may be integers, fractions, or zero and must be determined experimentally.

It is important to note that the exponents of the rate law are *not* necessarily equal to the stoichiometric coefficients in the overall reaction equation. (The exponents *are* equal to the stoichiometric coefficients of the rate-determining step. If one of the reactants or products in this step is an intermediate not included in the overall reaction, then calculating the rate law in terms of the original reactants is more complex.)

The **overall order of a reaction** (or the **reaction order**) is defined as the sum of the exponents, here equal to $x + y$.

a. **Experimental determination of rate law**
The values of k, *x*, and *y* in the rate law equation (rate = $k\,[A]^x\,[B]^y$) must be determined experimentally for a given reaction at a given temperature. The rate is usually measured as a function of the **initial** concentrations of the reactants, A and B.

Example: Given the data in Table 5.1, find the rate law for the following reaction at 300 K.

$$A + B \rightarrow C + D$$

Table 5.1

Trial	$[A]_{initial}$(M)	$[B]_{initial}$(M)	$r_{initial}$(M/sec)
1	1.00	1.00	2.0
2	1.00	2.00	8.1
3	2.00	2.00	15.9

DAT Synopsis

The exponents in the rate law are not equal to the stoichiometric coefficients unless the reaction actually occurs via a single step mechanism. Also note that product concentrations never appear in a rate law. Do not confuse a rate law with an equilibrium expression.

DAT Synopsis

One can determine the overall reaction order directly from the units of k. For instance, if we are given that $k = 1.2\ M^{-2}sec^{-1}$, then the reaction must be third order overall, since $(M^{-2}sec^{-1})(M^3)$ = rate in Ms^{-1}.

Solution: First, look for two trials in which the concentrations of all but one of the substances are held constant.

a) In trials 1 and 2, the concentration of A is kept constant, while the concentration of B is doubled. The rate increases by a factor of 8.1/2.0, approximately 4. Write down the rate expression of the two trials.

Trial 1: $r_1 = k[A]^x [B]^y = k(1.00)^x (1.00)^y$

Trial 2: $r_2 = k[A]^x [B]^y = k(1.00)^x (2.00)^y$

Divide the second equation by the first:

$$\frac{r_2}{r_1} = \frac{8.1}{2.0} = \frac{k(1.00)^x (2.00)^y}{k(1.00)^x (1.00)^y} = (2.00)^y$$

$$4 = (2.00)^y$$

$$y = 2$$

b) In trials 2 and 3, the concentration of B is kept constant, while the concentration of A is doubled; the rate is increased by a factor of 15.9/8.1, approximately 2. The rate expression of the two trials are as follows:

Trial 2: $r_2 = k(1.00)^x (2.00)^y$

Trial 3: $r_3 = k(2.00)^x (2.00)^y$

Divide the second equation by the first:

$$\frac{r_3}{r_2} = \frac{15.9}{8.1} = \frac{k(2.00)^x (2.00)^y}{k(1.00)^x (2.00)^y} = (2.00)^x$$

$$2 = (2.00)^x$$

$$x = 1$$

So $r = k[A] [B]^2$.

The order of the reaction with respect to A is 1 and with respect to B is 2; the overall reaction order is $1 + 2 = 3$.

To calculate k, substitute the values from any one of the above trials into the rate law, for Example,

$$2.0 \text{ M/sec} = k \times 1.00 \text{ M} \times (1.00 \text{ M})^2$$

$$k = 2.0 \text{ M}^{-2} \text{ sec}^{-1}$$

Therefore, the rate law is $r = 2.0 \text{ M}^{-2} \text{ sec}^{-1} [A][B]^2$

DAT Synopsis

The temperature, 300 K, doesn't enter into the calculation of the rate law; it is reported in the initial data just to make the results meaningful, since the rates of most reactions are temperature dependent.

3. Reaction Orders

Chemical reactions are often classified on the basis of kinetics as zero-order, first-order, second-order, mixed-order, or higher-order reactions. The general reaction a A + b B $\rightarrow$ c C + d D will be used in the discussion below.

a. Zero-order reactions

A zero-order reaction has a constant rate, which is independent of the reactants' concentrations. Thus, the rate law is rate = k, where k has units of $Msec^{-1}$.

b. First-order reactions

A first-order reaction (order = 1) has a rate proportional to the concentration of one reactant.

$$\text{rate} = k[A] \text{ or rate} = k[B]$$

First-order rate constants have units of sec^{-1}.

The classic example of a first-order reaction is the process of radioactive decay. The concentration of radioactive substance A at any time t can be expressed mathematically as

$$[A_t] = [A_o] e^{-kt}$$

where $[A_o]$ = initial concentration of A

$[A_t]$ = concentration of A at time t

k = rate constant

t = elapsed time

The half-life ($t_{1/2}$) of a reaction is the time needed for the concentration of the radioactive substance to decrease to one-half of its original value. Half-lives can be calculated from the rate law as follows:

$$t_{1/2} = \ln 2/k = 0.693/k$$

where k is the first-order rate constant.

c. Second-order reactions

A second-order reaction (order = 2) has a rate proportional to the product of the concentration of two reactants or to the square of the concentration of a single reactant; for example, rate = $k[A]^2$, rate = $k[B]^2$ or rate = k[A][B]. The units of second-order rate constants are $M^{-1} sec^{-1}$.

d. Higher-order reactions

A higher-order reaction has an order greater than 2.

Bridge to Organic Chemistry

Simple substitution reactions are common in organic chemistry, and the most widely accepted mechanisms of such reactions are those known as S_N1 (first order) and S_N2 (second order).

An organic chemist trying to determine whether a particular substitution reaction is occurring by one of these mechanisms would probably carry out an experimental rate law determination as described in this chapter.

For more on S_N1 and S_N2 reactions, see Organic Chemistry, chapter 4.

e. **Mixed-order reactions**
    A mixed-order reaction has a fractional order (e.g., rate = $k[A]^{1/3}$).

4. **Efficiency of Reactions**
    a. **Collision theory of chemical kinetics**
        For a reaction to occur, molecules must collide with each other. The **collision theory of chemical kinetics** states that the rate of a reaction is proportional to the number of collisions per second between the reacting molecules.

        Not all collisions, however, result in a chemical reaction. An **effective collision** (one that leads to the formation of products) occurs only if the molecules collide with correct orientation and sufficient force to break the existing bonds and form new ones. The minimum energy of collision necessary for a reaction to take place is called the **activation energy, E_a,** or the **energy barrier.** Only a fraction of colliding particles have enough kinetic energy to exceed the activation energy. This means that only a fraction of all collisions are effective. The rate of a reaction can therefore be expressed as follows:

        $$rate = fZ$$

        where Z is the total number of collisions occurring per second and f is the fraction of collisions that are effective.

    b. **Transition state theory**
        When molecules collide with sufficient energy, they form a **transition state** in which the old bonds are weakened and the new bonds are beginning to form. The transition state then dissociates into products, and the new bonds are fully formed. For a reaction $A_2 + B_2 \rightarrow 2AB$, the change along the reaction coordinate (a measure of the extent to which the reaction has progressed from reactants to products) can be represented as shown in Figure 5.1.

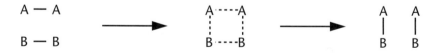

Figure 5.1

The **transition state,** also called the **activated complex,** has greater energy than either the reactants or the products and is denoted by the symbol ‡. The activation energy is required to bring the reactants to this energy level. Once an activated complex is formed, it can either dissociate into the products or revert to reactants without any additional energy input. Transition states are distinguished from intermediates in that, existing as they do at energy maxima, transition states do not have a finite lifetime.

A **potential energy diagram** illustrates the relationship among the activation energy, the heats of reaction, and the potential energy of the system. The most important factors in such diagrams are the **relative** energies of the products and reactants. The **enthalpy change** of the reaction (ΔH) is the difference between the potential energy of the products and the potential energy of the reactants (see "States and State Functions" in chapter 6). A negative enthalpy change indicates an exothermic reaction (where heat is given off), and a positive enthalpy change indicates an endothermic reaction (where heat is absorbed). The activated complex exists at the top of the energy barrier. The difference in potential energies between the activated complex and the reactants is the activation energy of the forward reaction; the difference in potential energies between the activated complex and the products is the activation energy of the reverse reaction.

For example, consider the formation of HCl from H_2 and Cl_2. Figure 5.2, which gives the energy profile of the reaction

$$H_2 + Cl_2 \rightleftharpoons 2\,HCl$$

shows that the reaction is exothermic. The potential energy of the products is less than the potential energy of the reactants; heat is evolved, and the heat of reaction is negative.

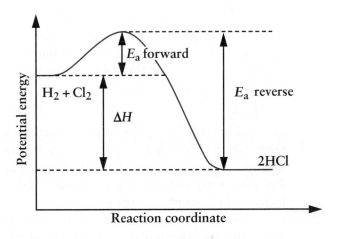

Figure 5.2

The thermodynamic properties of reactions are discussed further in chapter 6.

5. **Factors Affecting Reaction Rate**

The rate of a chemical reaction depends upon the individual species undergoing reaction and upon the reaction environment. The rate of reaction will increase if either of the following occurs: an increase in the number of effective collisions or a stabilization of the activated complex compared to the reactants.

a. **Reactant concentrations**

The greater the concentrations of the reactants (the more particles per unit volume), the greater will be the number of effective collisions per unit time. Therefore, the reaction rate will increase for all but zero-order reactions. For reactions occurring in the gaseous state, the partial pressures of the reactants can serve as a measure of concentration (see "Dalton's Law of Partial Pressures" in chapter 7).

b. **Temperature**

For nearly all reactions, the reaction rate will increase as the temperature of the system increases. Since the temperature of a substance is a measure of the particles' average kinetic energy, increasing the temperature increases the average kinetic energy of the molecules. Consequently, the proportion of molecules having energies greater than E_a (thus capable of undergoing reaction) increases with higher temperature.

c. **Medium**

The rate of a reaction may also be affected by the medium in which it takes place. Certain reactions proceed more rapidly in aqueous solution, whereas other reactions may proceed more rapidly in benzene. The state of the medium (liquid, solid, or gas) can also have a significant effect.

d. **Catalysts**

Catalysts are substances that increase reaction rate without themselves being consumed; they do this by lowering the activation energy. Catalysts are important in biological systems and in industrial chemistry; enzymes are biological catalysts. Catalysts may increase the frequency of collision between the reactants; change the relative orientation of the reactants, making a higher percentage of collisions effective; donate electron density to the reactants; or reduce intramolecular bonding within reactant molecules. Figure 5.3 compares the energy profiles of catalyzed and uncatalyzed reactions.

DAT Synopsis

As a rule of thumb, the rate of a reaction (for most but not all reactions) will approximately double for each 10°C increase in temperature.

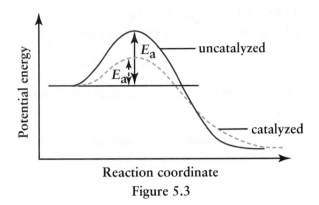

Figure 5.3

The energy barrier for the catalyzed reaction is much lower than the energy barrier for the uncatalyzed reaction. Note that the rates of both the forward and the reverse reactions are increased by catalysis, since E_a of the forward and reverse reactions is lowered by the same amount. Therefore, the presence of a catalyst causes the reaction to proceed more quickly toward equilibrium.

EQUILIBRIUM
A. THE DYNAMIC CONCEPT OF EQUILIBRIUM

So far, reaction rates have been discussed under the assumption that the reactions were **irreversible** (i.e., only proceeded in one direction) and that the reactions proceeded to completion. However, a **reversible** reaction often does not proceed to completion, because (by definition) the products can react to reform the reactants. This is particularly true of reactions occurring in closed systems, where products are not allowed to escape. When there is no **net** change in the concentrations of the products and reactants during a reversible chemical reaction, equilibrium exists. This is not to say that a reaction in equilibrium is static; change continues to occur in both the forward and reverse directions. Equilibrium can be thought of as a balance between the two reaction directions.

Consider the following reaction:

$$A \rightleftharpoons B$$

At equilibrium, the concentrations of A and B are constant, yet the reactions $A \rightarrow B$ and $B \rightarrow A$ continue to occur at equal rates.

B. LAW OF MASS ACTION

Consider the following **one-step** reaction:

$$2A \rightleftharpoons B + C$$

Since the reaction occurs in one step, the rates of the forward and reverse reaction are given by

$$\text{rate}_f = k_f[A]^2 \text{ and rate}_r = k_r[B] [C]$$

When $\text{rate}_f = \text{rate}_r$, equilibrium is achieved. Since the rates are equal, it can be stated that

$$k_f[A]^2 = k_f[B][C] \text{ or } \frac{k_f}{k_r} = \frac{[B][C]}{[A]^2}$$

Since k_f and k_r are both constants, this equation may be rewritten:

$$K_c = \frac{[B][C]}{[A]^2} \qquad \text{(see below for the general equation)}$$

where K_c is called the **equilibrium constant**, and the subscript c indicates that it is in terms of concentration (when dealing with gases, the equilibrium constant is referred to as K_p, and the subscript p indicates that it is in terms of pressure). For dilute solutions, K_c and K_{eq} are used interchangeably; the symbol K is also often used, though it is not completely correct to do so.

While the forward and reverse reaction rates are equal at equilibrium, the molar concentrations of the reactants and products usually are not equal. This means that the forward and reverse rate constants, k_f and k_r, are also usually unequal. For the **one-step** reaction described above,

$$k_f [A]^2 = k_r[B][C]$$

$$k_f = k_r\left(\frac{[B][C]}{[A]^2}\right)$$

In a reaction of more than one step, the equilibrium constant for the overall reaction is found by multiplying together the equilibrium constants for each step of the reaction. When this is done, the equilibrium constant for the overall reaction is equal to the concentrations of products divided by reactants in the overall reaction, each raised to its stoichiometric coefficient. The forward and reverse rate constants for any step n are designated k_n and k_{-n} respectively. For example, if the reaction

$$a A + b B \rightleftharpoons c C + d D$$

occurs in three steps, then

$$k_c = \frac{k_1 k_2 k_3}{k_{-1} k_{-2} k_{-3}} \quad \text{will equal} \quad \frac{[C]^c [D]^d}{[A]^a [B]^b}.$$

This expression is known as the **Law of Mass Action**.

Example: What is the expression for the equilibrium constant for the following reaction?

$$3\ H_2\ (g) + N_2\ (g) \rightleftharpoons 2\ NH_3\ (g)$$

Solution: $K_c = \dfrac{[NH_3]^2}{[H_2]^3 [N_2]}$

The **reaction quotient**, Q, is a measure of the degree to which a reaction has gone to completion. Q_c is equal to

$$\frac{[C]^c [D]^d}{[A]^a [B]^b}$$

Q_c is a constant only at equilibrium, when it is equal to K_c.

C. PROPERTIES OF THE EQUILIBRIUM CONSTANT

The equilibrium constant, K_{eq}, has the following characteristics:

- Pure solids and liquids do not appear in the equilibrium constant expression.
- K_{eq} is characteristic of a given system at a given temperature.
- If the value of K_{eq} is very large compared to 1, an equilibrium mixture of reactants and products will contain very little of the reactants compared to the products.
- If the value of K_{eq} is very small compared to 1 (i.e., less than 0.1), an equilibrium mixture of reactants and products will contain very little of the products compared to the reactants.
- If the value of K_{eq} is close to 1, an equilibrium mixture of products and reactants will contain approximately equal amounts of reactants and products.

D. LE CHÂTELIER'S PRINCIPLE

The French chemist Henry Louis Le Châtelier stated that a system to which a stress is applied tends to change so as to relieve the applied stress. This rule, known as **Le Châtelier's principle,** is used to determine the direction in which a reaction at equilibrium will proceed when subjected to a stress, such as a change in concentration, pressure, temperature, or volume.

1. **Changes in Concentration**

Increasing the concentration of a species will tend to shift the equilibrium away from the species that is added to re-establish its equilibrium concentration, and vice versa. For example, in the reaction

$$A + B \rightleftharpoons C + D$$

if the concentration of A and/or B is increased, the equilibrium will shift towards (or favor production of) C and D. Conversely, if the concentration of C and/or D is increased, the equilibrium will shift away from the production of C and D, favoring production of A and B. Similarly, decreasing the concentration of a species will tend to shift the equilibrium towards the production of that species. For example, if A and/or B is removed from the above reaction, the equilibrium will shift so as to favor increasing concentration of A and B.

This effect is often used in industry to increase the yield of a useful product or drive a reaction to completion. If D were constantly removed from the above reaction, the net reaction would produce more D and concurrently more C. Likewise, using an excess of the least expensive reactant helps to drive the reaction forward.

2. **Changes in Pressure or Volume**

In a system at constant temperature, a change in pressure causes a change in volume, and vice versa. Since liquids and solids are practically incompressible, a change in the pressure or volume of systems involving only these phases has little or no effect on their equilibrium. Reactions involving gases, however, may be greatly affected by changes in pressure or volume, since gases are highly compressible.

Pressure and volume are inversely related. An increase in the pressure of a system will shift the equilibrium so as to decrease the number of moles of gas present. This reduces the volume of the system and relieves the stress of the increased pressure. Consider the following reaction:

$$N_2 \ (g) + 3 \ H_2 \ (g) \rightleftharpoons 2 \ NH_3 \ (g)$$

The left side of the reaction has 4 moles of gaseous molecules, whereas the right side has only 2 moles. When the pressure of this system is increased, the equilibrium will shift so that the side of the reaction producing fewer moles is favored. Since there are fewer moles on the right, the equilibrium will shift towards the right. Conversely, if the volume of the same system is increased, its pressure immediately decreases, which, according to Le Châtelier's principle, leads to a shift in the equilibrium to the left.

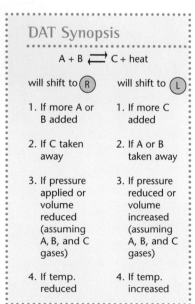

DAT Synopsis

$$A + B \rightleftharpoons C + heat$$

will shift to (R)   will shift to (L)

1. If more A or B added

2. If C taken away

3. If pressure applied or volume reduced (assuming A, B, and C gases)

4. If temp. reduced

1. If more C added

2. If A or B taken away

3. If pressure reduced or volume increased (assuming A, B, and C gases)

4. If temp. increased

3. **Changes in Temperature**

Changes in temperature also affect equilibrium. To predict this effect, heat may be considered as a product in an exothermic reaction and as a reactant in an endothermic reaction. Consider the following exothermic reaction:

$$A \rightleftharpoons B + heat$$

If this system were placed in an ice bath, its temperature would decrease, driving the reaction to the right to replace the heat lost. Conversely, if the system were placed in a boiling-water bath, the reaction equilibrium would shift to the left due to the increased "concentration" of heat.

Not only does a temperature change alter the position of the equilibrium, it also alters the numerical value of the equilibrium constant. In contrast, changes in the concentration of a species in the reaction, in the pressure, or in the volume will alter the position of the equilibrium without changing the numerical value of the equilibrium constant.

## 6

THERMOCHEMISTRY

All chemical reactions are accompanied by energy changes. Thermal, chemical, potential, and kinetic energies are all interconvertible, as they must obey the **Law of Conservation of Energy.** Energy changes determine whether reactions can occur and how easily they will do so. Thus, an understanding of **thermodynamics** is essential to an understanding of chemistry. In chemistry, thermodynamics helps determine whether a chemical reaction is **spontaneous** (i.e., if under a given set of conditions it can occur, by itself, without outside assistance). A spontaneous reaction may or may not proceed to completion, depending upon the rate of the reaction, which is determined by chemical kinetics (see chapter 5).

The application of thermodynamics to chemical reactions is called **thermochemistry.** Several thermodynamic definitions are very useful in thermochemistry. A **system** is the particular part of the universe being studied; everything outside the system is considered the **surroundings** or **environment**. A system may be

- **isolated:** It cannot exchange energy or matter with the surroundings, as with an insulated bomb reactor.
- **closed:** It can exchange energy but not matter with the surroundings, as with a steam radiator.
- **open:** It can exchange both matter and energy with the surroundings, as with a pot of boiling water.

A system undergoes a **process** when one or more of its properties changes. A process is associated with a change of state. An **isothermal** process occurs when the temperature of the system remains constant, an **adiabatic** process occurs when no heat exchange occurs, and an **isobaric** process occurs when the pressure of the system remains constant. Isothermal and isobaric processes are common, since it is usually easy to control temperature and pressure.

HEAT

A. DEFINITION

Heat is a form of energy that can easily transfer to or from a system, the result of a temperature difference between the system and its surroundings; this transfer will occur spontaneously from a warmer system to a cooler system. According to convention, heat absorbed by a system (from its surroundings) is considered positive, while heat lost by a system (to its surroundings) is considered negative.

Heat change is the most common energy change in chemical processes. Reactions that absorb heat energy are said to be **endothermic**, while those that release heat energy are said to be **exothermic**. Heat is commonly measured in **calories (cal)** or **joules (J)** and, more commonly, in kcal or kJ (1 cal = 4.184 J).

B. CALORIMETRY

Calorimetry measures heat changes. The terms **constant-volume calorimetry** and **constant-pressure calorimetry** are used to indicate the conditions under which the heat changes are measured. The heat (q) absorbed or released in a given process is calculated from this equation:

$$q = mc\Delta T$$

where m is the mass, c is the **specific heat**, and ΔT is the change in temperature.

1. Constant-Volume Calorimetry

In constant-volume calorimetry, the volume of the container holding the reacting mixture does not change during the course of the reaction. The heat of reaction is measured using a device called a bomb calorimeter. This apparatus consists of a steel bomb into which the reactants are placed. The bomb is immersed in an insulated container containing a known amount of water. The reactants are electrically ignited, and heat is absorbed or evolved as the reaction proceeds. The heat of the reaction, q_{rxn}, can be determined as follows.

Since no heat enters or leaves the system, the net heat change for the system is zero; therefore, the heat change for the reaction is compensated for by the heat change for the water and the bomb, which is easy to measure.

$$q_{system} = q_{rxn} + q_{water} + q_{steel} = 0$$

Thus:
$$q_{rxn} = -(q_{water} + q_{steel})$$
$$= -(m_{water}\, c_{water}\, \Delta T + m_{steel}\, c_{steel}\, \Delta T)$$

Note that the overall system, as defined, is adiabatic, since no net heat gain or loss occurs. However, the heat exchange between the various components makes it possible to determine the heat of reaction.

STATES AND STATE FUNCTIONS

The state of a system is described by the macroscopic properties of the system. Examples of macroscopic properties include temperature (T), pressure (P), and volume (V). When the state of a system changes, the values of the properties also change. Properties whose magnitude depends only on the initial and final states of the system, and not on the path of the change (how the change was accomplished), are known as **state functions**. Pressure, temperature, and volume are important state functions. Other examples are **enthalpy (H), entropy (S), free energy (G)** (all discussed below) and **internal energy (E or U)**. Although independent of path, state functions are not necessarily independent of one another.

A set of **standard conditions** (25°C and 1 atm) is normally used for measuring the enthalpy, entropy, and free energy of a reaction. A substance in its most stable form under standard conditions is said to be in its **standard state**. Examples of substances in their standard states include hydrogen as $H_2(g)$, water as $H_2O(\ell)$, and salt as $NaCl(s)$. The changes in enthalpy, entropy, and free energy that occur when a reaction takes place under standard conditions are called the **standard enthalpy**, **standard entropy**, and **standard free energy** changes respectively and are symbolized by $\Delta H°$, $\Delta S°$, and $\Delta G°$.

> **DAT Synopsis**
>
> Standard conditions in thermodynamics must not be confused with standard temperature and pressure (STP) in gas law calculations. (See chapter 7.)

A. ENTHALPY

Most reactions in the lab occur under constant pressure (at 1 atm, in open containers). To express heat changes at constant pressure, chemists use the term **enthalpy (H)**. The change in enthalpy (ΔH) of a process is equal to the heat absorbed or evolved by the system at constant pressure. The enthalpy of a process depends only on the enthalpies of the initial and final states, *not* on the path. Thus, to find the enthalpy change of a reaction, ΔH_{rxn}, one must subtract the enthalpy of the reactants from the enthalpy of the products:

$$\Delta H_{rxn} = H_{products} - H_{reactants}$$

A positive ΔH corresponds to an endothermic process, and a negative ΔH corresponds to an exothermic process.

Unfortunately, it is not possible to measure H directly; only ΔH can be measured and, even then, only for certain fast and spontaneous processes. Thus, several standard methods have been developed to calculate ΔH for any process.

1. **Standard Heat of Formation**

   The enthalpy of formation of a compound, $\Delta H°_f$, is the enthalpy change that would occur if one mole of a compound were formed directly from its elements in their standard states. Note that $\Delta H°_f$ of an element in its standard state is zero. The $\Delta H°_f$'s of most known substances are tabulated.

2. **Standard Heat of Reaction**

    The standard heat of a reaction, $\Delta H°_{rxn}$, is the hypothetical enthalpy change that would occur if the reaction were carried out under standard conditions (i.e., when reactants in their standard states are converted to products in their standard states at 298 K). It can be expressed as follows:

    $$\Delta H°_{rxn} = \text{(sum of } \Delta H°_f \text{ of products)} - \text{(sum of } \Delta H°_f \text{ of reactants)}$$

3. **Hess's Law**

    Hess's Law states that enthalpies of reactions are additive. When thermochemical equations (chemical equations for which energy changes are known) are added to give the net equation for a reaction, the corresponding heats of reaction are also added to give the net heat of reaction. Because enthalpy is a state function, the enthalpy of a reaction does not depend on the path taken but only on the initial and final states. For example, consider this reaction:

    $$Br_2\,(\ell) \rightarrow Br_2\,(g) \qquad \Delta H = (31 \text{ kJ/mol})(1 \text{ mol}) = 31 \text{ kJ}$$

    The enthalpy change of the above reaction, called the **heat of vaporization, $\Delta H°_{vap}$**, will always be 31 kJ/mol, provided that the same initial and final states, $Br_2(\ell)$ and $Br_2(g)$ respectively, exist at standard conditions. $Br_2(\ell)$ could instead be decomposed to Br atoms and then recombined to form $Br_2(g)$, but since the net reaction is the same, the change in enthalpy will always be the same.

    $$
    \begin{array}{lll}
    Br_2\,(\ell) & \rightarrow 2\ Br\,(g) & \Delta H_1 \\
    2\ Br\,(g) & \rightarrow Br_2\,(g) & \Delta H_2 \\
    \hline
    Br_2\,(\ell) & \rightarrow Br_2\,(g) & \Delta H = \Delta H_1 + \Delta H_2 = 31 \text{ kJ}
    \end{array}
    $$

    Example: Given the following thermochemical equations,

    a) $C_3H_8\,(g) + 5\ O_2\,(g) \rightarrow 3\ CO_2\,(g) + 4\ H_2O\,(\ell)$ $\Delta H_a = -2220.1$ kJ
    b) $C\,(graphite) + O_2\,(g) \rightarrow CO_2\,(g)$ $\Delta H_b = -393.5$ kJ
    c) $H_2\,(g) + 1/2\ O_2\,(g) \rightarrow H_2O\,(\ell)$ $\Delta H_c = -285.8$ kJ

    calculate ΔH for this reaction:

    d) $3\ C\,(graphite) + 4\ H_2\,(g) \rightarrow C_3H_8\,(g)$

    Solution: Equations a, b, and c must be combined to obtain equation d. Since equation d contains only C, H_2, and C_3H_8, we must eliminate O_2, CO_2, and H_2O from the first three equations. Equation a is reversed to get C_3H_8 on the product side.

DAT Synopsis

The various ΔH's used in calculations need not be for actual, measurable processes. Often, values such as those found in tables of heats of formation have been calculated via Hess's Law and can now be used for further calculations.

---

e) $3\ CO_2 + (g) + 4\ H_2O + (\ell) \rightarrow C_3H_8\ (g) + 5\ O_2\ (g)$ $\Delta H_e = 2220.1$ kJ

Next, equation b is multiplied by 3 (this gives equation f) and c by 4 (this gives equation g). The following addition is done to obtain the required equation d: 3b + 4c + e.

f) $3\ CO_2\ (g) + 4\ H_2O\ (\ell) \rightarrow C_3H_8\ (g) + 5\ O_2$ $\qquad \Delta H_e = 2220.1$ kJ

g) $3 \times [C\ (graphite) + O_2\ (g) \rightarrow CO_2\ (g)]$ $\qquad \Delta H_f = 3 \times -393.5$ kJ

h) $4 \times [H_2\ (g) + \dfrac{1}{2}O_2\ (g) \rightarrow H_2O\ (\ell)]$ $\qquad \Delta H_g = 4 \times -285.8$ kJ

$\overline{3\ C\ (graphite) + 4\ H_2\ (g) \rightarrow C_3H_8\ (g)}$ $\qquad \Delta H_d = -103.6$ kJ

where $\Delta H_d = \Delta H_e + \Delta H_f + \Delta H_g$.

It is important to note that the reverse of any reaction has an enthalpy of the same magnitude as that of the forward reaction, but its sign is opposite.

4. **Bond Dissociation Energy**

Heats of reaction are related to changes in energy associated with the breakdown and formation of chemical bonds. **Bond energy,** or **bond dissociation energy,** is an average of the energy required to break a particular type of bond in one mole of gaseous molecules. It is tabulated as the positive value of the energy absorbed as the bonds are broken. For example:

$$H_2\ (g) \rightarrow 2H\ (g) \qquad \Delta H = 436\ kJ$$

A molecule of H_2 gas is cleaved to produce two gaseous, unassociated hydrogen atoms. For each mole of H_2 gas cleaved, roughly 436 kJ of energy is absorbed by the system. The reaction is therefore endothermic. For bonds found in other than diatomic molecules, many compounds have been measured and the energy requirements averaged. For example, the C–H bond dissociation energy one would find in a table (415 kJ/mol) was compiled from measurements on thousands of different organic compounds. (See the Organic Chemistry section.)

Bond energies can be used to estimate enthalpies of reactions. The enthalpy change of a reaction is given by

ΔH_{rxn} = (ΔH of bonds broken) + (ΔH of bonds formed)

= total energy input – total energy released

Example: Calculate the enthalpy change for the following reaction:

$$C\ (s) + 2\ H_2\ (g) \rightarrow CH_4\ (g) \qquad \Delta H = ?$$

> ## DAT Synopsis
>
> Since it takes energy to pull two atoms apart, bond breakage is always endothermic. Bond formation is the reverse process and, thus, must always be exothermic.

Bond dissociation energies of H–H and C–H bonds are 436 kJ/mol and 415 kJ/mol, respectively. ΔH_f of C (g) = 715 kJ/mol.

Solution: CH_4 is formed from free elements in their standard states (C in solid and H_2 in gaseous state).

Thus here, $\Delta H_{rxn} = \Delta H_f$.

The reaction can be written as three steps:

a) C (s) → C (g) ΔH_1

b) 2 [H_2 (g) → 2 H (g)] $2\Delta H_2$

c) C (g) + 4 H (g) → CH_4 (g) ΔH_3

and $\Delta H_f = [\Delta H_1 + 2\Delta H_2] + [\Delta H_3]$.

$$\Delta H_1 \quad = \quad \Delta H_f\,C(g) = 715 \text{ kJ/mol}$$

ΔH_2 is the energy required to break the H–H bond of one mole of H_2,

so

$$\Delta H_2 \quad = \quad \text{bond energy of } H_2$$
$$= \quad 436 \text{ kJ/mol}$$

ΔH_3 is the energy released when 4 C–H bonds are formed,

so

$$\Delta H_3 \quad = \quad -(4 \times \text{bond energy of C–H})$$
$$= \quad -(4 \times 415 \text{ kJ/mol})$$
$$= \quad -1{,}660 \text{ kJ/mol}$$

[**Note:** Since energy is released when bonds are formed, ΔH_3 is negative.]

Therefore:

$$\Delta H_{rxn} = \Delta H_f \quad = [715 + 2(436)] - (1{,}660) \text{ kJ/mol}$$
$$= -73 \text{ kJ/mol}$$

5. **Heats of Combustion**

   One more type of standard enthalpy change that is often used is the standard heat of combustion, $\Delta H°_{comb}$. As stated earlier, a requirement for relatively easy measurement of ΔH is that the reaction be fast and spontaneous; combustion generally fits this description. The reactions used in the C_3H_8 (g) example above were combustion reactions, and the corresponding values ΔH_a, ΔH_b, and ΔH_c were thus heats of combustion.

B. ENTROPY

Entropy (*S*) is a measure of the disorder, or randomness, of a system. The units of entropy are energy/temperature, commonly J/K or cal/K. The greater the order in a system, the lower the entropy; the greater the disorder or randomness, the higher the entropy. At any given temperature, a solid will have lower entropy than a gas, because individual molecules in the gaseous state are moving randomly, while individual molecules in a solid are constrained in place. Entropy is a state function, so a change in entropy depends only on the initial and final states:

$$\Delta S = S_{final} - S_{initial}$$

A change in entropy is also given by

$$\Delta S = \frac{q_{rev}}{T}$$

where q_{rev} is the heat added to the system undergoing a reversible process (a process that proceeds with infinitesimal changes in the system's conditions) and *T* is the absolute temperature.

A standard entropy change for a reaction, $\Delta S°$, is calculated using the standard entropies of reactants and products:

$$\Delta S°_{rxn} = (\text{sum of } S°_{products}) - (\text{sum of } S°_{reactants})$$

The second law of thermodynamics states that all spontaneous processes proceed such that the entropy of the system plus its surroundings (i.e., the entropy of the universe) increases:

$$\Delta S_{universe} = \Delta S_{system} + \Delta S_{surroundings} > 0$$

A system reaches its maximum entropy at **equilibrium,** a state in which no observable change takes place as time goes on. For a reversible process, $\Delta S_{universe}$ is zero:

$$\Delta S_{universe} = \Delta S_{system} + \Delta S_{surroundings} = 0$$

A system will spontaneously tend towards an equilibrium state if left alone.

C. GIBBS FREE ENERGY

1. Spontaneity of Reaction

The thermodynamic state function, **G** (known as the **Gibbs free energy**), combines the two factors that affect the spontaneity of a reaction—changes in enthalpy, ΔH, and changes in entropy, ΔS. The change in the free energy of a system, ΔG, represents the maximum amount of energy released by a process, occurring at constant temperature and pressure, that is available to perform useful work. ΔG is defined by this equation:

$$\Delta G = \Delta H - T\Delta S$$

where T is the absolute temperature and $T\Delta S$ represents the total amount of heat absorbed by a system when its entropy increases reversibly.

In the equilibrium state, free energy is at a minimum. A process can occur spontaneously if the Gibbs function decreases (i.e., $\Delta G < 0$).

1. If ΔG is negative, the reaction is spontaneous.

2. If ΔG is positive, the reaction is not spontaneous.

3. If ΔG is zero, the system is in a state of equilibrium;

   thus, $\Delta G = 0$ and $\Delta H = T\Delta S$.

Because the temperature is always positive (i.e., in Kelvins), the effects of the signs of ΔH and ΔS and the effect of temperature on spontaneity can be summarized as follows:

ΔH	ΔS	Outcome
−	+	spontaneous at all temperatures
+	−	nonspontaneous at all temperatures
+	+	spontaneous only at high temperatures
−	−	spontaneous only at low temperatures

It is very important to note that the **rate** of a reaction depends on the **activation energy**, not the ΔG.

2. **Standard Free Energy**

Standard free energy, $\Delta G°$, is defined as the ΔG of a process occurring at 25°C and 1 atm pressure, and for which the concentrations of any solutions involved are 1 M. The standard free energy of formation of a compound, $\Delta G°_f$, is the free-energy change that occurs when 1 mol of a compound in its standard state is formed from its elements in their standard states under standard conditions. The standard free energy of formation of any element in its most stable form (and, therefore, its standard state) is zero. The standard free energy of a reaction, $\Delta G°_{rxn}$, is the free energy change that occurs when that reaction is carried out under standard state conditions (i.e., when the reactants in their standard states are converted to the products in their standard states, at standard conditions of T and P). For example: Conversion of C(*diamond*) to C(*graphite*) is spontaneous under standard conditions. However, its rate is so slow that the rxn is never observed.

$$\Delta G°_{rxn} = \text{(sum of } \Delta G°_f \text{ of products)} - \text{(sum of } \Delta G°_f \text{ of reactants)}$$

DAT Synopsis

For any given nonspontaneous reaction or process, the reverse reaction or process will be spontaneous.

DAT Synopsis

Recall that thermodynamics and kinetics are separate topic areas. In thermodynamics, *spontaneous* does not necessarily mean *instantaneous*.

DAT Synopsis

Note the similarity of this equation to Hess's Law. Almost any state function could be substituted for ΔG here.

3. **Reaction Quotient**

$\Delta G°_{rxn}$ can also be derived from the equilibrium constant for the equation:

$$\Delta G° = -RT \ln K_{eq}$$

where K_{eq} is the equilibrium constant, R is the gas constant, and T is the temperature in K.

Once a reaction commences, however, the standard state conditions no longer hold. K_{eq} must be replaced by another parameter, the *reaction quotient* (**Q**). For the reaction $a \text{ A} + b \text{ B} \rightleftharpoons c \text{ C} + d \text{ D}$,

$$Q = \frac{[C]^c \, [D]^d}{[A]^a \, [B]^b}$$

Likewise, ΔG must be used in place of $\Delta G°$. The relationship between the two is as follows:

$$\Delta G = \Delta G° + RT \ln Q$$

where R is the gas constant and T is the temperature in K.

4. **Examples**
   a. **Vaporization of water at one atmosphere pressure**

$$H_2O \, (\ell) + \text{heat} \rightarrow H_2O \, (g)$$

When water boils, hydrogen bonds (H-bonds) are broken. Energy is absorbed (the reaction is endothermic), and thus ΔH is positive. Entropy increases as the closely packed molecules of the liquid become the more randomly moving molecules of a gas; thus, $T\Delta S$ is also positive. Since ΔH and $T\Delta S$ are each positive, the reaction will proceed spontaneously only if $T\Delta S > \Delta H$. This is true only at temperatures above 100°C. Below 100°C, ΔG is positive, and the water remains a liquid. At 100°C, $\Delta H = T\Delta S$ and $\Delta G = 0$: An equilibrium is established between water and water vapor. The opposite is true when water vapor condenses. H-bonds are formed, and energy is released; the reaction is exothermic (ΔH is negative) and entropy decreases, since a liquid is forming from a gas ($T\Delta S$ is negative). Condensation will be spontaneous only if $\Delta H < T\Delta S$. This is the case at temperatures below 100°C. Above 100°C, $T\Delta S$ is more negative than H, ΔG is positive, and condensation is not spontaneous. Again, at 100°C, an equilibrium is established.

DAT Synopsis

This all makes good sense since you know that 100°C is the boiling point of water.

b. The combustion of C_6H_6 (benzene)

$$2\ C_6H_6\ (\ell) + 15\ O_2\ (g) \rightarrow 12\ CO_2\ (g) + 6\ H_2O\ (g) + \text{heat}$$

In this case, heat is released (ΔH is negative) as the benzene burns and the entropy is increased ($T\Delta S$ is positive), because two gases (18 moles total) have greater entropy than a gas and a liquid (15 moles gas and 2 liquid). ΔG is negative, and the reaction is spontaneous.

THE GAS PHASE

Matter can exist in three different physical forms, called **phases** or **states: gas, liquid,** and **solid.** Liquids and solids will be discussed in chapter 8.

The gaseous phase, the subject of this chapter, is the simplest to understand, since all gases display similar behavior and follow similar laws regardless of their identity. The atoms or molecules in a gaseous sample move rapidly and are far apart from each other. In addition, only very weak intermolecular forces exist between gas particles; this results in certain characteristic physical properties, such as the ability to expand to fill any volume and to take on the shape of a container. Furthermore, gases are easily, though not infinitely, compressible.

The state of a gaseous sample is generally defined by four variables: pressure (P), volume (V), temperature (T), and number of moles (n). Gas pressures are usually expressed in units of atmospheres (atm) or millimeters of mercury (mm Hg or torr), which are related as follows:

$$1 \text{ atm} = 760 \text{ mm Hg} = 760 \text{ torr}$$

Volume is generally expressed in liters (L) or milliliters (mL). The temperature of a gas is usually given in Kelvin (K, *not* °K). Gases are often discussed in terms of **standard temperature and pressure (STP),** which refers to conditions of 273.15 K (0°C) and 1 atm.

Note: It is important not to confuse **STP** with **standard conditions**—the two standards involve different temperatures and are used for different purposes. STP (0°C or 273 K) is generally used for gas law calculations; standard conditions (25°C or 298 K) is used when measuring standard enthalpy, entropy, Gibbs free energy, and voltage.

IDEAL GASES

When examining the behavior of gases under varying conditions of temperature and pressure, scientists speak of ideal gases. An ideal gas represents a hypothetical gas whose molecules have no intermolecular forces and occupy no volume. Although gases actually deviate from this idealized behavior, at relatively low pressures (atmospheric pressure) and high temperatures, many gases behave in a nearly ideal fashion. Therefore, the assumptions used for ideal gases can be applied to real gases with reasonable accuracy.

A. BOYLE'S LAW

Experimental studies performed by Robert Boyle in 1660 led to the formulation of Boyle's Law. His work showed that for a given gaseous sample held at constant temperature (isothermal conditions), the volume of the gas is inversely proportional to its pressure:

$$PV = k \text{ or } P_1V_1 = P_2V_2$$

where k is a proportionality constant and the subscripts 1 and 2 represent two different sets of conditions. A plot of pressure versus volume for a gas is shown in Figure 7.1.

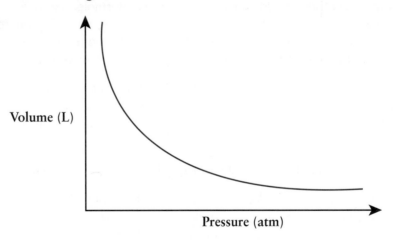

Figure 7.1

Example: Under isothermal conditions, what would be the volume of a 1 L sample of helium after its pressure is changed from 12 atm to 4 atm?

Solution:

$$P_1 = 12 \text{ atm} \qquad P_2 = 4 \text{ atm}$$

$$V_1 = 1 \text{ L} \qquad V_2 = x$$

$$P_1V_1 = P_2V_2$$

$$12 \text{ atm } (1 \text{ L}) = 4 \text{ atm } (x)$$

$$\frac{12}{4}\text{L} = x$$

$$x = 3 \text{ L}$$

B. LAW OF CHARLES AND GAY-LUSSAC

The Law of Charles and Gay-Lussac, or simply Charles' Law, was developed during the early 19th century. The law states that at constant pressure, the volume of a gas is directly proportional to its absolute temperature. The absolute temperature is the temperature expressed in Kelvin, which can be calculated from the expression $T_K = T_{°C} + 273.15$.

$$\frac{V}{T} = k \ \text{ or } \ \frac{V_1}{T_1} = \frac{V_2}{T_2}$$

where k is a constant and the subscripts 1 and 2 represent two different sets of conditions. A plot of temperature versus volume is shown in Figure 7.2.

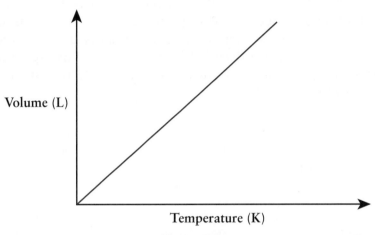

Figure 7.2

> **DAT Synopsis**
>
> While the temperature of 0 K cannot be physically attained, curves such as this one were originally used to figure out its location.

Example: If the absolute temperature of 2 L of gas at constant pressure is changed from 283.15 K to 566.30 K, what would be the final volume?

Solution: $T_1 = 283.15$ K $V_1 = 2$ L

$T_2 = 566.30$ K $V_2 = x$

$$\frac{V_1}{T_1} = \frac{V_2}{T_2}$$

$$\frac{2 \text{ L}}{283.15 \text{ K}} = \frac{x}{566.30 \text{ K}}$$

$$x = \frac{2 \text{ L}(566.30 \text{ K})}{283.15 \text{K}}$$

$$x = 4 \text{ L}$$

C. AVOGADRO'S PRINCIPLE

In 1811, Amedeo Avogadro proposed that for all gases at a constant temperature and pressure, the volume of the gas will be directly proportional to the number of moles of gas present; therefore, all gases have the same number of moles in the same volume.

$$\frac{n}{V} = k \text{ or } \frac{n_1}{V_1} = \frac{n_2}{V_2}$$

The subscripts 1 and 2 once again apply to two different sets of conditions with the same temperature and pressure.

D. IDEAL GAS LAW

The ideal gas law combines the relationships outlined in Boyle's Law, Charles' Law, and Avogadro's Principle to yield an expression that can be used to predict the behavior of a gas. The ideal gas law shows the relationship among four variables that define a sample of gas—pressure (P), volume (V), temperature (T), and number of moles (n)—and is represented by the equation

$$PV = nRT$$

The constant R is known as the **gas constant.** Under STP conditions (273.15 K and 1 atmosphere), 1 mole of gas was shown to have a volume of 22.4 L. Substituting these values into the ideal gas equation gave R = 8.21×10^{-2} L • atm/(mol • K).

The gas constant may be expressed in many other units: Another common value is 8.314 J/(K • mol), which is derived when SI units of pascals (for pressure) and cubic meters (for volume) are substituted into the ideal gas law. **When carrying out calculations based on the ideal gas law, it is important to choose a value of R that matches the units of the variables.**

Example: What volume would 12 g of helium occupy at 20°C and a pressure of 380 mm Hg?

Solution: The ideal gas law can be used, but first, all of the variables must be converted to yield units that will correspond to the expression of the gas constant as 0.0821 L • atm/(mol • K).

$$P = 380 \text{ mm Hg} \times \frac{1 \text{ atm}}{760 \text{ mm Hg}} = 0.5 \text{ atm}$$

$$T = 20°C + 273.15 = 293.15 \text{ K}$$

$$n = 12 \text{ g He} \times \frac{1 \text{ mol He}}{4.0 \text{ g}} = 3 \text{ mol He}$$

Substitute to the ideal gas equation:

$PV = nRT$

$(0.5 \text{ atm})(V) = (3 \text{ mol})(0.0821 \text{ L} \bullet \text{atm}/(\text{mol} \bullet \text{K})(293.15 \text{ K})$

$V = 144.4 \text{ L}$

In addition to standard calculations to determine the pressure, volume, or temperature of a gas, the ideal gas law may be used to determine the **density** and molar mass of the gas.

1. **Density**

   Density is defined as the mass per unit volume of a substance and, for gases, is usually expressed in units of g/L. By rearrangement, the ideal gas equation can be used to calculate the density of a gas.

   $$PV = nRT$$

   where $\quad n = \dfrac{m}{MM} \quad \dfrac{\text{(mass in g)}}{\text{(molar mass)}}$

   therefore $\quad PV = \dfrac{m}{MM} RT$

   and $\quad d = \dfrac{m}{V} \quad \dfrac{P(MM)}{RT}$

> **DAT Synopsis**
>
> For a point of comparison, you can quickly calculate the density of a simple gas at STP. For example, helium (4.0 g/mol divided by 22.4 L/mol) has a density of about 0.2 g/L, while carbon dioxide (44 g/mol over 22.4 L/mol) is about 2 g/L.

Another way to find the density of a gas is to start with the volume of a mole of gas at STP, 22.4 L; calculate the effect of pressure and temperature on the volume; and finally calculate the density by dividing the mass by the new volume. The following equation, derived from Boyle's and Charles' Laws, is used to relate changes in the temperature, volume, and pressure of a gas:

$$\frac{P_1 V_1}{T_1} = \frac{P_2 V_2}{T_2}$$

where the subscripts 1 and 2 refer to the two states of the gas (at STP and under the actual conditions). To calculate a change in volume, the equation is rearranged as follows:

$$V_2 = V_1 \left(\frac{P_1}{P_2} \right) \left(\frac{T_2}{T_1} \right)$$

V_2 is then used to find the density of the gas under nonstandard conditions.

$$d = \frac{m}{V_2}$$

If you *visualize* how the changes in pressure and temperature affect the volume of the gas, this can serve as a check to be sure you have not accidentally confused the pressure or temperature value that belongs in the numerator with the one that belongs in the denominator.

Example: What is the density of HCl gas at 2 atm and 45°C?

Solution: At STP, a mole of gas occupies 22.4 liters. Since the increase in pressure to 2 atm decreases volume, 22.4 L must be multiplied by $\left(\dfrac{1\,\text{atm}}{2\,\text{atm}}\right)$. And since the increase in temperature increases volume, the temperature factor will be $\left(\dfrac{318\,\text{K}}{273\,\text{K}}\right)$.

$$V_2 = \left(\frac{22.4\,\text{L}}{\text{mol}}\right)\left(\frac{1\,\text{atm}}{2\,\text{atm}}\right)\left(\frac{318\,\text{K}}{273\,\text{K}}\right) = \frac{13.0\,\text{L}}{\text{mol}}$$

$$d = \left(\frac{36\,\text{g/mol}}{13.0\,\text{L/mol}}\right) = 2.77\,\text{g/L}$$

2. **Molar Mass**

Sometimes the identity of a gas is unknown, and the molar mass (see "Molecules and Moles" in chapter 4) must be determined in order to identify it. Using the equation for density derived from the ideal gas law, the molar mass of a gas can be determined experimentally as follows. The pressure and temperature of a gas contained in a bulb of a given volume are measured, and the weight of the bulb plus sample is found. Then, the bulb is evacuated, and the empty bulb is weighed. The weight of the bulb plus sample minus the weight of the bulb yields the weight of the sample. Finally, the density of the sample is determined by dividing the weight of the sample by the volume of the bulb. The density at STP is calculated. The molecular weight is then found by multiplying the number of grams per liter by 22.4 liters per mole.

Example: What is the molar mass of a 2 L sample of gas that weighs 8 g at a temperature of 15°C and a pressure of 1.5 atm?

$$d = \frac{8\,\text{g}}{2\,\text{L}} \quad \text{at 15°C and 1.5 atm}$$

$$V_{STP} = (2\,\text{L})\left(\frac{273\,\text{K}}{288\,\text{K}}\right)\left(\frac{1.5\,\text{atm}}{1\,\text{atm}}\right) = 2.84\,\text{L}$$

$$\frac{8\,\text{g}}{2.84\,\text{L}} = 2.82\,\text{g/L at STP}$$

$$\left(\frac{2.82\,\text{g}}{\text{L}}\right)\left(\frac{22.4\,\text{L}}{\text{mol}}\right) = 63.2\,\text{g/mol}$$

REAL GASES

In general, the ideal gas law is a good approximation of the behavior of real gases, but all real gases deviate from ideal gas behavior to some extent, particularly when the gas atoms or molecules are forced into close proximity under high pressure and at low temperature so that molecular volume and intermolecular attractions become significant.

A. DEVIATIONS DUE TO PRESSURE

As the pressure of a gas increases, the particles are pushed closer and closer together. As the condensation pressure for a given temperature is approached, intermolecular attraction forces become more and more significant until the gas condenses into the liquid state (see "Phase Equilibria" in chapter 8).

At moderately high pressure (a few hundred atmospheres), a gas's volume is less than would be predicted by the ideal gas law due to intermolecular attraction. At extremely high pressure, the size of the particles becomes relatively large compared to the distance between them, and this causes the gas to take up a larger volume than would be predicted by the ideal gas law.

B. DEVIATIONS DUE TO TEMPERATURE

As the temperature of a gas is decreased, the average velocity of the gas molecules decreases, and the attractive intermolecular forces become increasingly significant. As the condensation temperature is approached for a given pressure, intermolecular attractions eventually cause the gas to condense to a liquid state (see "Phase Equilibria" in Chapter 8).

As the temperature of a gas is reduced towards its condensation point (which is the same as its boiling point), intermolecular attraction causes the gas to have a smaller volume than would be predicted by the ideal gas law. The closer the temperature of a gas is to its boiling point, the less ideal is its behavior.

DALTON'S LAW OF PARTIAL PRESSURES

When two or more gases are found in one vessel without chemical interaction, each gas will behave independently of the other(s). Therefore, the pressure exerted by each gas in the mixture will be equal to the pressure that gas would exert if it were the only one in the container. The pressure exerted by each individual gas is called the **partial pressure** of that gas. In 1801, John Dalton derived an expression, now known as **Dalton's Law of Partial Pressures**, which states that the total pressure of a gaseous mixture is equal to the sum of the partial pressures of the individual components. The equation is

$$P_T = P_A + P_B + P_C + \dots$$

The partial pressure of a gas is related to its mole fraction and can be determined using the following equations:

$$P_A = P_T x_A$$

where
$$x_A = \frac{n_A}{n_T} \left(\frac{\text{moles of A}}{\text{total moles}} \right)$$

Example: A vessel contains 0.75 mol of nitrogen, 0.20 mol of hydrogen, and 0.05 mol of fluorine at a total pressure of 2.5 atm. What is the partial pressure of each gas?

First calculate the mole fraction of each gas.

$$x_{N_2} = \frac{0.75 \text{ mol}}{1.0 \text{ mol}} = 0.75 \quad x_{H_2} = \frac{0.20 \text{ mol}}{1.0 \text{ mol}} = 0.20 \quad x_{F_2} = \frac{0.05 \text{ mol}}{1.0 \text{ mol}} = 0.05$$

Then calculate the partial pressure.

$$P_A = x_A P_T$$

$$P_{N_2} = (2.5 \text{ atm})(0.75) \qquad P_{H_2} = (2.5 \text{ atm})(0.20) \qquad P_{F_2} = (2.5 \text{ atm})(0.05)$$
$$= 1.875 \text{ atm} \qquad\qquad = 0.5 \text{ atm} \qquad\qquad = 0.125 \text{ atm}$$

KINETIC MOLECULAR THEORY OF GASES

As indicated by the gas laws, all gases show similar physical characteristics and behavior. A theoretical model to explain the behavior of gases was developed during the second half of the 19th century. The combined efforts of Boltzmann, Maxwell, and others led to a simple explanation of gaseous molecular behavior based on the motion of individual molecules. This model is called the **Kinetic Molecular Theory of Gases.** Like the gas laws, this theory was developed in reference to ideal gases, although it can be applied with reasonable accuracy to real gases as well.

A. ASSUMPTIONS OF THE KINETIC MOLECULAR THEORY

1. Gases are made up of particles whose volumes are negligible compared to the container volume.
2. Gas atoms or molecules exhibit no intermolecular attractions or repulsions.
3. Gas particles are in continuous, random motion, undergoing collisions with other particles and the container walls.
4. Collisions between any two gas particles are elastic, meaning that there is no overall gain or loss of energy.
5. The average kinetic energy of gas particles is proportional to the absolute temperature of the gas, and it is the same for all gases at a given temperature.

B. APPLICATIONS OF THE KINETIC MOLECULAR THEORY OF GASES

1. Average Molecular Speeds

According to the kinetic molecular theory of gases, the average kinetic energy of a gas particle is proportional to the absolute temperature of the gas:

$$KE = \frac{1}{2}\,mv^2 = \frac{3}{2}\,kT$$

where k is the Boltzmann constant. The typical speed of a gas molecule is proportional to the square root of the absolute temperature.

A **Maxwell-Boltzmann distribution curve** shows the distribution of speeds of gas particles at a given temperature. Figure 7.3 shows a distribution curve of molecular speeds at two temperatures, T_1 and T_2, where $T_2 > T_1$. Notice that the bell-shaped curve flattens and shifts to the right as the temperature increases, indicating that at higher temperatures, more molecules are moving at high speeds.

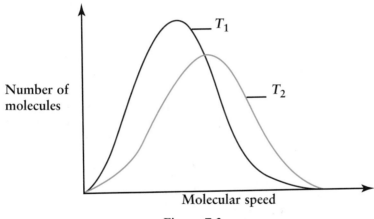

Figure 7.3

> **DAT Synopsis**
>
> Like kinetic energy, the average molecular speed is constant at a given temperature.

Real-World Analogy

Isotopic Enhancement: one common application of Graham's Law is in the separation of isotopes (chapter 1), and an example is the enrichment of uranium for nuclear reactors. Isotopes cannot be separated by normal chemical means, since they differ only in their masses and in their nuclear behavior.

Most of the naturally occurring atoms of uranium are uranium-238, while a few are the uranium-235 isotopes used as the fuel of nuclear fission reactors. Uranium reacts with molecular fluorine under the proper conditions to form gaseous uranium(VI) fluoride, $UF_6(g)$. If a large sample of $UF_6(g)$ is allowed to effuse partially into an evacuated container, the lighter molecules, $^{235}UF_6(g)$, will effuse faster, and the sample collected in the second container will thus contain a higher percentage of the U-235 isotope, while the sample remaining in the original container will contain a higher percentage of the $^{238}UF_6(g)$. The small difference in the masses of $^{235}UF_6(g)$ and $^{238}UF_6(g)$ makes for a small difference in the rates of effusion. Therefore, the procedure described above must be repeated many times before the collected $^{235}UF_6(g)$ can be reduced (see chapter 11) to metallic U-235 in sufficient isotopic purity to be used as a nuclear fuel.

2. Graham's Law of Diffusion and Effusion

a. Diffusion

Diffusion occurs when gas molecules diffuse through a mixture. Diffusion accounts for the fact that an open bottle of perfume can quickly be smelled across a room. The kinetic molecular theory of gases predicted that heavier gas molecules diffuse more slowly than lighter ones because of their differing average speeds. In 1832, Thomas Graham showed mathematically that under isothermal and isobaric conditions, the rates at which two gases diffuse are inversely proportional to the square root of their molar masses. Thus,

$$\frac{r_1}{r_2} = \left(\frac{MM_2}{MM_1}\right)^{\frac{1}{2}} = \sqrt{\frac{MM_2}{MM_1}}$$

where r_1 and MM_1 represent the diffusion rate and molar mass of gas 1 and r_2 and MM_2 represent the diffusion rate and molar mass of gas 2.

b. Effusion

Effusion is the flow of gas particles under pressure from one compartment to another through a small opening. Graham used the kinetic molecular theory of gases to show that for two gases at the same temperature, the rates of effusion are proportional to the average speeds. He then expressed the rates of effusion in terms of molar mass and found that the relationship is the same as that for diffusion:

$$\frac{r_1}{r_2} = \left(\frac{MM_2}{MM_1}\right)^{\frac{1}{2}}$$

PHASES AND PHASE CHANGES

When the attractive forces between molecules (i.e., van der Waals forces) overcome the kinetic energy that keeps them apart, the molecules move closer together such that they can no longer move about freely, entering the **liquid** or **solid** phase. Because of their smaller volume relative to gases, liquids and solids are often referred to as the **condensed phases**.

LIQUIDS

In a liquid, atoms or molecules are held close together with little space between them. As a result, liquids have definite volumes and cannot easily be expanded or compressed. However, the molecules can still move around and are in a state of relative disorder. Consequently, the liquid can change shape to fit its container, and its molecules are able to **diffuse** and **evaporate**.

One of the most important properties of liquids is their ability to mix, both with each other and with other phases, to form **solutions** (see chapter 9). The degree to which two liquids can mix is called their **miscibility**. Oil and water are almost completely **immiscible;** that is, their molecules tend to repel each other due to their polarity difference. Oil and water normally form separate layers when mixed, with oil on top because it is less dense. Under extreme conditions, such as violent shaking, two immiscible liquids can form a fairly homogeneous mixture called an **emulsion.** Although they look like solutions, emulsions are actually mixtures of discrete particles too small to be seen distinctly.

SOLIDS

In a solid, the attractive forces between atoms, ions, or molecules are strong enough to hold them rigidly together; thus, the particles' only motion is vibration about fixed positions, and the kinetic energy of solids is predominantly vibrational energy. As a result, solids have definite shapes and volumes.

A solid may be **crystalline** or **amorphous**. A crystalline solid, such as NaCl, possesses an ordered structure; its atoms exist in a specific, three-dimensional geometric arrangement with repeating patterns of atoms, ions, or molecules. An amorphous solid, such as glass, has no ordered three-dimensional arrangement, although the molecules are also fixed in place.

Most solids are crystalline in structure. The two most common forms of crystals are **metallic** and **ionic** crystals.

Ionic solids are aggregates of positively and negatively charged ions; there are no discrete molecules. The physical properties of ionic solids include high melting points, high boiling points, and poor electrical conductivity in the solid phase. These properties are due to the compounds' strong electrostatic interactions, which also cause the ions to be relatively immobile. Ionic structures are given by empirical formulas that describe the ratio of atoms in the lowest possible whole numbers. For example, the empirical formula $BaCl_2$ gives the ratio of barium to chloride within the crystal.

Metallic solids consist of metal atoms packed together as closely as possible. Metallic solids have high melting and boiling points as a result of their strong covalent attractions. Pure metallic structures (consisting of a single element) are usually described as layers of spheres of roughly similar radii.

The repeating units of crystals (both ionic and metallic) are represented by **unit cells.** There are many types of unit cells. We will now consider only the three cubic unit cells: **simple cubic, body-centered cubic,** and **face-centered cubic** (see Figure 8.1).

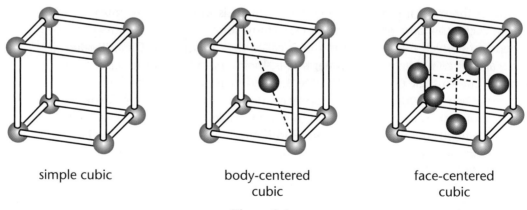

simple cubic   body-centered   face-centered
                             cubic   cubic

Figure 8.1

Atoms are represented as points but are actually adjoining spheres (see Figure 8.2). Each unit cell is surrounded by similar units. In the ionic unit cell, the spaces between points (anions) are filled with other ions (cations).

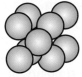

simple cubic

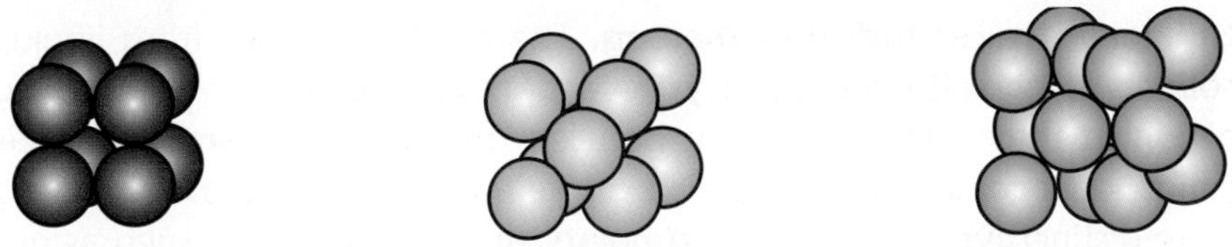

body-centered cubic

face-centered cubic

Figure 8.2

PHASE EQUILIBRIA

In an isolated system, phase changes (solid to liquid to gas) are reversible, and an equilibrium exists between phases. For example, at 1 atm and 0°C in an isolated system, an ice cube floating in water is in equilibrium. Some of the ice may absorb heat and melt, but an equal amount of water will release heat and freeze. Thus, the relative amounts of ice and water remain constant.

A. GAS-LIQUID EQUILIBRIUM

The temperature of a liquid is related to the average kinetic energy of the liquid molecules; however, the kinetic energy of the molecules will vary. A few molecules near the surface of the liquid may have enough energy to leave the liquid phase and escape into the gaseous phase. This process is known as **evaporation** (or **vaporization**). Each time the liquid loses a high-energy particle, the temperature of the remaining liquid decreases; thus, evaporation is a cooling process. Given enough kinetic energy, the liquid will completely evaporate.

If a cover is placed on a beaker of liquid, the escaping molecules are trapped above the solution. These molecules exert a countering pressure, which forces some of the gas back into the liquid phase; this process is called **condensation.** Atmospheric pressure acts on a liquid in a similar fashion as a solid lid. As evaporation and condensation proceed, an equilibrium is reached in which the rates of the two processes become equal. Once this equilibrium is reached, the pressure that the gas exerts over the liquid is called the **vapor pressure** of the liquid. Vapor pressure increases as temperature increases, since more molecules have sufficient kinetic energy to escape into the gas phase. The temperature at which the vapor pressure of the liquid equals the external pressure is called the **boiling point.**

B. LIQUID-SOLID EQUILIBRIUM

The liquid and solid phases can also coexist in equilibrium (e.g., the ice-water mixture discussed above). Even though the atoms or molecules of a solid are confined to definite locations, each atom or molecule can undergo motions about some equilibrium position. These motions (vibrations) increase when heat is applied. If atoms or molecules in the solid phase absorb enough energy in this fashion, the solid's three-dimensional structure breaks down, and the liquid phase begins. The transition from solid to liquid is called **fusion** or **melting.** The reverse process, from liquid to solid, is called **solidification, crystallization,** or **freezing.** The temperature at which these processes occur is called the **melting point** or **freezing point,** depending on the direction of the transition. Whereas pure crystals have distinct, very sharp melting points, amorphous solids, such as glass, tend to melt over a larger range of temperatures due to their less-ordered molecular distribution.

C. GAS-SOLID EQUILIBRIUM

A third type of phase equilibrium is that between a gas and a solid. When a solid goes directly into the gas phase, the process is called **sublimation.** Dry ice (solid CO_2) sublimes; the absence of the liquid phase makes it a convenient refrigerant. The reverse transition, from the gaseous to the solid phase, is called **deposition.**

D. THE GIBBS FUNCTION

The thermodynamic criterion for each of the above equilibria is that the change in Gibbs free energy must equal zero; $\Delta G = 0$. For an equilibrium between a gas and a solid,

$$\Delta G = \ G(g) - G(s),$$
$$\text{so } G(g) = \ G(s) \text{ at equilibrium.}$$

The same is true of the Gibbs functions for the other two equilibria.

PHASE DIAGRAMS
A. SINGLE COMPONENT

A standard **phase diagram** depicts the phases and phase equilibria of a substance at defined temperatures and pressures. In general, the gas phase is found at high temperature and low pressure, the solid phase is found at low temperature and high pressure, and the liquid phase is found at high temperature and high pressure. A typical phase diagram is shown in Figure 8.3.

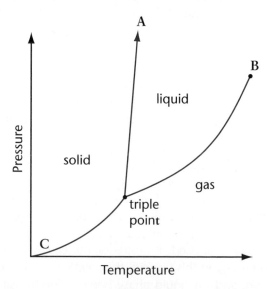

Figure 8.3

The three phases are demarcated by lines indicating the temperatures and pressures at which two phases are in equilibrium. Line A represents freezing/melting, line B evaporation/condensation, and line C sublimation/deposition. The intersection of the three lines is called the **triple point**. At this temperature and pressure, unique for a given substance, all three phases are in equilibrium. The point at B is known as the **critical point**, the temperature and pressure above which no distinction between liquid and gas is possible.

B. MULTIPLE COMPONENTS

The phase diagram for a mixture of two or more components (Figure 8.4) is complicated by the requirement that the composition of the mixture, as well as the temperature and pressure, must be specified. Consider a solution of two liquids, A and B. The vapor above the solution is a mixture of the vapors of A and B. The pressures exerted by vapor A and vapor B on the solution are the vapor pressures that each exerts above its individual liquid phase. **Raoult's Law** (described below) enables one to determine the relationship between the vapor pressure of vapor A and the concentration of liquid A in the solution.

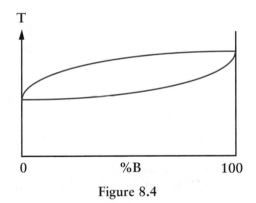

Figure 8.4

COLLIGATIVE PROPERTIES

Colligative properties are physical properties derived solely from the number of particles present, not the nature of those particles. These properties are usually associated with dilute solutions (see "Concentration" in chapter 9).

A. FREEZING-POINT DEPRESSION

Pure water (H_2O) freezes at 0°C; however, for every mole of solute particles dissolved in 1 L of water, the freezing point is lowered by 1.86°C. This is because the solute particles interfere with the process of crystal formation that occurs during freezing; the solute particles lower the temperature at which the molecules can align themselves into a crystalline structure.

The formula for calculating this **freezing-point depression** is

$$\Delta T_f = K_f m$$

where ΔT_f is the freezing-point depression, K_f is a proportionality constant characteristic of a particular solvent, and m is the molality of the solution (mol solute/kg solvent; see chapter 9). The K_f for water—which you do not need to memorize—is $1.86°Cm^{-1}$. Each solvent has its own characteristic K_f.

B. BOILING-POINT ELEVATION

A liquid boils when its vapor pressure equals the atmospheric pressure. If the vapor pressure of a solution is lower than that of the pure solvent, more energy (and consequently a higher temperature) will be required before its vapor pressure equals atmospheric pressure. The extent to which the boiling point of a solution is raised relative to that of the pure solvent is given by the following formula:

$$\Delta T_b = K_b m$$

where ΔT_b is the boiling-point elevation, K_b is a proportionality constant characteristic of a particular solvent, and m is the molality of the solution. The K_b for water is $0.51°Cm^{-1}$.

C. OSMOTIC PRESSURE

Consider a container separated into two compartments by a semipermeable membrane (which, by definition, selectively permits the passage of certain molecules). One compartment contains pure water, while the other contains water with dissolved solute. The membrane allows water but not solute to pass through. Because substances tend to flow, or **diffuse**, from higher to lower concentrations (which increases entropy), water will diffuse from the compartment containing pure water to the compartment containing the water-solute mixture. This net flow will cause the water level in the compartment containing the solution to rise above the level in the compartment containing pure water.

Because the solute cannot pass through the membrane, the concentrations of solute in the two compartments can never be equal. However, the pressure exerted by the water level in the solute-containing compartment will eventually oppose the influx of water; thus, the water level will rise only to the point at which it exerts a sufficient pressure to counterbalance the tendency of water to flow across the membrane. This pressure is defined as the **osmotic pressure (Π)** of the solution, and, it is given by this formula:

$$\Pi = MRT$$

where M is the molarity of the solution (see chapter 9), R is the ideal gas constant, and T is the temperature on the Kelvin scale. This equation clearly shows that molarity and osmotic pressure are directly proportional (i.e., as the concentration of the solution increases, the osmotic pressure also increases). Thus, the osmotic pressure depends only on the amount of solute, not its identity.

D. VAPOR-PRESSURE LOWERING (RAOULT'S LAW)

When solute B is added to pure solvent A, the vapor pressure of A above the solvent decreases (see Figure 8.4). If the vapor pressure of A above pure solvent A is designated by P°_A and the vapor pressure of A above the solution containing B is P_A, the vapor pressure decreases as follows:

$$\Delta P = P^{\circ}_A - P_A$$

In the late 1800s, the French chemist François Marie Raoult determined that this vapor pressure decrease is also equivalent to

$$\Delta P = x_B P^{\circ}_A$$

where x_B is the mole fraction of the solute B in solvent A. Since $x_B = 1 - x_A$ and $\Delta P = P^{\circ}_A - P_A$, substitution into the above equation leads to the common form of Raoult's Law:

$$P_A = x_A P^{\circ}_A$$

Similarly, the expression for the vapor pressure of the solute in solution (assuming it is volatile) is given by

$$P_B = x_B P^{\circ}_B$$

Raoult's Law holds only when the attraction between molecules of the different components of the mixture is equal to the attraction between the molecules of any one component in its pure state. When this condition does not hold, the relationship between mole fraction and vapor pressure will deviate from Raoult's Law. Solutions that obey Raoult's Law are called **ideal solutions.**

SOLUTIONS

Solutions are **homogeneous** (everywhere the same) mixtures of substances that combine to form a single phase, generally the liquid phase. Many important chemical reactions, both in the laboratory and in nature, take place in solution (including almost all reactions in living organisms).

NATURE OF SOLUTIONS

A solution consists of a **solute** (e.g., NaCl, NH$_3$, or C$_{12}$H$_{22}$O$_{11}$) dispersed (dissolved) in a **solvent** (e.g., H$_2$O or benzene). The solvent is the component of the solution whose phase remains the same after mixing. If the two substances are already in the same phase, the solvent is the component present in greater quantity. Solute molecules move about freely in the solvent and can interact with other molecules or ions; consequently, chemical reactions occur easily in solution.

A. SOLVATION

The interaction between solute and solvent molecules is known as solvation or **dissolution**; when water is the solvent, the interaction is called **hydration**, and the resulting solution is known as an **aqueous solution**. Solvation is possible when the attractive forces between solute and solvent are stronger than those between the solute particles. For example, when NaCl dissolves in water, its component ions dissociate from one another and become surrounded by water molecules. Because water is polar, ion-dipole interactions can occur between the Na$^+$ and Cl$^-$ ions and the water molecules. For nonionic solutes, solvation involves van der Waals forces between the solute and solvent molecules. The general rule is that like dissolves like; ionic and polar solutes are soluble in polar solvents, and nonpolar solutes are soluble in nonpolar solvents.

B. SOLUBILITY

The solubility of a substance is the maximum amount of that substance that can be dissolved in a particular solvent at a particular temperature. When this maximum amount of solute has been added, the solution is in equilibrium and is said to be **saturated**; if more solute is added, it will not dissolve. For example, at 18°C, a maximum of 83 g of glucose (C$_6$H$_{12}$O$_6$)

267

DAT Synopsis

Note that *dilute* is a relative term.

will dissolve in 100 mL of H_2O. Thus, the solubility of glucose is 83 g/100 mL. If more glucose is added, it will remain in solid form, precipitating to the bottom of the container. A solution in which the proportion of solute to solvent is small is said to be **dilute**, and one in which the proportion is large is said to be **concentrated**.

C. AQUEOUS SOLUTIONS

The most common class of solutions is the aqueous solutions, in which the solvent is water. The aqueous state is denoted by the symbol *aq*. In discussing the chemistry of aqueous solutions, it is useful to know how soluble various salts are in water; this information is given by the solubility rules below.

1. All salts of alkali metals are water soluble.
2. All salts of the ammonium ion (NH_4^+) are water soluble.
3. All chlorides, bromides, and iodides are water soluble, with the exceptions of Ag^+, Pb^{2+}, and Hg_2^{2+}.
4. All salts of the sulfate ion (SO_4^{2-}) are water soluble, with the exceptions of Ca^{2+}, Sr^{2+}, Ba^{2+}, and Pb^{2+}.
5. All metal oxides are insoluble, with the exception of the alkali metals and CaO, SrO, and BaO, all of which hydrolyze to form solutions of the corresponding metal hydroxides.
6. All hydroxides are insoluble, with the exception of the alkali metals and Ca^{2+}, Sr^{2+}, and Ba^{2+}.
7. All carbonates (CO_3^{2-}), phosphates (PO_4^{2-}), sulfides (S^{2-}), and sulfites (SO_3^{2-}) are insoluble, with the exception of the alkali metals and ammonium.

IONS

Ionic solutions are of particular interest to chemists because certain important types of chemical interactions—acid-base reactions and oxidation-reduction reactions, for instance—take place in ionic solutions. Ions and their properties in solution will be introduced here; the chemical reactions mentioned are discussed in detail in chapter 10, Acids and Bases, and chapter 11, Redox Reactions and Electrochemistry.

A. CATIONS AND ANIONS

Ionic compounds are made up of **cations** and **anions**, where a cation is a positive ion and an anion is a negative ion. The nomenclature of ionic compounds is based on the names of the component ions.

1. For elements (usually metals) that can form more than one positive ion, the charge is indicated by a Roman numeral in parentheses following the name of the element.

Fe^{2+} Iron (II)	Cu^+ Copper (I)
Fe^{3+} Iron (III)	Cu^{2+} Copper (II)

2. An older but still commonly used method is to add the endings **-ous** or **-ic** to the root of the Latin name of the element to represent the ions with lesser or greater charge, respectively.

Fe^{2+} Ferrous Cu^+ Cuprous
Fe^{3+} Ferric Cu^{2+} Cupric

3. Monatomic anions are named by dropping the ending of the name of the element and adding **-ide.**

H^- Hydride S^{2-} Sulfide
F^- Fluoride N^{3-} Nitride
O^{2-} Oxide P^{3-} Phosphide

4. Many polyatomic anions contain oxygen and are, therefore, called **oxyanions.** When an element forms two oxyanions, the name of the one with less oxygen ends in **-ite**, and the one with more oxygen ends in **-ate.**

NO_2^- Nitrite SO_3^{2-} Sulfite
NO_3^- Nitrate SO_4^{2-} Sulfate

5. When the series of oxyanions contains four oxyanions, prefixes are also used. **Hypo-** and **per-** are used to indicate less oxygen and more oxygen, respectively.

ClO^- Hypochlorite
ClO_2^- Chlorite
ClO_3^- Chlorate
ClO_4^- Perchlorate

6. Polyatomic anions often gain one or more H^+ ions to form anions of lower charge. The resulting ions are named by adding the word **hydrogen** or **dihydrogen** to the front of the anion's name. An older method uses the prefix **bi-** to indicate the addition of a single hydrogen ion.

HCO_3^- Hydrogen carbonate or bicarbonate
HSO_4^- Hydrogen sulfate or bisulfate
$H_2PO_4^-$ Dihydrogen phosphate

B. ION CHARGES

Metals, which are found in the left part of the periodic table, generally form positive ions, whereas nonmetals, which are found in the right part of the periodic table, generally form negative ions. Note, however, the existence of anions that contain metallic elements (e.g., MnO_4^- [permanganate] and CrO_4^{2-} [chromate]). All elements in a given group tend to form monatomic ions with the same charge. Thus ions of alkali metals (Group I) usually form cations with a single positive charge, the alkaline earth metals (Group II) form cations with a double positive charge, and the halides (Group VII) form anions with a single negative charge. Though other main group elements follow this trend, the intermediate electronegativity of such elements (making them less likely to form ionic compounds) and the transition from metallic to nonmetallic character complicates the picture.

C. ELECTROLYTES

The electrical conductivity of aqueous solutions is governed by the presence and concentration of ions in solution. For example, pure water does not conduct an electrical current well, since the concentrations of hydrogen and hydroxide ions are very small. Solutes whose solutions are conductive are called electrolytes. A solute is considered a **strong electrolyte** if it dissociates completely into its constituent ions. Examples of strong electrolytes include ionic compounds, such as NaCl and KI, and molecular compounds with highly polar covalent bonds that dissociate into ions when dissolved, such as HCl in water. A **weak electrolyte**, on the other hand, ionizes or hydrolyzes incompletely in aqueous solution, and only some of the solute is present in ionic form. Examples include acetic acid and other weak acids, ammonia and other weak bases, and $HgCl_2$. Many compounds do not ionize at all in aqueous solution, retaining their molecular structure in solution, which usually limits their solubility. These compounds are called **nonelectrolytes** and include many nonpolar gases and organic compounds, such as oxygen and sugar.

CONCENTRATION
A. UNITS OF CONCENTRATION

Concentration denotes the amount of solute dissolved in a solvent. The concentration of a solution is most commonly expressed as **percent composition by mass, mole fraction, molarity, molality,** or **normality.**

1. Percent Composition by Mass

The percent composition by mass (%) of a solution is the mass of the solute divided by the mass of the solution (solute plus solvent), multiplied by 100.

Example: What is the percent composition by mass of a salt water solution if 100 g of the solution contains 20 g of NaCl?

Solution:

$$\frac{20 \text{ g NaCl}}{100 \text{ g}} \times 100 = 20\% \text{ NaCl solution}$$

2. **Mole Fraction**

   The mole fraction (x) of a compound is equal to the number of moles of the compound divided by the total number of moles of all species within the system. The sum of the mole fractions in a system will always equal 1.

   Example: If 92 g of glycerol is mixed with 90 g of water, what will be the mole fractions of the two components? (MW of H_2O = 18; MW of $C_3H_8O_3$ = 92).

   Solution:

   $$90 \text{ g water} = 90 \text{ g} \times \frac{1 \text{ mol}}{18 \text{ g}} = 5 \text{ mol}$$

   $$92 \text{ g glycerol} = 92 \text{ g} \times \frac{1 \text{ mol}}{92 \text{ g}} = 1 \text{ mol}$$

   $$\text{Total mol} = 5 + 1 = 6 \text{ mol}$$

   $$x_{water} = \frac{5 \text{ mol}}{6 \text{ mol}} = 0.833$$

   $$x_{glycerol} = \frac{1 \text{ mol}}{6 \text{ mol}} = 0.167$$

   $$x_{water} + x_{glycerol} = 0.833 + 0.167 = 1.000$$

3. **Molarity**

   The molarity (m) of a solution is the number of moles of solute per liter of **solution**. Solution concentrations are usually expressed in terms of molarity. Molarity depends on the volume of the solution, not on the volume of solvent used to prepare the solution.

DAT Synopsis

For dilute solutions, the volume of the solution is approximately equal to the volume of solvent used.

Example: If enough water is added to 11 g of $CaCl_2$ to make 100 mL of solution, what is the molarity of the solution?

Solution:

$$\frac{11 \text{ g } CaCl_2}{110 \text{g } CaCl_2 \text{ / mol } CaCl_2} = 0.10 \text{ mol } CaCl_2$$

$$100 \text{ mL} \times \frac{1L}{1,000 \text{ mL}} = 0.10 \text{ L}$$

$$\text{molarity} = \frac{0.10 \text{ mol}}{0.10 \text{ L}} = 1.0 \text{ M}$$

4. Molality

The molality (m) of a solution is the number of moles of solute per kilogram of **solvent**. For dilute aqueous solutions at 25°C, the molality is approximately equal to the molarity, because the density of water at this temperature is 1 kilogram per liter. But note that this is an approximation and true only for **dilute aqueous** solutions.

Example: If 10 g of NaOH are dissolved in 500 g of water, what is the molality of the solution?

Solution:

$$\frac{10 \text{ g NaOH}}{40 \text{g NaOH / mol NaOH}} = 0.25 \text{ mol NaOH}$$

$$500 \text{ g} \times \frac{1 \text{ Kg}}{1,000 \text{g}} = 0.50 \text{ Kg}$$

$$\text{molality} = \frac{0.25 \text{ mol}}{0.50 \text{ Kg}} = 0.50 \text{ mol / Kg} = 0.50 m$$

5. Normality

The normality (N) of a solution is equal to the number of gram equivalent weights of solute per liter of solution. A gram equivalent weight, or equivalent, is a measure of the reactive capacity of a molecule (see "Molecules and Moles" in chapter 4).

To calculate the normality of a solution, we must know for what purpose the solution is being used, because it is the concentration of the reactive species with which we are concerned. Normality is unique among concentration units in that it is reaction dependent. For example, a 1 molar solution of sulfuric acid would be 2 normal for acid-base reactions (because each mole of sulfuric acid is 2 moles of H^+ ions) but is only 1 normal for a sulfate precipitation reaction (because each mole of sulfuric acid only provides 1 mole of sulfate ions).

B. DILUTION

A solution is diluted when solvent is added to a solution of high concentration to produce a solution of lower concentration. The concentration of a solution after dilution can be conveniently determined using this equation:

$$M_i V_i = M_f V_f$$

where M is molarity, V is volume, and the subscripts i and f refer to initial and final values, respectively.

Example: How many mL of a 5.5 M NaOH solution must be used to prepare 300 mL of a 1.2 M NaOH solution?

Solution : $5.5 \text{ M} \times V_i = 1.2\text{M} \times 0.3 \text{ L}$

$$V_i = \frac{1.2\text{M} \times 0.3 \text{ L}}{5.5 \text{ M}}$$

$$V_i = 0.065\text{L} = 65 \text{ mL}$$

SOLUTION EQUILIBRIA

The process of solvation, like other reversible chemical and physical changes, tends towards an equilibrium. Immediately after solute has been introduced into a solvent, most of the change taking place is dissociation, because no dissolved solute is initially present. However, according to Le Châtelier's Principle, as solute dissociates, the reverse reaction (precipitation of the solute) also begins to occur. Eventually an equilibrium is reached, with the rate of solute dissociation equal to the rate of precipitation, and the net concentration of the dissociated solute remains unchanged regardless of the amount of solute added.

An ionic solid introduced into a polar solvent dissociates into its component ions. The dissociation of such a solute in solution may be represented by

$$A_m B_n \text{ (s)} \rightleftharpoons m A^{n+} \text{ (aq)} + n B^{m-} \text{ (aq)}$$

A. THE SOLUBILITY PRODUCT CONSTANT

A slightly soluble ionic solid exists in equilibrium with its saturated solution. In the case of AgCl, for example, the solution equilibrium is as follows:

$$AgCl \text{ (s)} \rightleftharpoons Ag^+ \text{ (aq)} + Cl^- \text{ (aq)}$$

The **ion product**, I.P., of a compound in solution is defined as follows:

$$\text{I.P.} = [A^{n+}]^m [B^{m-}]^n$$

The same expression for a saturated solution at equilibrium defines the **solubility product constant, K_{sp}.**

$$K_{sp} = [A^{n+}]^m[B^{m-}]^n \text{ in a saturated solution}$$

However, I.P. is defined with respect to initial concentrations and does not necessarily represent either an equilibrium or a saturated solution, while K_{sp} does; at any point other than at equilibrium, the ion product is often referred to as Q_{sp}.

Each salt has its own distinct K_{sp} at a given temperature. If at a given temperature a salt's I.P. is equal to its K_{sp}, the solution is saturated, and the rate at which the salt dissolves equals the rate at which it precipitates out of solution. If a salt's I.P. exceeds its K_{sp}, the solution is supersaturated (holding more salt than it should be able to at a given temperature) and unstable. If the supersaturated solution is disturbed by adding more salt, other solid particles, or jarring the solution by a sudden decrease in temperature, the solid salt will precipitate until I.P. equals the K_{sp}. If I.P. is less than K_{sp}, the solution is unsaturated and no precipitate will form.

DAT Synopsis

If $Q_{sp} > K_{sp}$, precipitation will occur.

If $Q_{sp} < K_{sp}$, dissolution can continue until the solution is saturated.

If $Q = K$, solution is at equilibrium.

Example: The solubility of $Fe(OH)_3$ in an aqueous solution was determined to be 4.5×10^{-10} mol/L. What is the value of the K_{sp} for $Fe(OH)_3$?

Solution: The molar solubility (the solubility of the compound in mol/L) is given as 4.5×10^{-10} M. The equilibrium concentration of each ion can be determined from the molar solubility and the balanced dissociation reaction of $Fe(OH)_3$. The dissociation reaction is

$$Fe(OH)_3 \ (s) \rightleftharpoons Fe^{3+} \ (aq) + 3OH^- \ (aq)$$

Thus, for every mol of $Fe(OH)_3$ that dissociates, 1 mol of Fe^{3+} and 3 mol of OH^- are produced. Since the solubility is 4.5×10^{-10} M, the K_{sp} can be determined as follows:

$$K_{sp} = [Fe^{3+}][OH^-]^3$$

$$[OH^-] = 3[Fe^{3+}]; \qquad [Fe^{3+}] = 4.5 \times 10^{-10}M$$

$$K_{sp} = [Fe^{3+}](3[Fe^{3+}])^3 = 27[Fe^{3+}]^4$$

$$K_{sp} = (4.5 \times 10^{-10})[3(4.5 \times 10^{-10})]^3 = 27(4.5 \times 10^{-10})^4$$

$$K_{sp} = 1.1 \times 10^{-36}$$

DAT Synopsis

Every slightly soluble salt of general formula MX_3 will have $K_{sp} = 27x^4$, where x is the molar solubility.

Example: What are the concentrations of each of the ions in a saturated solution of $PbBr_2$, given that the K_{sp} of $PbBr_2$ is 2.1×10^{-6}? If 5 g of $PbBr_2$ are dissolved in water to make 1 L of solution at 25°C, would the solution be saturated, unsaturated, or supersaturated?

Solution: The first step is to write out the dissociation reaction:

$$PbBr_2 \ (s) \rightleftharpoons Pb^{2+} \ (aq) + 2Br^- \ (aq)$$

$$K_{sp} = [Pb^{2+}][Br^-]^2$$

Let x = the concentration of Pb^{2+}. Then $2x$ = the concentration of Br⁻ in the saturated solution at equilibrium (since $[Br^-]$ is two times $[Pb^{2+}]$).

$$(x)(2x)^2 = 4x^3$$

$$2.1 \times 10^{-6} = 4x^3$$

Solving for x, the concentration of Pb^{2+} in a saturated solution is 8.07×10^{-3} M, and the concentration of Br⁻ $(2x)$ is 1.61×10^{-2} M.

Next, we convert 5 g of $PbBr_2$ into moles:

$$5 \ g \times \frac{1 \ mol \ PbBr_2}{367 \ g} = 1.36 \times 10^{-2} \ mol$$

1.36×10^{-2} mol of $PbBr_2$ is dissolved in 1 L of solution, so the concentration of the solution 1.36×10^{-2} M. Since this is higher than the concentration of a saturated solution, this solution would be supersaturated.

DAT Synopsis

Every slightly soluble salt of general formula MX_2 will have $K_{sp} = 4x^3$, where x is the molar solubility.

B. FACTORS AFFECTING SOLUBILITY

The solubility of a substance varies depending on the temperature of the solution, the solvent, and, in the case of a gas-phase solute, the pressure. Solubility is also affected by the addition of other substances to the solution.

The solubility of a salt is considerably reduced when it is dissolved in a solution that already contains one of its ions, rather than in a pure solvent. For example, if a salt such as CaF_2 is dissolved in a solution already containing Ca^{2+} ions, the dissociation equilibrium will shift toward the production of the solid salt. This reduction in solubility, called the **common ion effect,** is another example of Le Châtelier's Principle.

Example: The K_{sp} of AgI in aqueous solution is 1×10^{-16} mol/L. If a 1×10^{-5} M solution of $AgNO_3$ is saturated with AgI, what will be the final concentration of the iodide ion?

Solution: The concentration of Ag^+ in the original $AgNO_3$ solution will be 1×10^{-5} mol/L. After AgI is added to saturation, the iodide concentration can be found by this formula:

$$1 \times 10^{-16} = [Ag^+][I^-]$$

$$= (1 \times 10^{-5})[I^-]$$

$$[I^-] = 1 \times 10^{-11} \text{ mol/L}$$

If the AgI had been dissolved in pure water, the concentration of both Ag^+ and I^- would have been 1×10^{-8} mol/L. The presence of the common ion, silver, at a concentration 1,000 times higher than what it would normally be in a silver iodide solution, has reduced the iodide concentration to one thousandth of what it would have been otherwise. An additional 1×10^{-11} mol/L of silver will, of course, dissolve in solution along with the iodide ion, but this will not significantly affect the final silver concentration, which is much higher.

DAT Synopsis

Every slightly soluble salt of general formula MX will have $K_{sp} = x^2$, where x is the molar solubility.

## 10

ACIDS AND BASES

Many important reactions in chemical and biological systems involve two classes of compounds called **acids** and **bases**. Acids and bases cause color changes in certain compounds called **indicators**, which may be in solution or on paper. A particular common indicator is **litmus paper**, which turns red in acidic solution and blue in basic solution. A more extensive discussion of the chemical properties of acids and bases is outlined below.

DEFINITIONS

A. ARRHENIUS DEFINITION

The first definitions of acids and bases were formulated by Svante Arrhenius towards the end of the 19th century. Arrhenius defined an acid as a species that produces H^+ (a proton) in an aqueous solution and a base as a species that produces OH^- (a hydroxide ion) in an aqueous solution. These definitions, though useful, fail to describe acidic and basic behavior in nonaqueous media.

B. BRØNSTED-LOWRY DEFINITION

A more general definition of acids and bases was proposed independently by Johannes Brønsted and Thomas Lowry in 1923. A Brønsted-Lowry acid is a species that donates protons, while a Brønsted-Lowry base is a species that accepts protons. For example, NH_3 and Cl^- are both Brønsted-Lowry bases because they accept protons. However, they cannot be called Arrhenius bases since in aqueous solution, they do not dissociate to form OH^-. The advantage of the Brønsted-Lowry concept of acids and bases is that it is not limited to aqueous solutions.

Brønsted-Lowry acids and bases always occur in pairs, called **conjugate acid-base pairs.** The two members of a conjugate pair are related by the transfer of a proton. For example, H_3O^+ is the conjugate acid of the base H_2O, and NO_2^- is the conjugate base of HNO_2:

$$H_3O^+ (aq) \rightleftharpoons H_2O (aq) + H^+ (aq)$$

$$HNO_2 (aq) \rightleftharpoons NO_2^- (aq) + H^+ (aq)$$

C. LEWIS DEFINITION

At approximately the same time as Brønsted and Lowry, Gilbert Lewis also proposed definitions of acids and bases. Lewis defined an acid as an electron-pair acceptor and a base as an electron-pair donor. Lewis's are the most inclusive definitions. Just as every Arrhenius acid is a Brønsted-Lowry acid, every Brønsted-Lowry acid is also a Lewis acid (and likewise for bases). However, the Lewis definition encompasses some species not included within the Brønsted-Lowry definition. For example, BCl_3 and $AlCl_3$ can each accept an electron pair and are therefore Lewis acids, despite their inability to donate protons.

NOMENCLATURE OF ARRHENIUS ACIDS

The name of an acid is related to the name of the parent anion (the anion that combines with H^+ to form the acid). Acids formed from anions whose names end in **-ide** have the prefix **hydro-** and the ending **-ic**.

F^-	Fluoride	HF	Hydrofluoric acid
Br^-	Bromide	HBr	Hydrobromic acid

Acids formed from oxyanions are called **oxyacids**. If the anion ends in **-ite** (less oxygen), then the acid will end with **-ous acid**. If the anion ends in **-ate** (more oxygen), then the acid will end with **-ic acid**. Prefixes in the names of the anions are retained. Some examples:

ClO^-	Hypochlorite	HClO	Hypochlorous acid
ClO_2^-	Chlorite	$HClO_2$	Chlorous acid
ClO_3^-	Chlorate	$HClO_3$	Chloric acid
ClO_4^-	Perchlorate	$HClO_4$	Perchloric acid
NO_2^-	Nitrite	HNO_2	Nitrous acid
NO_3^-	Nitrate	HNO_3	Nitric acid

PROPERTIES OF ACIDS AND BASES
A. HYDROGEN ION EQUILIBRIA (pH AND pOH)

Hydrogen ion concentration, [H+], is generally measured as **pH**, where

$$pH = -\log[H^+] = \log(1/[H^+])$$

Likewise, hydroxide ion concentration, [OH−], is measured as **pOH**, where

$$pOH = -\log[OH^-] = \log(1/[OH^-])$$

In any aqueous solution, the H_2O solvent dissociates slightly:

$$H_2O(\ell) \rightleftharpoons H^+(aq) + OH^-(aq)$$

This dissociation is an equilibrium reaction and is, therefore, described by a constant, K_w, **the water dissociation constant.**

$$K_w = [H^+][OH^-] = 10^{-14}$$

Rewriting this equation in logarithmic form gives this:

$$pH + pOH = 14$$

In pure H_2O, [H+] is equal to [OH−], since for every mole of H_2O that dissociates, one mole of H+ and one mole of OH− are formed. A solution with equal concentrations of H+ and OH− is neutral and has a pH of 7($-\log 10^{-7} = 7$). A pH below 7 indicates a relative excess of H+ ions and, therefore, an acidic solution; a pH above 7 indicates a relative excess of OH− ions and, therefore, a basic solution.

Math Note: Estimating p-Scale Values

A useful skill for various problems involving acids and bases, as well as their corresponding buffer solutions, is the ability to convert pH, pOH, pK_a, and pK_b quickly into nonlogarithmic form and vice versa.

When the original value is a power of ten, the operation is relatively simple; changing the sign on the exponent gives the corresponding p-scale value directly. For example:

If [H+] = 0.001, or 10^{-3}, then pH = 3.

If $K_b = 1.0 \times 10^{-7}$, then $pK_b = 7$.

More difficulty arises (in the absence of a calculator) when the original value is not an exact power of 10; exact calculation would be excessively onerous, but a simple method of approximation exists. If the nonlogarithmic value is written in proper scientific notation, it will look like $n \times 10^{-m}$, where n is a number between 1 and 10. The log of this product can be written as $\log(n \times 10^{-m}) = -m + \log n$, and the negative log is thus $m - \log n$. Now, since n is a number between 1 and 10, its logarithm will be a fraction between 0 and 1. Thus, $m - \log n$ will be between $m - 1$ and m.

Further, the larger n is, the larger the fraction log x will be and, therefore, the closer to $m - 1$ our answer will be.

> Example: If $K_a = 1.8 \times 10^{-5}$, then $pK_a = 5 - \log 1.8$. Since 1.8 is small, its log will be small, and the answer will be closer to 5 than to 4. (The actual answer is 4.74.)

B. STRONG ACIDS AND BASES

Strong acids and bases are those that completely dissociate into their component ions in aqueous solution. For example, when NaOH is added to water, it dissociates completely:

$$NaOH(s) + \text{excess } H_2O(\ell) \rightarrow Na^+ (aq) + OH^- (aq)$$

Hence, in a 1 M solution of NaOH, complete dissociation gives 1 mole of OH^- ions per liter of solution.

$$pH = 14 - (-\log[OH^-]) = 14 + \log[1] = 14$$

Virtually no undissociated NaOH remains. Note that the $[OH^-]$ contributed by the dissociation of H_2O is considered to be negligible in this case. The contribution of OH^- and H^+ ions from the dissociation of H_2O can be neglected only if the concentration of the acid or base is greater than 10^{-7} M. For example, the pH of a 1×10^{-8} M HCl solution (HCl is a strong acid) might appear to be 8, since $\{-\log (1 \times 10^{-8})\} = 8$. However, a pH of 8 is in the basic pH range, and an HCl solution is not basic. The discrepancy arises from the fact that at low HCl concentrations, H^+ from the dissociation of water does contribute significantly to the total $[H^+]$. The $[H^+]$ from the dissociation of water is less than 1×10^{-7} M due to the common ion effect. The total concentration of H^+ can be calculated from

$$K_w = (x + 1 \times 10^{-8})(x) = 1.0 \times 10^{-14}, \text{ where } x = [H^+] = [OH^-] \text{ (both from the dissociation of water molecules).}$$

Solving for x gives $x = 9.5 \times 10^{-8}$ M,

so $[H^+]_{total} = (9.5 \times 10^{-8} + 1 \times 10^{-8})$ M $= 1.05 \times 10^{-7}$ M

and pH $= -\log (1.05 \times 10^{-7}) = 6.98$, slightly less than 7, as should be expected for a very dilute, yet acidic, solution.

Strong acids commonly encountered in the laboratory include $HClO_4$ (perchloric acid), HNO_3 (nitric acid), H_2SO_4 (sulfuric acid), and HCl (hydrochloric acid). Commonly encountered strong bases include NaOH (sodium hydroxide), KOH (potassium hydroxide), and other soluble hydroxides of Group IA and IIA metals. Calculation of the pH and pOH of strong acids and bases assumes complete dissociation of the acid or base in solution: $[H^+]$ = normality of strong acid and $[OH^-]$ = normality of strong base.

C. WEAK ACIDS AND BASES

Weak acids and bases are those that only partially dissociate in aqueous solution. A weak monoprotic acid, HA, in aqueous solution will achieve the following equilibrium after dissociation (H_3O^+ is equivalent to H^+ in aqueous solution):

$$HA\ (aq) + H_2O\ (\ell) \rightleftharpoons H_3O^+\ (aq) + A^-\ (aq)$$

The **acid dissociation constant, K_a**, is a measure of the degree to which an acid dissociates.

$$K_a = \frac{[H_3O^+][A^-]}{[HA]}$$

The weaker the acid, the smaller the K_a. Note that K_a does not contain an expression for the pure liquid, water.

A weak monovalent base, BOH, undergoes dissociation to give B^+ and OH^-. The **base dissociation constant, K_b**, is a measure of the degree to which a base dissociates. The weaker the base, the smaller its K_b. For a monovalent base, K_b is defined as follows:

$$K_b = \frac{[B^+][OH^-]}{[BOH]}$$

A **conjugate acid** is defined as the acid formed when a base gains a proton. Similarly, a **conjugate base** is formed when an acid loses a proton. For example, in the HCO_3^-/CO_3^{2-} conjugate acid/base pair, CO_3^{2-} is the conjugate base, and HCO_3^- is the conjugate acid:

$$HCO_3^-\ (aq) \rightleftharpoons H^+\ (aq) + CO_3^{2-}\ (aq)$$

To find the K_a of the conjugate acid HCO_3^-, the reaction with water must be considered:

$$HCO_3^-\ (aq) + H_2O\ (\ell) \rightleftharpoons H_3O^+\ (aq) + CO_3^{2-}\ (aq)$$

Likewise, for the K_b of CO_3^{2-},

$$CO_3^{2-}\ (aq) + H_2O\ (\ell) \rightleftharpoons HCO_3^-\ (aq) + OH^-\ (aq)$$

In a conjugate acid/base pair formed from a weak acid, the conjugate base is generally stronger than the conjugate acid. Thus, for HCO_3^- and CO_3^{2-}, the reaction of CO_3^{2-} (the conjugate base) in water to produce HCO_3^- (the conjugate acid) and OH^- occurs to a greater extent (i.e., is more favorable) than the reverse reaction.

DAT Synopsis

As a weak acid or base, the effect on pH will always be less than that of a strong acid or base of the same concentration. For example, before calculating the pH of a 0.01 M solution of acetic acid, $K_a = 1.8 \times 10^{-5}$, recognize that it will be higher than that of a 0.01 M solution of a strong acid like HCl; since the pH of 0.01 M HCl is 2, the pH of 0.01 M acetic acid must be greater than 2.

The equilibrium constants for these reactions are as follows:

$$K_a = \frac{[H^+][CO_3^{2-}]}{[HCO_3^-]} \text{ and } K_b = \frac{[HCO_3^-][OH^-]}{[CO_3^{2-}]}$$

Adding the two reactions shows that the net reaction is simply the dissociation of water:

$$H_2O \ (\ell) \rightleftharpoons H^+ \ (aq) + OH^- \ (aq)$$

The equilibrium constant for this net reaction is $K_w = [H^+][OH^-]$, which is the product of K_a and K_b. Thus, if the dissociation constant either for an acid or for its conjugate base is known, then the dissociation constant for the other can be determined, using this equation:

$$K_a \times K_b = K_w = 1 \times 10^{-14}$$

Thus K_a and K_b are inversely related. In other words, if K_a is large (the acid is strong), then K_b will be small (the conjugate base will be weak), and vice versa.

D. APPLICATIONS OF K_a AND K_b

To calculate the concentration of H+ in a 2.0 M aqueous solution of acetic acid, CH_3COOH (Ka = 1.8×10^{-5}), first write the equilibrium reaction:

$$CH_3COOH \ (aq) \rightleftharpoons H^+ \ (aq) + CH_3COO^- \ (aq)$$

Next, write the expression for the acid dissociation constant:

$$K_a = \frac{[H^+][CH_3COO^-]}{[CH_3COOH]} = 1.8 \times 10^{-5}$$

Since acetic acid is a weak acid, the concentration of CH_3COOH at equilibrium is equal to its initial concentration, 2.0 M, less the amount dissociated, x. Likewise $[H^+] = [CH_3COO^-] = x$, since each molecule of CH_3COOH dissociates into one H+ ion and one CH_3COO^- ion. Thus, the equation can be rewritten as follows:

$$K_a = \frac{[x][x]}{[2.0-x]} = 1.8 \times 10^{-5}$$

We can approximate that $2.0 - x \approx 2.0$, since acetic acid is a weak acid and only slightly dissociates in water. This simplifies the calculation of x:

$$K_a = \frac{[x][x]}{[2.0]} = 1.8 \times 10^{-5}$$
$$x = 6.0 \times 10^{-3} \text{ M}$$

The fact that $[x]$ is so much less than the initial concentration of acetic acid (2.0 M) validates the approximation; otherwise, it would have been necessary to solve for x using the quadratic formula. (A rule of thumb is that the approximation is valid as long as x is less than 5 percent of the initial concentration.)

SALT FORMATION

Acids and bases may react with each other, forming a salt and (often, but not always) water, in what is termed a **neutralization reaction** (see "Neutralization Reaction" in chapter 4). For example:

$$HA + BOH \rightarrow BA + H_2O$$

The salt may precipitate out or remain ionized in solution, depending on its solubility and the amount produced. Neutralization reactions generally go to completion. The reverse reaction, in which the salt ions react with water to give back the acid or base, is known as **hydrolysis.**

Four combinations of strong and weak acids and bases are possible:

1. strong acid + strong base: e.g., $HCl + NaOH \rightarrow NaCl + H_2O$
2. strong acid + weak base: e.g., $HCl + NH_3 \rightarrow NH_4Cl$
3. weak acid + strong base: e.g., $HClO + NaOH \rightarrow NaClO + H_2O$
4. weak acid + weak base: e.g., $HClO + NH_3 \rightleftharpoons NH_4ClO$

The products of a reaction between equal concentrations of a strong acid and a strong base are a salt and water. The acid and base neutralize each other, so the resulting solution is neutral (pH = 7), and the ions formed in the reaction do not react with water. The product of a reaction between a strong acid and a weak base is also a salt, but usually no water is formed since weak bases are usually not hydroxides. However, in this case, the cation of the salt will react with the water solvent, reforming the weak base. This reaction constitutes hydrolysis. For example:

$$HCl \text{ } (aq) + NH_3 \text{ } (aq) \rightleftharpoons NH_4^+ \text{ } (aq) + Cl^- \text{ } (aq) \text{ Reaction I}$$

$$NH_4^+ \text{ } (aq) + H_2O \text{ } (aq) \rightleftharpoons NH_3 \text{ } (aq) + H_3O^+ \text{ } (aq) \text{ Reaction II}$$

NH_4^+ is the conjugate acid of a weak base (NH_3) and is, therefore, stronger than the conjugate base (Cl^-) of the strong acid HCl. NH_4^+ will thus react with OH^-, reducing the concentration of OH^-. There will thus be an excess of H^+, which will lower the pH of the solution.

On the other hand, when a weak acid reacts with a strong base, the solution is basic due to the hydrolysis of the salt to reform the acid with the concurrent formation of hydroxide ion from the hydrolyzed water molecules. The pH of a solution containing a weak acid and a weak base depends on the relative strengths of the reactants. For example, the acid HClO has a $K_a = 3.2 \times 10^{-8}$, and the base NH_3 has a $K_b = 1.8 \times 10^{-5}$. Thus, an aqueous solution of HClO and NH_3 is basic since K_a for HClO is less than K_b for NH_3.

POLYVALENCE AND NORMALITY

The relative acidity or basicity of an aqueous solution is determined by the relative concentrations of **acid** and **base equivalents.** An acid equivalent is equal to one mole of H^+ (or H_3O^+) ions; a base equivalent is equal to one mole of OH^- ions. Some acids and bases are polyvalent; that is, each mole of the acid or base liberates more than one acid or base equivalent. For example, the diprotic acid H_2SO_4 undergoes the following dissociation in water:

$$H_2SO_4\ (aq) \rightarrow H^+\ (aq) + HSO_4^-\ (aq)$$

$$HSO_4^-\ (aq) \rightleftharpoons H^+\ (aq) + SO_4^{2-}\ (aq)$$

One mole of H_2SO_4 can thus produce 2 acid equivalents (2 moles of H^+). The acidity or basicity of a solution depends upon the concentration of acidic or basic equivalents that can be liberated. The quantity of acidic or basic capacity is directly indicated by the solution's normality (see "Concentration" in chapter 9). Since each mole of H_3PO_4 can liberate 3 moles (equivalents) of H^+, a 2 M H_3PO_4 solution would be 6 N (6 normal).

Another useful measurement is equivalent weight. For example, the gram molecular weight of H_2SO_4 is 98 g/mol. Since each mole liberates 2 acid equivalents, the gram equivalent weight of H_2SO_4 would be $\frac{98}{2} = 49\,g$; that is, the dissociation of 49 g of H_2SO_4 would release 1 acid equivalent. Common polyvalent acids include H_2SO_4, H_3PO_4, and H_2CO_3.

AMPHOTERIC SPECIES

An **amphoteric,** or **amphiprotic,** species is one that can act either as an acid or a base, depending on its chemical environment. In the Brønsted–Lowry sense, an amphoteric species can either gain or lose a proton. Water is the most common example. When water reacts with a base, it behaves as an acid:

$$H_2O + B^- \rightleftharpoons HB + OH^-$$

When water reacts with an acid, it behaves as a base:

$$HA + H_2O \rightleftharpoons H_3O^+ + A^-$$

The partially dissociated conjugate base of a polyprotic acid is usually amphoteric (e.g., HSO_4^- can either gain an H^+ to form H_2SO_4 or lose an H^+ to form SO_4^{2-}). The hydroxides of certain metals (e.g., Al, Zn, Pb, and Cr) are also amphoteric. Furthermore, species that can act as either oxidizing or reducing agents (see "Oxidation-Reduction Reactions" in chapter 11) are considered to be amphoteric as well, since by accepting or donating electron pairs, they act as Lewis acids or bases, respectively.

TITRATION AND BUFFERS

Titration is a procedure used to determine the molarity of an acid or base. This is accomplished by reacting a known volume of a solution of unknown concentration with a known volume of a solution of known concentration. When the number of acid equivalents equals the number of base equivalents added, or vice versa, the **equivalence point** is reached. It is important to emphasize that, while a strong acid/strong base titration will have an equivalence point at pH 7, the equivalence point need not always occur at pH 7. Also, when titrating polyprotic acids or bases, there are several equivalence points, as each acidic or basic species is titrated separately (see "Polyprotic Acids and Bases" later in this chapter).

The equivalence point in a titration is estimated in two common ways: either by using a graphical method, plotting the pH of the solution as a function of added titrant by using a **pH meter** (e.g., Figure 10.1), or by watching for a color change of an added **indicator.** Indicators are weak organic acids or bases that have different colors in their undissociated and dissociated states. Indicators are used in low concentrations and, therefore, do not significantly alter the equivalence point. The point at which the indicator actually changes color is not the equivalence point but is called the **end point**. If the titration is performed well, the volume difference (and therefore the error) between the end point and the equivalence point is usually small and may be either corrected for or ignored.

A. STRONG ACID AND STRONG BASE

Consider the titration of 10 mL of a 0.1 N solution of HCl with a 0.1 N solution of NaOH. Plotting the pH of the reaction solution versus the quantity of NaOH added gives the curve shown in Figure 10.1.

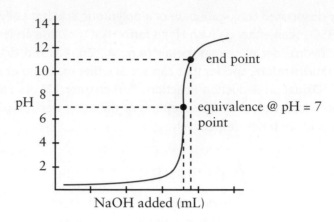

Figure 10.1. Titration of HCl with NaOH

Because HCl is a strong acid and NaOH is a strong base, the equivalence point of the titration will be at pH 7, and the solution will be neutral. Note that the end point shown is close to, but not exactly equal to, the equivalence point; selection of a better indicator—say, one that changes colors at pH 8—would have given a better approximation.

In the early part of the curve (when little base has been added), the acidic species predominates, so the addition of small amounts of base will not appreciably change either the [OH⁻] or the pH. Similarly, in the last part of the titration curve (when an excess of base has been added), the addition of small amounts of base will not change the [OH⁻] significantly, and the pH remains relatively constant. The addition of base most alters the concentrations of H⁺ and OH⁻ near the equivalence point, and thus the pH changes most drastically in that region.

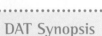
B. WEAK ACID AND STRONG BASE

Titration of a weak acid, HA, with a strong base produces the titration curve shown in Figure 10.2.

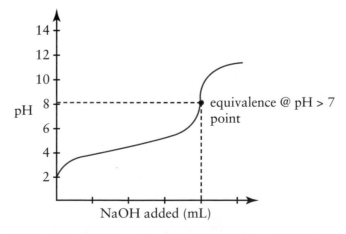

Figure 10.2. Titration of a Weak Acid, HA, with NaOH

Comparing Figure 10.2 with Figure 10.1 shows that the initial pH of the weak acid solution is greater than the initial pH of the strong acid solution. The pH changes most significantly early on in the titration, and the equivalence point is in the basic range.

C. BUFFERS

A **buffer solution** consists of a mixture of a weak acid and its salt (which consists of its conjugate base and a cation) or a mixture of a weak base and its salt (which consists of its conjugate acid and an anion). Two examples of buffers are a solution of acetic acid (CH_3COOH) and its salt, sodium acetate ($CH_3COO^-Na^+$), and a solution of ammonia (NH_3) and its salt, ammonium chloride ($NH_4^+Cl^-$). Buffer solutions have the useful property of resisting changes in pH when small amounts of acid or base are added.

Consider a buffer solution of acetic acid and sodium acetate:

$$CH_3COOH \rightleftharpoons H^+ + CH_3COO^-$$

When a small amount of NaOH is added to the buffer, the OH^- ions from the NaOH react with the H^+ ions present in the solution; subsequently, more acetic acid dissociates (equilibrium shifts to the right), restoring the $[H^+]$. Thus, an increase in $[OH^-]$ does not appreciably change pH. Likewise, when a small amount of HCl is added to the buffer, H^+ ions from the HCl react with the acetate ions to form acetic acid. Thus, $[H^+]$ is kept relatively constant, and the pH of the solution is relatively unchanged.

The **Henderson-Hasselbalch equation** is used to estimate the pH of a solution in the buffer region where the concentrations of the species and its conjugate are present in approximately equal concentrations. For a weak acid buffer solution,

$$pH = pk_a + \log \frac{[\text{conjugate base}]}{[\text{weak acid}]}$$

Note that when [conjugate base] = [weak acid] (in a titration, halfway to the equivalent point), the pH = pK_a because the log 1 = 0. Likewise, for a weak base buffer solution,

$$pOH = pk_b + \log \frac{[\text{conjugate acid}]}{[\text{weak base}]}$$

and pOH = pK_b when [conjugate acid] = [weak base].

D. POLYPROTIC ACIDS AND BASES

The titration curve for a polyprotic acid or base looks different than that for a monoprotic acid or base. Figure 10.3 shows the titration of Na_2CO_3 with HCl in which the polyprotic acid H_2CO_3 is the ultimate product.

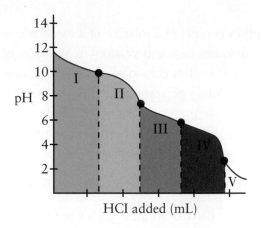

Figure 10.3. Titration of Na_2CO_3 with HCl

In region I, little acid has been added, and the predominant species is CO_3^{2-}. In region II, more acid has been added, and the predominant species are CO_3^{2-} and HCO_3^- in relatively equal concentrations. The flat part of the curve is the first buffer region, corresponding to the pK_a of HCO_3^- ($K_a = 5.6 \times 10^{-11}$ implies $pK_a = 10.25$).

Region III contains the equivalence point, at which all of the CO_3^{2-} is titrated to HCO_3^-. As the curve illustrates, a rapid change in pH occurs at the equivalence point; in the latter part of region III, the predominant species is HCO_3^-.

In region IV, the acid has neutralized approximately half of the HCO_3^-, and now H_2CO_3 and HCO_3^- are in roughly equal concentrations. This flat region is the second buffer region of the titration curve, corresponding to the pK_a of H_2CO_3 ($K_a = 4.3 \times 10^{-7}$ implies $pK_a = 6.37$). In region V, the equivalence point for the entire titration is reached, as all of the HCO_3^-, is converted to H_2CO_3. Again, a rapid change in pH is observed near the equivalence point as acid is added.

## 11

REDOX REACTIONS AND ELECTROCHEMISTRY

Electrochemistry is the study of the relationships between chemical reactions and electrical energy. **Electrochemical reactions** include spontaneous reactions that produce electrical energy and nonspontaneous reactions that use electrical energy to produce a chemical change. Both types of reactions always involve a transfer of electrons with conservation of charge and mass.

OXIDATION-REDUCTION REACTIONS
A. OXIDATION AND REDUCTION

The law of conservation of charge states that an electrical charge can be neither created nor destroyed. Thus, an isolated loss or gain of electrons cannot occur; **oxidation** (loss of electrons) and **reduction** (gain of electrons) must occur simultaneously, resulting in an electron transfer called a **redox reaction**. An **oxidizing agent** causes another atom in a redox reaction to undergo oxidation and is itself reduced. A **reducing agent** causes the other atom to be reduced and is itself oxidized.

B. ASSIGNING OXIDATION NUMBERS

It is important, of course, to know which atom is oxidized and which is reduced. **Oxidation numbers** are assigned to atoms in order to keep track of the redistribution of electrons during a chemical reaction. From the oxidation numbers of the reactants and products, it is possible to determine how many electrons are gained or lost by each atom. The oxidation number of an atom in a compound is assigned according to the following rules:

1. **The oxidation number of free elements is zero.** For example, the atoms in N_2, P_4, S_8, and He all have oxidation numbers of zero.

2. **The oxidation number for a monatomic ion is equal to the charge of the ion.** For example, the oxidation numbers for Na^+, Cu^{2+}, Fe^{3+}, Cl^-, and N^{3-} are +1, +2, +3, −1, and −3, respectively.

3. **The oxidation number of each Group IA element in a compound is +1. The oxidation number of each Group IIA element in a compound is +2.**

KAPLAN) EXCLUSIVE

OIL RIG stands for "Oxidation Is Loss, Reduction Is Gain"—of electrons, that is.

Alternatively, reduction is just what it sounds like: reduction of charge.

4. **The oxidation number of each Group VIIA element in a compound is –1, except when combined with an element of higher electronegativity.** For example, in HCl, the oxidation number of Cl is –1; in HOCl, however, the oxidation number of Cl is +1.

5. **The oxidation number of hydrogen is –1 in compounds with less electronegative elements than hydrogen (Groups IA and IIA).** Examples include NaH and CaH_2. The more common oxidation number of hydrogen is +1.

6. **In most compounds, the oxidation number of oxygen is –2.** This is not the case, however, in molecules such as OF_2. Here, because F is more electronegative than O, the oxidation number of oxygen is +2. Also, in peroxides such as BaO_2, the oxidation number of O is –1 instead of –2 because of the structure of the peroxide ion, $[O–O]^{2-}$. (Note that Ba, a Group IIA element, can not be a +4 cation.)

7. **The sum of the oxidation numbers of all the atoms present in a neutral compound is zero. The sum of the oxidation numbers of the atoms present in a polyatomic ion is equal to the charge of the ion.** Thus, for SO_4^{2-}, the sum of the oxidation numbers must be –2.

Example: Assign oxidation numbers to the atoms in the following reaction in order to determine the oxidized and reduced species and the oxidizing and reducing agents.

$$SnCl_2 + PbCl_4 \rightarrow SnCl_4 + PbCl_2$$

Solution: All these species are neutral, so the oxidation numbers of each compound must add up to zero. In $SnCl_2$, since there are two chlorines present and chlorine has an oxidation number of –1, Sn must have an oxidation number of +2. Similarly, the oxidation number of Sn in $SnCl_4$ is +4; the oxidation number of Pb is +4 in $PbCl_4$ and +2 in $PbCl_2$. Notice that the oxidation number of Sn goes from +2 to +4; it loses electrons and thus is oxidized, making it the reducing agent. Since the oxidation number of Pb has decreased from +4 to +2, it has gained electrons and been reduced. Pb is the oxidizing agent. The sum of the charges on both sides of the reaction is equal to zero, so charge has been conserved.

DAT Synopsis

The conventions of formula writing put cation first and anion second. Thus NaH implies H^-, while HCl implies H^+.

KAPLAN EXCLUSIVE

An oxidizing agent causes something else to oxidize. Conversely, a reducing agent causes something else to reduce.

C. BALANCING REDOX REACTIONS

By assigning oxidation numbers to the reactants and products, one can determine how many moles of each species are required for conservation of charge and mass, which is necessary to balance the equation. To balance a redox reaction, both the net charge and the number of atoms must be equal on both sides of the equation. The most common method for balancing redox equations is the **half-reaction method**, also known as the **ion-electron method**, in which the equation is separated into two half-reactions—the oxidation part and the reduction part. Each half-reaction is balanced separately, and they are then added to give a balanced overall reaction. Consider a redox reaction between $KMnO_4$ and HI in an acidic solution:

$$MnO_4^- + I^- \rightarrow I_2 + Mn^{2+}$$

Step 1: Separate the two half-reactions.

$$I^- \rightarrow I_2$$

$$MnO_4^- \rightarrow Mn^{2+}$$

Step 2: Balance the atoms of each half-reaction. First, balance all atoms except H and O. Next, in an acidic solution, add H_2O to balance the O atoms and then add H^+ to balance the H atoms. (In a basic solution, use OH^- and H_2O to balance the O's and H's.)

To balance the iodine atoms, place a coefficient of two before the I^- ion.

$$2\,I^- \rightarrow I_2$$

For the permanganate half-reaction, Mn is already balanced. Next, balance the oxygens by adding $4H_2O$ to the right side.

$$MnO_4^- \rightarrow Mn^{2+} + 4H_2O$$

Finally, add H^+ to the left side to balance the 4 H_2Os. These two half-reactions are now balanced.

$$MnO_4^- + 8\,H^+ \rightarrow Mn^{2+} + 4H_2O$$

Step 3: Balance the charges of each half-reaction. The reduction half-reaction must consume the same number of electrons as are supplied by the oxidation half. For the oxidation reaction, add 2 electrons to the right side of the reaction:

$$2\,I^- \rightarrow I_2 + 2e^-$$

For the reduction reaction, a charge of +2 must exist on both sides. Add 5 electrons to the left side of the reaction to accomplish this:

$$5\ e^- + 8\ H^+ + MnO_4^- \rightarrow Mn^{2+} + 4\ H_2O$$

Next, both half-reactions must have the same number of electrons so that they will cancel. Multiply the oxidation half by 5 and the reduction half by 2.

$$5(2I^- \rightarrow I_2 + 2e^-)$$

$$2(5e^- + 8H^+ + MnO_4^- \rightarrow Mn^{2+} + 4\ H_2O)$$

Step 4: Add the half-reactions:

$$10\ I^- \rightarrow 5\ I_2 + 10\ e^-$$

$$16\ H^+ + 2\ MnO_4^- + 10\ e^- \rightarrow 2\ Mn^{2+} + 8\ H_2O$$

The final equation is this:

$$10\ I^- + 10\ e^- + 16\ H^+ + 2\ MnO_4^- \rightarrow 5\ I_2 + 2\ Mn^{2+} + 10\ e^- + 8\ H_2O$$

To get the overall equation, cancel out the electrons and any H_2Os, H^+s, or OH^-s that appear on both sides of the equation.

$$10\ I^- + 16\ H^+ + 2\ MnO_4^- \rightarrow 5\ I_2 + 2\ Mn^{2+} + 8\ H_2O$$

Step 5: Finally, confirm that mass and charge are balanced. There is a +4 net charge on each side of the reaction equation, and the atoms are stoichiometrically balanced.

ELECTROCHEMICAL CELLS

Electrochemical cells are contained systems in which a redox reaction occurs. There are two types of electrochemical cells, **galvanic cells** (also known as **voltaic cells**) and **electrolytic cells**. Spontaneous reactions occur in galvanic cells, and nonspontaneous reactions in electrolytic cells. Both types contain **electrodes** at which oxidation and reduction occur. For all electrochemical cells, the electrode at which oxidation occurs is called the **anode**, and the electrode where reduction occurs is called the **cathode**.

A. GALVANIC CELLS

A redox reaction occurring in a **galvanic cell** has a negative ΔG and is therefore a **spontaneous reaction**. Galvanic cell reactions supply energy and are used to do work. This energy can be harnessed by placing the oxidation and reduction half-reactions in separate containers called **half-cells**. The half-cells are then connected by an apparatus that allows for the flow of electrons.

A common example of a galvanic cell is the Daniell cell. shown in Figure 11.1.

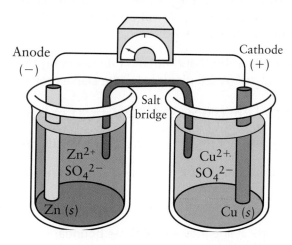

Figure 11.1. Daniell Cell

In the Daniell cell, a zinc bar is placed in an aqueous $ZnSO_4$ solution, and a copper bar is placed in an aqueous $CuSO_4$ solution. The anode of this cell is the zinc bar where Zn (s) is oxidized to Zn^{2+} (aq). The cathode is the copper bar, and it is the site of the reduction of Cu^{2+} (aq) to Cu (s). The half-cell reactions are written as follows:

$$Zn\ (s) \rightarrow Zn^{2+}\ (aq) + 2e^- \rightarrow (anode)$$

$$Cu^{2+}\ (aq) + 2e \rightarrow Cu\ (s) \rightarrow (cathode)$$

If the two half-cells were not separated, the Cu^{2+} ions would react directly with the zinc bar, and no useful electrical work would be obtained. To complete the circuit, the two solutions must be connected. Without connection, the electrons from the zinc oxidation half reaction would not be able to get to the copper ions; thus, a wire (or other conductor) is necessary. If only a wire were provided for this electron flow, the reaction would soon cease anyway, because an excess negative charge would build up in the solution surrounding the cathode, and an excess positive charge would build up in the solution surrounding the anode. This charge gradient is dissipated by the presence of a **salt bridge**, which permits the exchange of cations and anions. The salt bridge contains an inert electrolyte, usually KCl or NH_4NO_3, whose ions will not react with the electrodes or with the ions in solution. At the same time, the anions from the salt bridge (e.g., Cl-) diffuse from the salt bridge of the Daniell cell into the $ZnSO_4$ solution to balance out the charge of the newly created Zn^{2+} ions, and the cations of the salt bridge (e.g., K+) flow into the $CuSO_4$ solution to balance out the charge of the SO_4^{2-} ions left in solution when the Cu^{2+} ions deposit as copper metal.

During the course of the reaction, electrons flow from the zinc bar (anode) through the wire and the voltmeter toward the copper bar (cathode).

The anions (Cl⁻) flow externally (via the salt bridge) into the $ZnSO_4$, and the cations (K^+) flow into the $CuSO_4$. This flow depletes the salt bridge and, along with the finite quantity of Cu^{2+} in the solution, accounts for the relatively short lifetime of the cell.

A **cell diagram** is a shorthand notation representing the reactions in an electrochemical cell. A cell diagram for the Daniell cell is as follows:

$$\text{Zn } (s) \mid Zn^{2+}(x\text{M SO}_4^{2-}) \parallel Cu^{2+}(y\text{M SO}_4^{2-}) \mid \text{Cu } (s)$$

The following rules are used in constructing a cell diagram:

1. The reactants and products are always listed from left to right in the form:
$$\text{anode} \mid \text{anode solution} \parallel \text{cathode solution} \mid \text{cathode}$$

2. A single vertical line indicates a phase boundary.
3. A double vertical line indicates the presence of a salt bridge or some other type of barrier.

B. ELECTROLYTIC CELLS

A redox reaction occurring in an **electrolytic cell** has a positive ΔG and is therefore **nonspontaneous**. In **electrolysis**, electrical energy is required to induce reaction. The oxidation and reduction half-reactions are usually placed in one container.

Michael Faraday was the first to define certain quantitative principles governing the behavior of electrolytic cells. He theorized that the amount of chemical change induced in an electrolytic cell is directly proportional to the number of moles of electrons that are exchanged during a redox reaction. The number of moles exchanged can be determined from the balanced half-reaction. In general, for a reaction which involves the transfer of n electrons per atom,

$$M^{n+} + n\, e^- \rightarrow M\ (s)$$

One mole of M (s) will be produced if n moles of electrons are supplied.

The number of moles of electrons needed to produce a certain amount of M (s) can now be related to a measurable electrical property. One electron carries a charge of 1.6×10^{-19} coulombs (C). The charge carried by one mole of electrons can be calculated by multiplying this number by Avogadro's number, as follows:

$$(1.6 \times 10^{-19})(6.022 \times 10^{23}) = 96{,}487 \text{ C/mol e}^-$$

This number is called **Faraday's constant**, and one **faraday (F)** is equivalent to the amount of charge contained in one mole of electrons (1 F = 96,487 coulombs, or J/V).

An example of an electrolytic cell, in which molten NaCl is electrolyzed to form Cl_2 (g) and Na (l), is given in Fugure 11.2.

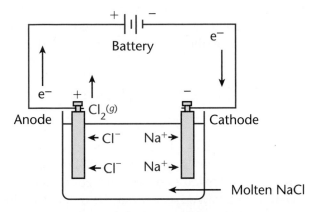

Figure 11.2. Example of an Electrolytic Cell

In this cell, Na^+ ions migrate towards the cathode, where they are reduced to Na (ℓ). Similarly, Cl^- ions migrate towards the anode, where they are oxidized to Cl_2 (g). This cell is used in industry as the major means of sodium and chlorine production. Note that sodium is a liquid at the temperature of molten NaCl; it is also less dense than the molten salt and thus is easily removed as it floats to the top of the reaction vessel.

C. ELECTRODE CHARGE DESIGNATIONS

The anode of an **electrolytic cell** is considered **positive**, since it is attached to the positive pole of the battery and so attracts anions from the solution. The anode of a **galvanic cell**, on the other hand, is considered **negative**, because the **spontaneous** oxidation reaction that takes place at the galvanic cell's anode is the original source of that cell's negative charge (i.e., is the source of electrons). In spite of this difference in designating charge, oxidation takes place at the anode in both types of cells, and electrons always flow through the wire from the anode to the cathode.

In a galvanic cell, charge is spontaneously created as electrons are released by the oxidizing species at the anode; since this is the source of electrons, the anode of a galvanic cell is considered the negative electrode.

In an electrolytic cell, electrons are forced through the cathode, where they encounter the species which is to be reduced. Here it is the cathode that is providing electrons, and thus the cathode of an electrolytic cell is considered the negative electrode. Alternatively, one can think of the cathode as the electrode attached to the negative pole of the battery (or other power source) used for the electrolysis.

In either case, a simple mnemonic is that the CAThode attracts the CATions. In the Daniell cell, for example, the electrons created at the anode as the zinc oxidizes travel through the wire to the copper half-cell, where they attract copper(II) cations to the cathode.

> **DAT Synopsis**
>
> In an electrolytic cell, the anode is positive, and the cathode is negative. In a galvanic cell, the anode is negative, and the cathode is positive. However, in both types of cells, reduction occurs at the cathode, and oxidation occurs at the anode.

One common topic in which this distinction arises is electrophoresis, a technique often used to separate amino acids based on their isoelectronic points, or pI's (see Organic Chemistry, chapter 15). The positively charged amino acids (i.e., those that are protonated at the pH of the solution) will migrate towards the cathode; negatively charged amino acids (i.e., those that are deprotonated at the solution pH migrate instead towards the anode.

REDUCTION POTENTIALS AND THE ELECTROMOTIVE FORCE
A. REDUCTION POTENTIALS

Sometimes when electrolysis is carried out in an aqueous solution, water, rather than the solute, is oxidized or reduced. For example, if an aqueous solution of NaCl is electrolyzed, water may be reduced at the cathode to produce H_2 (g) and OH^- ions, instead of Na^+ being reduced to Na (s), as occurs in the absence of water. The species in a reaction that will be oxidized or reduced can be determined from the **reduction potential** of each species, defined as the tendency of a species to acquire electrons and be reduced. Each species has its own intrinsic reduction potential; the more positive the potential, the greater the species' tendency to be reduced.

A reduction potential is measured in volts (V) and is defined relative to the **standard hydrogen electrode (SHE)**, which is arbitrarily given a potential of 0.00 volts. **Standard reduction potential, ($E°$)**, is measured under **standard conditions**: 25°C, a 1 M concentration for each ion participating in the reaction, a partial pressure of 1 atm for each gas that is part of the reaction, and metals in their pure state. The relative reactivities of different half-cells can be compared to predict the direction of electron flow. A higher $E°$ means a greater tendency for reduction to occur, while a lower $E°$ means a greater tendency for oxidation to occur.

Example: Given the following half-reactions and $E°$ values, determine which species would be oxidized and which would be reduced.

$Ag^+ + e \rightarrow Ag$ (s) $E° = +0.80$ V

$Tl^+ + e- \rightarrow Tl$ (s) $E° = -0.34$ V

Solution: Ag^+ would be reduced to Ag (s) and Tl (s) would be oxidized to Tl^+, since Ag^+ has the higher $E°$. Therefore, the reaction equation would be

$Ag^+ + Tl$ (s) $\rightarrow Tl^+ + Ag$ (s)

which is the sum of the two spontaneous half-reactions.

It should be noted that reduction and oxidation are opposite processes. Therefore, to obtain the oxidation potential of a given half-reaction, the reduction half-reaction and the sign of the reduction potential are both reversed. For instance, from the example above, the oxidation half-reaction and oxidation potential of Tl (*s*) are as follows:

$$Tl\ (s) \rightarrow Tl^+ + e^- \qquad E° = +0.34\ V$$

B. THE ELECTROMOTIVE FORCE

Standard reduction potentials are also used to calculate the **standard electromotive force (emf or $E°_{cell}$)** of a reaction, the difference in potential between two half-cells. The emf of a reaction is determined by adding the standard reduction potential of the reduced species and the standard oxidation potential of the oxidized species. When adding standard potentials, do *not* multiply by the number of moles oxidized or reduced.

$$emf = E°_{red} + E°_{ox} \qquad \text{(Equation 1)}$$

The standard emf of a galvanic cell is positive, while the standard emf of an electrolytic cell is negative.

Example: Given that the standard reduction potentials for Sm^{3+} and $[RhCl_6]^{3-}$ are –2.41 V and +0.44 V, respectively, calculate the emf of the following reaction:

$$Sm^{3+} + Rh + 6\ Cl^- \rightarrow [RhCl_6]^{3-} + Sm$$

Solution: First, determine the oxidation and reduction half-reactions. As written, the Rh is oxidized, and the Sm^{3+} is reduced. Thus, the Sm^{3+} reduction potential is used as is, while the reverse reaction for Rh, $[RhCl_6]^{3-} \rightarrow Rh + 6\ Cl^-$, applies, and the oxidation potential of $[RhCl_6]^{3-}$ must be used. Then, using Equation 1, the emf can be calculated to be (–2.41 V) + (–0.44 V) = –2.85 V. The cell is thus electrolytic as written. From this result, it is evident that the reaction would proceed spontaneously to the left, in which case the Sm would be oxidized, while $[RhCl_6]^{3-}$ would be reduced.

THERMODYNAMICS OF REDOX REACTIONS

A. EMF AND GIBBS FREE ENERGY

The thermodynamic criterion for determining the spontaneity of a reaction is ΔG, Gibbs free energy, the maximum amount of useful work produced by a chemical reaction. In an electrochemical cell, the work done is dependent on the number of coulombs and the energy available. Thus, ΔG and emf are related as follows:

$$\Delta G = -nFE_{cell} \qquad \text{(Equation 2)}$$

where n is the number of moles of electrons exchanged, F is Faraday's constant, and E_{cell} is the emf of the cell. **Keep in mind that if Faraday's constant is expressed in coulombs (J/V), then ΔG must be expressed in J, not kJ.**

If the reaction takes place under standard conditions (25°C, 1 atm pressure, and all solutions at 1M concentration), then the ΔG is the standard Gibbs free energy and E_{cell} is the standard cell potential. The above equation then becomes

$$\Delta G° = -nFE°_{cell} \qquad \text{(Equation 3)}$$

B. THE EFFECT OF CONCENTRATION ON EMF

Thus far, only the calculations for the emf of cells in unit concentrations (all the ionic species present have a molarity of 1, and all gases are at a pressure of 1 atm) have been discussed. However, concentration does have an effect on the emf of a cell: emf varies with the changing concentrations of the species involved. It can also be determined by the use of the **Nernst equation:**

$$E_{cell} = E°_{cell} - (RT/nF)(\ln Q)$$

Q is the reaction quotient for a given reaction. For example, in this reaction,

$$a\,A + b\,B \rightarrow c\,C + d\,D$$

the reaction quotient would be

$$Q = \frac{[C]^c\,[D]^d}{[A]^a\,[B]^b}$$

The emf of a cell can be measured by a **voltmeter**. A **potentiometer** is a kind of voltmeter that draws no current and gives a more accurate reading of the difference in potential between two electrodes.

C. EMF AND THE EQUILIBRIUM CONSTANT (KEQ)

For reactions in solution, $\Delta G°$ can be determined in another manner, as follows:

$$\Delta G° = -RT \ln K_{eq} \qquad \text{(Equation 4)}$$

where R is the gas constant 8.314 J/(K•mol), T is the temperature in K, and K_{eq} is the equilibrium constant for the reaction.

If Equations 3 and 4 are combined, then

$$\Delta G° = -nFE°_{cell} = -RT \ln K_{eq}$$

or simply

$$nFE°_{cell} = RT \ln K_{eq} \qquad \text{(Equation 5)}$$

If the values for n, T, and K_{eq} are known, then the $E°_{cell}$ for the redox reaction can be readily calculated.

Flashback

Recall that if ΔG is positive, the reaction is not spontaneous; if ΔG is negative, the reaction is spontaneous.

DAT Synopsis

ΔG is negative if and only if emf is positive.

A very positive E_{cell} means a very negative ΔG.

DAT Synopsis

If $E°_{cell}$ is positive, then ln K is positive. This means that K must be greater than 1 and that the equilibrium must lie toward the right (i.e., products are favored).

NUCLEAR PHENOMENA

The subject of this chapter is the nucleus and nuclear phenomena. It begins with a review of some of the standard terminology used in nuclear chemistry and physics. The concept of binding energy and the equivalent concept of the mass defect are then introduced. Briefly, an amount of energy, called the **binding energy**, is required to break up a given nucleus into its constituent protons and neutrons. That energy is converted to mass via Einstein's $E = mc^2$, resulting in a larger mass for the constituent protons and neutrons than that of the original nucleus, the difference being called the **mass defect**. The remainder of the chapter is concerned with a brief discussion of nuclear reactions (**fission** and **fusion**) and an extended treatment of **radioactive decay**, which itself is presented in two distinct parts. The first deals with the four types of radioactive decay and a discussion of the reaction equations that describe them. The second covers the general problem of determining the number of nuclei that have not decayed as a function of time, along with the associated concept of the half-life of a decay process.

NUCLEI

At the center of an atom lies its nucleus, consisting of one or more **nucleons** (protons or neutrons) held together with considerably more energy than the energy needed to hold electrons in orbit around the nucleus. The radius of the nucleus is about 100,000 times smaller than the radius of the atom. Some common nuclear properties are the following:

A. ATOMIC NUMBER (Z)

Z is always an integer and is equal to the **number of protons** in the nucleus. Each element has a unique number of protons; therefore, the atomic number Z identifies the element. Z is used as a presubscript to the chemical symbol in **isotopic notation**. The chemical symbols and the atomic numbers of all the elements are given in the periodic table.

DAT Synopsis

Each element is defined by its atomic number Z (number of protons in the nucleus).

ATOMIC NUMBERS OF THE CHEMICAL ELEMENTS

Atomic number Z	Chemical symbol	Element name
1	H	hydrogen
2	He	helium
3	Li	lithium
.	.	.
.	.	.
92	U	uranium
.	.	.
.	.	.
.	.	.

B. MASS NUMBER (A)

A is an integer equal to the total **number of nucleons** (neutrons and protons) in a nucleus. Let N represent the number of neutrons in a nucleus. The equation relating A, N, and Z is simply:

$$A = N + Z$$

In isotopic notation, A appears as a presuperscript to the chemical symbol.

Examples: $^{1}_{1}H$ —a single proton; the nucleus of ordinary hydrogen

$^{4}_{2}He$ —the nucleus of ordinary helium, consisting of 2 protons and 2 neutrons. It is also known as an alpha particle (α-particle).

$^{235}_{92}U$ —a fissionable form of uranium, consisting of 92 protons and 143 neutrons

C. ISOTOPE

The nucleus of a given element can have different numbers of neutrons and, hence, different mass numbers. For a nucleus of a given element with a given number of protons (atomic number Z), the various nuclei with different numbers of neutrons are called **isotopes** of that element. The term *isotope* is also used in a generic sense to refer to any nucleus. The term **radionuclide** is another generic term used to refer to any radioactive isotope, especially those used in **nuclear medicine.**

> **DAT Synopsis**
> Protons and neutrons are both referred to as nucleons.

> **DAT Synopsis**
> All isotopes of a given element have the same value of Z, but different values of N and A.

Example: The three isotopes of hydrogen are these:

$^{1}_{1}$H — a single proton; the nucleus of ordinary hydrogen

$^{2}_{1}$H — a proton and a neutron together, often called a **deuteron;** the nucleus of one type of heavy hydrogen called **deuterium**

$^{3}_{1}$H — a proton and two neutrons together, often called a **triton;** the nucleus of a heavier type of heavy hydrogen called **tritium**

D. ATOMIC MASS AND ATOMIC MASS UNIT

Atomic mass is most commonly measured in **atomic mass units** (abbreviated amu or simply u). By definition, 1 amu is exactly one-twelfth the mass of the neutral carbon-12 atom (not just the nucleus—the atom includes the nucleus and all 6 electrons). In terms of more familiar mass units,

$$1 \text{ amu} = 1.66 \times 10^{-27} \text{ kg} = 1.66 \times 10^{-24} \text{ g}$$

E. ATOMIC WEIGHT

Because isotopes exist, atoms of a given element can have different masses. The atomic weight refers to a weighted average of the **masses** (not the weights) of an element. The average is weighted according to the natural abundances of the various isotopic species of an element. The atomic weight can be measured in amu.

Example: 99.985499% of hydrogen occurs in the common ^{1}H isotope with a mass of 1.00782504 u. About 0.0142972% occurs as deuterium with a mass (including the electron) of 2.01410 u, and about 0.0003027% occurs as tritium with a mass of 3.01605 u. The atomic weight of hydrogen A_r(H) is the sum of the mass of each isotope multiplied by its natural abundance (x):

$$A_r(H) = m_{1H}x_{1H} + m_{2H}x_{2H} + m_{3H}x_{3H}$$
$$= (1.00782504)(0.99985499)$$
$$+ (2.01410)(0.000142972)$$
$$+ (3.01605)(0.000003027)$$
$$= 1.00797 \text{ amu}$$

NUCLEAR BINDING ENERGY AND MASS DEFECT

Every nucleus (other than $^{1}_{1}$H) has a smaller mass than the combined mass of its constituent protons and neutrons. The difference is called the **mass defect.** Scientists had difficulty explaining why this mass defect occurred until Einstein discovered the equivalence of matter and energy, embodied by the equation $E = mc^2$. The mass defect is a result of matter that has been converted to

> **DAT Synopsis**
> Atomic weight really means mass, not weight.

> **DAT Synopsis**
> The mass of a nucleus is always less than the combined masses of its constituent protons and neutrons.

energy. This energy, called **binding energy,** holds the nucleons together in the nucleus. (Note: The binding energy per nucleon peaks at iron, which implies that iron is the most stable atom. In general, intermediate-sized nuclei are more stable than large and small nuclei.)

The mass defect and binding energy of ^{4}He are calculated in the following example.

> **DAT Synopsis**
>
> Energy necessary to break up a nucleus into constituent nucleons is binding energy. It is analogous to ionization energy needed to break up a hydrogen atom into a proton and electron.

Example: Measurements of the atomic mass of a neutron and a proton yield these results:

$$proton = 1.00728 \text{ amu}$$
$$neutron = 1.00867 \text{ amu}$$

A measurement of the atomic mass of a ^{4}He nucleus yields this:

$$^4He = 4.00260 \text{ amu}$$

^{4}He consists of 2 protons and 2 neutrons, which should theoretically give a ^{4}He mass of

$$Z(m_p) + N(m_n) = 2(1.00728) + 2(1.00867)$$
$$= 4.03190 \text{ amu}$$

What is the mass defect and binding energy of this nucleus?

Solution: The difference, $4.03190 - 4.00260 = 0.02930$ amu, is the mass defect for ^{4}He and is interpreted as the conversion of mass into the binding energy of the nucleus. The rest energy of 1 amu is 932 MeV, so using $E = mc^2$, we find that $c^2 = 932$ MeV/amu. Therefore, the binding energy of ^{4}He is

$$B.E. = \Delta mc^2$$
$$= (0.02930)(932)$$
$$= 27.3 \text{ MeV}$$

NUCLEAR REACTIONS AND DECAY

> **DAT Synopsis**
>
> Fusion: Combine smaller nuclei into larger nucleus.
>
> Fission: Split larger nucleus into smaller nuclei.
>
> Both fusion and fission release energy since initial mass > final mass.

Nuclear reactions, such as fusion, fission, and radioactive decay, involve either combining or splitting the nuclei of atoms. Since the binding energy per nucleon is greatest for intermediate-sized atoms, when small atoms combine or large atoms split, a great amount of energy is released.

A. FUSION

Fusion occurs when small nuclei combine into a larger nucleus. As an example, many stars, including the sun, power themselves by fusing four hydrogen nuclei to make one helium nucleus. By this method, the sun produces 4×10^{26} J every second. Here on earth, researchers are trying to find ways to use fusion as an alternative energy source.

B. FISSION

Fission is a process in which a large nucleus splits into smaller nuclei. Spontaneous fission rarely occurs. However, by the absorption of a low-energy neutron, fission can be induced in certain nuclei. Of special interest are those fission reactions that release more neutrons, since these other neutrons will cause other atoms to undergo fission. This in turn releases more neutrons, creating a **chain reaction.** Such induced fission reactions power commercial nuclear electric-generating plants.

> Example: A fission reaction occurs when uranium-235 (U-235) absorbs a low-energy neutron, briefly forming an excited state of U-236, which then splits into xenon-140, strontium-94, and x more neutrons. In isotopic notation form the reactions are

$$\,^{235}_{92}\text{U} + \,^{1}_{0}\text{n} \longrightarrow \,^{236}_{92}\text{U} \longrightarrow \,^{140}_{54}\text{Xe} + \,^{94}_{38}\text{Sr} + x\,^{1}_{0}\text{n}$$

How many neutrons are produced in the last reaction?

> Solution: The question is asking "What is x?" By treating each arrow as an equal sign, the problem is simply asking to balance the last "equation." The mass numbers (A) on either side of each arrow must be equal. This is an application of **nucleon** or **baryon number conservation,** which says that the total number of neutrons plus protons remains the same, even if neutrons are converted to protons and vice versa, as they are in some decays. Since $235 + 1 = 236$, the first arrow is indeed balanced. To find the number of neutrons, solve for x in the last equation (arrow):

$$236 = 140 + 94 + x$$
$$x = 236 - 140 - 94$$
$$= 2$$

So two neutrons are produced in this reaction. These neutrons are free to go on and be absorbed by more ^{235}U and cause more fissioning, and the process continues in a chain reaction. Note that it really was not necessary to know that the intermediate state $^{236}_{92}$U was formed.

Some radioactive nuclei may be induced to fission via more than one **decay channel** or **decay mode.** For example, a different fission reaction may occur when uranium-235 absorbs a slow neutron and then immediately splits into barium-139, krypton-94, and three more neutrons with no intermediate state:

$$\,^{236}_{92}\text{U} + \,^{1}_{0}\text{n} \longrightarrow \,^{139}_{56}\text{Ba} + \,^{94}_{36}\text{Kr} + 3\,^{1}_{0}\text{n}$$

> **DAT Synopsis**
>
> A chain reaction means that each fission produces at least one more fission.

> **DAT Synopsis**
>
> Total mass number, A, remains unchanged in nuclear reactions.

C. RADIOACTIVE DECAY

Radioactive decay is a naturally occurring spontaneous decay of certain nuclei accompanied by the emission of specific particles. It could be classified as a certain type of fission. Radioactive decay problems are of three general types:

1. The integer arithmetic of particle and isotope species
2. Radioactive half-life problems
3. The use of exponential decay curves and decay constants

1. **Isotope Decay Arithmetic and Nucleon Conservation**

    Let the letters X and Y represent nuclear isotopes, and let us further consider the three types of decay particles and how they affect the mass number and atomic number of the **parent isotope** $^A_Z X$ and the resulting **daughter isotope** $^{A'}_{Z'} Y$ in the decay:

    $$^A_Z X \longrightarrow {}^{A'}_{Z'} Y + \text{emitted decay particle}$$

    a. **Alpha decay** is the emission of an α-particle, which is a ^{4}He nucleus that consists of two protons and two neutrons. The alpha particle is very massive (compared to a beta particle) and doubly charged. Alpha particles interact with matter very easily; hence, they do not penetrate shielding (such as lead sheets) very far.

    The emission of an α-particle means that the daughter's atomic number Z will be 2 less than the parent's atomic number, and the daughter's mass number will be 4 less than the parent's mass number. This can be expressed in two simple equations:

    $$\alpha \textbf{ decay}$$
    $$Z_{\text{daughter}} = Z_{\text{parent}} - 2$$
    $$A_{\text{daughter}} = A_{\text{parent}} - 4$$

    The generic alpha decay reaction is then:

    $$^A_Z X \longrightarrow {}^{A-4}_{Z-2} Y + \alpha$$

    Example: Suppose a parent X alpha decays into a daughter Y such that

    $$^{238}_{92} X \longrightarrow {}^{A'}_{Z'} Y + \alpha$$

    What are the mass number (A') and atomic number (Z') of the daughter isotope Y?

DAT Synopsis

....

The parent nucleus undergoes radioactive decay to produce the daughter nucleus.

DAT Synopsis

....

An α-particle is a helium nucleus with 2 protons and 2 neutrons (i.e., ^{4}He).

Solution: Since $\alpha = {}^{4}_{2}\text{He}$, balancing the mass numbers and atomic numbers is all that needs to be done:

$$238 = A' + 4$$
$$A' = 234$$
$$92 = Z' + 2$$
$$Z' = 90$$

So $A' = 234$ and $Z' = 90$. Note that it was not necessary to know the chemical species of the isotopes to do this problem. However, it would have been possible to look at the periodic table and see that $Z = 92$ means X is uranium-238 (${}^{238}_{92}\text{U}$) and that $Z = 90$ means Y is thorium-234 (${}^{234}_{90}\text{Th}$).

b. **Beta decay** is the emission of a β-particle, which is an electron given the symbol e⁻ or β⁻. Electrons do not reside in the nucleus but are emitted by the nucleus when a neutron in the nucleus decays into a proton and a β⁻ (and an antineutrino). Since an electron is singly charged and about 1,836 times lighter than a proton, the beta radiation from radioactive decay is more penetrating than alpha radiation. In some cases of induced decay, a positively charged antielectron known as a **positron** is emitted. The positron is given the symbol e⁺ or β⁺.

> **DAT Synopsis**
>
> A β⁻-particle is also called a β-particle and is just an electron.

β⁻ decay means that a neutron disappears and a proton takes its place. Hence, the parent's mass number is unchanged, and the parent's atomic number is increased by 1. In other words, the daughter's A is the same as the parent's, and the daughter's Z is one more than the parent's.

In positron decay, a proton (instead of a neutron as in β⁻ decay) splits into a positron and a neutron. Therefore, a β⁺ decay means that the parent's mass number is unchanged and the parent's atomic number is decreased by 1. In other words, the daughter's A is the same as the parent's, and the daughter's Z is one less than the parent's. In equation form:

> **DAT Synopsis**
>
> A β⁺-particle is a positron, which is a particle with same mass as electron but opposite charge.

β⁻ decay

$$Z_{\text{daughter}} = Z_{\text{parent}} + 1$$
$$A_{\text{daughter}} = A_{\text{parent}}$$

β⁺ decay

$$Z_{\text{daughter}} = Z_{\text{parent}} - 1$$
$$A_{\text{daughter}} = A_{\text{parent}}$$

> **DAT Synopsis**
>
> For both types of β-decay, A is unchanged, because you either change a neutron into a proton (β⁻-decay) or a proton into a neutron (β⁺-decay).

The generic negative beta decay reaction is as follows:

$$\ce{^{A}_{Z}X} \longrightarrow \ce{^{A}_{Z+1}Y} + \beta^-$$

The generic positive beta decay reaction is

$$\ce{^{A}_{Z}X} \longrightarrow \ce{^{A}_{Z-1}Y} + \beta^+$$

Example: Suppose a cobalt-60 nucleus beta-decays:

$$\ce{^{60}Co} \longrightarrow \ce{^{A'}_{Z'}Y} + e^-$$

What is the element Y, and what are A' and Z'?

Solution: Again, balance mass numbers:

$$60 = A' + 0$$
$$A' = 60$$

Now balance the atomic numbers, taking into account that cobalt has 27 protons (you learn this by consulting the periodic table) and that there is one more proton on the right-hand side:

$$27 = Z' - 1$$
$$Z' = 28$$

By looking at the periodic table, one finds that $Z' = 28$ is nickel:

$$Y = \ce{^{60}_{28}Ni}$$

c.   **Gamma decay** is the emission of γ–particles, which are high-energy photons. They carry no charge and simply lower the energy of the emitting (parent) nucleus without changing the mass number or the atomic number. In other words, the daughter's A is the same as the parent's, and the daughter's Z is the same as the parent's.

$$\gamma \textbf{ decay}$$

$$Z_{\text{parent}} = Z_{\text{daughter}}$$
$$A_{\text{parent}} = A_{\text{daughter}}$$

The generic gamma decay reaction is thus

$$\ce{^{A}_{Z}X}^* \longrightarrow \ce{^{A}_{Z}X} + \gamma$$

Example: Suppose a parent isotope $^{A}_{Z}X$ emits a β^- and turns into an excited state of the isotope $^{A'}_{Z'}Y*$, which then γ decays to $^{A''}_{Z''}Y$, which in turn α decays to $^{A'''}_{Z'''}W$. If W is ^{60}Fe, what is $^{A}_{Z}X$?

Solution: Since the final daughter in this chain of decay is given, it will be necessary to work backward through the reactions. By looking at the periodic table, one finds that W = Fe means $Z''' = 26$; hence, the last reaction is the following α decay:

$$^{A''}_{Z''}Y \longrightarrow {}^{60}_{26}Fe + {}^{4}_{2}He$$

By balancing the atomic numbers, you find

$$Z'' = 26 + 2 = 28$$

A balancing of the mass numbers implies

$$A'' = 60 + 4 = 64$$

The second-to-last reaction is a γ decay, which simply releases energy from the nucleus but does not alter the atomic number or the mass number of the parent. That is, $Z' = Z'' = 28$, and $A' = A'' = 64$. So the second reaction is

$$^{64}_{28}Y* \longrightarrow {}^{64}_{28}Y + \gamma$$

The first reaction was a β^+ decay that must have looked like this:

$$^{A}_{Z}X \longrightarrow {}^{64}_{28}Y* + e^+$$

Again, balance the atomic numbers:

$$Z = 28 + 1 = 29$$

You carry out a balancing of mass numbers by taking into account that a proton has disappeared on the left and reappeared as a neutron on the right, leaving mass number unchanged:

$$A = 64 + 0 = 64$$

By looking at the periodic table, you find that $Z = 29$ means that X is Cu. Since $A = 64$, that means that the solution is

$$^{A}_{Z}X = {}^{64}_{29}Cu$$

While the problem did not ask for it, it is possible again to look at the periodic table to find that $Z' = Z'' = 28$ means $Y^* = Y = Ni$. The total chain of decays can be written as follows:

$$^{64}_{29}Cu \longrightarrow {}^{64}_{28}Ni^* + \beta^+$$

$$^{64}_{28}Ni^* \longrightarrow {}^{64}_{28}Ni + \gamma$$

$$^{64}_{28}Ni \longrightarrow {}^{60}_{26}Fe + \alpha$$

d. **Electron capture**

Certain unstable radionuclides are capable of capturing an inner (K or L shell) electron that combines with a proton to form a neutron. The atomic number is now one less than the original, but the mass number remains the same. Electron capture is a rare process that is perhaps best thought of as an inverse β^- decay.

2. **Radioactive Decay Half-Life ($T_{1/2}$)**

In a collection of a great many identical radioactive isotopes, the **half-life** ($T_{1/2}$) of the sample is the time it takes for half of the sample to decay.

Example: If the half-life of a certain isotope is 4 years, what fraction of a sample of that isotope will remain after 12 years?

Solution: If 4 years is one half-life, then 12 years is three half-lives. During the first half-life—the first 4 years—half of the sample will have decayed. During the second half-life (years 4 to 8), half of the remaining half will decay, leaving one-fourth of the original. During the third and final period (years 8 to 12), half of the remaining fourth will decay, leaving one-eighth of the original sample. Thus, the fraction remaining after 3 half-lives is $(1/2)^3$ or $(1/8)$.

3. **Exponential Decay**

Let n be the number of radioactive nuclei that have not yet decayed in a sample. It turns out that the **rate** at which the nuclei decay ($\Delta n/\Delta t$) is proportional to the number that remain (n). This suggests the following equation:

$$\frac{\Delta n}{\Delta t} = -\lambda n$$

where λ is known as the **decay constant**. The solution of this equation tells us how the number of radioactive nuclei changes with time.

> **DAT Synopsis**
>
> (fraction of original nuclei remaining after n half-lives) = $(1/2)^n$.

The solution is known as an **exponential decay**:

$$n = n_0 e^{-\lambda t}$$

where n_0 is the number of undecayed nuclei at time $t = 0$. (The decay constant is related to the half-life by $\lambda = \dfrac{\ln 2}{T_{1/2}} = \dfrac{0.693}{T_{1/2}}$.)

Example: If at time $t = 0$ there is a 2 mole sample of radioactive isotopes of decay constant 2 (hour)$^{-1}$, how many nuclei remain after 45 minutes?

Solution: Since 45 minutes is 3/4 of an hour, the exponent is

$$\lambda t = 2\frac{3}{4} = \frac{6}{4} = \frac{3}{2}$$

The exponential factor will be a number smaller than 1:

$$e^{-\lambda t} = e^{-3/2} = 0.22$$

So only 0.22 or 22 percent of the original two-mole sample will remain. To find n_0, we can multiply the number of moles we have by the number of particles per mole (Avogadro's number):

$$n_0 = 2(6.02 \times 10^{23}) = 1.2 \times 10^{24}$$

From the equation that describes exponential decay, you can calculate the number that remain after 45 minutes:

$$n = n_0 e^{-\lambda t}$$
$$= (1.2 \times 10^{24})(0.22)$$
$$= 2.6 \times 10^{23} \text{ particles}$$

ORGANIC CHEMISTRY

NOMENCLATURE

Nomenclature, the set of accepted conventions for naming compounds, is crucial to a discussion of organic chemistry. The rules of nomenclature presented in this chapter are for general cases only. More specific examples will be discussed in the chapters dealing with particular types of compounds.

You may see specific nomenclature questions on the DAT such as "Name the following compound," or "Which structure represents the following named compound?" But more importantly, nomenclature represents the basic language of organic chemistry. If you don't know it, you may feel as though you're taking a test in a foreign language—which, in a way, you would be!

> **DAT Synopsis**
>
> You must memorize the names of the four simplest alkanes:
> - Meth-
> - Eth-
> - Prop-
> - But-

ALKANES

Alkanes are the simplest organic molecules, consisting only of carbon and hydrogen atoms held together by single bonds.

A. STRAIGHT-CHAIN ALKANES

The names of the four simplest alkanes are

CH_4	CH_3CH_3	$CH_3CH_2CH_3$	$CH_3CH_2CH_2CH_3$
methane	ethane	propane	butane

The names of the longer-chain alkanes consist of prefixes derived from the Greek root for the number of carbon atoms, with the ending **-ane**.

C_5H_{12} = **pent**ane C_9H_{20} = **non**ane
C_6H_{14} = **hex**ane $C_{10}H_{22}$ = **dec**ane
C_7H_{16} = **hept**ane $C_{11}H_{24}$ = **undec**ane
C_8H_{18} = **oct**ane $C_{12}H_{26}$ = **dodec**ane

These prefixes are applicable to more complex organic molecules and should be memorized.

> **DAT Synopsis**
>
> All straight-chain alkanes have the general formula C_nH_{2n+2} (n is an integer).

> **DAT Synopsis**
>
> Straight-chain alkanes are fat soluble (i.e., nonpolar).

B. BRANCHED-CHAIN ALKANES

The International Union of Pure and Applied Chemistry (IUPAC) has proposed a set of simple rules for naming complex molecules. This basic system can be used to name all classes of organic compounds. Throughout these notes, the IUPAC names will be listed as the primary name, and common names will appear in parentheses.

1. **Find the longest chain in the compound.**
   The longest continuous carbon chain within the compound is taken as the backbone. If there are two or more chains of equal length, the most highly substituted chain takes precedence. The longest chain may not be obvious from the structural formula as it is drawn. For example, the backbone shown in Figure 1.1 is an octane (it contains eight carbon atoms).

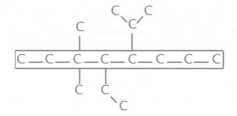

Figure 1.1

2. **Number the chain.**
   Number the chain from one end in such a way that the lowest set of numbers is obtained for the substituents.

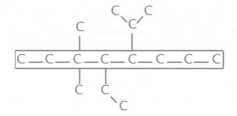

NOT

Figure 1.2

3. **Name the substituents.**
   Substituents are named according to their appropriate prefix with the ending **-yl**. More complex substituents are named as derivatives of the longest chain in the group.

CH_3-	CH_3CH_2-	$CH_3CH_2CH_2-$
methyl	ethyl	*n*-propyl

The prefix *n*- in the above example indicates an unbranched ("normal") compound. There are special names for some common branched alkanes, and these are usually used in the naming of substituents.

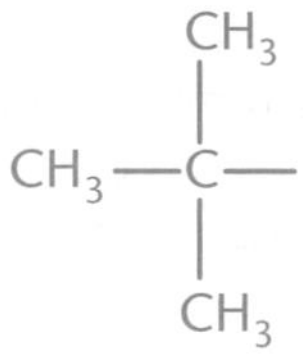

t-butyl

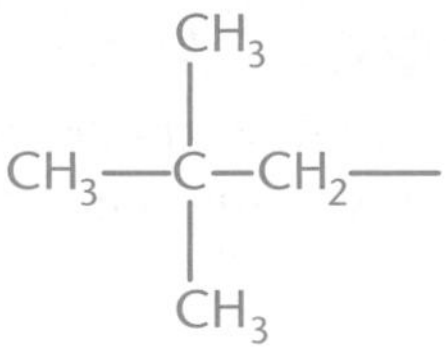

neopentyl

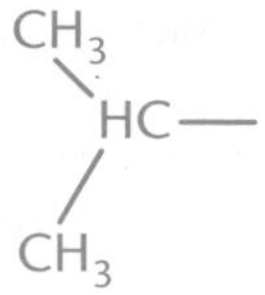

isopropyl

DAT Synopsis

You should memorize these common structures.

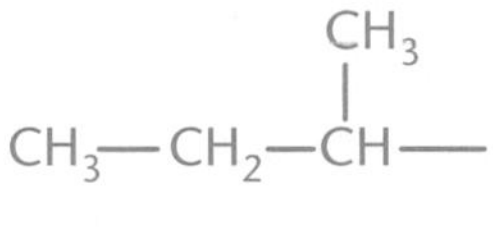

sec-butyl

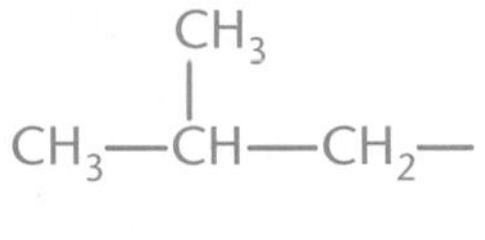

isobutyl

Figure 1.3

If there are two or more equivalent groups, the prefixes **di-**, **tri-**, **tetra-**, etc. are used.

4. **Assign a number to each substituent.**
   Each substituent is assigned a number to identify its point of attachment to the principal chain. If the prefixes **di-**, **tri-**, **tetra-**, etc. are used, a number is still necessary for each individual group.

5. **Complete the name.**
   List the substituents in alphabetical order with their corresponding numbers. Prefixes such as di-, tri-, etc. as well as the hyphenated prefixes (*tert-* [or *t-*], *sec-*, *n-*) are ignored in alphabetizing. In contrast, **cyclo-**, **iso-**, and **neo-** are considered part of the group name and are alphabetized. Commas should be placed between numbers, and dashes should be placed between numbers and words. Figure 1.4 shown an example.

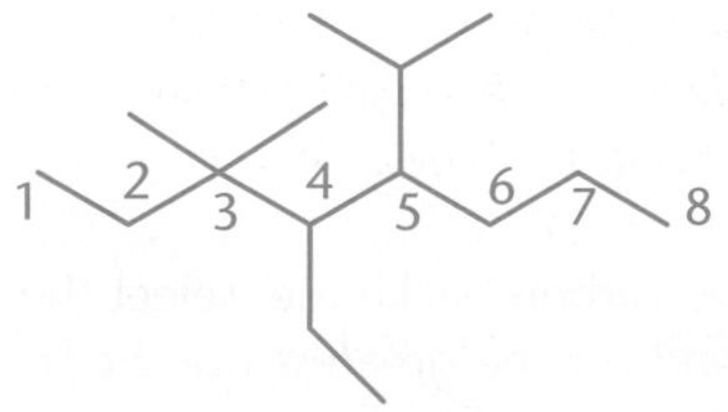

4-ethyl-5-isopropyl-3,3-dimethyl octane

Figure 1.4

You may also need to indicate the isomer you are describing—e.g., *cis* or *trans*, *R* or *S*, etc. Isomers will be discussed in detail in chapter 2.

C. CYCLOALKANES

Alkanes can form rings. These are named according to the number of carbon atoms in the ring with the prefix **cyclo-**.

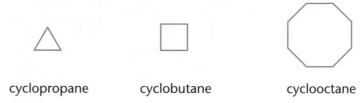

cyclopropane   cyclobutane   cyclooctane

Figure 1.5

Substituted cycloalkanes are named as derivatives of the parent cycloalkane. The substituents are named, and the carbon atoms are numbered around the ring *starting from the point of greatest substitution*. Again, the goal is to provide the lowest series of numbers, as in rule number 2 above.

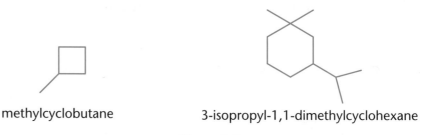

methylcyclobutane   3-isopropyl-1,1-dimethylcyclohexane

Figure 1.6

MORE COMPLICATED MOLECULES

Organic molecules that are more complicated than simple alkanes can also be named using this five-step process, with a few additional considerations.

MULTIPLE BONDS
A. ALKENES

Alkenes (or **olefins**) are compounds containing carbon-carbon double bonds. The nomenclature rules are essentially the same as for alkanes, except that the ending **-ene** is used rather than **-ane**. (Exceptions: The common names *ethylene* and *propylene,* are used preferentially over the IUPAC names *ethene* and *propene*).

When identifying the carbon backbone, select the longest chain that contains the double bond (or the greatest number of double bonds, if more than one is present).

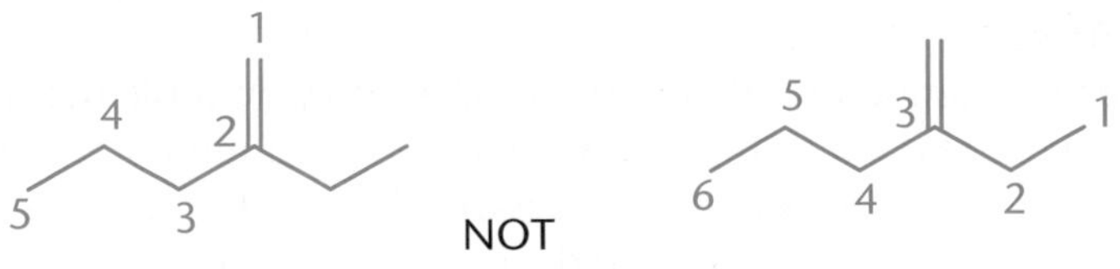

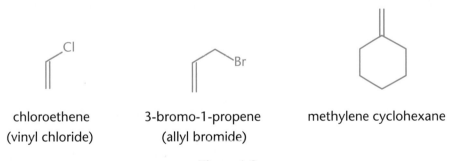

NOT

Figure 1.7

Number the backbone so that the double bond receives the lowest number possible. Remember that multiple double bonds must be named using the prefixes di-, tri-, etc. and that each must receive a number. Also, you may need to name the configurational isomer (*cis/trans*, *Z/E*). This topic will be discussed further in chapter 2.

Substituents are named as they are for alkanes, and their positions are specified by the number of the backbone carbon atom to which they are attached.

Frequently, an alkene group must be named as a substituent. In these cases, the systematic names may be used, but common names are more popular. **Vinyl-** derivatives are monosubstituted ethylenes (**ethenyl-**), and **allyl**-derivatives are propylenes substituted at the C3 position (**2-propenyl**). **Methylene** refers to the –CH_2 group.

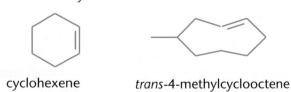

| chloroethene | 3-bromo-1-propene | methylene cyclohexane |
| (vinyl chloride) | (allyl bromide) | |

Figure 1.8

B. CYCLOALKENES

Cycloalkenes are named like cycloalkanes but with the suffix **-ene** rather than **-ane**. If there is only one double bond and no other substituents, a number is not necessary.

cyclohexene   *trans*-4-methylcyclooctene

Figure 1.9

C. ALKYNES

Alkynes are compounds that possess carbon-carbon triple bonds. The suffix **-yne** replaces *-ane* in the parent alkane. The position of the triple bond is indicated by a number when necessary. The common name for ethyne is **acetylene,** and this name is used almost exclusively.

> **DAT Synopsis**
>
> Regardless of how they are drawn, triple bonds are linear.

$HC\equiv CH$

ethyne
(acetylene)

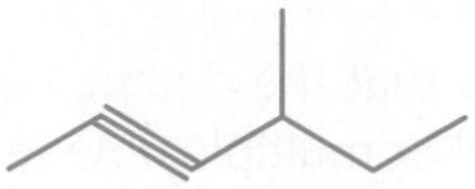

4-methyl-2-hexyne

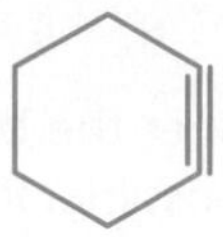

cyclohexyne

Figure 1.10

SUBSTITUTED ALKANES

A. HALOALKANES

Compounds that contain a halogen substituent are named. The appendages are numbered and alphabetized as alkyl groups are treated. Notice that the presence of the halide does not dramatically affect the numbering of the chain—you should still proceed so that substituents receive the lowest possible numbers. Figure 1.11 shows two examples.

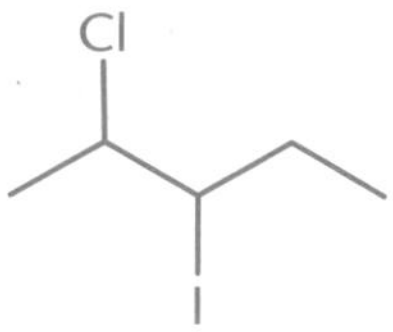

2-chloro-3-iodopentane

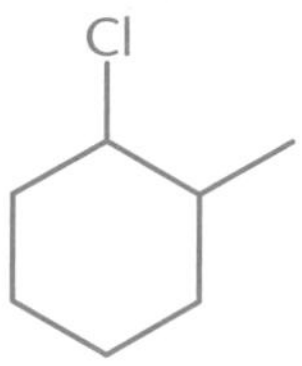

1-chloro-2-methylcyclohexane

Figure 1.11

Alternatively, the haloalkane may be named as an **alkyl halide.** In this system, chloroethane is called **ethyl chloride**. Other examples are shown in Figure 1.12.

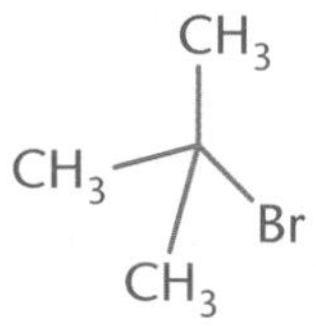

2-bromo-2-methylpropane
(*t*-butyl bromide)

2-iodopropane
(isopropyl iodide)

Figure 1.12

B. ALCOHOLS

In the IUPAC system, **alcohols** are named by replacing the *-e* of the corresponding alkane with **-ol**. The chain is numbered so that the carbon attached to the hydroxyl group (–OH) receives the lowest number possible. In compounds that possess a multiple bond and a hydroxyl group, numerical priority is given to the carbon attached to the –OH.

> **DAT Synopsis**
>
> –OH has priority over a multiple bond when numbering the chain.

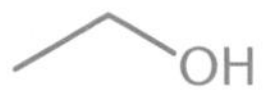

ethanol

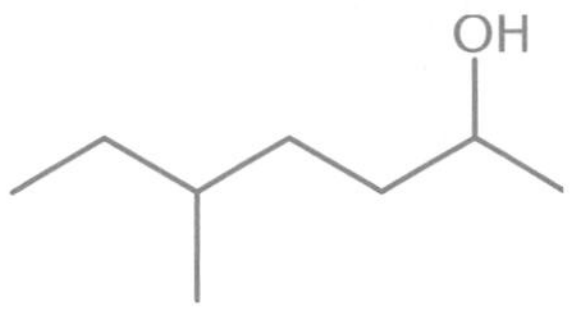

5-methyl-2-heptanol

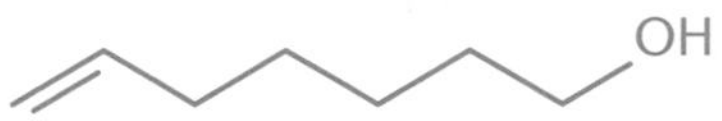

hept-6-en-1-ol

Figure 1.13

A common system of nomenclature exists for alcohols in which the name of the alkyl group is combined with the word *alcohol*. These common names are used for simple alcohols. For example, methanol may be named "methyl alcohol," while 2-propanol may also be named "isopropyl alcohol."

Molecules with two hydroxyl groups are called **diols** (or **glycols**) and are named with the suffix **-diol**. Two numbers are necessary to locate the two functional groups. Diols with hydroxyl groups on adjacent carbons are referred to as **vicinal**, and diols with hydroxyl groups on the same carbon are **geminal**. Geminal diols (also called **hydrates**) are not commonly observed because they spontaneously lose water **(dehydrate)** to produce carbonyl compounds (containing C=O; see chapter 8).

> **DAT Synopsis**
>
> Ethers may have the prefix *alkoxy–* or be given a common name (e.g., ethyl methyl ether).

C. ETHERS

In the IUPAC system, **ethers** are named as derivatives of alkanes, and the larger alkyl group is chosen as the backbone. The ether functionality is specified as an **alkoxy-** prefix, indicating the presence of an ether (*-oxy-*), and the corresponding smaller alkyl group (*alk-*). The chain is numbered to give the ether the lowest position. Common names for ethers are frequently used. They are derived by naming the two alkyl groups in alphabetical order and adding the word *ether*. The generic term *ether* refers to diethyl ether, a commonly used solvent.

For **cyclic ethers**, numbering of the ring begins at the oxygen and proceeds to provide the lowest numbers for the substituents. Three-membered rings are termed **oxiranes** by IUPAC, although they are commonly called **epoxides**.

DAT Synopsis

Cyclic ethers with three members are *epoxides*.

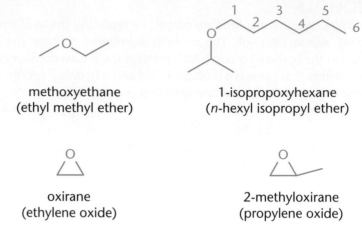

methoxyethane
(ethyl methyl ether)

1-isopropoxyhexane
(*n*-hexyl isopropyl ether)

oxirane
(ethylene oxide)

2-methyloxirane
(propylene oxide)

Figure 1.14

tetrahydrofuran
(THF)

Figure 1.15

D. ALDEHYDES AND KETONES

Aldehydes are named according to the longest chain containing the aldehyde functional group. The suffix **-al** replaces the *-e* of the corresponding alkane. The carbonyl carbon receives the lowest number, although numbers are not always necessary since, by definition, an aldehyde is terminal and receives the number 1.

n-butanal

5,5-dimethylhexanal

Figure 1.16

DAT Synopsis

An aldehyde is a terminal functional group: It defines the C–1 of the backbone.

The common names *formaldehyde*, *acetaldehyde*, and *propionaldehyde* are used almost exclusively instead of the IUPAC names *methanal*, *ethanal*, and *propanal*, respectively.

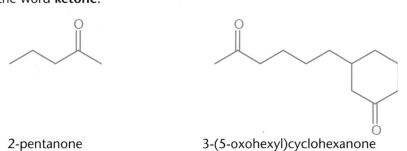

methanal
(formaldehyde)

ethanal
(acetaldehyde)

propanal
(propionaldehyde)

Figure 1.17

Ketones are named analogously, with **-one** as a suffix. The carbonyl group has to be assigned the lowest possible number. In complex molecules, the carbonyl group can be named as a prefix with the term **oxo-**. Alternatively, the individual alkyl groups may be listed in alphabetical order, followed by the word **ketone**.

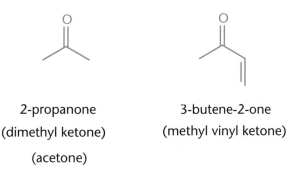

2-pentanone

3-(5-oxohexyl)cyclohexanone

2-propanone
(dimethyl ketone)
(acetone)

3-butene-2-one
(methyl vinyl ketone)

Figure 1.18

A commonly used alternative to the numerical designation of substituents is to term the carbon atom adjacent to the carbonyl carbon as α and the carbon atoms successively along the chain as β, γ, δ, etc. This system is encountered with dicarbonyl compounds and halocarbonyl compounds.

E. CARBOXYLIC ACIDS

Carboxylic acids are named with the ending **-oic** and the word **acid** replacing the *-e* ending of the corresponding alkane. Carboxylic acids are terminal functional groups and, like aldehydes, are numbered one (1). The common names formic acid (methanoic acid), acetic acid (ethanoic acid), and propionic acid (propanoic acid) are used almost exclusively.

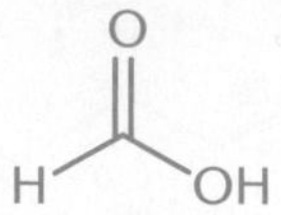

| methanoic acid | ethanoic acid | propanoic acid |
| (formic acid) | (acetic acid) | (propionic acid) |

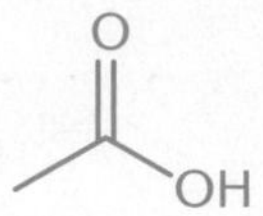

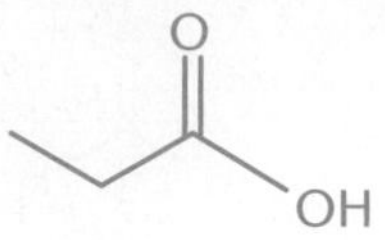

Figure 1.19

F. AMINES

The longest chain attached to the nitrogen atom is taken as the backbone. For simple compounds, name the alkane and replace the final *e* with *amine*. More complex molecules are often named using the prefix *amino-*.

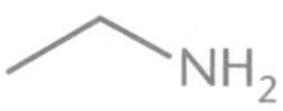

ethanamine 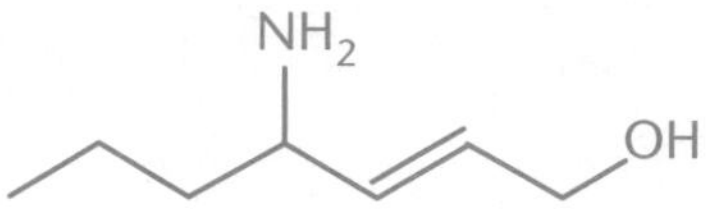   4-aminohept-2-en-1-ol

Figure 1.20

To specify the location of an additional alkyl group that is attached to the nitrogen, the prefix *N-* is used, as shown in Figure 1.21.

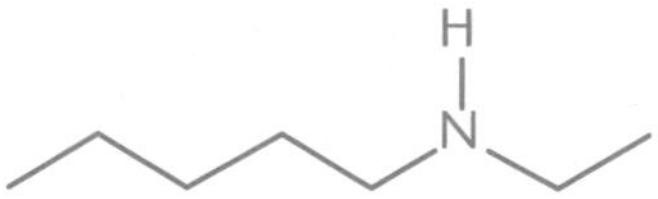

N-ethylpentanamine

(ethylpentylamine)

Figure 1.21

DAT Synopsis

When additional alkyl groups are attached to the nitrogen, use the prefix *N-*.

SUMMARY OF FUNCTIONAL GROUPS

Table 1.1 lists the major functional groups you need to know.

Table 1.1

Functional Group	Structure	IUPAC Prefix	IUPAC Suffix
Carboxylic acid	$R-\overset{O}{\underset{OH}{C}}$	carboxy-	-oic acid
Ester	$R-\overset{O}{\underset{OR}{C}}$	alkoxycarbonyl-	-oate
Acyl halide	$R-\overset{O}{\underset{X}{C}}$	halocarbonyl-	-oyl halide
Amide	$R-\overset{O}{\underset{NH_2}{C}}$	amido-	-amide
Nitrile/Cyanide	$RC\equiv N$	cyano-	-nitrile
Aldehyde	$R-\overset{O}{\underset{H}{C}}$	oxo-	-al
Ketone	$R-\overset{O}{\underset{R}{C}}$	oxo-	-one
Alcohol	ROH	hydroxy-	-ol
Thiol	RSH	sulfhydryl-	-thiol
Amine	RNH_2	amino-	-amine
Imine	$R_2C=NR'$	imino-	-imine
Ether	ROR	alkoxy-	-ether
Sulfide	R_2S	alkylthio-	
Halide	-I, -Br, -Cl, -F	halo-	
Nitro	RNO_2	nitro-	
Azide	RN_3	azido-	
Diazo	RN_2^+	diazo-	

DAT Synopsis

More complex molecules can also be named with the same five steps, with a few additional considerations:

1. Multiple bonds should be on the main carbon backbone whenever possible.
2. –OH is a high-priority functional group, placed above multiple bonds in numbering.
3. Haloalkanes, ethers, and ketones are often given common names (e.g., methyl chloride, ethyl methyl ether, diethyl ketone).
4. Aldehydes and carboxylic acids are terminal functional groups. If present, they define C–1 of the carbon chain (taking precedence over hydroxy, –OH, or multiple bonds).
5. Remember to specify the isomer, if relevant (such as *cis* or *trans*, *R* or *S*, etc.).

## 2

ISOMERS

Isomers are chemical compounds that have the same molecular formula but differ in structure—that is, in their atomic connectivity, rotational orientation, or three-dimensional position of their atoms. Isomers may be extremely similar, sharing most or all of their physical and chemical properties, or they may be very different.

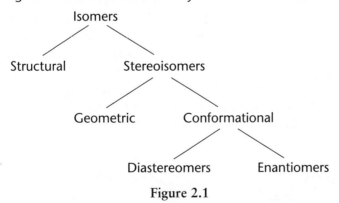

Note that geometric isomers are actually a class of diastereomers.

Figure 2.1

STRUCTURAL ISOMERISM

Structural isomers are compounds that share only their molecular formula. Because their atomic connections may be completely different, they often have very different chemical and physical properties (such as melting point, boiling point, solubility, etc.). For example, five different structures exist for compounds with the formula C_6H_{14}.

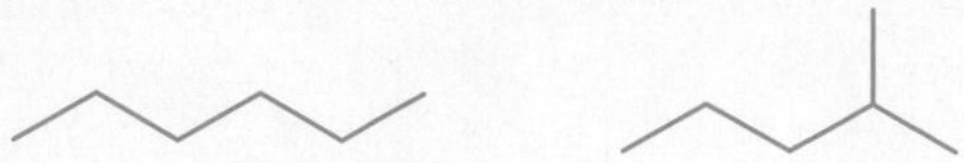

n-hexene 2-methylpentane

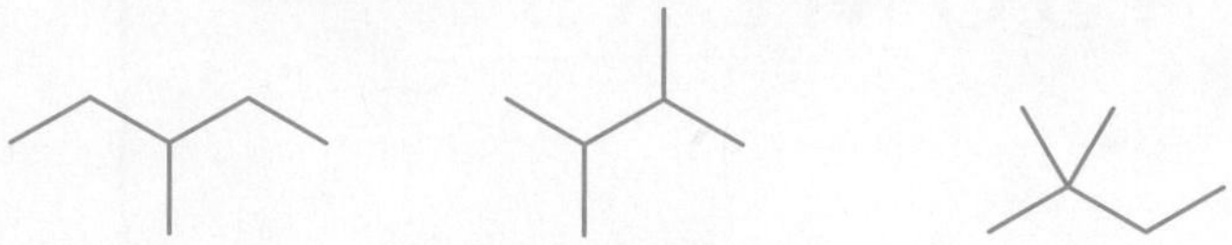

3-methylpentane 2,3-methylpentane 2,2-methylpentane

Figure 2.2

All have the same formula, but they differ in their carbon framework and in the number and type of atoms bonded to each other.

STEREOISOMERISM

> **DAT Synopsis**
>
> Stereoisomers have the same atomic connections, but the atoms are arranged differently in space.

Stereoisomers are compounds that differ from each other only in the way that their atoms are oriented in space. Geometric isomers; enantiomers, diastereomers, and *meso* compounds; and conformational isomers all fall under this heading.

A. GEOMETRIC ISOMERS

> **DAT Synopsis**
>
> Geometric isomers differ in their arrangement of atoms around a double bond. They may have different physical properties, such as melting and boiling points. However, they tend to have quite similar chemical reactivity.

Geometric isomers are compounds that differ in the position of substituents attached to a double bond. If two substituents are on the same side, the double bond is called ***cis***. If they are on opposite sides, it is a ***trans*** double bond.

For compounds with polysubstituted double bonds, the situation can be confusing, and an alternative method of naming is employed. The highest-priority substituent attached to each double-bonded carbon has to be determined: The higher the atomic number, the higher the priority, and if the atomic numbers are equal, priority is determined by the substituents of these atoms. The alkene is called (Z) (from German *zusammen*, meaning together) if the two highest-priority substituents on each carbon lie on the same side of the double bond and (E) (from German *entgegen*, meaning opposite) if they are on opposite sides.

> **KAPLAN EXCLUSIVE**
>
> Z = zame zide (same side)
>
> E = epposite (opposite sides)

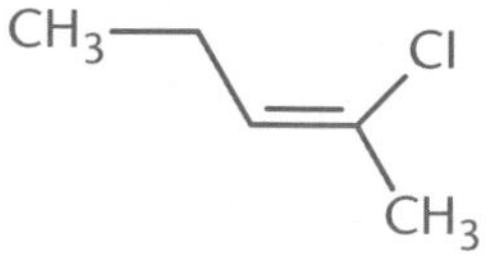

(Z)-2-chloro-2-pentene

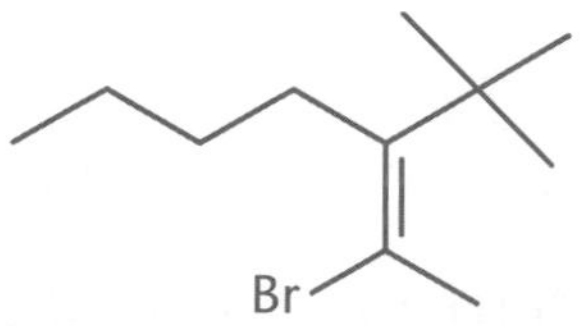

(E)-2-bromo-3-*t*-butyl-2-heptene

Figure 2.3

B. CHIRALITY

An object that is not superimposable upon its mirror image is called **chiral**. Familiar chiral objects are your right and left hands. Although essentially identical, they differ in their ability to fit into a right-handed glove. They are mirror images of each other yet cannot be superimposed. **Achiral** objects are mirror images that can be superimposed; for example, the letter *A* is identical to its mirror image and therefore achiral.

DAT Synopsis

Chirality = handedness. Nonsuperimposable mirror images exist—like your right and left hands.

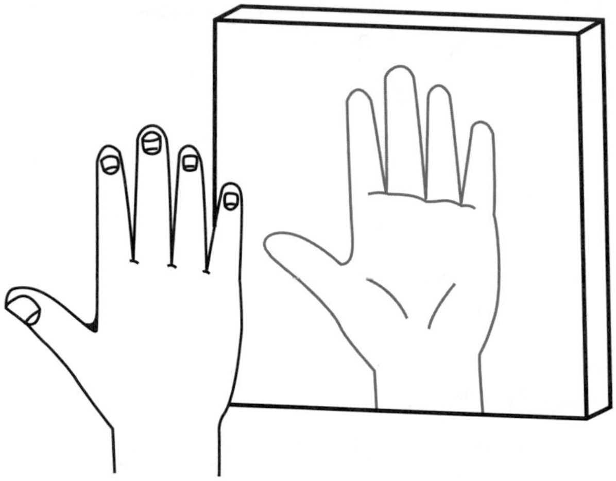

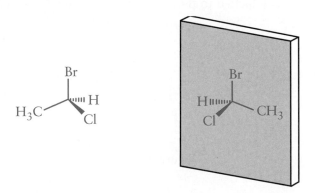

Figure 2.4

In organic chemistry, chirality is most frequently encountered when carbon atoms have four different substituents. Such a carbon atom is called *asymmetric* because it lacks a plane or point of symmetry. For example, the C–1 carbon atom in 1-bromo-1-chloroethane has four different substituents. The molecule is chiral because it is not superimposable on its mirror image. Chiral objects that are nonsuperimposable mirror images are called **enantiomers** and are a specific type of stereoisomer.

DAT Synopsis

A carbon must have four different substituents to be a chiral center.

Figure 2.5

A carbon atom with only three different substituents, such as 1,1-dibromoethane, has a plane of symmetry and is therefore achiral. A simple 180° rotation along the *y*-axis allows the compound to be superimposed upon its mirror image.

DAT Synopsis

Rotating a molecule in space does not change its chirality.

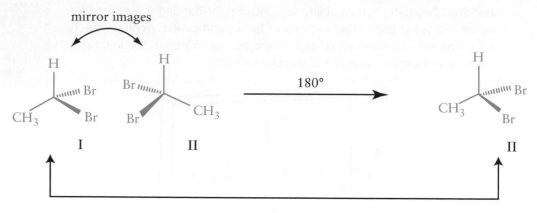

mirror images

I   II   180°   II

Superimposable

Figure 2.6

1. **Relative and Absolute Configuration**

   The **configuration** is the spatial arrangement of the atoms or groups of a stereoisomer. The **relative configuration** of a chiral molecule is its configuration in relation to another chiral molecule. The **absolute configuration** of a chiral molecule describes the spatial arrangement of these atoms or groups. There is a set sequence to determine the absolute configuration of a molecule at a single chiral center.

   Step 1:

   Assign priority to the four substituents, looking only at the first atom that is directly attached to the chiral center. Higher atomic number takes precedence over lower atomic number. If the atomic numbers are equal, then priority is determined by the substituents attached to these atoms. See the example in Figure 2.7.

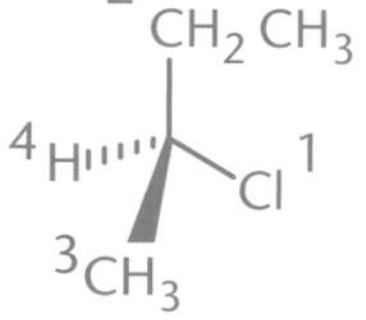

Figure 2.7

Step 2:

Orient the molecule in space so that the line of sight proceeds down the bond from the asymmetric carbon atom (the chiral center) to the substituent with lowest priority. The three substituents with highest priority should radiate from the asymmetric atom like the spokes of a wheel.

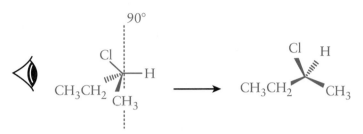

Figure 2.8

Step 3:

Proceeding from highest priority (#1) on down, determine the order of substituents around the wheel as either clockwise or counterclockwise. If the order is clockwise, the asymmetric atom is called **R** (from Latin *rectus,* meaning right). If it is counterclockwise, it is called **S** (from Latin *sinister,* meaning left).

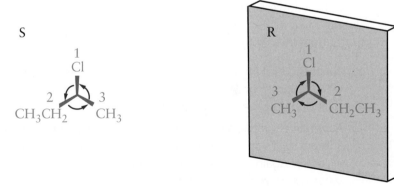

Figure 2.9

Step 4:

Provide a full name for the compound. The terms *R* and *S* are put in parentheses and separated from the rest of the name by a dash. If there is more than one asymmetric carbon, location is specified by a number preceding the *R* or *S* within the parentheses, without a dash.

2. Fischer Projections

A three-dimensional molecule can be conveniently represented in two dimensions in a **Fischer projection**. In this system, horizontal lines indicate bonds that project out from the plane of the page, while vertical lines indicate bonds behind the plane of the page. The point of intersection of the lines represents a carbon atom. They can be interconverted by interchanging any two pairs of substituents or by rotating the projection in the plane of the page by 180°. If only one pair of substituents is interchanged, or if the molecule is rotated by 90°, the mirror image of the original compound is obtained.

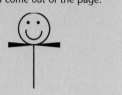

Figure 2.10

This provides another way to determine the chirality at a chiral center. If the lowest-priority substituent is on the vertical axis, it is already pointing away from you. Simply picture moving from #1 → #2 → #3, and you'll be able to name the center.

However, if the lowest-priority substituent is on the horizontal axis, it is pointing towards you, so the situation is trickier. Here are some ways to handle this situation:

1) Go ahead and imagine rotating from #1 → #2 → #3. Obtain a designation (*R* or *S*). The *true* designation will be the opposite of what you have just obtained.

2) Alternatively, make a single switch—move the low-priority substituent so that it is on the vertical axis. Obtain the designation (*R* or *S*). Again, the *true* designation will be the opposite of what you have just obtained.

3) Another approach is to make two switches or interconversions—that is, move the low-priority atom to the vertical axis and "trade" some other pair of atoms at the same time. This new molecule has the same configuration as the molecule you started with. So you can go ahead and determine the correct designation right away.

3. Optical Activity

Enantiomers have identical chemical and physical properties with one exception: **optical activity**. A compound is optically active if it has the ability to rotate plane-polarized light. Ordinary light is unpolarized. It consists of waves vibrating in all possible planes perpendicular to its direction of motion. A polarizer allows light waves oscillating only in a particular direction to pass, producing plane-polarized light.

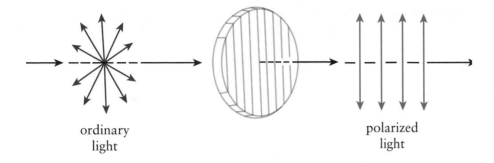

ordinary
light

polarized
light

Figure 2.11

If plane-polarized light is passed through an optically active compound, the orientation of the plane is rotated by an angle α. The enantiomer of this compound will rotate light by the same amount but in the opposite direction. A compound that rotates the plane of polarized light to the right, or clockwise (from the point of view of an observer seeing the light approach), is **dextrorotatory** and is indicated by (+). A compound that rotates light toward the left, or counterclockwise, is **levorotatory** and is labeled (–). The direction of rotation cannot be determined from the structure of a molecule and must be determined experimentally.

The amount of rotation depends on the number of molecules that a light wave encounters. This depends on two factors: the concentration of the optically active compound and the length of the tube through which the light passes. Chemists have set standard conditions of 1 g/ml for concentration and 1 dm for length to compare the optical activities of different compounds. Rotations measured at different concentrations and tube lengths can be converted to a standardized **specific rotation** (α) using the following equation:

$$\text{specific rotation } ([\alpha]) = \frac{\text{observed rotation}(\alpha)}{\text{concentration (g/ml)} \times \text{length (dm)}}$$

A **racemic mixture**, or **racemic modification**, is a mixture of equal concentrations of both the (+) and (–) enantiomers. The rotations cancel each other and no optical activity is observed.

C. OTHER CHIRAL COMPOUNDS

1. Diastereomers

For any molecule with n chiral centers, there are 2^n possible stereoisomers. Thus, if a compound has two chiral carbon atoms, it has four possible stereoisomers (see Figure 2.12).

Bridge

This equation can be rewritten as

$$\alpha = [\alpha] \times \text{conc} \times \text{length}$$

Notice how similar this equation is to Beer's Law. (See chapter 13.)

DAT Synopsis

A racemic mixture displays no optical activity.

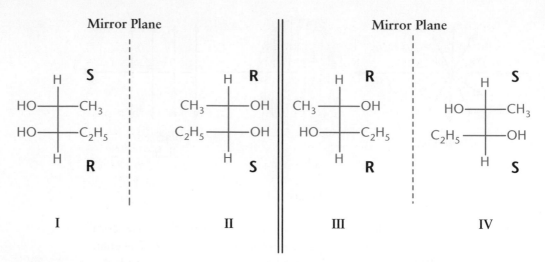

Figure 2.12

DAT Synopsis

Diastereomers may have different physical properties (such as solubility) and can therefore be separated by physical means.

I and II are mirror images of each other and are therefore enantiomers. Similarly, III and IV are enantiomers. However, I and III are not. They are stereoisomers that are not mirror images, so they are called **diastereomers**. Notice that other combinations of nonmirror image stereoisomers are also diastereomeric. Hence I and IV, II and III, I and III, and II and IV are all pairs of diastereomers.

DAT Synopsis

Meso compounds have a mirror image that is superimposable. Thus, they are not optically active.

KAPLAN EXCLUSIVE

MeSo compounds have a Mirror plane of Symmetry.

2. ***Meso* Compounds**

The criterion for optical activity of a molecule containing a single chiral center is that it has no plane of symmetry. The same applies to a molecule with two or more chiral centers. If a plane of symmetry exists, the molecule is not optically active, even though it possesses chiral centers. Such a molecule is called a *meso* compound. Figure 2.13 shows some examples.

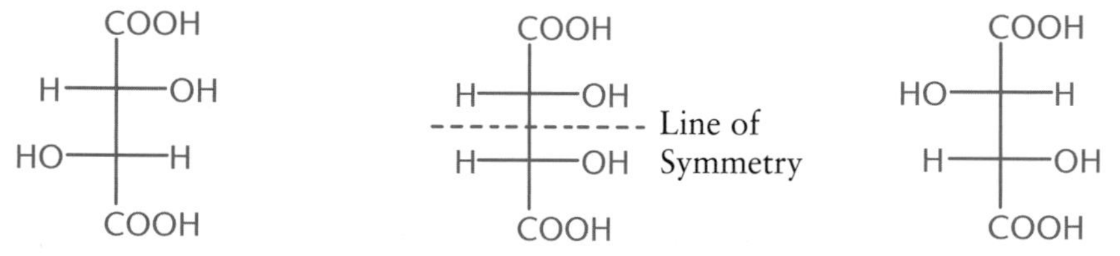

L-tartaric acid *Meso*-tartaric acid *D*-tartaric acid

Figure 2.13

DAT Synopsis

See chapter 14 for explanation of *D* versus. *L* configurations.

D- and *L*-tartaric acid are both optically active, but *meso*-tartaric acid has a plane of symmetry and is not optically active. Although *meso*-tartaric acid has two chiral carbon atoms, the lack of optical activity is a function of the molecule as a whole.

D. CONFORMATIONAL ISOMERISM

Conformational isomers are compounds that differ only by rotation about one or more single bonds. Essentially, these isomers represent the same compound in a slightly different position—analogous to a person who may be either standing up or sitting down. These different conformations can be seen when the molecule is depicted in a **Newman projection,** in which the line of sight extends along a carbon-carbon bond axis. The conformations are encountered as the molecule is rotated about this axis. The classic example for demonstrating conformational isomerism in a straight chain is *n*-butane. In a Newman projection, the line of sight extends through the C2–C3 bond axis.

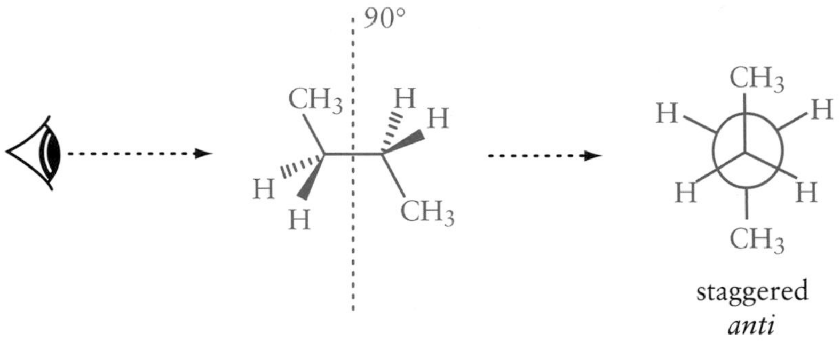

staggered
anti

Figure 2.14

1. **Straight-Chain Conformations**
   The most stable conformation is when the two methyl groups (C1 and C4) are oriented 180° from each other. There is no overlap of atoms along the line of sight (besides C2 and C3), so the molecule is said to be in a **staggered** conformation. Specifically, it is called the *anti* conformation, because the two methyl groups are antiperiplanar to each other. This particular orientation is very stable and thus represents an energy minimum because all atoms are far apart, minimizing repulsive steric interactions.

   The other type of staggered conformation, called *gauche,* occurs when the two methyl groups are 60° apart. To convert from the *anti* to the *gauche* conformation, the molecule must pass through an **eclipsed** conformation, in which the two methyl groups are 120° apart and overlap with the H atoms on the adjacent carbon. When the two methyl groups overlap with each other, the molecule is said to be **totally eclipsed** and is in its highest energy state.

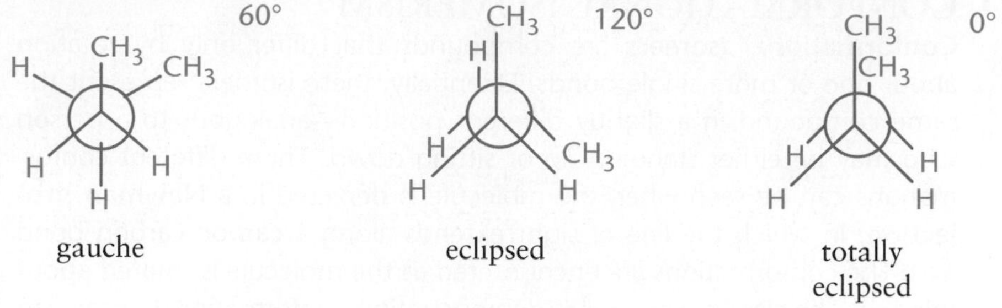

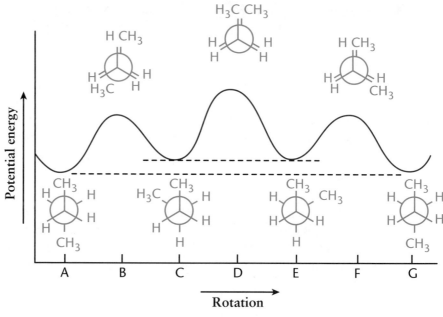

Figure 2.15

DAT Synopsis

Notice that the *anti* isomer has the lowest energy, while the totally eclipsed isomer has the highest energy.

A plot of potential energy versus the degree of rotation about the C2–C3 bond shows the relative minima and maxima the molecule encounters throughout its various conformations.

Figure 2.16

It is important to note that these barriers are rather small (3–4 kcal/mol) and are easily overcome at room temperature. Very low temperatures will slow conformational interconversion. If the molecules do not possess sufficient energy to cross the energy barrier, they may not rotate at all.

2. **Cyclic Conformations**
   a. **Strain energies**

   In cycloalkanes, ring strain arises from three factors: angle strain, torsional strain, and nonbonded strain. Angle strain results when bond angles deviate from their ideal values, torsional strain results when cyclic molecules must assume conformations that have eclipsed interactions, and nonbonded strain (van der Waals repulsion) results when atoms or groups compete for the same space. To alleviate these three types of strain, cycloalkanes attempt to adopt nonplanar conformations. Cyclobutane puckers into a slight V shape; cyclopentane adopts what is called the **envelope** conformation; and cyclohexane exists mainly in three conformations called the **chair**, the **boat**, and the **twist** or **skew-boat** (see Figure 2.17).

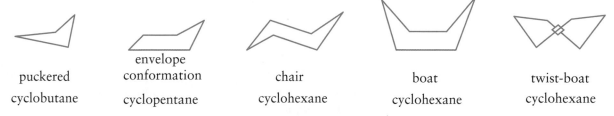

| puckered cyclobutane | envelope conformation cyclopentane | chair cyclohexane | boat cyclohexane | twist-boat cyclohexane |

Figure 2.17. Conformations of Cyclic Hydrocarbons

b. **Cyclohexane**
   i. **Unsubstituted**
   The most stable conformation of cyclohexane is the chair conformation. In this conformation, all three types of strain are eliminated. The hydrogen atoms that are perpendicular to the plane of the ring are called axial, and those parallel are called equatorial. The axial-equatorial orientations alternate around the ring.

   The boat conformation is adopted when the chair "flips" and converts to another chair. In such a process, hydrogen atoms that were equatorial become axial, and vice versa, in the new chair. In the boat conformation, all of the atoms are eclipsed, creating a high-energy state. To avoid this strain, the boat can twist into a slightly more stable form called the twist or skew-boat conformation.

   ii. **Monosubstituted**
   The interconversion between the two chairs can be slowed or even prevented if a sterically bulky group is attached to the ring. The equatorial position is favored over the axial position because of steric repulsion with other axial substituents. Hence, a large group, such as *t*-butyl, can lock the molecule in one conformation.

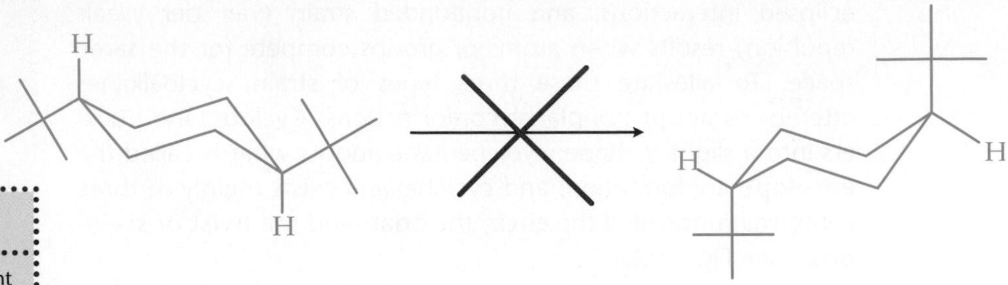

DAT Synopsis

A bulky substituent can prevent the ring from adapting certain conformations.

Figure 2.18

iii. Disubstituted

Different isomers can exist for disubstituted cycloalkanes. If both substituents are located on the same side of the ring, the molecule is called *cis*; if the two groups are on opposite sides of the ring, it is called *trans*.

DAT Synopsis

Cis and *trans* apply to cycloalkanes too!

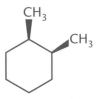

cis-1,2-dimethylcyclohexane

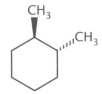

trans-1,2-dimethylcyclohexane

Figure 2.19

In *trans*-1,4-dimethylcyclohexane, both of the methyl groups are equatorial in one chair conformation and axial in the other, but in either case, they point in opposite directions relative to the plane of the ring.

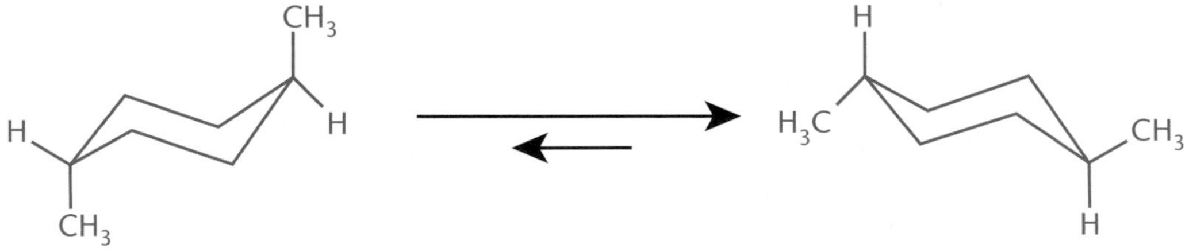

trans-1,4-dimethylcyclohexane

Figure 2.20

## 3

BONDING

As we discussed in General Chemistry chapter 3, there are two types of chemical bonds: **ionic**, in which an electron is transferred from one atom to another, and **covalent**, in which pairs of electrons are shared between two atoms. In organic chemistry, it is important to understand the details of covalent bonding, as these play a crucial role in determining the properties and reactions of organic compounds.

ATOMIC ORBITALS

The first three quantum numbers, n, ℓ, and m, describe the size, shape, and number of the atomic orbitals an element possesses. The number n, which can equal 1, 2, 3, . . . , corresponds to the energy levels in an atom and is essentially a measure of size. Within each electron shell, there can be several types of orbitals (s, p, d, f, g, . . . corresponding to the quantum numbers $\ell = 0$, 1, 2, 3, 4, . . .).

Each type of atomic orbital has a specific shape. An s-orbital is spherical and symmetrical, centered around the nucleus. A p-orbital is composed of two lobes located symmetrically about the nucleus and contains a **node** (an area where the probability of finding an electron is zero). A d-orbital is composed of four symmetrical lobes and contains two nodes. Both d- and f-orbitals are complex in shape and are rarely encountered in organic chemistry (refer to General Chemistry chapters 1 and 3).

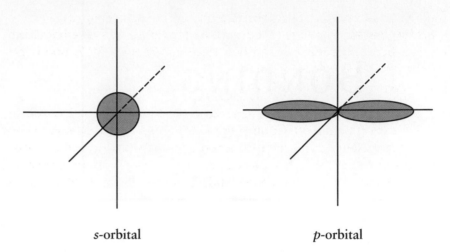

s-orbital   *p*-orbital

Figure 3.1

MOLECULAR ORBITALS

A. SINGLE BONDS

Two atomic orbitals can be combined to form what is called a **molecular orbital (MO)**. Molecular orbitals are obtained mathematically by adding the wave functions of the atomic orbitals. If the signs of the wave functions are the same, a lower-energy **bonding orbital** is produced. If the signs are different, a higher-energy **antibonding orbital** is produced. This is represented schematically by the addition of two *s*-orbitals. Two *p*-orbitals or one *p*- and one *s*-orbital can also be combined in a similar fashion.

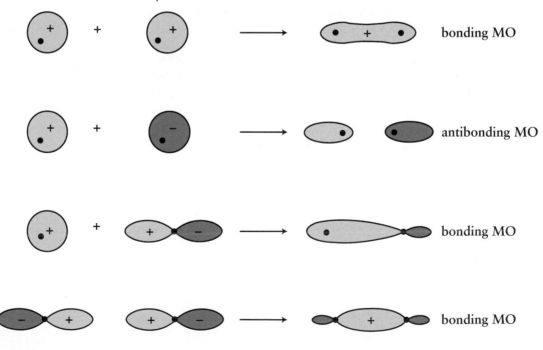

Figure 3.2

When a molecular orbital is formed by head-to-head overlap, as in Figure 3.2, the resulting bond is called a **sigma (σ) bond**. All single bonds are sigma bonds, accommodating two electrons. Shorter single bonds are stronger than longer single bonds.

B. DOUBLE AND TRIPLE BONDS

When two p-orbitals overlap in a parallel fashion, a bonding MO is formed called a **pi (π) bond**. When both a sigma and a pi bond exist between two atoms, a **double bond** is formed. When a sigma bond and two pi bonds exist, a **triple bond** is formed. As can be seen in Figure 3.3, the overlap of the p-orbitals involved in a π bond hinder rotation about double and triple bonds.

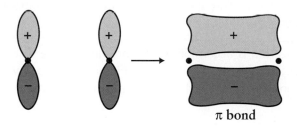

π bond

Figure 3.3

A pi bond cannot exist independently of a sigma bond. Only after the formation of a sigma bond will the p-orbitals of adjacent carbons be parallel, because without the bond, the three p-orbitals are orthogonal to one another.

In general, pi bonds are weaker than sigma bonds; it is possible to break one bond of a double bond, leaving a single bond intact.

HYBRIDIZATION

The carbon atom has the electron configuration $1s^2 2s^2 2p^2$ and, therefore, needs four electrons to complete its octet. A typical molecule formed by carbon is methane, CH_4. Experimentation shows that the four sigma bonds in methane are equal. This is inconsistent with the unsymmetrical distribution of valence electrons: two electrons in the 2s-orbital, one in the p_x-orbital, one in the p_y-orbital, and none in the p_z-orbital.

A. sp^3

The theory of **orbital hybridization** was developed to account for this discrepancy. Hybrid orbitals are formed by mixing different types of atomic orbitals. If one s-orbital and three p-orbitals are mathematically combined, the result is four sp^3-hybrid orbitals that have a new shape.

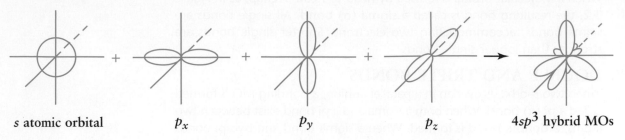

s atomic orbital p_x p_y p_z $4sp^3$ hybrid MOs

Figure 3.4

Bridge

VSEPR theory, which determines the shape of molecules, is discussed in General Chemistry chapter 3.

These four orbitals will point towards the vertices of a tetrahedron, minimizing repulsion. This explains the preferred tetrahedral geometry adopted by carbon.

The hybridization is accomplished by promoting one of the 2s electrons into the $2p_z$-orbital (see Figure 3.5). This produces four valence orbitals, each with one electron, which can be mathematically mixed to provide the hybrids.

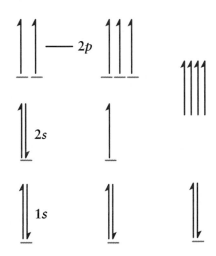

unhybridized ground state   unhybridized excited state   hybridized ground state

Figure 3.5

B. sp^2

Although carbon is most often found with sp^3 hybridization, there are other possibilities. If one s-orbital and two p-orbitals are mixed, three sp^2 hybrid orbitals are obtained.

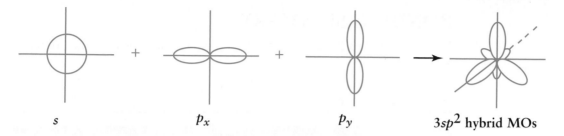

$$s \quad\quad\quad p_x \quad\quad\quad p_y \quad\quad\quad 3sp^2 \text{ hybrid MOs}$$

Figure 3.6

This occurs, for example, in ethylene. The third *p*-orbital of each carbon atom is left unhybridized and participates in the pi bond. The three *sp²* orbitals are 120° apart, allowing maximum separation. These orbitals participate in the formation of the C=C and C–H single bonds.

C. *sp*

If two *p*-orbitals are used to form a triple bond, and the remaining *p*-orbital is mixed with an *s*-orbital, two *sp* hybrid orbitals are obtained. They are oriented 180° apart, explaining the linear structure of molecules like acetylene.

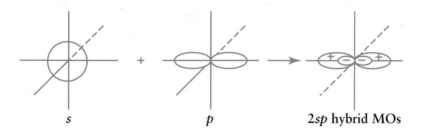

$$s \quad\quad\quad p \quad\quad\quad 2sp \text{ hybrid MOs}$$

Figure 3.7

BONDING SUMMARY

Tables 3.1 and 3.2 summarizes the major features of bonding in organic molecules.

Table 3.1

Bond Order	Component Bonds	Hybridization	Angles	Examples
single	sigma	sp^3	109.5°	C–C; C–H
double	sigma pi	sp^2	120°	C=C; C=O
triple	sigma pi pi	sp	180°	C≡C; C≡N

Table 3.2

	Hybridization	Bond Length	Bond Energy
C–C	sp^3	Largest	Lowest
C=C	sp^2	Medium	Medium
C≡C	sp	Shortest	Highest

## 4

ALKANES

Alkanes are fully saturated hydrocarbons, compounds consisting only of hydrogen and carbon atoms joined by single bonds. Their general formula is C_nH_{2n+2}, which means they have the maximum possible number of hydrogen atoms attached to each carbon atom.

Flashback

Refer to chapter 1 for the general rules of nomenclature for the alkanes.

NOMENCLATURE

Once again, be sure that you are familiar with the common, frequently encountered names, such as those shown in Figure 4.1.

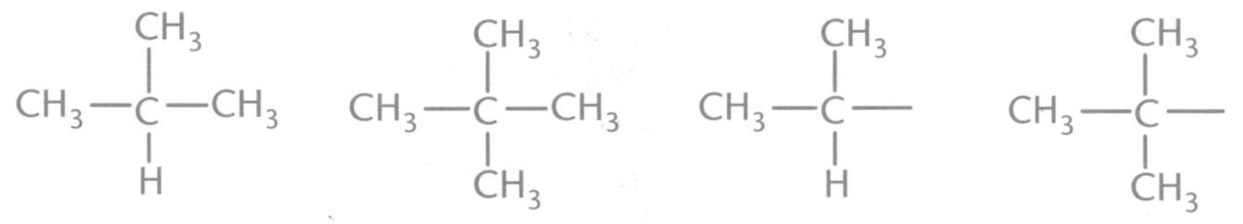

isobutane   neopentane   isopropyl   *t*-butyl

Figure 4.1

Carbon atoms can be characterized by the number of other carbon atoms to which they are directly bonded. A **primary** carbon atom (written as **1°**) is bonded to only one other carbon atom. A **secondary (2°)** carbon is bonded to two, a **tertiary (3°)** to three, and a **quaternary (4°)** to four other carbon atoms. In addition, hydrogen atoms attached to 1°, 2°, or 3° carbon atoms are referred to as 1°, 2°, or 3°, respectively.

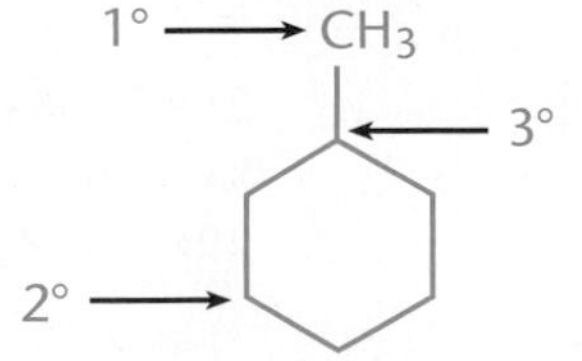

Figure 4.2

PHYSICAL PROPERTIES

The physical properties of alkanes vary in a regular manner. In general, as the molecular weight increases, the melting point, boiling point, and density also increase. At room temperature, the straight-chain compounds C_1 through C_4 are gases, C_5 through C_{16} are liquids, and the longer-chain compounds are waxes and harder solids. Branched molecules have slightly lower boiling and melting points than their straight-chain isomers. Greater branching reduces the surface area of a molecule, decreasing the weak intermolecular attractive forces (van der Waals forces). Hence, the molecules are held together less tightly, effectively lowering the boiling point. In addition, branched molecules are more difficult to pack into a tight, three-dimensional structure. This difficulty is reflected in the lower melting points of branched alkanes.

REACTIONS

A. FREE RADICAL HALOGENATION

One frequently encountered reaction of alkanes is **halogenations**, in which one or more hydrogen atoms are replaced by halogen atoms (Cl, Br, or I) via a **free-radical substitution** mechanism. These reactions involve three steps:

1. **Initiation**—Diatomic halogens are homolytically cleaved by either heat or light (hv), resulting in the formation of free radicals. Free radicals are neutral species with unpaired electrons (such as Cl• or $R_3C•$). They are extremely reactive and readily attack alkanes.

$$\text{Initiation: } X_2 \xrightarrow[\text{or } \Delta]{h\nu} 2X\bullet$$

2. **Propagation**—A propagation step is one in which a radical produces another radical that can continue the reaction. A free radical reacts with an alkane, removing a hydrogen atom to form HX and creating an alkyl radical. The alkyl radical can then react with X_2 to form an alkyl halide, generating X•.

$$\text{Propagation:} \quad X\bullet + RH \rightarrow HX + R\bullet$$
$$R\bullet + X_2 \rightarrow RX + X\bullet$$

3. **Termination**—Two free radicals combine with one another to form a stable molecule.

$$\text{Termination:} \quad 2X\bullet \rightarrow X_2$$
$$X\bullet + R\bullet \rightarrow RX$$
$$2R\bullet \rightarrow R_2$$

A single free radical can initiate many reactions before the reaction chain is terminated.

Larger alkanes have many hydrogens that the free radical can attack. Bromine radicals react fairly slowly and primarily attack the hydrogens on the carbon atom that can form the most stable free radical (i.e., the most substituted carbon atom).

$$\bullet CR_3 > \bullet CR_2H > \bullet CRH_2 > \bullet CH_3$$
$$3° > 2° > 1° > \text{methyl}$$

Thus, a tertiary radical is the most likely to be formed in a free-radical bromination reaction.

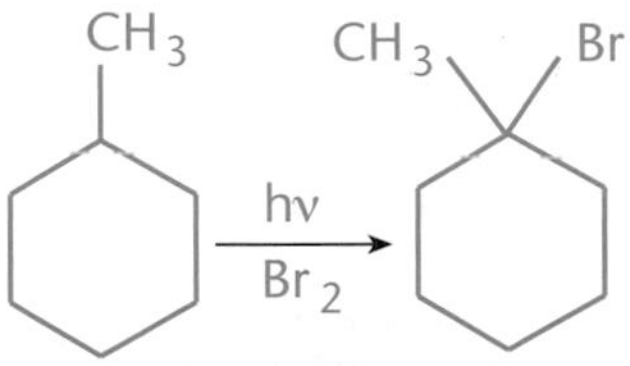

Figure 4.3

Free-radical chlorination is a more rapid process and, thus, depends not only on the stability of the intermediate but on the number of hydrogens present. Free-radical chlorination reactions are likely to replace primary hydrogens because of their abundance, despite the relative instability of primary radicals. Unfortunately, free-radical chlorination reactions produce mixtures of products and are preparatively useful only when just one type of hydrogen is present.

DAT Synopsis

Free radicals, as well as carbocations, follow the same patterns of stability:
3° > 2° > 1° > methyl

B. COMBUSTION

The reaction of alkanes with molecular oxygen, to form carbon dioxide, water, and heat, is a process of great practical importance. It is an unusual reaction because heat, not a chemical species, is generally the desired product. The reaction mechanism is very complex and is believed to proceed through a radical process. The equation for the complete **combustion** of propane is

$$C_3H_8 + 5O_2 \rightarrow 3CO_2 + 4H_2O + \text{heat}$$

Combustion is often incomplete, producing significant quantities of carbon monoxide instead of carbon dioxide. This frequently occurs, for example, in the burning of gasoline in an internal combustion engine.

Real-World Analogy

Nitrogen in the air is also often oxidized in the internal combustion engine. Various nitrogen oxides are major contributors to air pollution.

C. PYROLYSIS

Pyrolysis occurs when a molecule is broken down by heat. Pyrolysis, also called **cracking**, is most commonly used to reduce the average molecular weight of heavy oils and to increase the production of the more desirable volatile compounds. In the pyrolysis of alkanes, the C–C bonds are cleaved, producing smaller-chain alkyl radicals. These radicals can recombine to form a variety of alkanes:

$$CH_3CH_2CH_3 \xrightarrow{\Delta} CH_3\bullet + \bullet CH_2CH_3$$

$$2\ CH_3\bullet \longrightarrow CH_3CH_3$$

$$2\ \bullet CH_2CH_3 \longrightarrow CH_3CH_2CH_2CH_3$$

Figure 4.4

Alternatively, in a process called **disproportionation,** a radical transfers a hydrogen atom to another radical, producing an alkane and an alkene:

$$CH_3\bullet + \bullet CH_2CH_3 \rightarrow CH_4 + CH_2 = CH_2$$

Figure 4.5

SUBSTITUTION REACTIONS OF ALKYL HALIDES

Alkyl halides and indeed other substituted carbon atoms can take part in reactions known as **nucleophilic substitutions. Nucleophiles** ("nucleus lovers") are electron-rich species that are attracted to positively polarized atoms.

A. NUCLEOPHILES

1. Basicity

If the nucleophiles have the same attacking atom (for example, oxygen), then nucleophilicity is roughly correlated to basicity. In other words, the stronger the base, the stronger the nucleophile. For example, nucleophilic strength decreases in this order:

$$RO^- > HO^- > RCO_2^- > ROH > H_2O$$

2. Size and Polarizability

If the attacking atoms differ, nucleophilic ability doesn't necessarily correlate to basicity. In a protic solvent, large atoms tend to be better nucleophiles, as they can shed their solvent molecules and are more polarizable. Hence, nucleophilic strength decreases in this order:

$$CN^- > I^- > RO^- > HO^- > Br^- > Cl^- > F^- > H_2O$$

> **DAT Synopsis**
>
> In protic solvents (solvents capable of hydrogen bonding), larger atoms are better nucleophiles. In aprotic solvents, more basic atoms are better nucleophiles

In aprotic solvents, however, the nucleophiles are "naked"; they are not solvated. In this situation, nucleophilic strength is related to basicity. For example in DMSO, the order of nucleophilic strength is the same as base strength:

$$F^- > Cl^- > Br^- > I^-$$

Note that this is the opposite of what happens in polar solvents.

B. LEAVING GROUPS

The ease with which nucleophilic substitution takes place is also dependent on the leaving group. The best leaving groups are those that are weak bases, as these can accept an electron pair and dissociate to form a stable species. In the case of the halogens, therefore, this is the opposite of base strength:

$$I^- > Br^- > Cl^- > F^-$$

DAT Synopsis

Weak bases make good leaving groups.

C. S_N1 REACTIONS

S_N1 is the designation for **unimolecular nucleophilic substitution** reaction. It is called unimolecular because the rate of the reaction is dependent upon only one species. Generally, the rate-determining step is the dissociation of this species to form a stable, positively charged ion called a **carbocation** or **carbonium ion**.

1. **Mechanism of S_N1 Reactions**

    S_N1 reactions involve two steps: the dissociation of a molecule into a carbocation and a good leaving group, followed by the combination of the carbocation with a strong nucleophile.

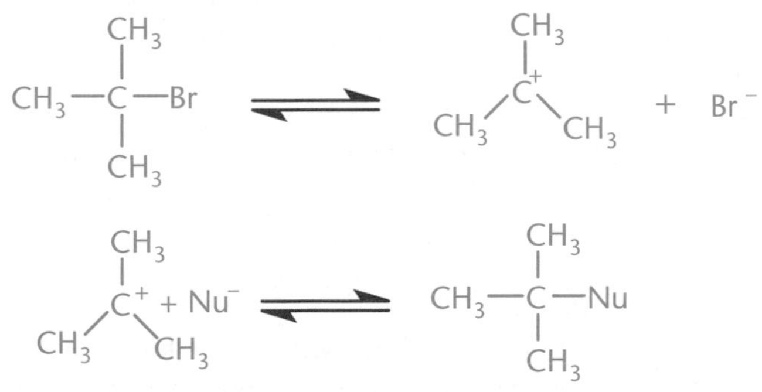

Figure 4.6

In the first step, a carbocation is formed. Carbocations are stabilized by polar solvents that have lone electron pairs to donate (e.g., water, acetone). Carbocations are also stabilized by charge delocalization. More highly substituted cations are therefore more stable. The order of stability for carbocations is as follows:

tertiary > secondary > primary > methyl

To get the desired product, the original substituent should be a better leaving group than the nucleophile, so that at equilibrium, RNu is the main product. Conditions are usually chosen so that the second step of the reaction is essentially irreversible.

Bridge

The kinetics of unimolecular reactions are first order. See General Chemistry chapter 5.

2. **Rate of S$_N$1 Reactions**

The rate at which a reaction occurs can never be greater than the rate of its slowest step. Such a step is termed the **rate-limiting** or **rate-determining step** of the reaction, because it limits the speed of the reaction. In an S$_N$1 reaction, the slowest step is the dissociation of the molecule to form a carbocation, a step that is energetically unfavorable. The formation of a carbocation is, therefore, the rate-limiting step of an S$_N$1 reaction. The only reactant in this step is the original molecule, so the rate of the entire reaction, under a given set of conditions, depends only on the concentration of this original molecule (a so-called **first-order reaction**). The rate is *not* dependent on the concentration or the nature of the nucleophile, because it plays no part in the rate-limiting step.

The rate of an S$_N$1 reaction can be increased by anything that accelerates the formation of the carbocation. The most important factors are as follows:

a. Structural factors: Highly substituted alkyl halides allow for distribution of the positive charge over a greater number of carbon atoms and thus form the most stable carbocations.

b. Solvent effects: Highly polar solvents are better at surrounding and isolating ions than are less polar solvents. Polar protic solvents, such as water, work best since solvation stabilizes the intermediate state.

c. Nature of the leaving group: Weak bases dissociate more easily from the alkyl chain and thus make better leaving groups, increasing the rate of carbocation formation.

D. S$_N$2 REACTIONS

The formation of a carbocation is not always favorable. Under certain conditions, substitution can proceed by a different mechanism, which does not involve a carbocation. An S$_N$2 (**bimolecular nucleophilic substitution**) reaction involves a nucleophile pushing its way into a compound while simultaneously displacing the leaving group. Its rate-determining, and only, step involves two molecules: the **substrate** and the nucleophile.

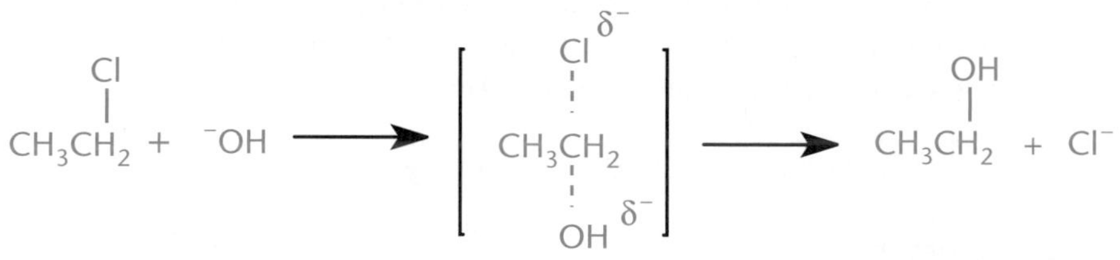

Figure 4.7

1. **Mechanism of S$_N$2 Reactions**
   In S$_N$2 reactions, the nucleophile actively displaces the leaving group. For this to occur, the nucleophile must be strong, and the reactant cannot be sterically hindered. The nucleophile attacks the reactant from the backside of the leaving group, forming a trigonal bipyramidal **transition state**. As the reaction progresses, the bond to the nucleophile strengthens while the bond to the leaving group weakens. The leaving group is displaced as the bond to the nucleophile becomes complete.

2. **Rate of S$_N$2 Reactions**
   The single step of an S$_N$2 reaction involves *two* reacting species: the substrate (the molecule with a leaving group, usually an alkyl halide) and the nucleophile. The concentrations of both therefore play a role in determining the rate of an S$_N$2 reaction; the two species must "meet" in solution, and raising the concentration of either will make such a meeting more likely. Since the rate of the S$_N$2 reaction depends on the concentration of two reactants, it follows **second-order kinetics**.

> **DAT Synopsis**
>
> An intermediate is distinct from a transition state. An intermediate is a well-defined species with a finite lifetime. On the other hand, a transition state is a theoretical structure used to define a mechanism.

> **Bridge**
>
> The kinetics of second-order reactions such as S$_N$2 are discussed in General Chemistry chapter 5.

E. S$_N$1 VERSUS S$_N$2

Certain reaction conditions favor one substitution mechanism over the other. It is also possible for both to occur in the same flask. Sterics, nucleophilic strength, leaving group ability, reaction conditions, and solvent effects are all important in determining which reaction will occur.

STEREOCHEMISTRY OF SUBSTITUTION REACTIONS

A. S$_N$1 STEREOCHEMISTRY

S$_N$1 reactions involve carbocation intermediates, which are approximately planar and therefore achiral.

> **DAT Synopsis**
>
> When you see H$^+$ above the arrow, think of cationic mechanisms such as S$_N$1.

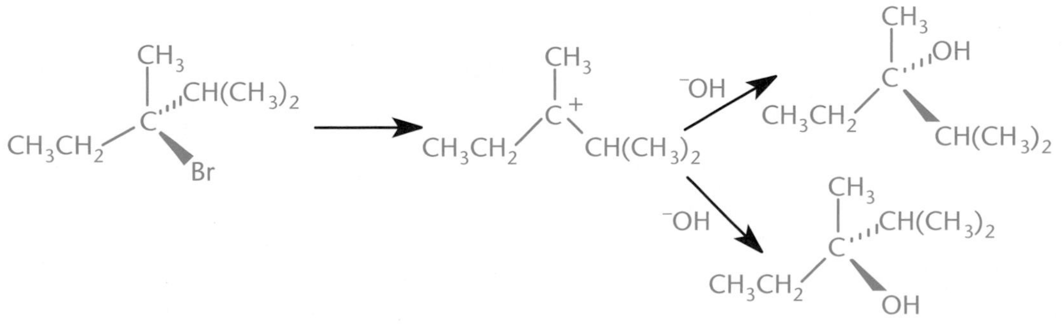

Figure 4.8

Flashback

Refer to chapter 2 for further discussion of optical activity.

If the original compound is optically active because of the reacting chiral center, then a racemic mixture will be produced. S_N1 reactions result in a loss of optical activity.

B. S_N2 STEREOCHEMISTRY

The single step of an S_N2 reaction involves a chiral transition state. Since the nucleophile attacks from one side of the central carbon and the leaving group departs from the opposite side, the reaction "flips" the bonds attached to the carbon.

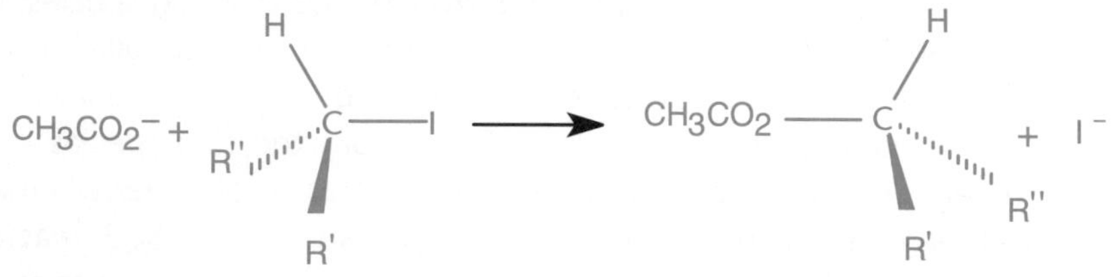

Figure 4.9

If the reactant is chiral, optical activity is usually retained; however, in the case of S_N2 reactions, an inversion of configuration occurs.

Figure 4.10 summarizes S_N1 and S_N2 reactions.

S_N1	S_N2
• 2 steps • Favored in polar protic solvents. • 3° > 2° > 1° > methyl • Rate = k[RX] • Racemic products • Favored with the use of bulky nucleophiles.	• 1 step • Favored in polar aprotic solvents. • 1° > 2° > 3° • Rate = k[Nu][RX] • Optically active/ inverted products

Figure 4.10

## 5

ALKENES AND ALKYNES

ALKENES

Alkenes are hydrocarbons that contain carbon-carbon double bonds. The general formula for a straight-chain alkene with one double bond is C_nH_{2n}. The degree of unsaturation (the number N of double bonds or rings) of a compound of molecular formula C_nH_m can be determined according to this equation:

$$N = \frac{1}{2}(2n + 2 - m)$$

Double bonds are considered functional groups, and alkenes are more reactive than the corresponding alkanes.

A. NOMENCLATURE

Alkenes, also called **olefins**, may be described by the terms *cis, trans, E,* and *Z*. The common names *ethylene, propylene,* and *isobutylene* are often used over the IUPAC names.

Flashback

Refer to chapter 1 for the general rules of nomenclature for alkenes.

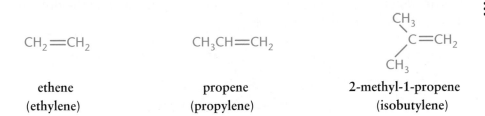

ethene
(ethylene)

propene
(propylene)

2-methyl-1-propene
(isobutylene)

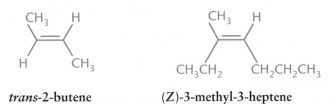

trans-2-butene

(Z)-3-methyl-3-heptene

Figure 5.1

B. PHYSICAL PROPERTIES

The physical properties of alkenes are similar to those of alkanes. For example, the melting and boiling points increase with increasing molecular weight and are similar in value to those of the corresponding alkanes. Terminal alkenes (or 1-alkenes) usually boil at a lower temperature than internal alkenes, and they can be separated by fractional distillation (see "Distillation" in chapter 12). *Trans*-alkenes generally have higher melting points than *cis*-alkenes because their higher symmetry allows better packing in the solid state. They also tend to have lower boiling points than *cis*-alkenes because they are less **polar**.

Polarity is a property that results from the asymmetrical distribution of electrons in a particular molecule. In alkenes, this distribution creates dipole moments that are oriented from the electropositive alkyl groups toward the electronegative alkene. In *trans*-2-butene, the two dipole moments are oriented in opposite directions and cancel each other. The compound possesses no net dipole moment and is not polar. On the other hand, *cis*-2-butene has a net dipole moment, resulting from addition of the two smaller dipoles. The compound is polar, and the additional intermolecular forces tend to raise the boiling point.

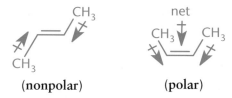

(nonpolar)   (polar)

Figure 5.2

The net dipole of alkene compound can grossly be assessed by the distribution of electrons across the molecule.

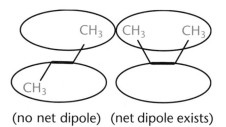

(no net dipole)   (net dipole exists)

Figure 5.3

C. SYNTHESIS

Alkenes can be synthesized in a number of different ways. The most common method involves **elimination reactions** of either alcohols or alkyl halides.

In these reactions the carbon skeleton loses HX (where X is a halide), or a molecule of water, to form a double bond:

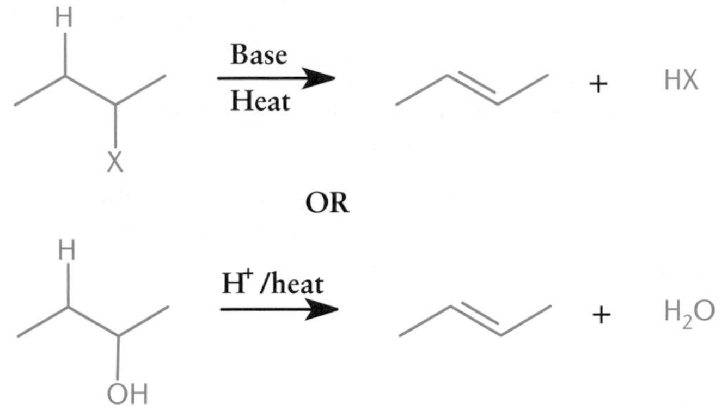

OR

Figure 5.4

Elimination occurs by two distinct mechanisms, unimolecular and bimolecular, which are referred to as **E1** and **E2**, respectively.

1. **Unimolecular Elimination**
   Unimolecular elimination, abbreviated E1, is a two-step process proceeding through a carbocation intermediate. The rate of reaction is dependent on the concentration of only one species, namely the substrate. The elimination of a leaving group and a proton results in the production of a double bond. In the first step, the leaving group departs, producing a carbocation. In the second step, a proton is removed by a base.

   E1 is favored by the same factors that favor S_N1: highly polar solvents, highly branched carbon chains, good leaving groups, and weak nucleophiles in low concentration. These mechanisms are therefore competitive, and directing a reaction toward either E1 or S_N1 alone is difficult, although high temperatures tend to favor E1.

2. **Bimolecular Elimination**
   Bimolecular elimination, termed E2, occurs in one step. Its rate is dependent on the concentration of two species, the substrate and the base. A strong base, such as the ethoxide ion ($C_2H_5O^-$), removes a proton, while a halide ion *anti* to the proton leaves, resulting in the formation of a double bond.

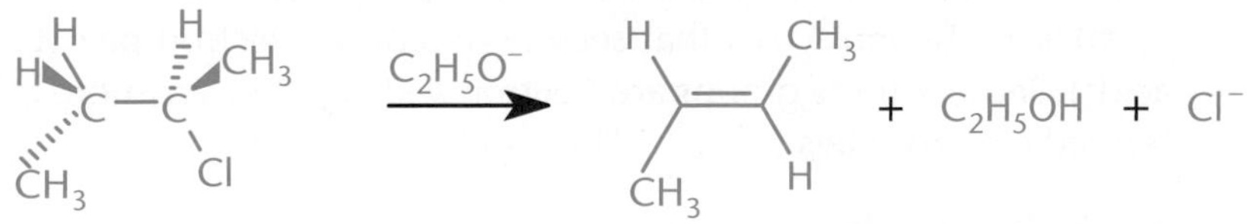

Figure 5.5

Often there are two possible products. In such cases, the more substituted double bond is formed preferentially.

Controlling E2 versus S_N2 is easier than controlling E1 versus S_N1.

- Steric hindrance does not greatly affect E2 reactions. Therefore, highly substituted carbon chains, which form the most stable alkenes, undergo E2 most easily and S_N2 rarely.

- A strong base favors E2 over S_N2. S_N2 is favored over E2 by weak Lewis bases (strong nucleophiles).

Other factors, such as the polarity of the solvent and branching of the carbon chain, can be modified to reduce the competition between E1 and S_N1 reactions.

D. REACTIONS

1. Reduction

Catalytic hydrogenation is the reductive process of adding molecular hydrogen to a double bond with the aid of a metal catalyst. Typical catalysts are platinum, palladium, and nickel (usually Raney nickel, a special powdered form), but occasionally rhodium, iridium, or ruthenium is used.

The reaction takes place on the surface of the metal. One face of the double bond is coordinated to the metal surface, and thus the two hydrogen atoms are added to the same face of the double bond. This type of addition is called *syn* addition.

> **DAT Synopsis**
>
> Reactions where one stereoisomer is favored are termed stereospecific reactions.

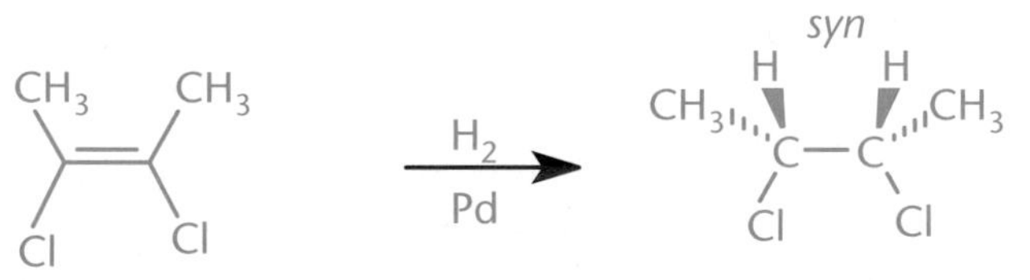

Figure 5.6

2. Electrophilic Additions

The π bond is somewhat weaker than the σ bond and can therefore be broken without breaking the σ bond. As a result, one can *add* compounds to double bonds while leaving the carbon skeleton intact. Though many different **addition reactions** exist, most operate via the same essential mechanism.

The electrons of the π bond are particularly exposed and are thus easily attacked by molecules that seek to accept an electron pair (Lewis acids). Because these groups are electron seeking, they are more often termed **electrophiles** (literally, "lovers of electrons").

a. Addition of HX

The electrons of the double bond act as a Lewis base and react with electrophilic HX molecules. The first step yields a carbocation intermediate after the double bond reacts with a proton. In the second step, the halide ion combines with the carbocation to give an alkyl halide. In cases where the alkene is asymmetrical, the initial protonation proceeds to produce the *most stable carbocation*. The proton will add to the less substituted carbon atom (the carbon atom with the most protons), since alkyl substituents stabilize carbocations. This phenomenon is called **Markovnikov's Rule**. An example is shown in Figure 5.7:

DAT Synopsis

Markovnikov's Rule refers to the addition of something (e.g., halide, hydroxyl group) to the most substituted carbon in the double bond.

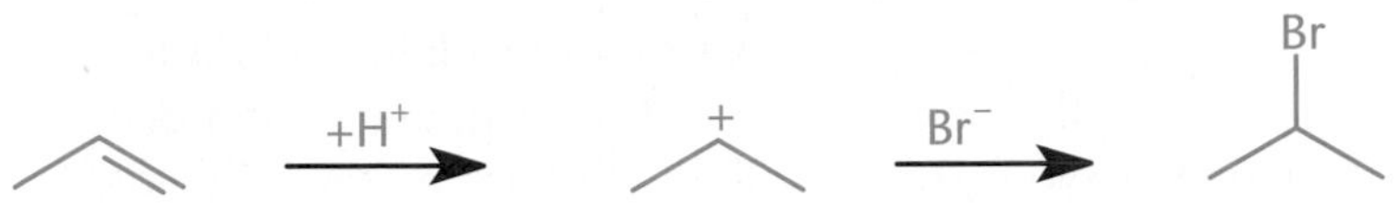

Figure 5.7

b. **Addition of X_2**

The addition of halogens to a double bond is a rapid process. It is frequently used as a diagnostic tool to test for the presence of double bonds. The double bond acts as a nucleophile and attacks an X_2 molecule, displacing X^-. The intermediate carbocation forms a **cyclic halonium ion**, which is then attacked by X^-, giving the dihalo compound. Note that this addition is *anti*, because the X^- attacks the cyclic halonium ion in a standard S_N2 displacement.

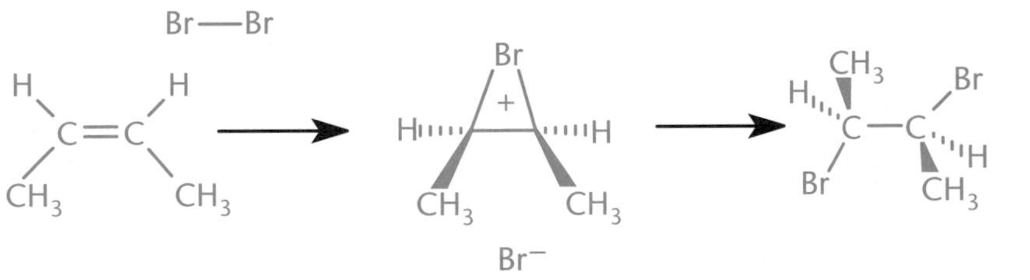

Anti addition

Figure 5.8

If the reaction is carried out in a nucleophilic solvent, the solvent molecules can compete in the displacement step, producing, for example, a **halo alcohol** (rather than the **dihalo** compound).

c. **Addition of H_2O**

Water can be added to alkenes under acidic conditions. The double bond is protonated according to Markovnikov's Rule, forming the most stable carbocation. This carbocation reacts with water, forming a protonated alcohol, which then loses a proton to yield the alcohol. The reaction is performed at low temperature because the reverse reaction is an acid-catalyzed **dehydration** favored by high temperatures.

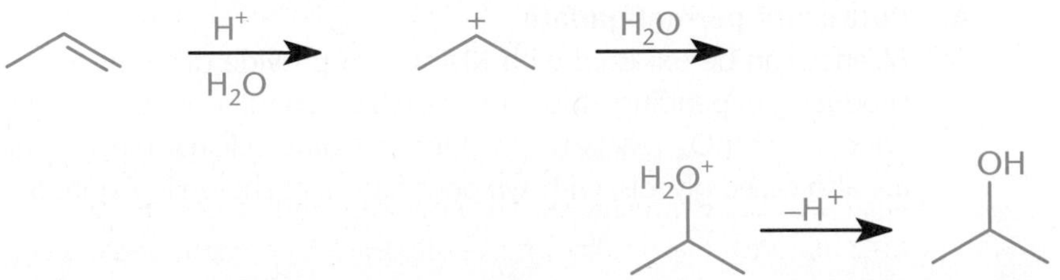

Figure 5.9

Direct addition of water is generally not useful in the laboratory because yields vary greatly with reaction conditions; therefore, this reaction is generally carried out indirectly using mercuric acetate, $Hg(CH_3COO)_2$.

3. **Free Radical Additions**

   An alternate mechanism exists for the addition of HX to alkenes, which proceeds through **free-radical intermediates** and occurs when peroxides, oxygen, or other impurities are present. Free-radical additions disobey the Markovnikov Rule because X• adds first to the double bond, producing the most stable free radical, whereas H+ adds first in standard electrophilic additions, producing the most stable carbocation. The reaction is useful for HBr but is not practical for HCl or HI, because the energetics are unfavorable.

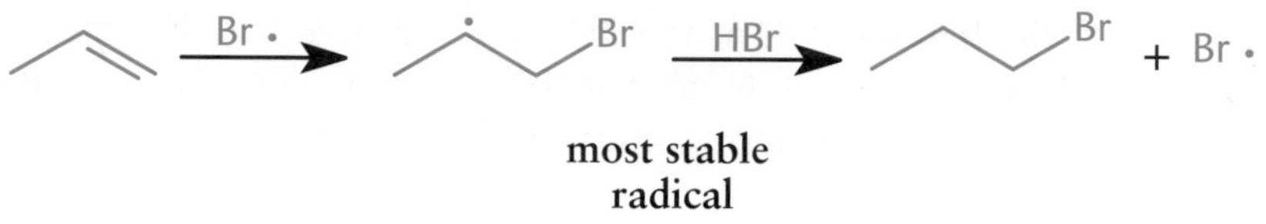

DAT Synopsis

When peroxides are present, expect free-radical reactions that do not follow Markovnikov's Rule.

most stable
radical

Figure 5.10

4. **Hydroboration**

   Diborane (B_2H_6) adds readily to double bonds. The boron atom is a Lewis acid and attaches to the less sterically hindered carbon atom. The second step is an oxidation-hydrolysis with peroxide and aqueous base, producing the alcohol with overall anti-Markovnikov, *syn* orientation.

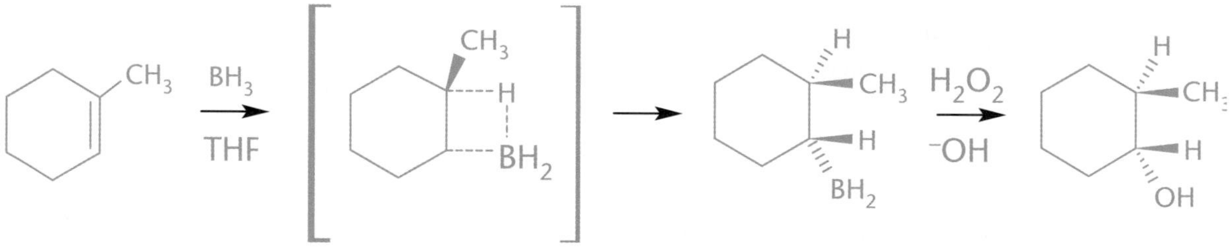

Figure 5.11

5. **Oxidation**
   a. **Potassium permanganate**

      Alkenes can be oxidized with $KMnO_4$ to provide different types of products, depending upon the reaction conditions. Cold, dilute, aqueous $KMnO_4$ reacts to produce 1,2 diols (vicinal diols), which are also called glycols, with *syn* orientation, as shown in Figure 5.12.

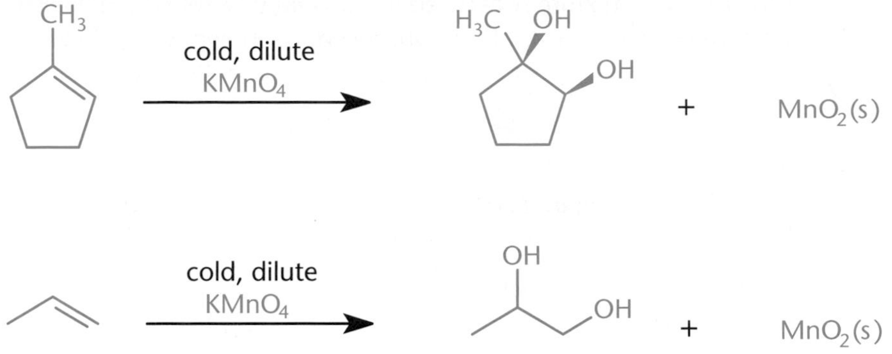

Figure 5.12

Bridge

As we see in General Chemistry chapter 11, the reaction $Mn^{7+} + 3e^- \rightarrow Mn^{4+}$, is a reduction in the electrochemical sense. By default, the organic compound is oxidized. Note that in aqueous solutions, another reaction, $Mn^{7+} + 5e^- \rightarrow Mn^{2+}$, is more likely.

If a hot, basic solution of potassium permanganate is added to the alkene and then acidified, nonterminal alkenes are cleaved to form two molar equivalents of carboxylic acid, and terminal alkenes are cleaved to form a carboxylic acid and carbon dioxide. If the nonterminal double-bonded carbon is disubstituted, however, a ketone will be formed, as shown in Figure 5.13.

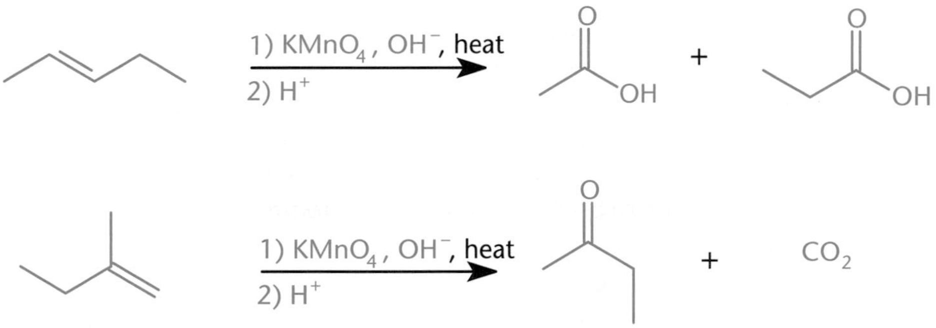

Figure 5.13

b. Ozonolysis

Treatment of alkenes with ozone followed by reduction with zinc and water results in cleavage of the double bond in the manner shown in Figure 5.14.

Figure 5.14

DAT Synopsis

1) $KMnO_4^-$, OH 2) H^+, heat $\rightarrow$: 1. cleavage 2. oxidation

1) O_3, CH_2Cl_2 2) Zn/H_2O $\rightarrow$: 1. cleavage only

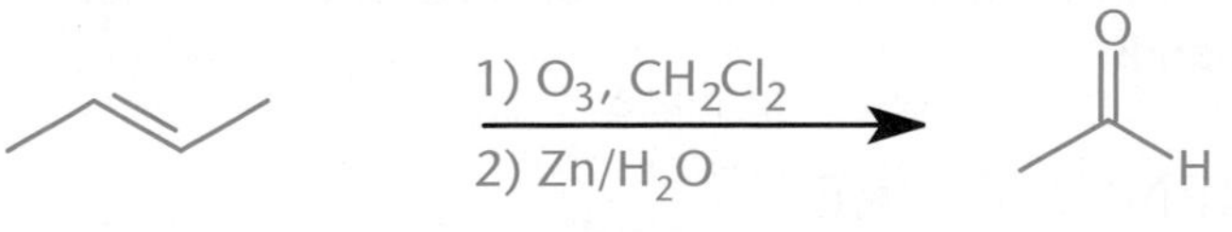

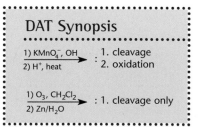

If the reaction mixture is reduced with sodium borohydride, $NaBH_4$, the corresponding alcohols are produced, as shown in Figure 5.15.

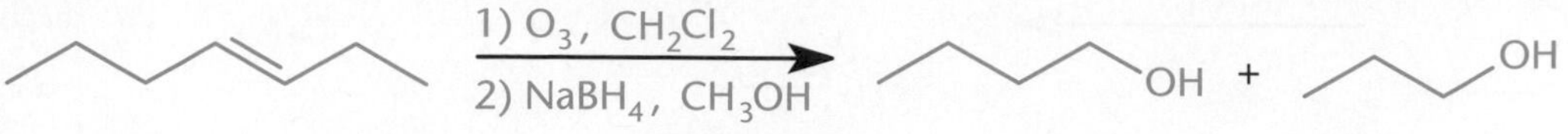

Figure 5.15

c. **Peroxycarboxylic acids**
Alkenes can be oxidized with peroxycarboxylic acids. Peroxyacetic acid (CH_3CO_3H) and *m*-chloroperoxybenzoic acid (mcpba) are commonly used. The products formed are **oxiranes** (also called **epoxides**), as shown in Figure 5.16.

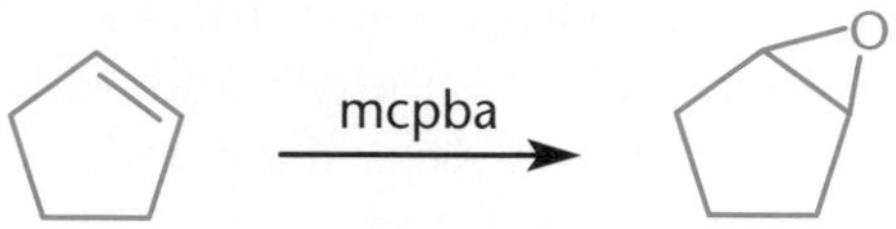

Figure 5.16

6. **Polymerization**
Polymerization is the creation of long, high-molecular-weight chains **(polymers)**, composed of repeating subunits (called **monomers**). Polymerization usually occurs through a radical mechanism, although anionic and even cationic polymerizations are commonly observed. A typical example is the formation of polyethylene from ethylene (ethene), which requires high temperatures and pressures (see Figure 5.17).

$$CH_2{=}CH_2 \xrightarrow[\text{high pressure}]{R\bullet,\ \text{heat}} RCH_2CH_2(CH_2CH_2)_nCH_2CH_2R$$

Figure 5.17

> **Flashback**
>
> Refer to chapter 1 for the general rules of nomenclature of alkynes.

ALKYNES

Alkynes are hydrocarbon compounds that possess one or more carbon-carbon triple bonds.

A. NOMENCLATURE

The suffix **-yne** is used, and the position of the triple bond is specified when necessary. A common exception to the IUPAC rules is ethyne, which is called *acetylene*. Frequently, compounds are named as derivatives of acetylene.

$$CH_3CH_2CH_2CHC\!\equiv\!CCH_3 \qquad CH\!\equiv\!CH \qquad CH_3C\!\equiv\!CH$$
$$\underset{Cl}{|}$$

4-chloro-2-heptyne	ethyne	propyne
	(acetylene)	(methylacetylene)

Figure 5.18

B. PHYSICAL PROPERTIES

The physical properties of the alkynes are similar to those of the analogous alkenes and alkanes. In general, the shorter-chain compounds are gases, boiling at somewhat higher temperatures than the corresponding alkenes. Internal alkynes, like alkenes, boil at higher temperatures than terminal alkynes.

Asymmetrical distribution of electron density causes alkynes to have dipole moments that are larger than those of alkenes but still small in magnitude. Thus, solutions of alkynes can be slightly polar.

Terminal alkynes are fairly acidic, having pKa's of approximately 25. This property is exploited in some of the reactions of alkynes, which will be discussed later.

C. SYNTHESIS

Triple bonds can be made by the elimination of two molecules of HX from a geminal or vicinal dihalide, as shown in Figure 5.19.

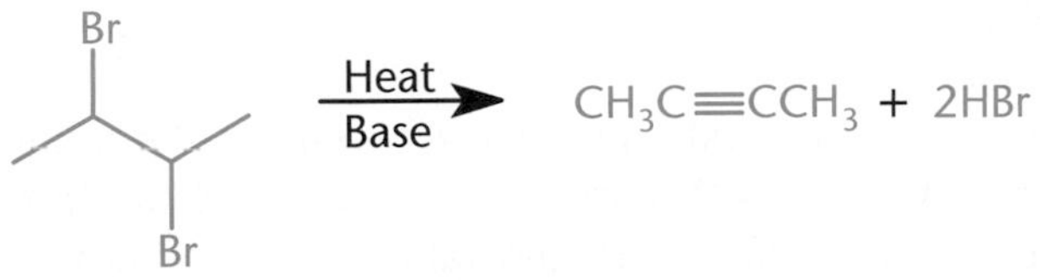

$$\xrightarrow[\text{Base}]{\text{Heat}}\quad CH_3C\!\equiv\!CCH_3 \;+\; 2HBr$$

Figure 5.19

This reaction is not always practical and requires high temperatures and a strong base. A more useful method adds an already existing triple bond into a particular carbon skeleton. A terminal triple bond is converted to a nucleophile by removing the acidic proton with strong base, producing an **acetylide ion**. This ion will perform nucleophilic displacements on alkyl halides at room temperature, as shown in Figure 5.20.

$$CH\!\equiv\!CH \xrightarrow{\;n\text{-BuLi}\;} CH\!\equiv\!C^-\,Li^+ \xrightarrow{\;CH_3Cl\;} CH\!\equiv\!CCH_3$$

Figure 5.20

D. REACTIONS

1. Reduction

Alkynes, just like alkenes, can be hydrogenated with a catalyst to produce alkanes. A more useful reaction stops the reduction after addition of just one equivalent of H_2, producing alkenes. This partial hydrogenation can take place in two different ways. The first uses **Lindlar's catalyst**, which is palladium on barium sulfate ($BaSO_4$) with quinoline, a poison that stops the reaction at the alkene stage. Because the reaction occurs on a metal surface, the product alkene is the *cis* isomer. The other method uses sodium in liquid ammonia below −33°C (the boiling point of ammonia) and produces the *trans* isomer of the alkene via a free radical mechanism (see Figure 5.21).

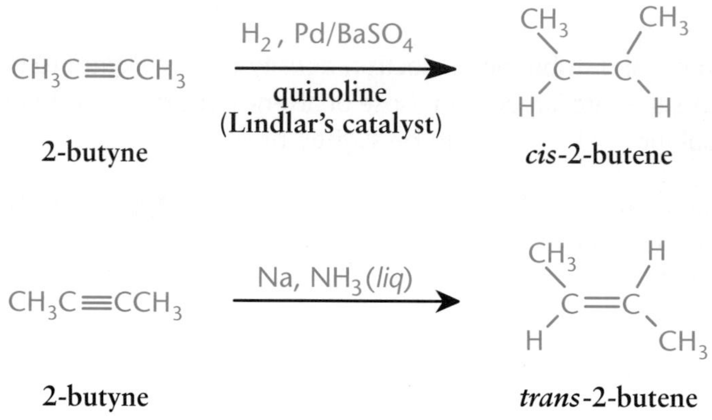

$$CH_3C\equiv CCH_3 \xrightarrow[\substack{\text{quinoline} \\ \text{(Lindlar's catalyst)}}]{H_2, \ Pd/BaSO_4}$$

2-butyne   *cis*-2-butene

$$CH_3C\equiv CCH_3 \xrightarrow{Na, \ NH_3(liq)}$$

2-butyne   *trans*-2-butene

Figure 5.21

2. Addition

a. Electrophilic

Electrophilic addition to alkynes occurs in the same manner as it does to alkenes. The reaction occurs according to Markovnikov's Rule. The addition can generally be stopped at the intermediate alkene stage, or it can be carried further. The examples in Figure 5.22 are illustrative.

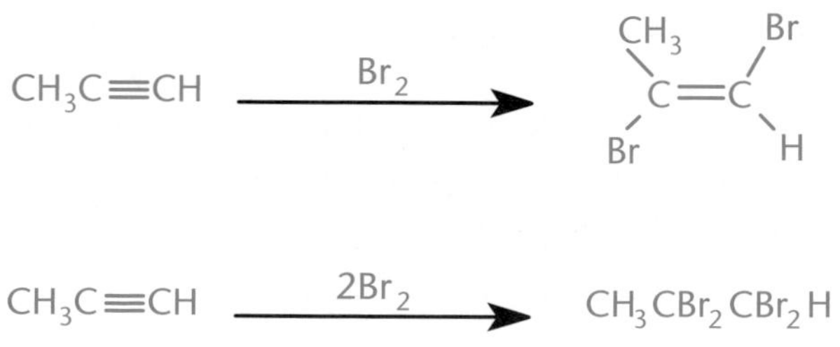

$$CH_3C\equiv CH \xrightarrow{Br_2}$$

$$CH_3C\equiv CH \xrightarrow{2Br_2} CH_3CBr_2CBr_2H$$

Figure 5.22

b. Free radical

Radicals add to triple bonds as they do to double bonds—with anti-Markovnikov orientation. The reaction product is usually the *trans* isomer, because the intermediate vinyl radical can isomerize to its more stable form.

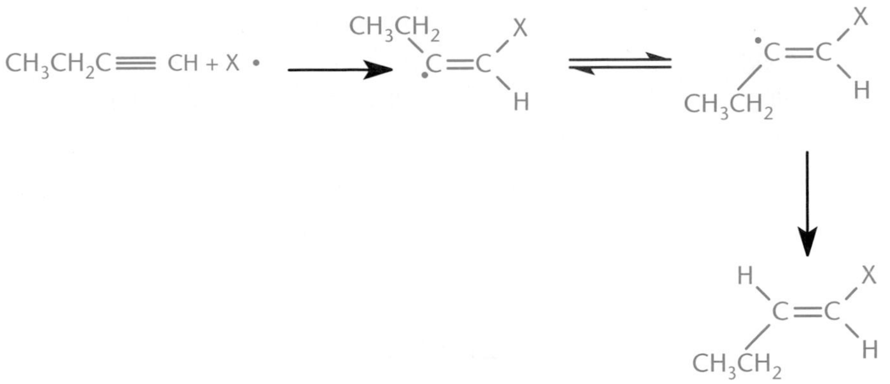

$$CH_3CH_2C \equiv CH + X \cdot \longrightarrow$$

Figure 5.23

3. Hydroboration

Addition of boron to triple bonds occurs by the same method as addition of boron to double bonds. Addition is *syn,* and the boron atom adds first. The boron atom can be replaced with a proton from acetic acid to produce a *cis* alkene, as shown in Figure 5.24.

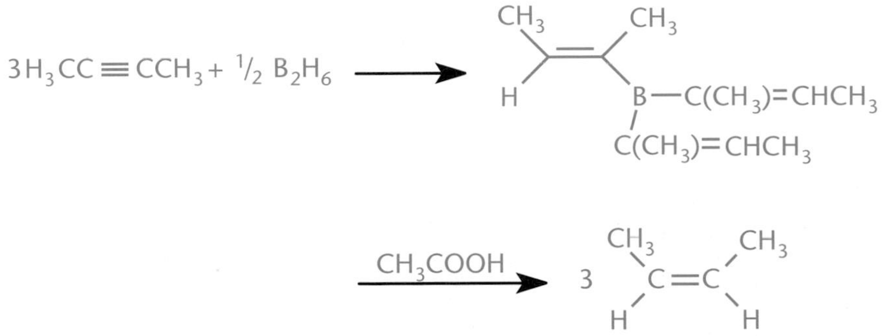

$$3H_3CC \equiv CCH_3 + \tfrac{1}{2} B_2H_6 \longrightarrow$$

$B-C(CH_3)=CHCH_3$
$C(CH_3)=CHCH_3$

$$\xrightarrow{CH_3COOH} \quad 3$$

Figure 5.24

With terminal alkynes, a disubstituted borane is used to prevent further boration of the vinylic intermediate to an alkane. The vinylic borane intermediate can be oxidatively cleaved with hydrogen peroxide (H_2O_2), creating an intermediate vinyl alcohol, which rearranges to the more stable carbonyl compound (via **keto-enol tautomerism;**) keto-enol tautomerisms will be discussed in chapter 8.

Free Radical (Hx)	anti-Markovnikov	1. Add X. 2. Add H.
Ions (Hx)	Markovnikov	1. Add H$^+$. 2. Add X$^-$.

Figure 5.25

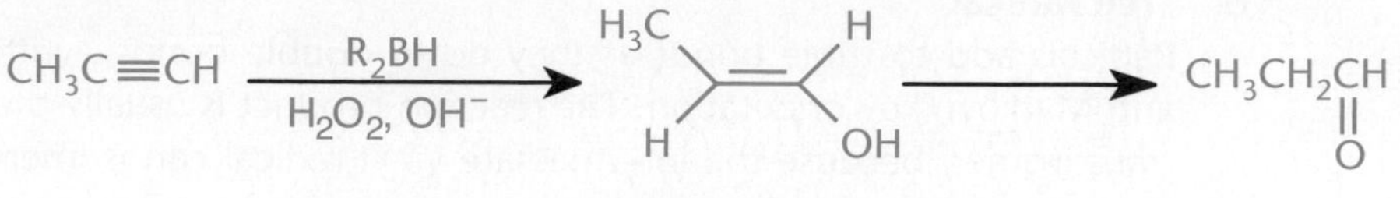

$$CH_3C \equiv CH \xrightarrow[\text{H}_2\text{O}_2,\ \text{OH}^-]{\text{R}_2\text{BH}} \ \begin{array}{c} H_3C \\ \end{array} \begin{array}{c} H \\ \\ OH \end{array} \longrightarrow CH_3CH_2CH{=}O$$

Figure 5.26

4. **Oxidation**

    Alkynes can be oxidatively cleaved with either basic potassium permangenate (followed by acidification) or ozone.

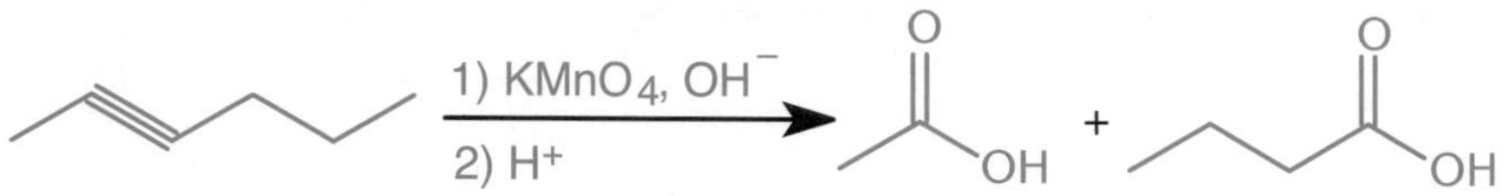

Figure 5.27

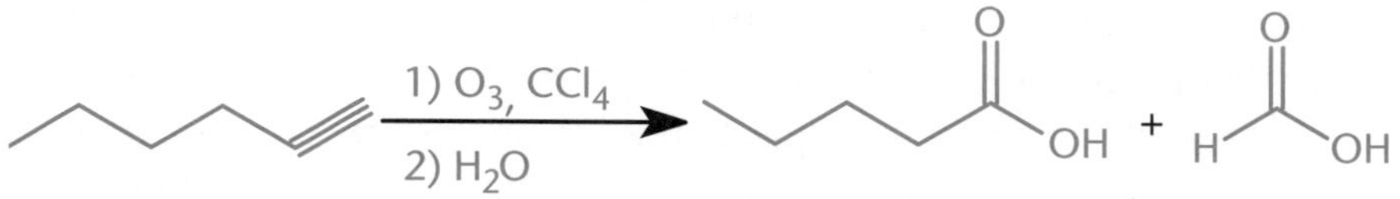

Figure 5.28

## 6

AROMATIC COMPOUNDS

The terms **aromatic** and **aliphatic,** meaning "fragrant" and "fatty," respectively, were used originally to distinguish types of organic compounds. The terms persist with new definitions. *Aromatic* now describes any unusually stable ring system. These compounds are cyclic, conjugated polyenes that possess $4n + 2$ pi electrons and adopt planar conformations to allow maximum overlap of the conjugated pi orbitals. *Aliphatic* describes all compounds that are not aromatic.

The criterion of $4n + 2$ pi electrons is known as **Hückel's Rule,** and it is an important indicator of aromaticity. In general, if a cyclic conjugated polyene follows Hückel's Rule, then it is an aromatic compound. Neutral compounds, anions, and cations may all be aromatic. Some typical aromatic compounds and ions are shown in Figure 6.1.

> **DAT Synopsis**
>
> *n* can be any nonnegative integer; thus, $4n + 2$ can be 2, 6, 10, 14, 18, etc.

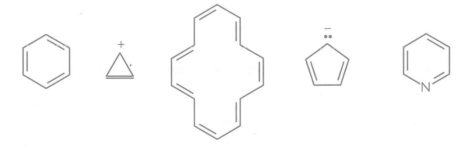

Figure 6.1

A cyclic, conjugated polyene that possesses $4n$ electrons is said to be **antiaromatic** (a cyclic, conjugated polyene that is destabilized). Some typical antiaromatic compounds are shown in Figure 6.2.

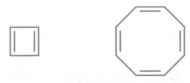

Figure 6.2

NOMENCLATURE

Aromatic compounds are referred to as **aryl** compounds, or **arenes,** and are represented by the symbol **Ar**. Aliphatic compounds are called **alkyl** and are represented by the symbol **R.** Common names exist for many mono- and di-substituted aromatic compounds.

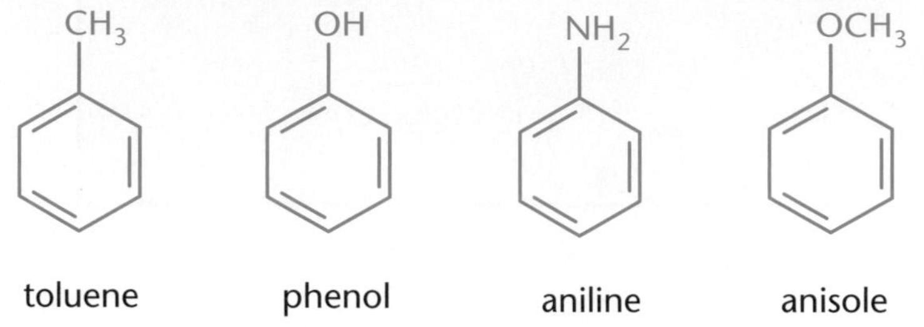
CH3
OH
NH2
OCH3
toluene
phenol
aniline
anisole

Figure 6.3

The benzene group is called a **phenyl** group **(Ph)** when named as a substituent. The term **benzyl** refers to a toluene molecule substituted at the methyl position.

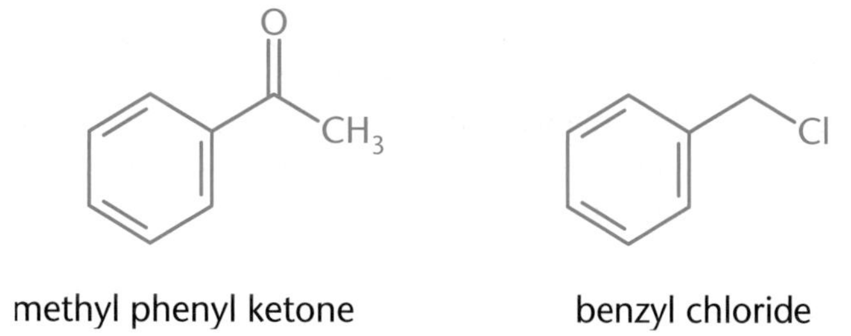
O
CH3
Cl
methyl phenyl ketone
benzyl chloride

Figure 6.4

Substituted benzene rings are named as alkyl benzenes, with the substituents numbered to produce the lowest sequence. A 1,2-disubstituted compound is called ***ortho***- or **o**-; a 1,3-disubstituted compound is called ***meta***- or ***m***-; and a 1,4-disubstituted compound is called ***para***- or ***p***-.

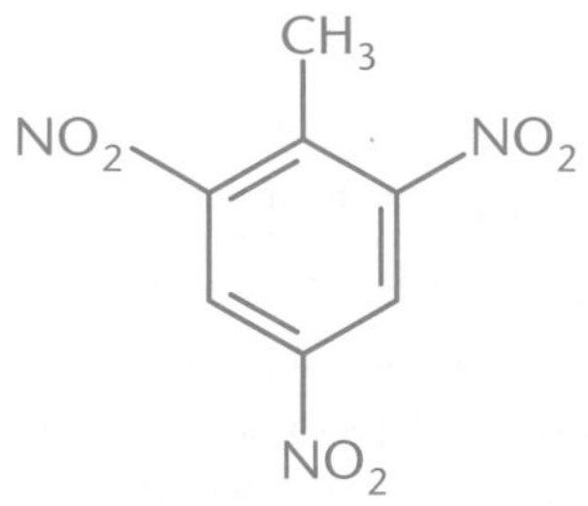

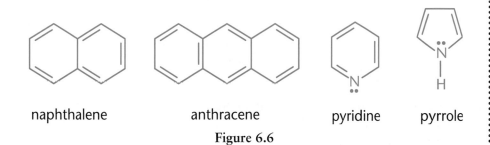

2,4,6-trinitrotoluene (TNT)

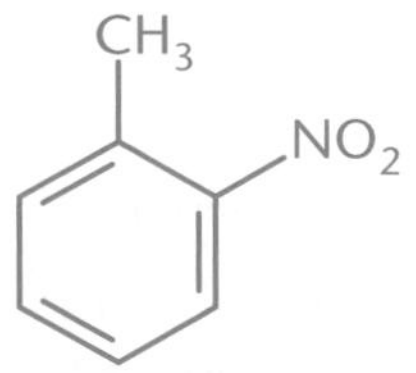

o-nitrotoluene

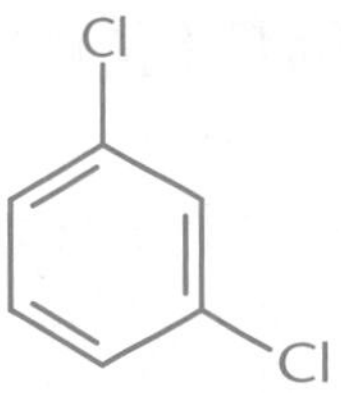

m-dichlorobenzene

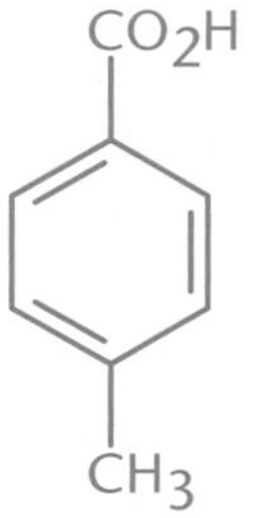

p-methylbenzoic acid

Figure 6.5

There are many polycyclic and heterocyclic aromatic compounds.

naphthalene

anthracene

pyridine

pyrrole

Figure 6.6

> **DAT Synopsis**
>
> The nonbonding electron pair in pyridine is in a nitrogen sp^2 orbital. This orbital is perpendicular to the *p*-orbitals around the ring and, therefore, is not involved in the conjugated pi system. On the other hand, the nonbonding pair in pyrrole is in a nitrogen sp^3 orbital parallel to the ring *p*-orbitals and, therefore, can participate in the delocalized pi system.

PROPERTIES

The physical properties of aromatic compounds are generally similar to those of other hydrocarbons. By contrast, chemical properties are significantly affected by aromaticity. The characteristic planar shape of benzene permits the ring's six pi orbitals to overlap, delocalizing the electron density. All six carbon atoms are sp^2 hybridized, and each of the six orbitals overlaps equally with its two neighbors. As a result, the delocalized electrons form two "pi electron clouds," one above and one below the plane of the ring. This delocalization stabilizes the molecule, making it fairly unreactive: In particular, benzene does not undergo addition reactions as do alkenes. The same holds true for other aromatic compounds, since the definition of an aromatic compound includes the condition that it have a delocalized pi electron system.

REACTIONS

A. ELECTROPHILIC AROMATIC SUBSTITUTION

The most important reaction of aromatic compounds is electrophilic aromatic substitution. In this reaction, an electrophile replaces a proton on an aromatic ring, producing a substituted aromatic compound. The most common examples are halogenation, sulfonation, nitration, and acylation.

1. Halogenation

Aromatic rings react with bromine or chlorine in the presence of a Lewis acid, such as $FeCl_3$, $FeBr_3$, or $AlCl_3$, to produce monosubstituted products in good yield. Reaction of fluorine and iodine with aromatic rings is less useful, as fluorine tends to produce multisubstituted products and iodine's lack of reactivity requires special conditions for the reaction to proceed.

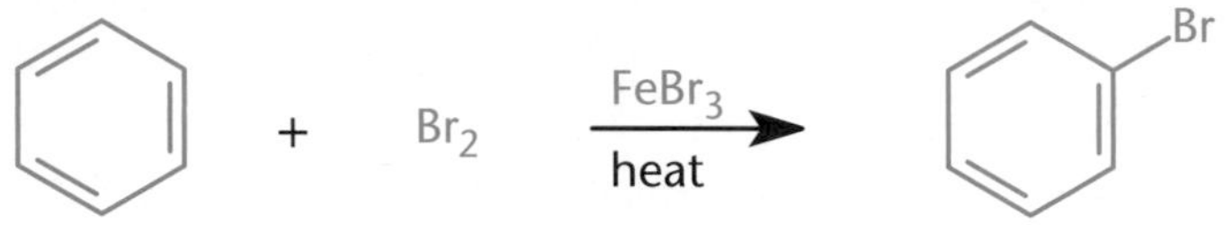

Figure 6.7

2. Sulfonation

Aromatic rings react with fuming sulfuric acid (a mixture of sulfuric acid and sulfur trioxide) to form sulfonic acids.

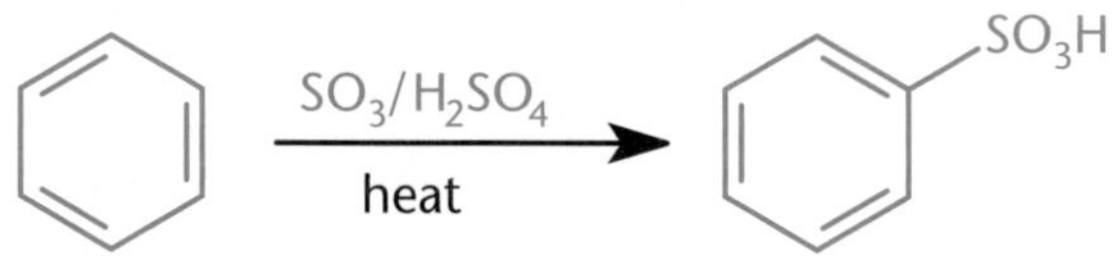

Figure 6.8

3. Nitration

The nitration of aromatic rings is another synthetically useful reaction. A mixture of nitric and sulfuric acids is used to create the nitronium ion, NO_2^+, a strong electrophile. This reacts with aromatic rings to produce nitro compounds.

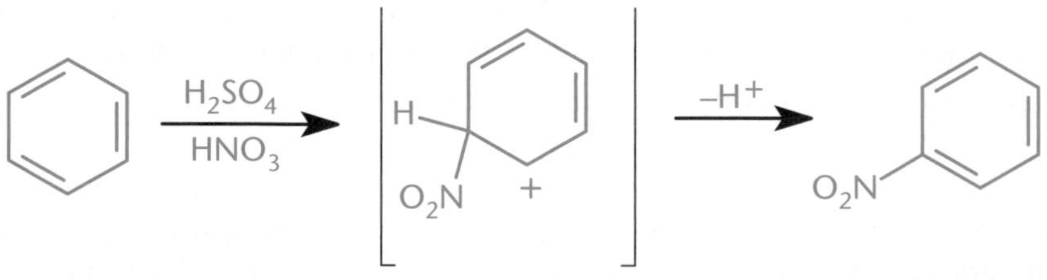

Figure 6.9

4. Acylation (Friedel-Crafts Reaction)

In a Friedel-Crafts acylation reaction, a carbocation electrophile, usually an acyl group, is incorporated into the aromatic ring. These reactions are usually catalyzed by Lewis acids, such as $AlCl_3$.

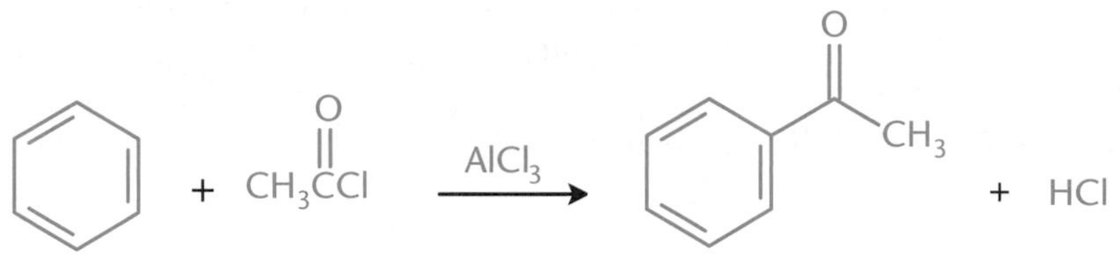

Figure 6.10

> **DAT Synopsis**
>
> Friedel-Crafts alkylation reactions can also occur, but these are less useful because the product is attacked faster than the starting material, leading to over-alkylation. (See substituent effects below.)

5. Substituent Effects

Substituents on an aromatic ring strongly influence the susceptibility of the ring to electrophilic aromatic substitution, and they also strongly affect what position on the ring an incoming electrophile is most likely to attack. Substituents can be grouped into three different classes according to whether substitution is enhanced (activating) or inhibited (deactivating) and where the reaction is likely to take place with respect to the group already present. These effects depend on whether the group tends to donate or withdraw electron density and how it does so; the specifics of these mechanisms will not be discussed here. Arranged in order of decreasing strength of the substituent effect, the three classes are listed below:

a. Activating, *ortho/para*-directing substituents (electron donating): NH_2, NR_2, OH, NHCOR, OR, OCOR, and R.

b. Deactivating, *ortho/para*-directing substituents (weakly electron withdrawing): F, Cl, Br, and I.

c. Deactivating, *meta*-directing substituents (electron withdrawing): NO_2, SO_3H, and carbonyl compounds, including COOH, COOR, COR, and CHO.

For example, when toluene undergoes electrophilic aromatic substitution, the methyl group directs substitution to occur at the *ortho* and *para* positions, as shown in Figure 6.11.

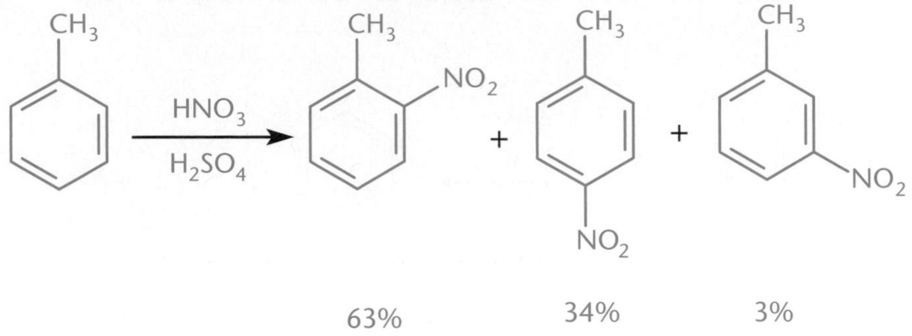

63%   34%   3%

Figure 6.11

B. REDUCTION

1. Catalytic Reduction

Benzene rings can be reduced by catalytic hydrogenation under vigorous conditions (elevated temperature and pressure) to yield cyclohexane. Ruthenium or rhodium on carbon are the most common catalysts; platinum or palladium may also be used.

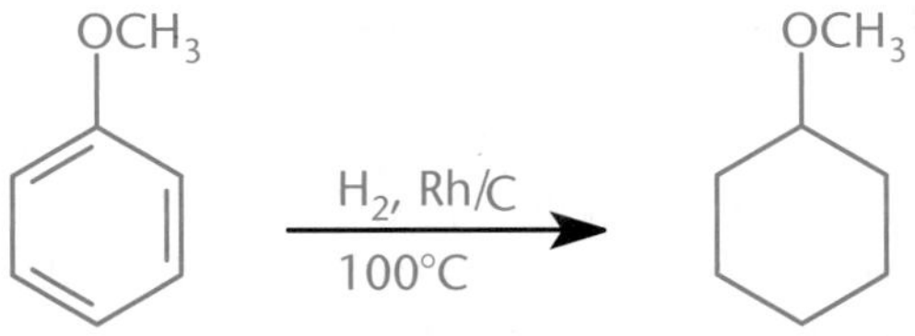

Figure 6.12

## 7

ALCOHOLS AND ETHERS

ALCOHOLS

Alcohols are compounds with the general formula **ROH.** The functional group **–OH** is called the **hydroxyl** group. An alcohol can be thought of as a substituted water molecule, with an alkyl group R replacing one H atom.

A. NOMENCLATURE

Alcohols are named in the IUPAC system by replacing the **-e** ending of the root alkane with the ending **-ol**. The carbon atom attached to the hydroxyl group must be included in the longest chain and receive the lowest possible number. Figure 7.1 shows some examples.

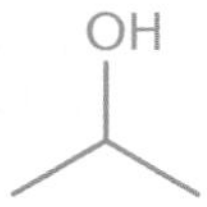

2-propanol

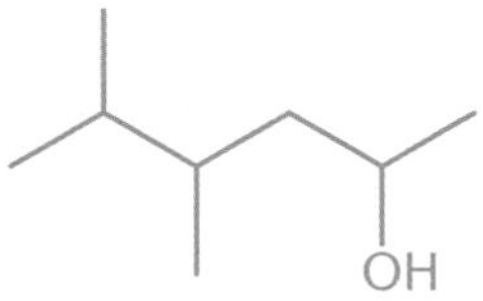

4,5-dimethyl-2-hexanol

Figure 7.1

Alternatively, the alkyl group can be named as a derivative, followed by the word *alcohol*.

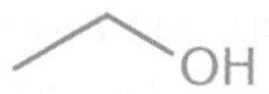

ethyl alcohol

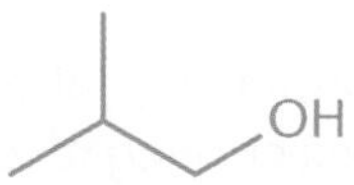

isobutyl alcohol

Figure 7.2

Compounds of the general formula ArOH, with a hydroxyl group attached to an aromatic ring, are called **phenols** (see chapter 6).

DAT Synopsis

The –OH group has high priority, so its C must be in the carbon backbone, with the lowest number possible.

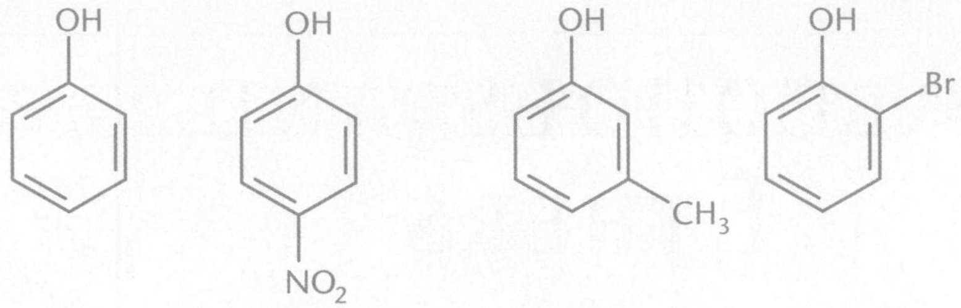

phenol *p*-nitrophenol *m*-cresol *o*-bromophenol
(*m*-methylphenol)

Figure 7.3

DAT Synopsis

Aromatic alcohols (ArOH) are called phenols. Resonance (through the ring) gives them special properties.

B. PHYSICAL PROPERTIES

The boiling points of alcohols are significantly higher than those of the analogous hydrocarbons due to **hydrogen bonding** (see General Chemistry chapter 3).

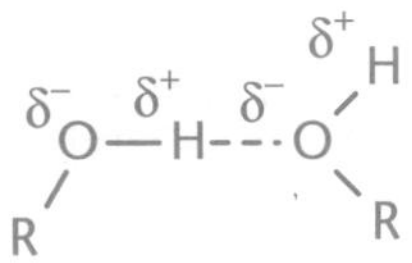

DAT Synopsis

Hydrogen bonding results in both elevated boiling points and better solubility in water

Figure 7.4

KAPLAN EXCLUSIVE

Hydrogen bonds form on the "phone"—the "FON"! (Fluorine, Oxygen, Nitrogen)

Molecules with more than one hydroxyl group show greater degrees of hydrogen bonding, as is evident from the boiling points shown in Figure 7.5.

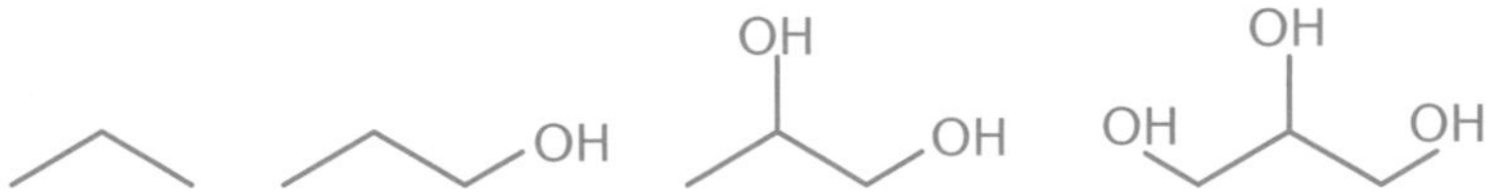

boiling point (°C)   −42.1   97.4   189.0   290.0

Figure 7.5

DAT Synopsis

Alcohols are weakly acidic:

ROH ⇌ RO⁻ + H⁺

Hydrogen bonding can also occur when hydrogen atoms are attached to other highly electronegative atoms, such as nitrogen and fluorine. HF has particularly strong hydrogen bonds, because the high electronegativity of fluorine causes the HF bond to be highly polarized.

The hydroxyl hydrogen atom is weakly acidic, and alcohols can dissociate into protons and alkoxy ions just as water dissociates into protons and hydroxide ions. pK_a values of several compounds are listed in Table 7.1.

Table 7.1

Dissociation		pK$_a$
$H_2O \rightleftharpoons$	$HO^- + H^+$	15.7
$CH_3OH \rightleftharpoons$	$CH_3O^- + H^+$	15.5
$C_2H_5OH \rightleftharpoons$	$C_2H_5O^- + H^+$	15.9
i-PrOH $\rightleftharpoons$	*i*-PrO$^-$ + H$^+$	17.1
t-BuOH $\rightleftharpoons$	*t*-BuO$^-$ + H$^+$	18.0
$CF_3CH_2OH \rightleftharpoons$	$CF_3CH_2O^- + H^+$	12.4
PhOH $\rightleftharpoons$	PhO$^-$ + H$^+$	≈10.0

Bridge

$pK_a = -\log K_a$

Strong acids have high K_a's and small pK_a's. Thus, phenol, which has the smallest pKa, is the most acidic (see General Chemistry chapter 10).

The hydroxyl hydrogens of phenols are more acidic than those of alcohols due to resonance structures that distribute the negative charge throughout the ring, thus stabilizing the anion. As a result, these compounds form intermolecular hydrogen bonds and have relatively high melting and boiling points. Phenol is slightly soluble in water (presumably due to hydrogen bonding), as are some of its derivatives. Phenols are much more acidic than aliphatic alcohols and can form salts with inorganic bases such as NaOH.

The presence of other substituents on the ring has significant effects on the acidity, boiling points, and melting points of phenols. As with other aromatic compounds, electron-withdrawing substituents increase acidity, and electron-donating groups decrease acidity.

DAT Synopsis

Acidity decreases as more alkyl groups are attached because the electron-donating alkyl groups destabilize the alkoxide anion. Electron-withdrawing groups stabilize the alkoxy anion, making the alcohol more acidic .

C. REVIEW

1. Key Reaction for Mechanisms for Alcohols and Ethers

As you read about synthesis of (and from) alcohols and ethers, you'll see the same basic reaction mechanisms recurring over and over. Rather than memorizing each reaction individually, try to think of them in broad categories. Focus on how the basic mechanism works and on how this particular reaction exemplifies it. The "Big Three" mechanisms for alcohols and ethers are:

DAT Synopsis

Charge likes to be spread out as widely as possible!

↑ acidity	resonance e$^-$ withdrawing
↓ acidity	e$^-$ donating

a. **S_N1, S_N2: nucleophilic substitution**

Example:

$$CH_3Br + OH^- \longrightarrow CH_3OH + Br^-$$

See chapter 4 for review.

b. **Electrophilic addition to a double bond**

Example:

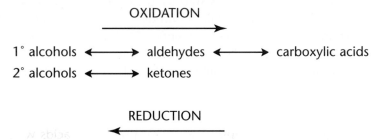

This and other reactions adding H_2O to double bonds are covered in chapter 4.

c. **Nucleophilic addition to a carbonyl**

Example:

This mechanism is discussed further in chapters 8–10.

Also, when thinking about alcohols, you should keep in mind their place on the oxidation-reduction continuum:

OXIDATION

→

1° alcohols ⟷ aldehydes ⟷ carboxylic acids

2° alcohols ⟷ ketones

REDUCTION

←

As you read about the individual reactions in which alcohols participate, try to fit them into this framework (possible for most reactions, though not all).

D. SYNTHESIS

Alcohols can be prepared from a variety of compounds. Methanol, also called wood alcohol, is obtained from the destructive distillation of wood. It is toxic and can cause blindness if ingested. Ethanol, or grain alcohol, is produced from the fermentation of sugars and can be metabolized by the body; however, in large enough quantities, it too is toxic.

1. Addition Reactions

Alcohols can be prepared via several reactions that involve addition of water to double bonds (discussed in "Alkenes: Reactions" in chapter 5). Alcohols can also be prepared from the addition of organometallic compounds to carbonyl groups (discussed in chapter 9).

KAPLAN EXCLUSIVE

More bonds to oxygen means more oxidized.

2. Substitution Reactions

Both S_N1 and S_N2 reactions can be used to produce alcohols under the proper conditions (discussed in "Substitution Reactions in Alkyl Halides" in chapter 4).

3. Reduction Reactions

Alcohols can be prepared from the reduction of aldehydes, ketones, carboxylic acids, or esters. Lithium aluminum hydride ($LiAlH_4$, or LAH) and sodium borohydride ($NaBH_4$) are the two most frequently used reducing reagents. LAH is more powerful and more difficult to work with, whereas $NaBH_4$ is more selective and easier to handle. For example, LAH will reduce carboxylic acids and esters, while $NaBH_4$ will not.

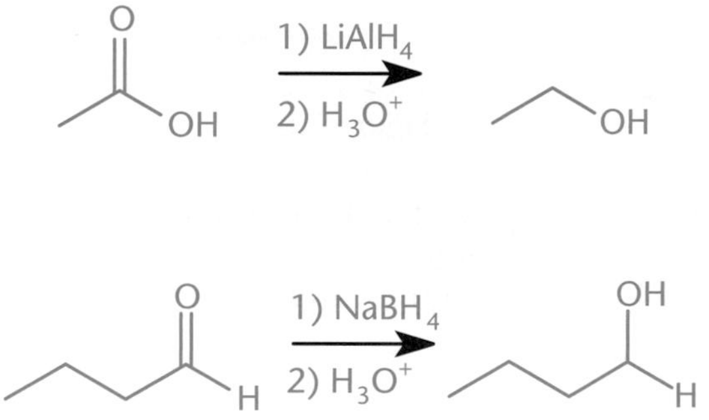

Figure 7.6

4. Phenol Synthesis

Phenols can be synthesized from arylsulfonic acids with hot NaOH. However, this reaction is useful only for phenol or its alkylated derivatives, as most functional groups are destroyed by the harsh reaction conditions.

A more versatile method of synthesizing phenols is via hydrolysis of diazonium salts.

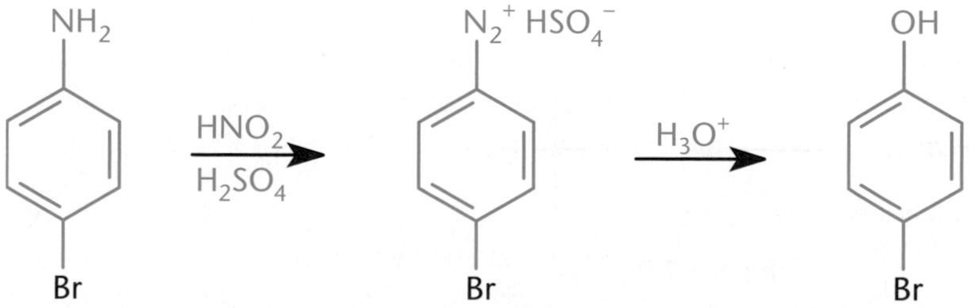

Figure 7.7

DAT Synopsis

Think of electrophilic addition of H_2O to a double bond, only this time it's in reverse—elimination.

E. REACTIONS

1. Elimination Reactions

Alcohols can be **dehydrated** in a strongly acidic solution (usually H_2SO_4) to produce alkenes. The mechanism of this dehydration reaction is E1, and it proceeds via the protonated alcohol.

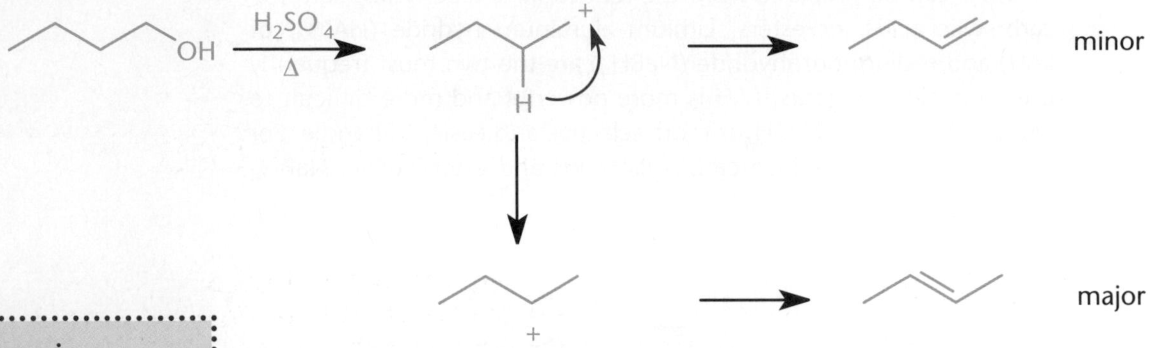

Figure 7.8

DAT Synopsis

In E1, you want to form the most stable (that is, most substituted) carbocation.

Notice from Figure 7.8 that two products are obtained, with the more stable alkene being the major product. This occurs via movement of a proton to produce the more stable 2° carbocation. This type of rearrangement is commonly encountered with carbocations.

DAT Synopsis

Alcohols can participate in S_N1/S_N2 reactions, but only if you turn the –OH into a better leaving group by one of the following methods:

— Protonate it.
— Convert to a tosylate.
— Form an inorganic ester.

2. Substitution Reactions

The displacement of hydroxyl groups in substitution reactions is rare because the hydroxide ion is a poor leaving group. If such a transformation is desired, the hydroxyl group must be made into a good leaving group. Protonating the alcohol makes water the leaving group, which is good for S_N1 reactions; even better, the alcohol can be converted into a tosylate (*p*-toluenesulfonate) group, which is an excellent leaving group for S_N2 reactions (see Figures 7.9a and 7.9b).

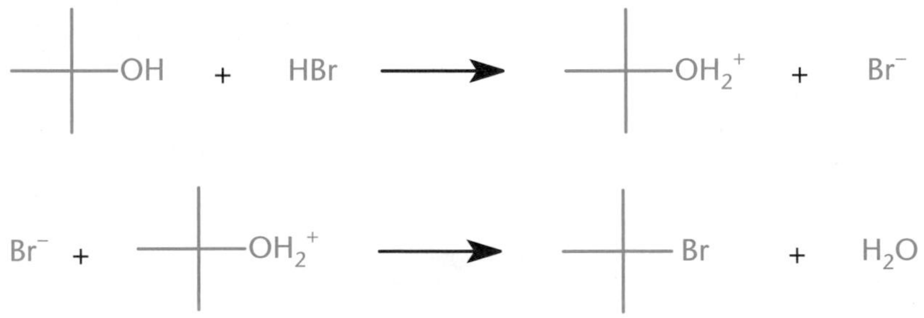

Figure 7.9a

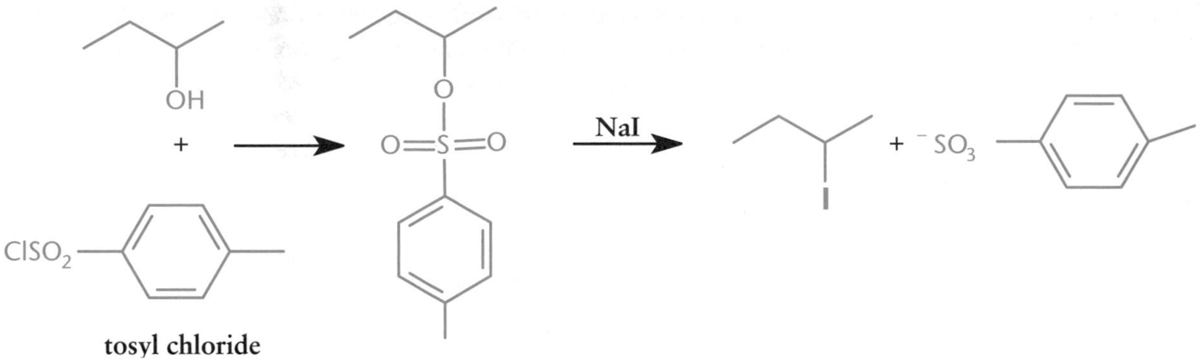

Figure 7.9b

A common method of converting alcohols into alkyl halides involves the formation of inorganic esters, which readily undergo S_N2 reactions. Alcohols react with thionyl chloride to produce an intermediate inorganic ester (a chlorosulfite) and HCl. The chloride ion of HCl displaces SO_2 and regenerates Cl^-, forming the desired alkyl chloride.

$$CH_3OH + SOCl_2 \longrightarrow CH_3OSOCl + HCl$$

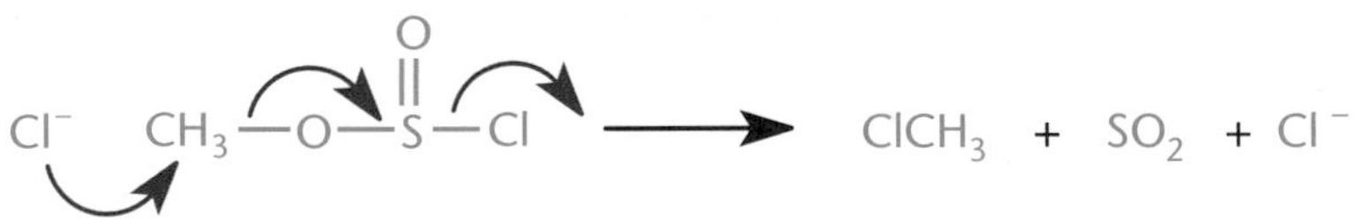

Figure 7.10

An analogous reaction, where the alcohol is treated with PBr_3 instead of thionyl chloride, produces alkyl bromides.

Phenols readily undergo electrophilic aromatic substitution reactions; because it has lone pairs that it can donate to the ring, the –OH group is a strongly activating, *ortho/para*-directing ring substituent (see "Reactions" in chapter 6).

DAT Synopsis

Phenols are good substrates for electrophilic aromatic substitution; the –OH is activating and *ortho/para* directing.

3. **Oxidation Reactions**
The oxidation of alcohols generally involves some form of chromium (VI) as the oxidizing agent, which is reduced to chromium (III) during the reaction. PCC (pyridinium chlorochromate, $C_5H_6NCrO_3Cl$) is commonly used as a mild oxidant. It converts primary alcohols to aldehydes without overoxidation to the acid. (In contrast, $KMnO_4$ is a very strong oxidizing agent that will take the alcohol all the way to the carboxylic acid.) It can also be used to form ketones from 2° alcohols. Tertiary alcohols cannot be oxidized for valence reasons.

DAT Synopsis

When you see a transition metal (such as Cr or Mn) with lots of oxygen (Cr_2O_7, CrO_3, MnO_4), think OXIDATION.

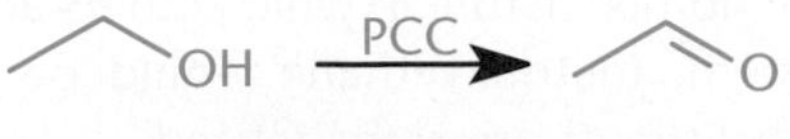

Figure 7.11

Another reagent used to oxidize secondary alcohols is alkali (either sodium or potassium) dichromate salt. This will also oxidize 1° alcohols to carboxylic acids.

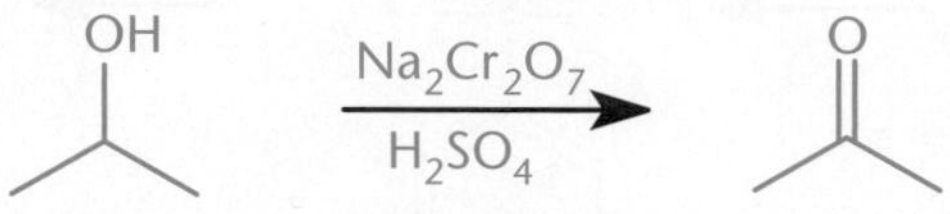

Figure 7.12

> **DAT Synopsis**
>
> Alcohols can be formed by and can participate in many of the key reaction mechanisms you've already seen:
>
> 1) S_N1, S_N2 (although –OH must be made into a better leaving group);
> 2) addition of H_2O to a double bond (including electrophilic addition) and reverse reactions such as E1 (see chapter 5);
> 3) nucleophilic addition to a carbonyl;
>
> 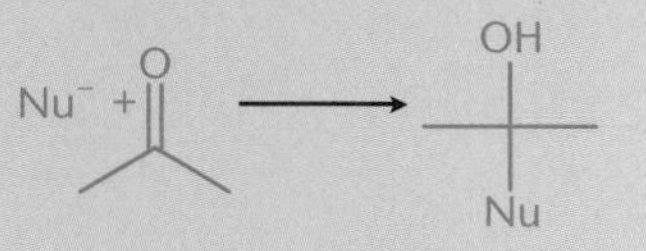
>
>
> 4) oxidation/reduction reactions.

A stronger oxidant is chromium trioxide, CrO_3. This is often dissolved with dilute sulfuric acid in acetone; the mixture is called Jones reagent. It oxidizes primary alcohols to carboxylic acids and secondary alcohols to ketones.

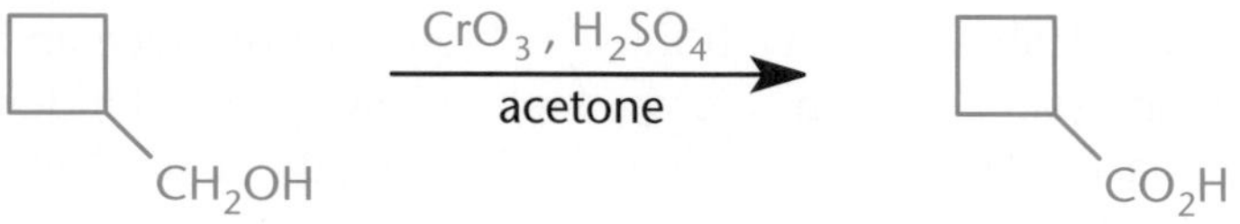

Figure 7.13

Treatment of phenols with oxidizing reagents produces compounds called quinones (2,5-cyclohexadiene-1,4-diones).

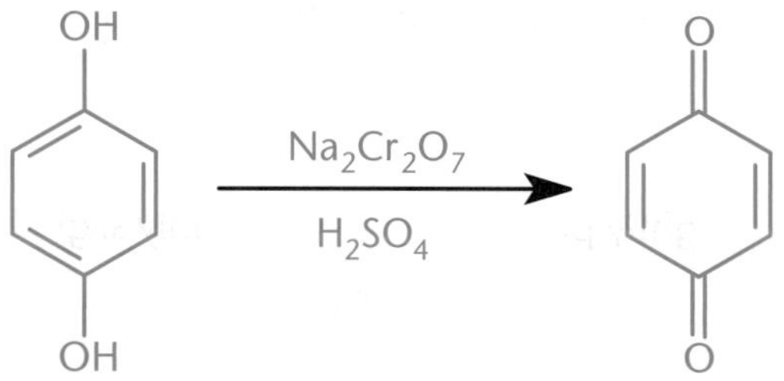

1,4-benzenediol **p-benzoquinone**

Figure 7.14

ETHERS

An ether is a compound with two alkyl (or aryl) groups bonded to an oxygen atom. The general formula for an ether is **ROR**. Ethers can be thought of as disubstituted water molecules. The most familiar ether is diethyl ether, once used as a medical anesthetic and still often used that way in the laboratory.

A. NOMENCLATURE

Ethers are named according to IUPAC rules as **alkoxyalkanes,** with the smaller chain as the prefix and the larger chain as the suffix. There is a common system of nomenclature in which ethers are named as alkyl alkyl ethers. In this system, methoxyethane would be named ethyl methyl ether. The alkyl substituents are alphabetized.

methoxyethane (ethyl methyl ether) — ethoxybenzene (ethyl phenyl ether)

Figure 7.15

Exceptions to these rules occur for cyclic ethers, for which many common names also exist.

> **DAT Synopsis**
>
> Remember that smaller rings have more angle strain, making them less stable.

oxirane (epoxide) — oxyethane — oxacyclopentane (tetrahydrofuran)

Figure 7.16

B. PHYSICAL PROPERTIES

Ethers do not undergo hydrogen bonding because they have no hydrogen atoms bonded to the oxygen atoms. Ethers therefore boil at relatively low temperatures compared to alcohols; in fact, they boil at approximately the same temperatures as alkanes of comparable molecular weight.

> **DAT Synopsis**
>
> There's no H on the phone "FON"—therefore, no H-bonds and lower boiling points than alcohols.

Ethers are only slightly polar and, therefore, only slightly soluble in water. They are rather inert to most organic reagents and are frequently used as solvents.

C. SYNTHESIS

The Williamson ether synthesis produces ethers from the reaction of metal alkoxides with primary alkyl halides or tosylates. The alkoxides behave as nucleophiles and displace the halide or tosylate via an S_N2 reaction, producing an ether.

> **DAT Synopsis**
>
> Look! It's S_N2 again! Therefore, you need a strong nucleophile (alkoxides are good) and an unhindered substrate (*not* bulky or highly substituted).

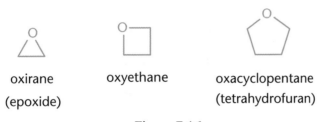

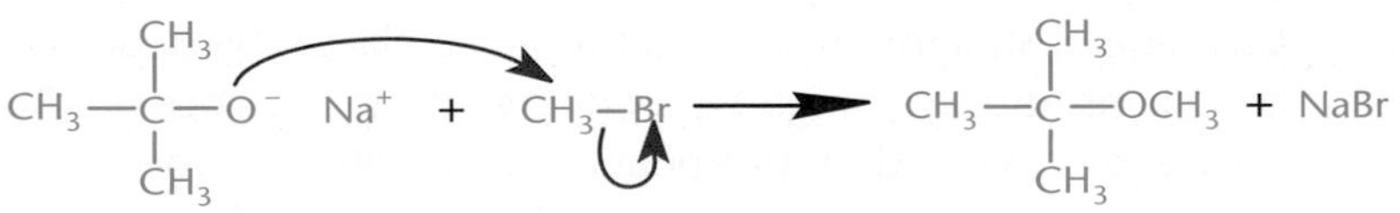

Figure 7.17

It is important to remember that alkoxides will attack only nonhindered halides. Thus, to synthesize a methyl ether, an alkoxide must attack a methyl halide; the reaction cannot be accomplished with methoxide ion attacking a hindered alkyl halide substrate.

The Williamson ether synthesis can also be applied to phenols. Relatively mild reaction conditions are sufficient, due to the phenols' acidity.

DAT Synopsis

More S_N2! This time, however, it's intramolecular—the nucleophile and leaving group are part of the same molecule.

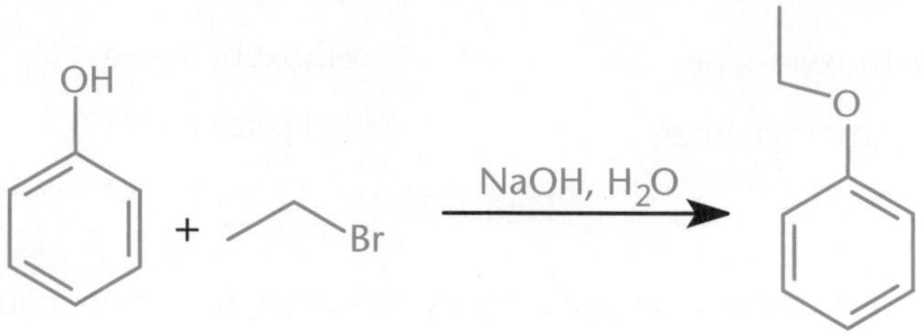

Figure 7.18

Cyclic ethers are prepared in a number of ways. Oxiranes can be synthesized by means of an internal S_N2 displacement.

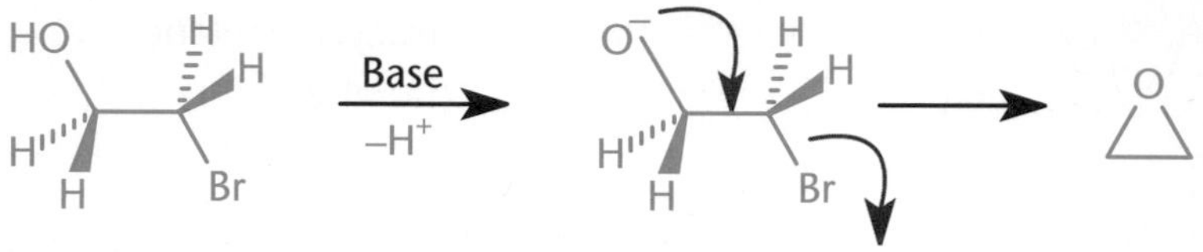

Figure 7.19

DAT Synopsis

Q: Why are intramolecular reactions favored?

A: Both rate and equilibrium are strongly affected by the reagent concentrations. In intramolecular reactions, the reagents "see" fairly high concentrations of one another—they're basically "tied together."

Oxidation of an alkene with a **peroxy acid** (general formula RCOOOH) such as mcpba (*m*-chloroperoxybenzoic acid) will also produce an oxirane.

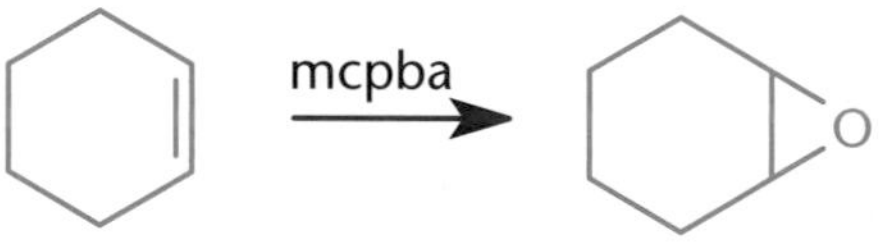

Figure 7.20

D. REACTIONS

1. Peroxide Formation

Ethers react with the oxygen in air to form highly explosive compounds called **peroxides** (general formula ROOR).

2. Cleavage

Cleavage of straight-chain ethers will take place only under vigorous conditions: usually at high temperatures in the presence of HBr or HI. Cleavage is initiated by protonation of the ether oxygen. The reaction then proceeds by an S_N1 or S_N2 mechanism, depending on the conditions and the structure of the ether. Although not shown in Figure 7.21, the alcohol products usually react with a second molecule of hydrogen halide to produce an alkyl halide.

DAT Synopsis

Remember, strong bases are poor leaving groups. Without protonation, the leaving group would be an alkoxide (strongly basic), and the reaction would be unlikely to proceed.

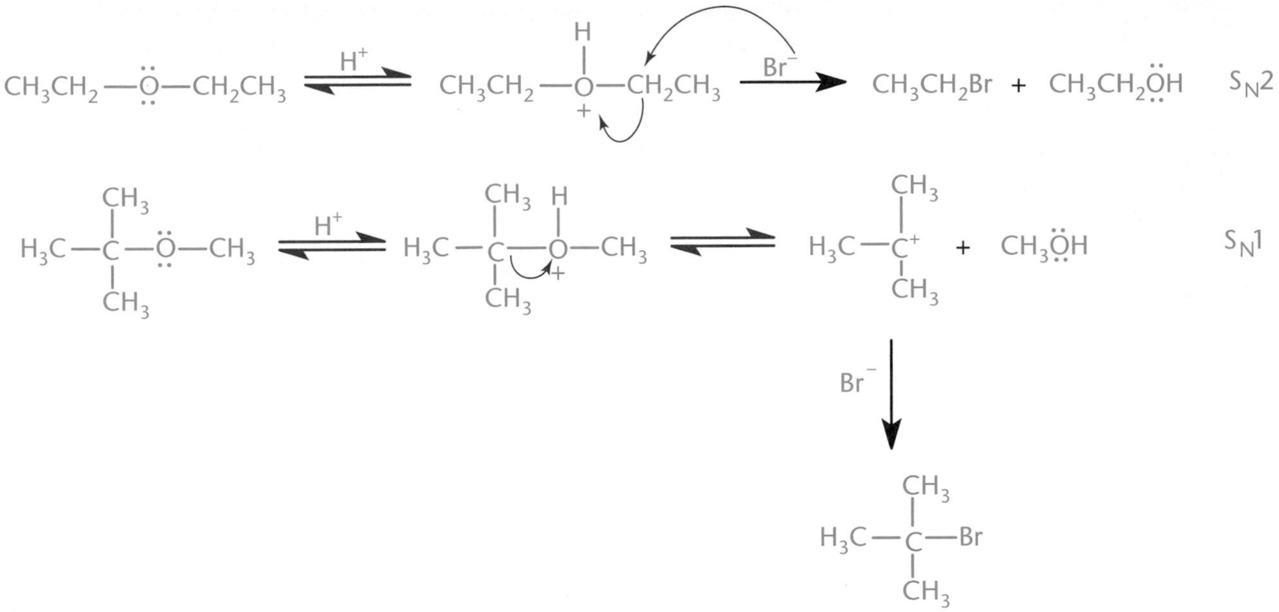

Figure 7.21

Since epoxides are highly strained cyclic ethers, they are susceptible to S_N2 reactions. Unlike straight-chain ethers, these reactions can be catalyzed by acid or base. In symmetrical epoxides, either carbon can be nucleophilically attacked, but in asymmetrical epoxides, the most substituted carbon is nucleophilically attacked in the presence of acid, and the least substituted carbon is attacked in the presence of base (see Figure 7.22).

DAT Synopsis

Cleavage of straight-chain ethers is acid-catalyzed. Cleavage of cyclic ethers can be acid- or base-catalyzed.

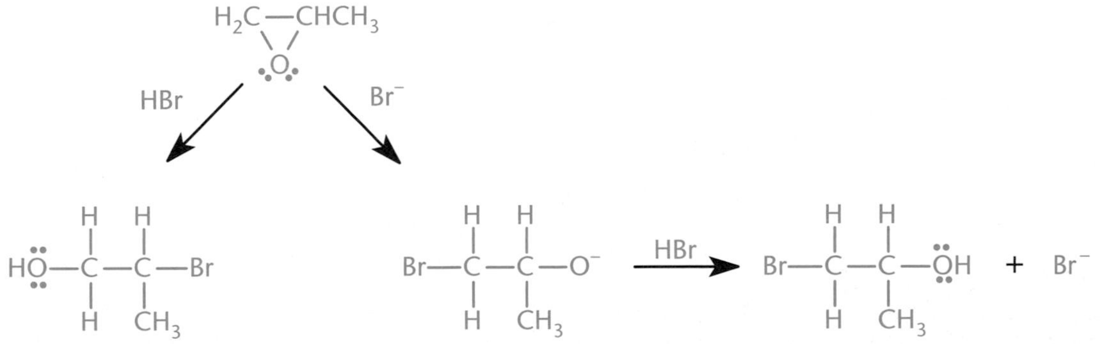

acid-catalyzed ring opening

base-catalyzed ring opening

Figure 7.22

Base-catalyzed cleavage has the most S_N2 character, so it occurs at the least hindered (least substituted) carbon. The basic environment provides the best nucleophile.

DAT Synopsis

Base-catalyzed cleavage has the most S_N2 character, while acid-catalyzed cleavage seems to have some S_N1 character.

In contrast, acid-catalyzed cleavage is thought to have some S_N1 character as well as some S_N2 character. The epoxide O can be protonated, making it a better leaving group. This gives the carbons a bit of positive charge. Since substitution stabilizes this charge (remember, 3° carbons make the best carbocations), the more substituted C becomes a good target for nucleophilic attack.

Don't let epoxides intimidate you; the same basic principles and reaction mechanisms apply, just as we've seen with more simple compounds.

## 8

ALDEHYDES AND KETONES

Aldehydes and **ketones** are compounds that contain the **carbonyl group, C=O,** a double bond between a carbon atom and an oxygen atom. A ketone has two alkyl or aryl groups bonded to the carbonyl, whereas an aldehyde has one alkyl group and one hydrogen (or, in the case of formaldehyde, two hydrogens) bonded to the carbonyl. The carbonyl group is one of the most important functional groups in organic chemistry. In addition to aldehydes and ketones, it is also found in carboxylic acids, esters, amides, and more complicated compounds.

NOMENCLATURE

In the IUPAC system, aldehydes are named with the suffix **-al**. The position of the aldehyde group does not need to be specified: It must occupy the terminal (C–1) position. Common names exist for the first five aldehydes: formaldehyde, acetaldehyde, propionaldehyde, butyraldehyde, and valeraldehyde (see Figure 8.1).

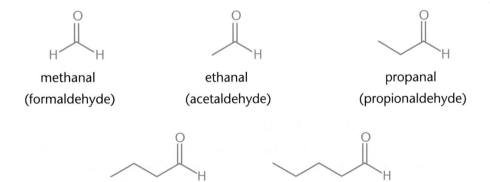

| methanal | ethanal | propanal |
| (formaldehyde) | (acetaldehyde) | (propionaldehyde) |

butanal (butyraldehyde)   pentanal (valeraldehyde)

Figure 8.1

In more complicated molecules, the suffix **-carbaldehyde** can be used. In addition, the aldehyde can be named as a functional group with the prefix **formyl-**.

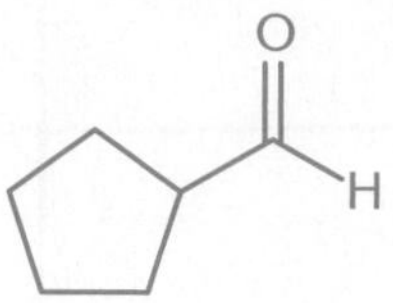

cyclopentanecarbaldehyde

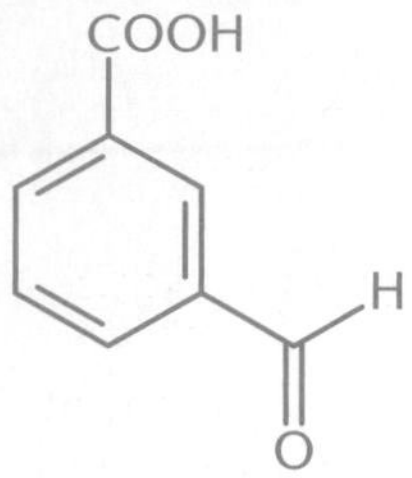

m-formylbenzoic acid

Figure 8.2

Ketones are named with the suffix **-one**. The location of the carbonyl group must be specified with a number, except in cyclic ketones, where it is assumed to occupy the number 1 position. The common system of naming **ketones** lists the two alkyl groups followed by the word *ketone*. When it is necessary to name the carbonyl as a substituent, the prefix **oxo-** is used.

> **DAT Synopsis**
>
> The carbonyl group has a dipole moment. Oxygen is more electronegative—it is an "electron hog," pulling the electrons away from the carbon.

2-propanone
(dimethyl ketone)
(acetone)

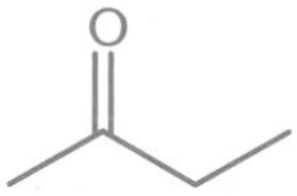

2-butanone
(ethyl methyl ketone)

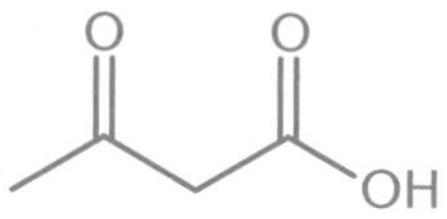

3-oxobutanoic acid

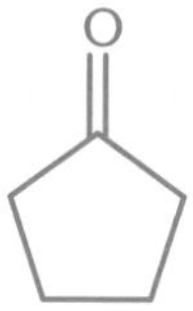

cyclopentanone

Figure 8.3

PHYSICAL PROPERTIES

The physical properties of aldehydes and ketones are governed by the presence of the carbonyl group. The dipole moments associated with the polar carbonyl groups align, causing an elevation in boiling point relative to the alkanes. This elevation is less than that in alcohols, since no hydrogen bonding is involved.

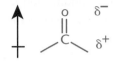

Figure 8.4

SYNTHESIS

There are numerous methods of preparing aldehydes and ketones; four of the most common are described below.

A. OXIDATION OF ALCOHOLS

An aldehyde can be obtained from the oxidation of a primary alcohol; a ketone can be obtained from a secondary alcohol. As mentioned in chapter 7, these reactions are usually performed with PCC, sodium or potassium dichromate, or chromium trioxide (Jones reagent).

B. OZONOLYSIS OF ALKENES

Double bonds can be oxidatively cleaved to yield aldehydes and/or ketones, typically with ozone. See chapter 5 for more details.

C. FRIEDEL-CRAFTS ACYLATION

This reaction, discussed in "Reactions" in chapter 6, produces ketones of the form R–CO–Ar.

REACTIONS

A. ENOLIZATION AND REACTIONS OF ENOLS

Protons alpha to carbonyl groups are relatively acidic ($pK_a \approx 20$) due to resonance stabilization of the conjugate base. A hydrogen atom that detaches itself from the alpha carbon has a finite probability of reattaching itself to the oxygen instead of the carbon. Therefore, aldehydes and ketones exist in solution as a mixture of two isomers, the familiar **keto** form and the **enol** form, representing the unsaturated alcohol (**ene** = the double bond, **ol** = the alcohol, so **ene** + **ol** = **enol**). The two isomers, which differ only in the placement of a proton, are called **tautomers**. The equilibrium between the tautomers lies far to the keto side. The process of interconverting from the keto to the enol tautomer is called **enolization**. Tautomers are structural isomers, *not* resonance structures.

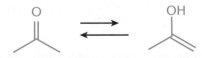

Figure 8.5

Enols are the necessary intermediates in many reactions of aldehydes and ketones. The enolate carbanion, which is nucleophilic, can be created with a strong base, such as lithium diisopropyl amide (LDA) or potassium hydride (KH). This nucleophilic carbanion reacts via S_N2 with α,β-unsaturated carbonyl compounds in reactions called **Michael additions**.

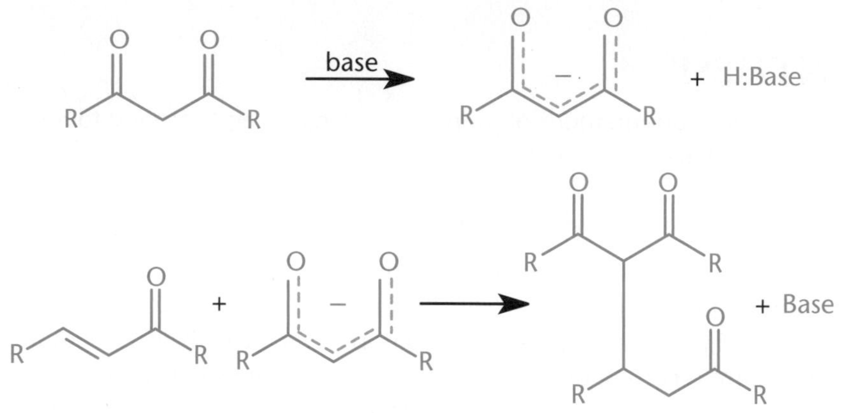

Figure 8.6

B. ADDITION REACTIONS

General Reaction Mechanism: Nucleophilic Addition to a Carbonyl

Many of the reactions of aldehydes and ketones share this general reaction mechanism. Rather than memorizing them all individually, focus on understanding the basic pattern. Then, you can learn how each reaction exemplifies it.

As shown in Figure 8.4, the C=O bond is polarized, with a partial positive charge on C and a partial negative charge on O. This makes the carbon ripe for nucleophilic attack.

DAT Synopsis

The carbonyl carbon is a good target for nucleophilic attack.

The nucleophile attacks, forming a bond to the C, which causes the π bond in the C=O to break. This generates a tetrahedral intermediate. If no good leaving group is present, the double bond cannot re-form, and the final product is nearly identical to the intermediate, except that usually the O^- will accept a proton to become a hydroxyl (–OH).

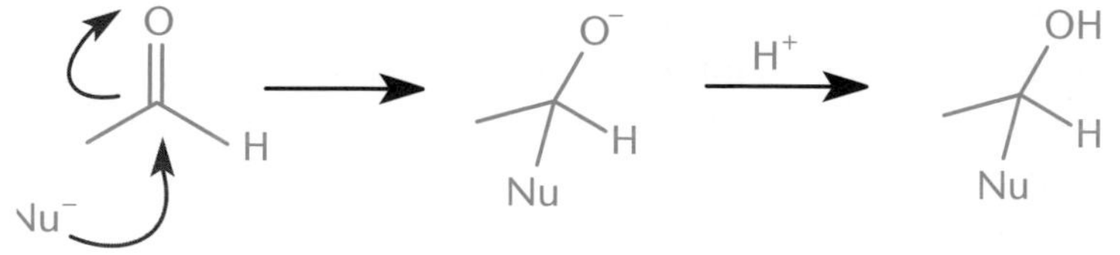

Figure 8.7

Although Figure 8.7 only shows nucleophilic addition to an aldehyde, this mechanism applies to ketones as well.

1. **Hydration**

   In the presence of water, aldehydes and ketones react to form *gem* diols (1,1-diols). In this case, water acts as the nucleophile attacking at the carbonyl carbon. This hydration reaction proceeds slowly; the rate may be increased by the addition of a small amount of acid or base.

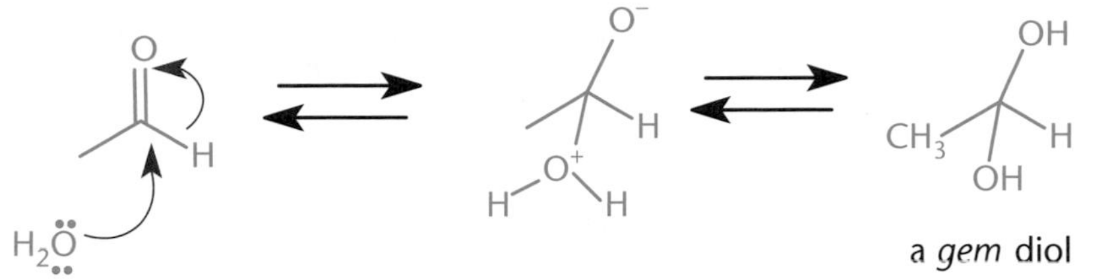

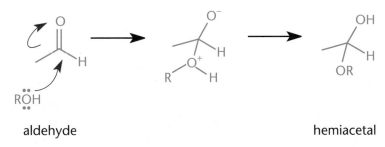

Figure 8.8

a *gem* diol

2. **Acetal and Ketal Formation**

   A reaction similar to hydration occurs when aldehydes and ketones are treated with alcohols. When one equivalent of alcohol (the nucleophile in this reaction) is added to an aldehyde or ketone, the product is a **hemiacetal** or a **hemiketal**, respectively. When two equivalents of alcohol are added, the product is an **acetal** or a **ketal**, respectively. The reaction mechanism is the same as for hydration and is catalyzed by anhydrous acid. Acetals and ketals, which are comparatively inert, are frequently used as protecting groups for carbonyl functionalities. They can easily be converted back to the carbonyl with aqueous acid.

aldehyde   hemiacetal

Figure 8.9

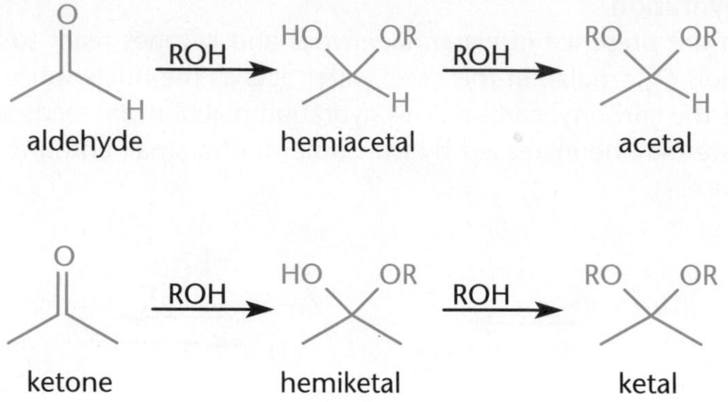

Figure 8.10

3. **Reaction with HCN**
   Aldehydes and ketones react with HCN (hydrogen cyanide) to produce stable compounds called **cyanohydrins**. HCN dissociates and the nucleophilic cyanide anion attacks the carbonyl carbon atom. Protonation of the oxygen produces the cyanohydrin. The cyanohydrin gains its stability from the newly formed C–C bond. (In contrast, when a carbonyl reacts with HCl, a weak C–Cl bond is formed, and the resulting chlorohydrin is unstable.)

> **DAT Synopsis**
>
> When CN^- is the nucleophile, cyanohydrins are formed.

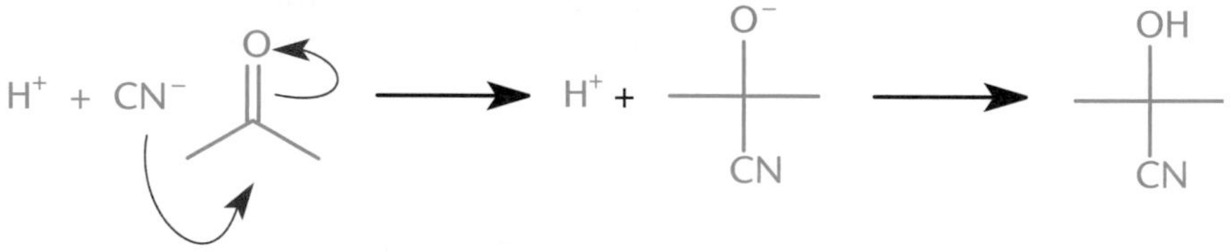

Figure 8.11

4. **Condensations with Ammonia Derivatives**
   Ammonia and some of its derivatives are nucleophiles and can add to carbonyl compounds. In the simplest case, ammonia adds to the carbon atom and water is lost, producing an **imine,** a compound with a nitrogen atom double-bonded to a carbon atom. (A reaction in which water is lost between two molecules is called a **condensation reaction**.)

   In this case, the first part of the reaction follows the mechanism of nucleophilic addition described above. However, after formation of a tetrahedral intermediate, this reaction proceeds further: The C=O double bond reforms, and a leaving group is kicked off. This mechanism is called nucleophilic *substitution* on a carbonyl and will be described in greater detail in chapter 9.

   Some common ammonia derivatives that react with aldehydes and ketones are hydroxylamine (H_2NOH), hydrazine (H_2NNH_2), and semicarbazide ($H_2NNHCONH_2$); these form oximes, hydrazones, and semicarbazones, respectively.

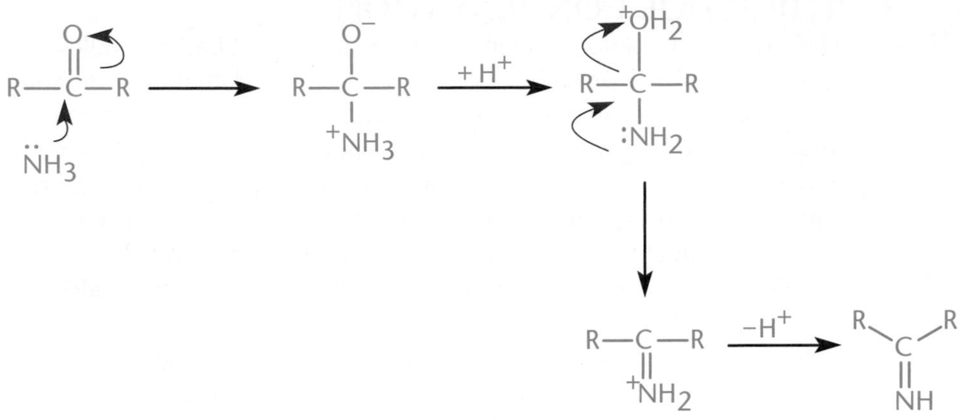

Figure 8.12

Don't worry too much about protons coming and going; there should be plenty in the solution, so you can transiently put them where needed to facilitate this reaction.

Examples of other potential nucleophiles and their respective products are shown in Figure 8.13.

> **DAT Synopsis**
>
> Nitrogen-containing compounds can be nucleophiles too.

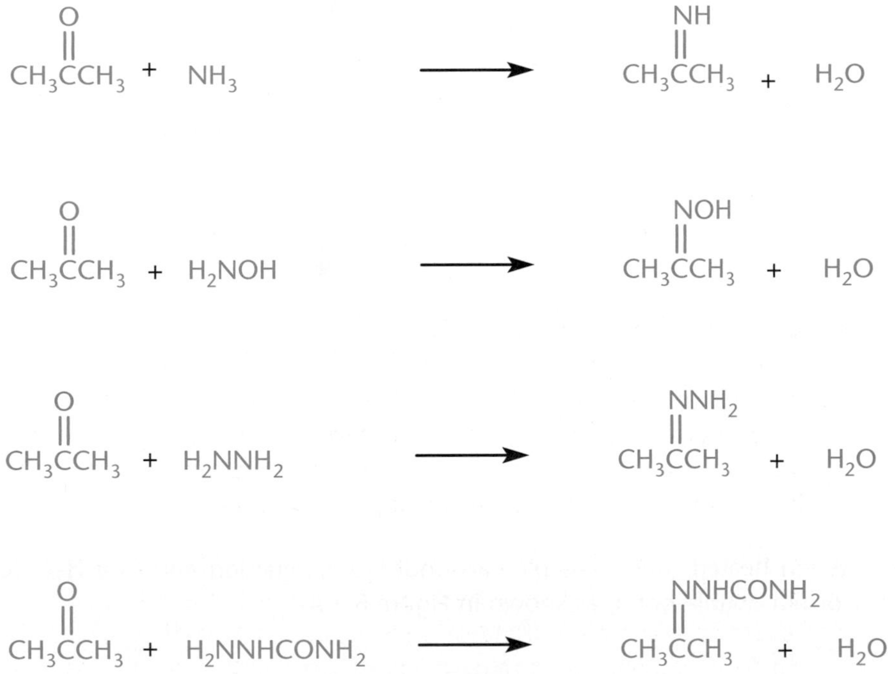

Figure 8.13

C. THE ALDOL CONDENSATION

The aldol condensation is an important reaction that basically follows the mechanism of nucleophilic addition to a carbonyl that was described above. In this case, an aldehyde acts both as nucleophile (enol form) and target (keto form.) When acetaldehyde (ethanal) is treated with base, an enolate ion is produced. This enolate ion, being nucleophilic, can react with the carbonyl group of another acetaldehyde molecule. The product is 3-hydroxybutanal, which contains both an alcohol and an aldehyde functionality. This type of compound is called an **aldol**, from **ald**ehyde and alco**hol**. With stronger base and higher temperatures, condensation occurs, producing an α,β-unsaturated aldehyde. This type of condensation reaction has become known as the **aldol condensation**.

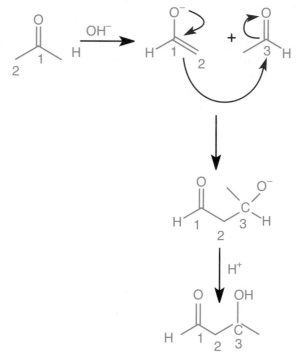

3-hydroxybutanal
(an aldol)

Figure 8.14a

When heated, this molecule can undergo elimination and lose H_2O to form a double bond, as shown in Figure 8.14b.

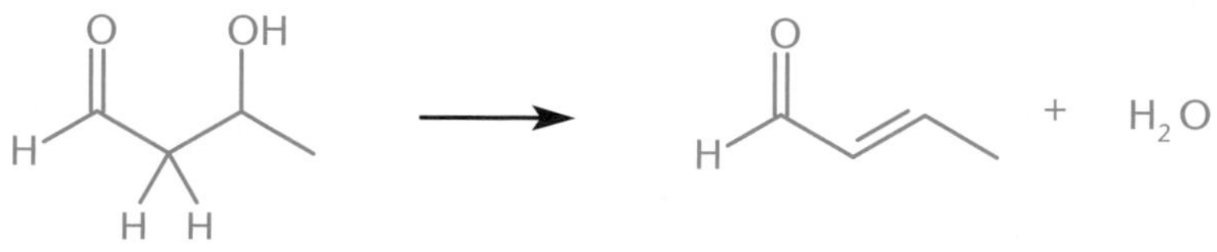

Figure 8.14b

The aldol condensation is most useful when only one type of aldehyde or ketone is present, since mixed condensations usually result in a mixture of products.

D. THE WITTIG REACTION

The **Wittig reaction** is a method of forming carbon-carbon double bonds by converting aldehydes and ketones into alkenes. The first step involves the formation of a phosphonium salt from the S_N2 reaction of an alkyl halide with the nucleophile triphenylphosphine, $(C_6H_5)_3P$. The phosphonium salt is then deprotonated (losing the proton α to the phosphorus) with a strong base, yielding a neutral compound called an **ylide** (pronounced "ill-id") or **phosphorane**. (The phosphorus atom may be drawn as pentavalent, utilizing the low-lying $3d$ atomic orbitals.)

> **DAT Synopsis**
>
> The Wittig reaction ultimately converts C=O to C=C.

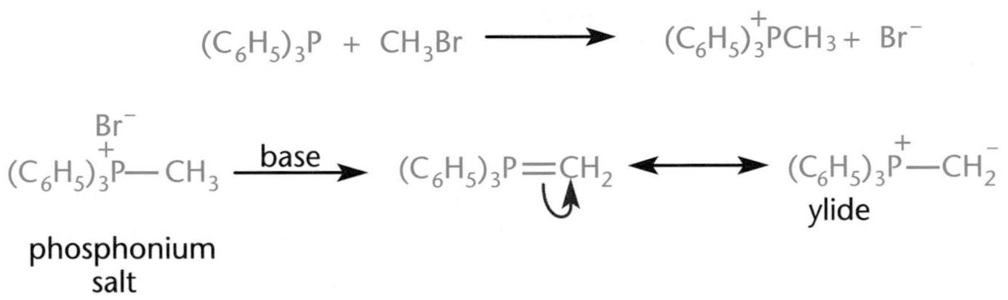

$$(C_6H_5)_3P + CH_3Br \longrightarrow (C_6H_5)_3\overset{+}{P}CH_3 + Br^-$$

Figure 8.15

Notice that an ylide is a type of carbanion and has nucleophilic properties. When combined with an aldehyde or ketone, an ylide attacks the carbonyl carbon, giving an intermediate called a **betaine**, which forms a four-membered ring intermediate called an oxaphosphetane. This decomposes to yield an alkene and triphenylphosphine oxide.

> **DAT Synopsis**
>
> The ylide can act as a nucleophile and attack the carbonyl.

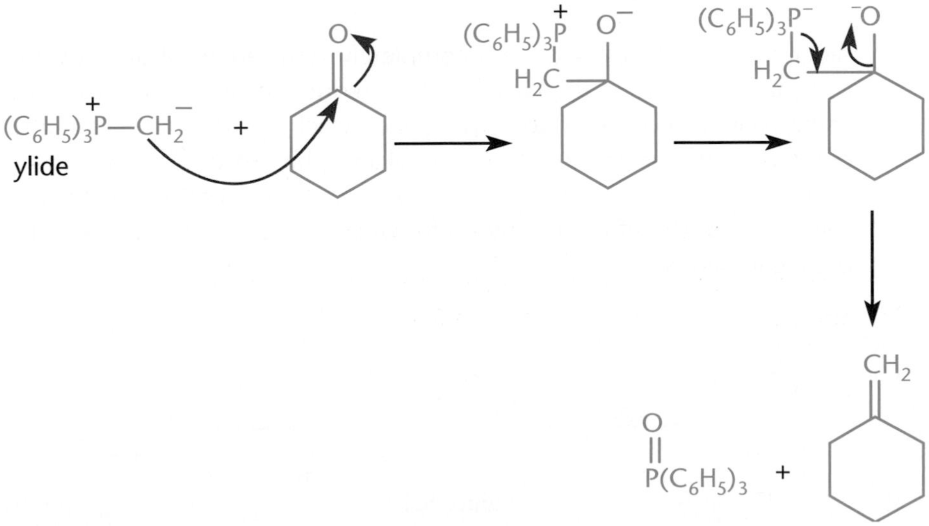

Figure 8.16

The decomposition reaction is driven by the strength of the phosphorus-oxygen bond that is formed.

E. OXIDATION AND REDUCTION

Aldehydes and ketones occupy the middle of the oxidation-reduction continuum. They are more oxidized than alcohols but less oxidized than carboxylic acids.

Aldehydes can be oxidized with a number of different reagents, such as $KMnO_4$, CrO_3, Ag_2O, or H_2O_2. The product of oxidation is a carboxylic acid.

Figure 8.17

> **DAT Synopsis**
>
> Aldehydes can be oxidized to carboxylic acids or reduced to alcohols.
>
> Ketones can be reduced to alcohols.

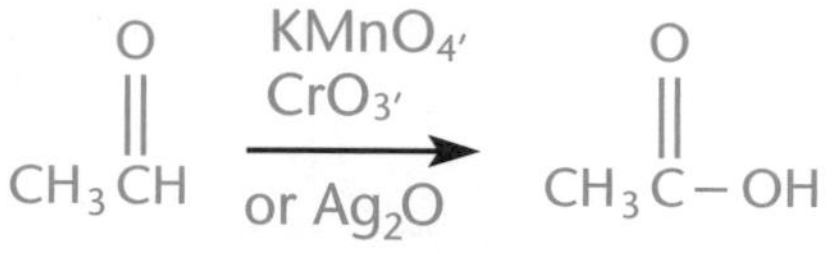

A number of reagents will reduce aldehydes and ketones to alcohols. The most common is lithium aluminum hydride (LAH); sodium borohydride ($NaBH_4$) is often used when milder conditions are needed.

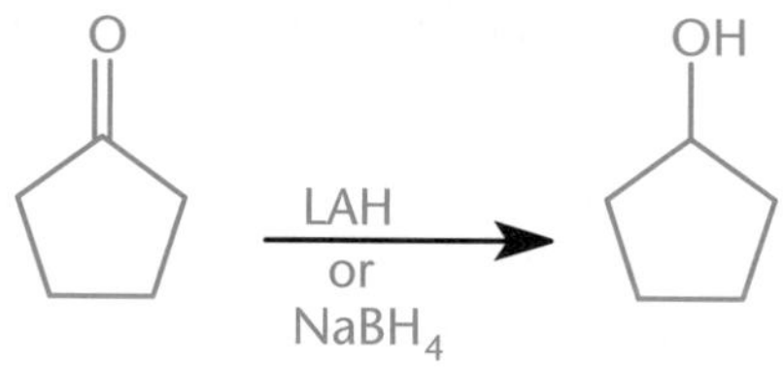

Figure 8.18

Aldehydes and ketones can be completely reduced to alkanes by two common methods. In the **Wolff-Kishner** reduction (see Figure 8.19), the carbonyl is first converted to a hydrazone, which releases molecular nitrogen (N_2) when heated and forms an alkane (the protons being abstracted from the solvent). The Wolff-Kishner reaction is performed in basic solution and, therefore, is only useful when the product is stable under basic conditions.

> **DAT Synopsis**
>
> Both aldehydes and ketones can be fully reduced to alkanes:
>
> — Wolff-Kishner (H_2NNH_2)
>
> — Clemmensen (Hg(Zn), HCl)

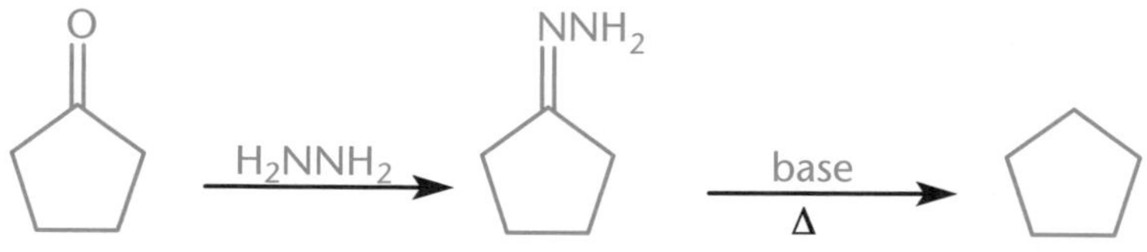

Figure 8.19

An alternative reduction not subject to this restriction is the **Clemmensen reduction** (see Figure 8.20), where an aldehyde or ketone is heated with amalgamated zinc in hydrochloric acid.

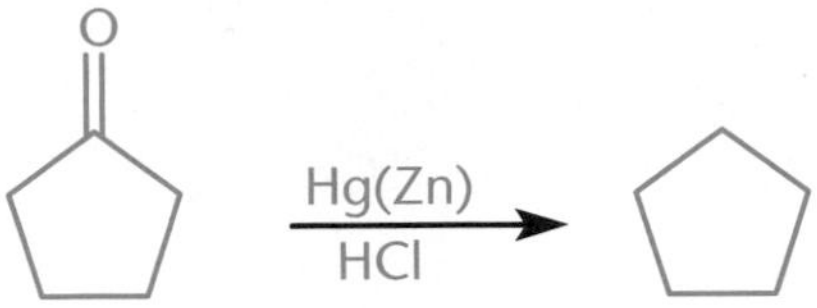

Figure 8.20

## 9

CARBOXYLIC ACIDS

Carboxylic acids are compounds that contain hydroxyl groups attached to carbonyl groups. This functionality is known as a **carboxyl group**. The hydroxyl hydrogen atoms are acidic, with pK_a values in the general range of 3 to 6. Carboxylic acids occur widely in nature and are synthesized by all living organisms.

NOMENCLATURE

In the IUPAC system of nomenclature, carboxylic acids are named by adding the suffix **-oic acid** to the alkyl root. The chain is numbered so that the carboxyl group receives the lowest possible number. Additional substituents are named in the usual fashion.

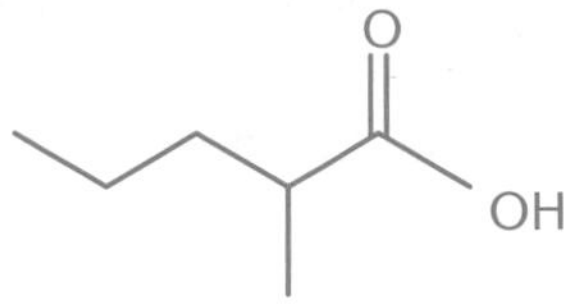

2-methylpentanoic acid 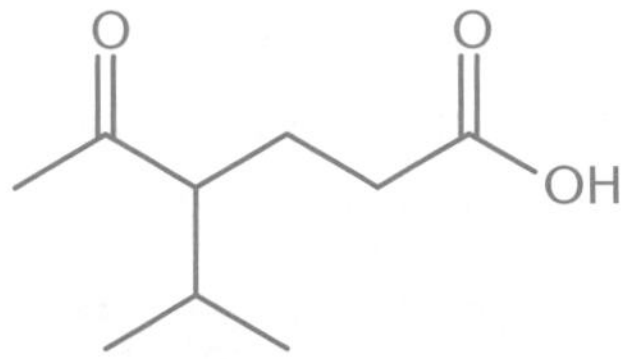   4-isopropyl-5-oxohexanoic acid

Figure 9.1

> ### DAT Synopsis
> This is a very high priority group! It determines C–1 of the carbon backbone, as well as the suffix (-oic acid).

Carboxylic acids were among the first organic compounds discovered. Their original names continue today in the common system of nomenclature. For example, formic acid (from Latin *formica*, meaning ant) was found in ants and butyric acid (from Latin *butyrum*, meaning butter) in rancid butter. The common and IUPAC names of the first three carboxylic acids are listed in Figure 9.2.

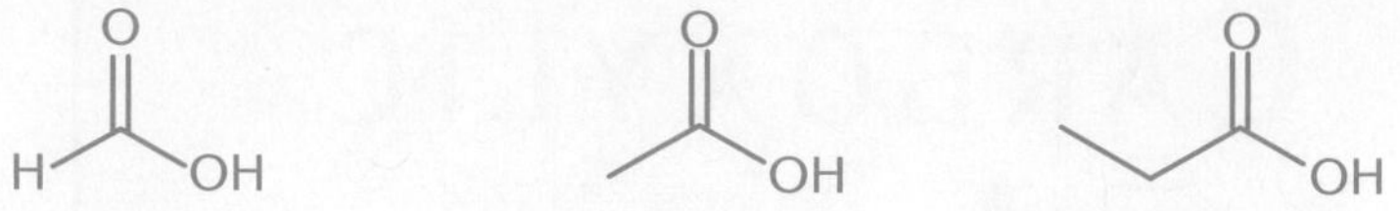

methanoic acid (formic acid) | ethanoic acid (acetic acid) | propanoic acid (propionic acid)

Figure 9.2

> **DAT Synopsis**
>
> Salts have the suffix *-ate* (e.g., sodium hexanoate).

Cyclic carboxylic acids are usually named as cycloalkane carboxylic acids. The carbon atom to which the carboxyl group is attached is numbered 1. Salts of carboxylic acids are named beginning with the cation, followed by the name of the acid with the ending **-ate** replacing **-ic acid**. Typical examples are shown in Figure 9.3.

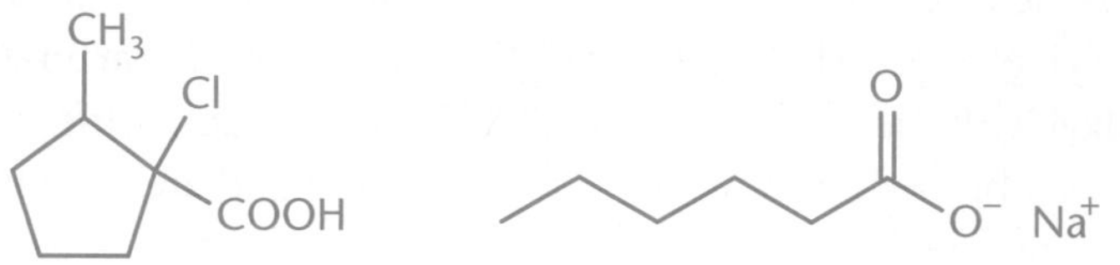

1-chloro-2-methylcyclopentane carboxylic acid | sodium hexanoate

Figure 9.3

Dicarboxylic acids—compounds with two carboxyl groups—are common in biological systems. The first six straight-chain terminal dicarboxylic acids are oxalic, malonic, succinic, glutaric, adipic, and pimelic acids. Their IUPAC names are ethanedioic acid, propanedioic acid, butanedioic acid, pentanedioic acid, hexanedioic acid, and heptanedioic acid.

PHYSICAL PROPERTIES

A. HYDROGEN BONDING

Carboxylic acids are polar and can form hydrogen bonds. As a result, carboxylic acids can form dimers: pairs of molecules connected by hydrogen bonds. The boiling points of carboxylic acids are, therefore, even higher than those of the corresponding alcohols. The boiling points follow the usual trend of increasing with molecular weight.

> **DAT Synopsis**
>
> Carboxylic acids are polar and can form hydrogen bonds. Their acidity is due to resonance stabilization and can be enhanced by adding electronegative groups or other potential resonance structures.

B. ACIDITY

The acidity of carboxylic acids is due to the resonance stabilization of the carboxylate anion (the conjugate base). When the hydroxyl proton dissociates from the acid, the negative charge left on the carboxylate group is delocalized between the two oxygen atoms.

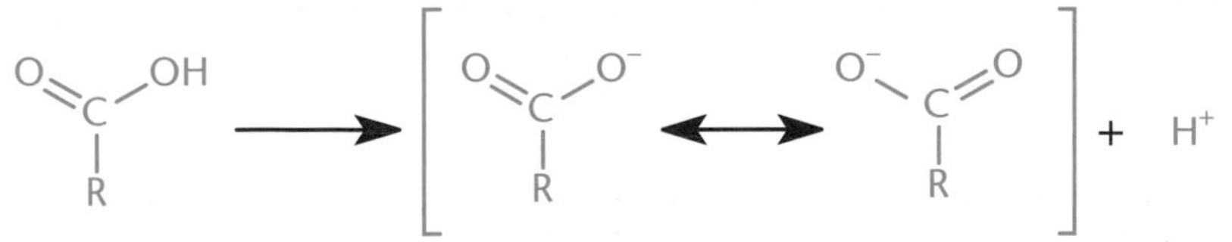

Figure 9.4

Substituents on carbon atoms adjacent to a carboxyl group can influence acidity. Electron-withdrawing groups, such as $-Cl$ or $-NO_2$, further delocalize the negative charge and increase acidity. Electron-donating groups, such as $-NH_2$ or $-OCH_3$, destabilize the negative charge, making the compound less acidic.

In dicarboxylic acids, one $-COOH$ group (which is electron withdrawing) influences the other, making the compound more acidic than the analogous monocarboxylic acid. The second carboxyl group is then influenced by the carboxylate anion. Ionization of the second group will create a doubly charged species in which the two negative charges repel each other. Since this is unfavorable, the second proton is less acidic than that of a monocarboxylic acid.

β-dicarboxylic acids are notable for the high acidity of the α-hydrogens located between the two carboxyl groups ($pK_a \sim 10$). Loss of this acidic hydrogen atom produces a carbanion that is stabilized by the electron-withdrawing effect of the two carboxyl groups (the same effect seen in β-ketoacids, $RC=OCH_2\ COOH$).

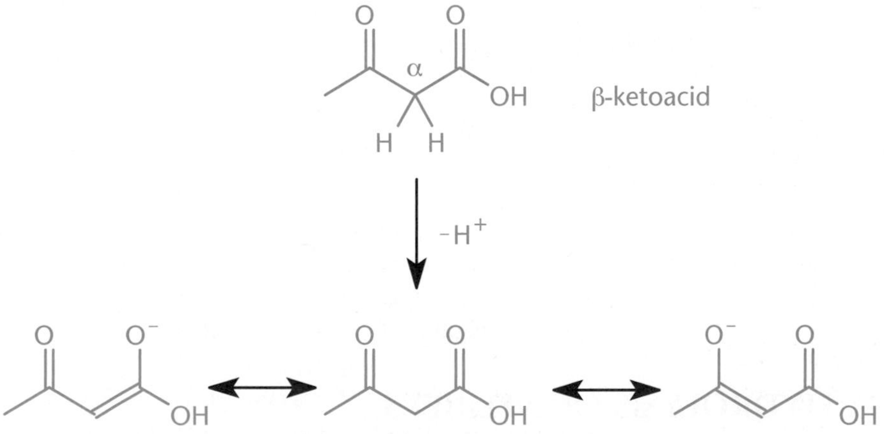

Figure 9.5

Similarly, the β-dicarboxylic acid also has acidic α hydrogens.

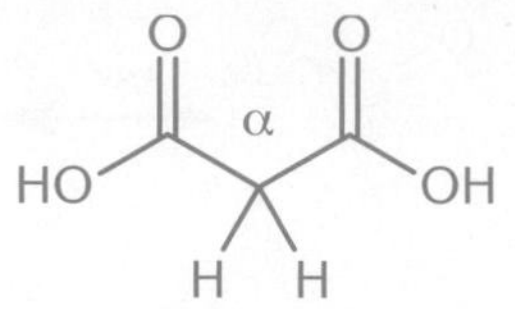

Figure 9.6

KAPLAN EXCLUSIVE

Carboxylic acids are the most oxidized.

SYNTHESIS

A. OXIDATION REACTIONS

Carboxylic acids can be prepared via oxidation of aldehydes, primary alcohols, and certain alkylbenzenes. The oxidant is usually potassium permanganate, $KMnO_4$. Note that secondary and tertiary alcohols cannot be oxidized to carboxylic acids because of valence limitations.

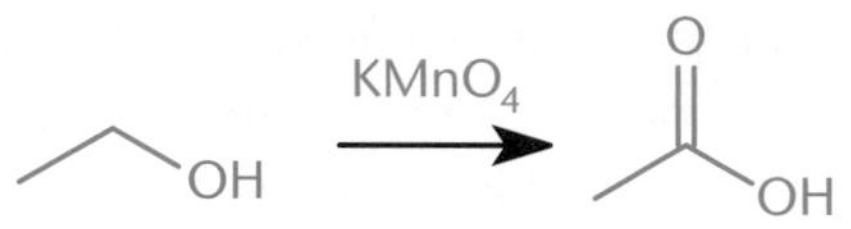

Figure 9.7

B. CARBONATION OF ORGANOMETALLIC REAGENTS

Organometallic reagents, such as Grignard reagents, react with carbon dioxide (CO_2) to form carboxylic acids. This reaction is useful for the conversion of tertiary alkyl halides into carboxylic acids, which cannot be accomplished through other methods. Note that this reaction adds one carbon atom to the chain.

DAT Synopsis

Both carbonation and hydrolysis *increase* the chain length by one carbon.

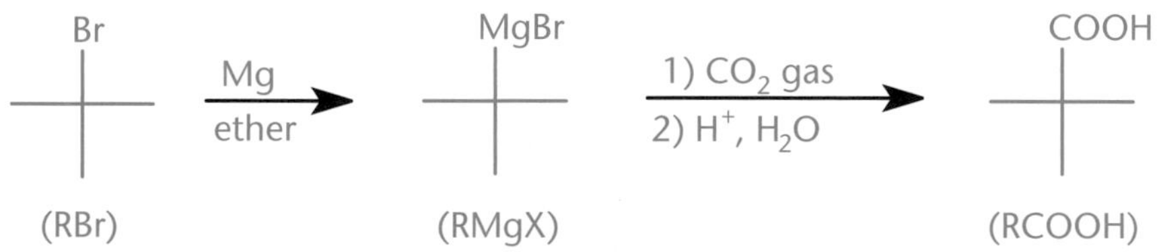

Figure 9.8

C. HYDROLYSIS OF NITRILES

Nitriles, also called cyanides, are compounds containing the functional group –CN. The cyanide anion CN^- is a good nucleophile and will displace primary and secondary halides in typical S_N2 fashion.

Nitriles can be hydrolyzed under either acidic or basic conditions. The products are carboxylic acids and ammonia (or ammonium salts).

$$CH_3Cl \longrightarrow CH_3CN \longrightarrow CH_3\overset{\overset{\displaystyle O}{\|}}{C}OH + NH_4^+$$

Figure 9.9

This allows for the conversion of alkyl halides into carboxylic acids. As in the carbonation reaction, an additional carbon atom is introduced. For instance, if the desired product is acetic acid, a possible starting material would be methyl iodide.

REACTIONS

A. SOAP FORMATION

When long-chain carboxylic acids react with sodium or potassium hydroxide, they form salts. These salts, called soaps, are able to solubilize nonpolar organic compounds in aqueous solutions because they possess both a nonpolar "tail" and a polar carboxylate "head," as shown in Figure 9.10.

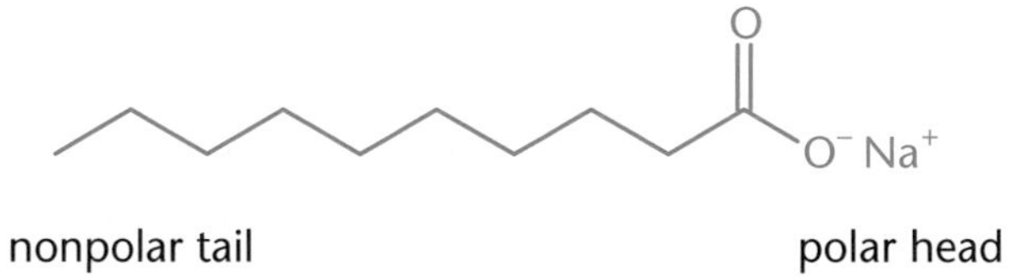

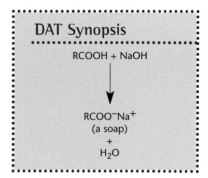

DAT Synopsis

RCOOH + NaOH

↓

RCOO⁻Na⁺
(a soap)
+
H_2O

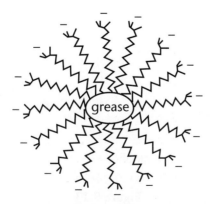

nonpolar tail   polar head

Figure 9.10

When placed in aqueous solution, soap molecules arrange themselves into spherical structures called **micelles**. The polar heads face outward, where they can be solvated by water molecules, and the nonpolar hydrocarbon chains are inside the sphere, protected from the solvent. Nonpolar molecules, such as grease, can dissolve in the hydrocarbon interior of the spherical micelle, while the micelle as a whole is soluble in water because of its polar shell (see Figure 9.11).

DAT Synopsis

nonpolar "tail" = hydrophobic.
polar "head" = hydrophilic.

Real–World Analogy

Notice the similarity between micelle formation and the assembly of the plasma membrane (made of phospholipids).

Figure 9.11

B. NUCLEOPHILIC SUBSTITUTION

Many of the reactions that carboxylic acids (and their derivatives) partici-pate in can be described by a single mechanism: nucleophilic substitution. This mechanism is very similar to nucleophilic addition to a carbonyl, shown in the preceding chapter. The key difference: Nucleophilic substi-tution concludes with re-formation of the C=O double bond and elimina-tion of a leaving group.

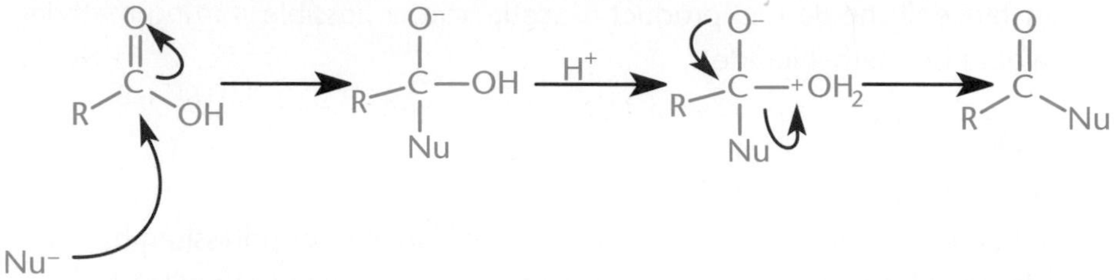

Figure 9.12

1. Reduction

Carboxylic acids occupy the most oxidized side of the oxidation-reduction continuum (see "Alcohols: Review" in chapter 7). Carboxylic acids are reduced with lithium aluminum hydride (LAH) to the corresponding alcohols. Aldehyde intermediates that may be formed in the course of the reaction are also reduced to the alcohol. The reaction occurs by nucle-ophilic addition of hydride to the carbonyl group.

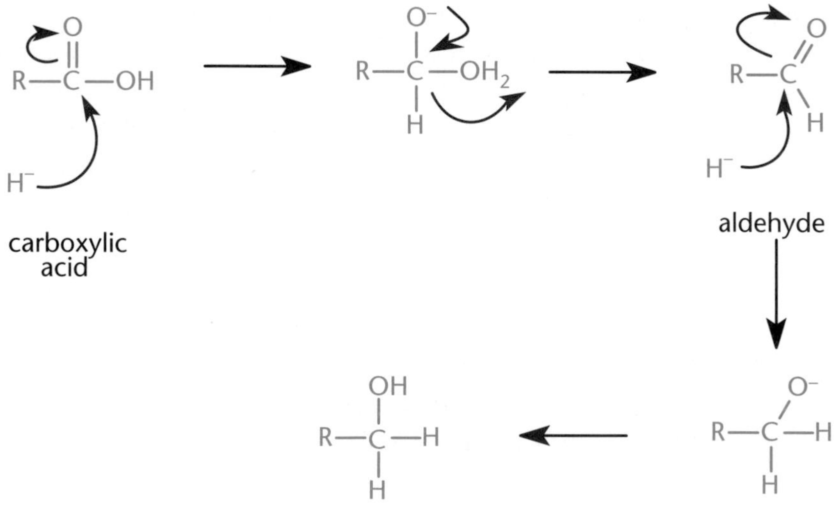

carboxylic acid

aldehyde

alcohol

Figure 9.13

2. Ester Formation

Carboxylic acids react with alcohols under acidic conditions to form esters and water. In acidic solution, the O on the C=O can become protonated. This accentuates the polarity of the bond, putting even more positive charge on the C and making it even more susceptible to nucleophilic attack. This condensation reaction occurs most rapidly with primary alcohols.

> **DAT Synopsis**
>
> Protonating the C=O makes the C even more ripe for nucleophilic attack.

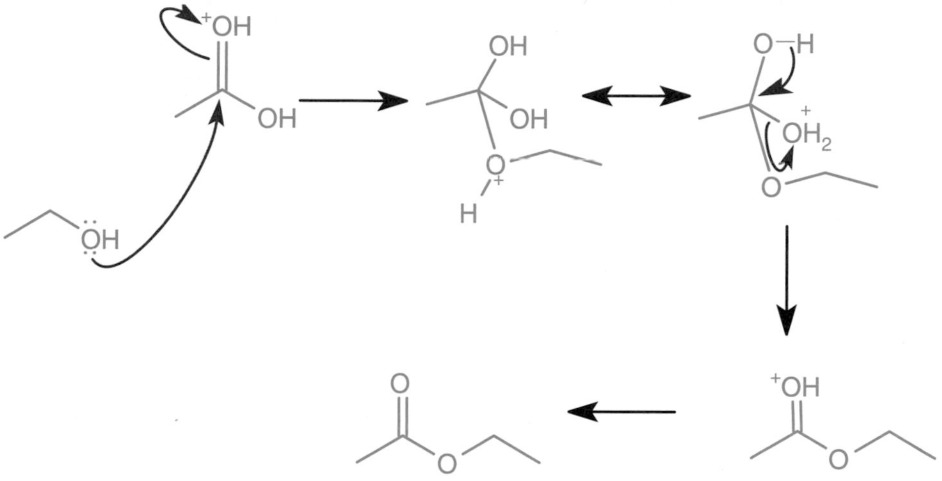

Figure 9.14

3. Acyl Halide Formation

Acyl halides, also called acid halides, are compounds with carbonyl groups bonded to halides. Several reagents can accomplish this transformation; thionyl chloride, $SOCl_2$, is the most common.

> **DAT Synopsis**
>
> Acid chlorides are among the highest-energy (least stable and most reactive) members of the carbonyl family.

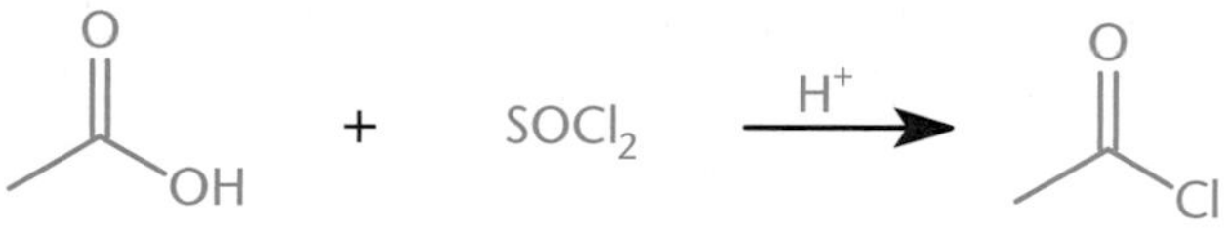

Figure 9.15

Acid chlorides are very reactive, as the greater electron-withdrawing power of the Cl^- makes the carbonyl carbon more susceptible to nucleophilic attack than the carbonyl carbon of a carboxylic acid. Thus, acid chlorides are frequently used as intermediates in the conversion of carboxylic acids to esters and amides.

DAT Synopsis

Key reactions include

- soap formation (e.g., when neutralized by NaOH or KOH);
- nucleophilic substitution;
- decarboxylation, in which CO_2 is lost.

C. DECARBOXYLATION

Carboxylic acids can undergo decarboxylation reactions, resulting in the loss of carbon dioxide.

1,3-dicarboxylic acids and other β-keto acids may spontaneously decarboxylate when heated. The carboxyl group is lost and replaced with a hydrogen. The reaction proceeds through a six-membered ring transition state. The enol initially formed tautomerizes to the more stable keto form (see Figure 9.16).

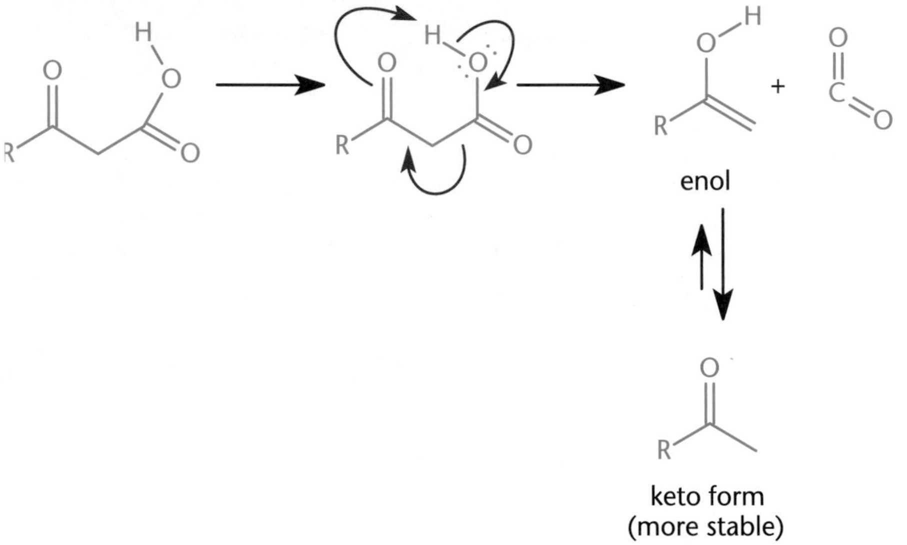

Figure 9.16

## 10

Carboxylic Acid Derivatives

Carboxylic acids can be converted into several types of derivatives: **acyl halides, anhydrides, amides,** and **esters**. These are compounds in which the –OH of the carboxyl group has been replaced with **–X, –OCOR, –NH_2,** or **–OR,** respectively. They readily undergo nucleophilic substitution reactions, including hydrolysis (H_2O as nucleophile), which produces the original carboxylic acid. They also undergo other additions and substitutions, including various interconversions between different acid derivatives. In general, the acyl halides are the most reactive of the carboxylic acid derivatives, followed by the anhydrides, the esters, and the amides.

DAT Synopsis

Order of reactivity:

acyl halides > anhydrides > esters > amides.

ACYL HALIDES

A. NOMENCLATURE

Acyl halides are also called **acid** or **alkanoyl halides**. (The acyl group is RCO–.) They are the most reactive of the carboxylic acid derivatives. They are named in the IUPAC system by changing the *-ic acid* ending of the carboxylic acid to **-yl halide**. Some typical examples are ethanoyl chloride (also called acetyl chloride), benzoyl chloride, and *n*-butanoyl bromide.

Flashback

Carboxylic acid nomenclature was discussed in chapter 9.

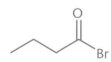

ethanoyl chloride (acetyl chloride) | benzoyl chloride | *n*-butanoyl bromide

Figure 10.1

DAT Synopsis

The most common acyl halide is acyl chloride, made with RCOOH + $SOCl_2$.

B. SYNTHESIS

The most common acyl halides are the acid chlorides, although acid bromides and iodides are occasionally encountered. They are prepared by reaction of the carboxylic acid with thionyl chloride, $SOCl_2$, producing SO_2 and HCl as side products. Alternatively, PCl_3 or PCl_5 (or PBr_3, to make an acid bromide) will accomplish the same transformation.

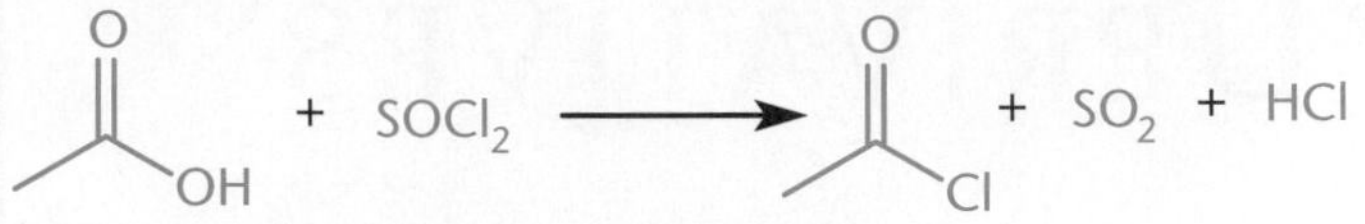

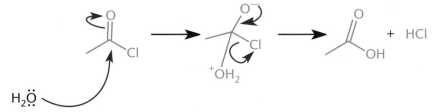

Figure 10.2

C. REACTIONS: NUCLEOPHILIC ACYL SUBSTITUTION

The following reactions of acyl halides proceed via the mechanism of nucleophilic substitution on a carbonyl, shown in detail in "Reactons" in chapter 9.

1. Hydrolysis

The simplest reaction of acid halides is their conversion back to carboxylic acids. They react very rapidly with water to form the corresponding acid, along with HCl, which is responsible for their irritating odor.

Figure 10.3

KAPLAN EXCLUSIVE

Hydrolysis = hydro + lysis, or cleavage by water.

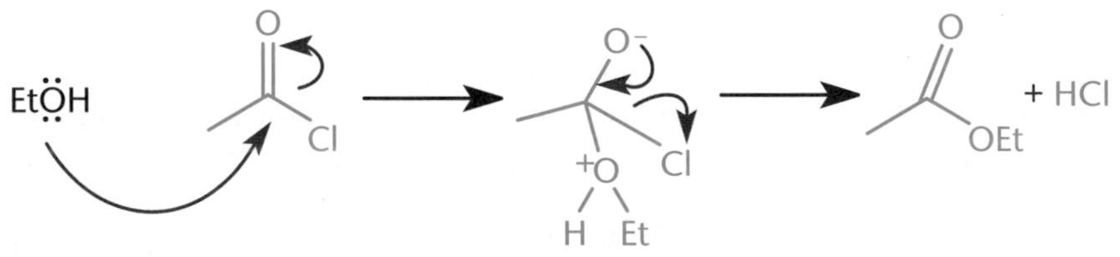

DAT Synopsis

1. Hydrolysis regenerates the carboxylic acid.
2. All carboxylic acid derivatives are susceptible to hydrolysis.

2. Conversion into Esters

Acyl halides can be converted into esters by reaction with alcohols. The same type of nucleophilic attack found in hydrolysis leads to the formation of a tetrahedral intermediate, with the hydroxyl oxygen as the nucleophile. Chloride is displaced, and HCl is released as the side-product.

Figure 10.4

3. Conversion into Amides

Acyl halides can be converted into amides (compounds of the general formula $RCONR_2$) by an analogous reaction with amines. Nucleophilic amines, such as ammonia, attack the carbonyl group, displacing chloride. The side product is ammonium chloride, formed from excess ammonia and HCl.

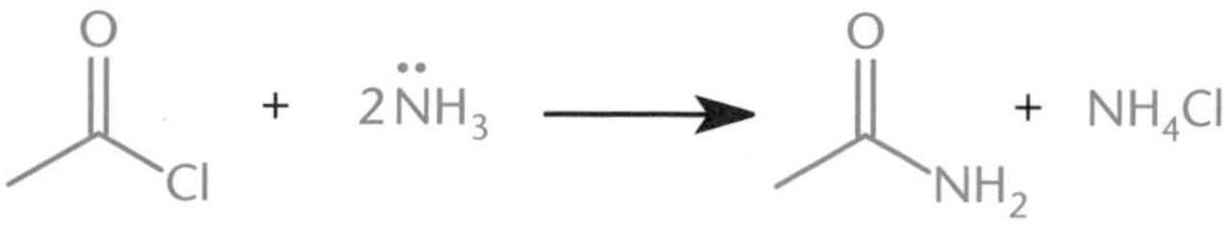

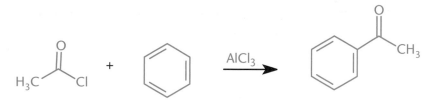

Figure 10.5

D. OTHER REACTIONS

1. Friedel-Crafts Acylation

Aromatic rings can be acylated in a Friedel-Crafts reaction. The mechanism is electrophilic aromatic substitution, and the attacking reagent is an acylium ion, formed by reaction of an acid chloride with $AlCl_3$ or another Lewis acid. The product is an alkyl aryl ketone.

Figure 10.6

Flashback

Friedel-Crafts reactions were discussed in chapter 6.

DAT Synopsis

The mechanism for the Friedel-Crafts acylation is electrophilic aromatic substitution.

2. Reduction

Acid halides can be reduced to alcohols or selectively reduced to the intermediate aldehydes. Catalytic hydrogenation in the presence of a "poison" like quinoline accomplishes the latter transformation. (Compare with Lindlar's catalyst, "Alkynes: Reactions" in chapter 5.)

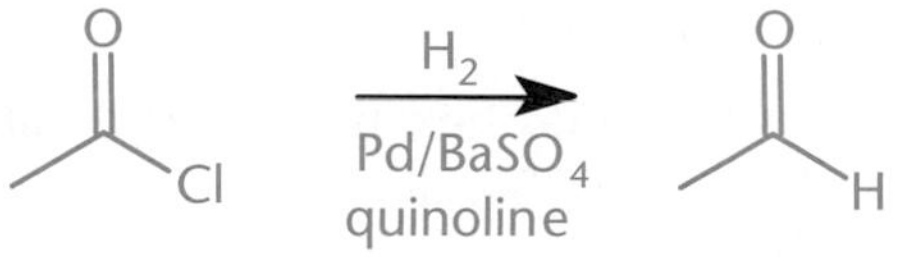

Figure 10.7

ANHYDRIDES

A. NOMENCLATURE

Anhydrides, also called **acid anhydrides**, are the condensation dimers of carboxylic acids with the general formula RCOOCOR. They are named by substituting the word **anhydride** for the word *acid* in an alkanoic acid. The most common and important anhydride is acetic anhydride, the dimer of acetic acid. Other common anhydrides, such as succinic, maleic, and phthalic anhydrides, are **cyclic anhydrides** arising from intramolecular condensation or dehydration of diacids (Figure 10.9).

KAPLAN EXCLUSIVE

Anhydride means "without water." Anhydrides are formed by two acid molecules condensing (losing water).

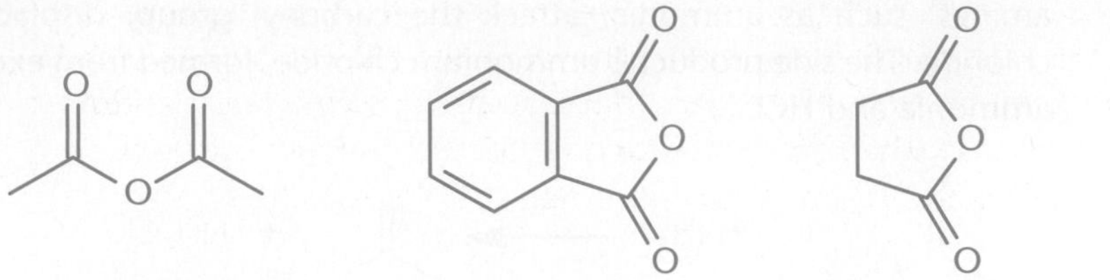

acetic anhydride
(ethanoic anhydride)

phthalic anhydride

succinic anhydride

Figure 10.8

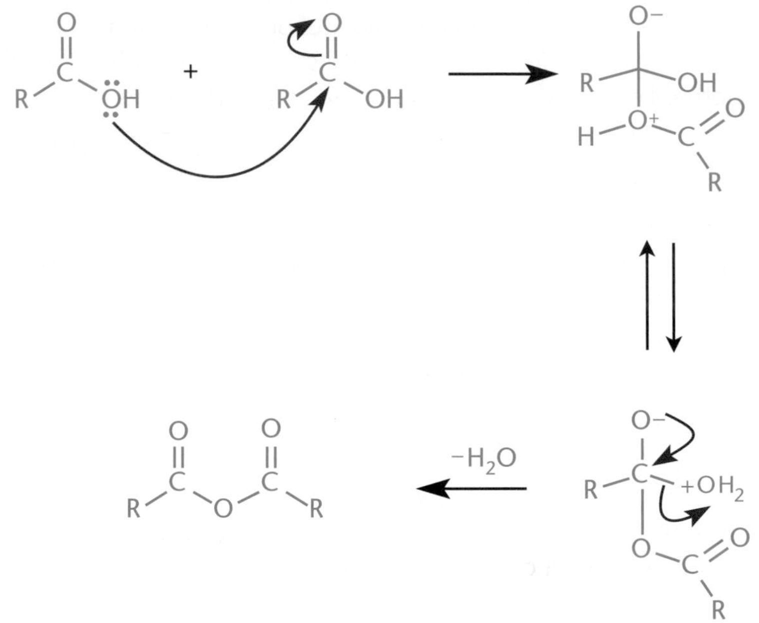

Figure 10.9. Condensation of Two Carboxylic Acid Molecules to Form an Anhydride

B. SYNTHESIS

Anhydrides can be synthesized by reaction of an acid chloride with a carboxylate salt.

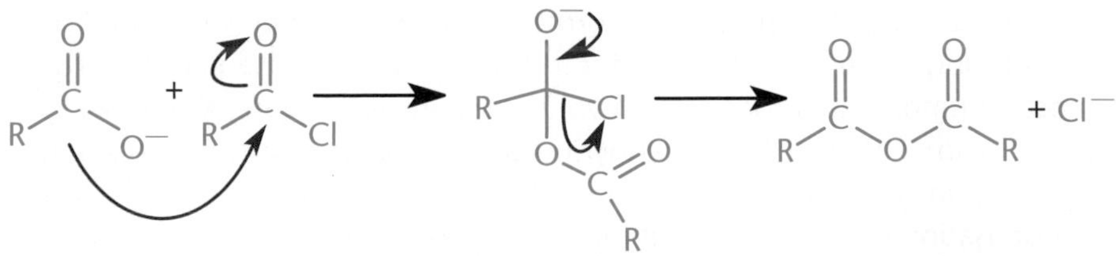

Figure 10.10. Reaction of Acid Chloride with Carboxylate Anion to Form an Anhydride

Certain cyclic anhydrides can be formed simply by heating carboxylic acids. The reaction is driven by the increased stability of the newly formed ring; hence, only five- and six-membered ring anhydrides are easily made. In this case, the hydroxyl of one –COOH moiety acts as a nucleophile, attacking the carbonyl on the other –COOH moiety.

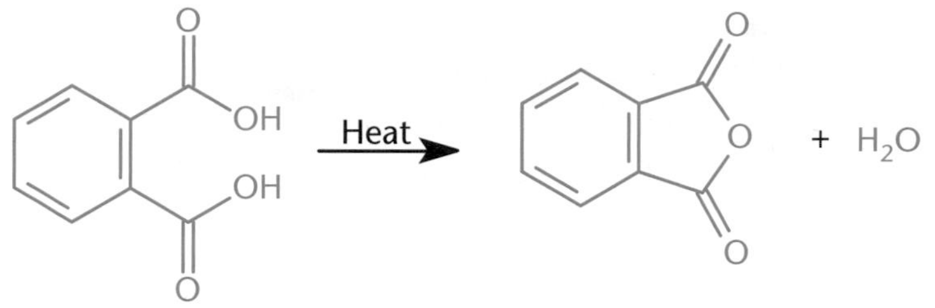

o-phtalic acid   phthalic anhydride

Figure 10.11

C. REACTIONS

Anhydrides react under the same conditions as acid chlorides, but since they are somewhat more stable, they are a bit less reactive. The reactions are slower and produce a carboxylic acid as the side product instead of HCl. Cyclic anhydrides are also subject to these reactions, which cause ring opening at the anhydride group along with formation of the new functional groups.

1. **Hydrolysis**

   Anhydrides are converted into carboxylic acids when exposed to water. Note that in the reaction shown in Figure 10.12, the leaving group is actually a carboxylic acid.

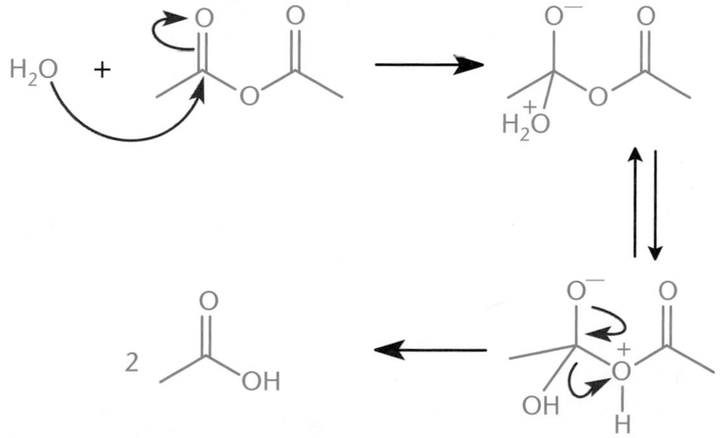

Figure 10.12

2. Conversion into Amides

Anhydrides are cleaved by ammonia, producing amides and ammonium carboxylates. Thus, as show in Figure 10.13, even though the leaving group is actually a carboxylic acid, the final products are an amide and the ammonium salt of a carboxylate anion.

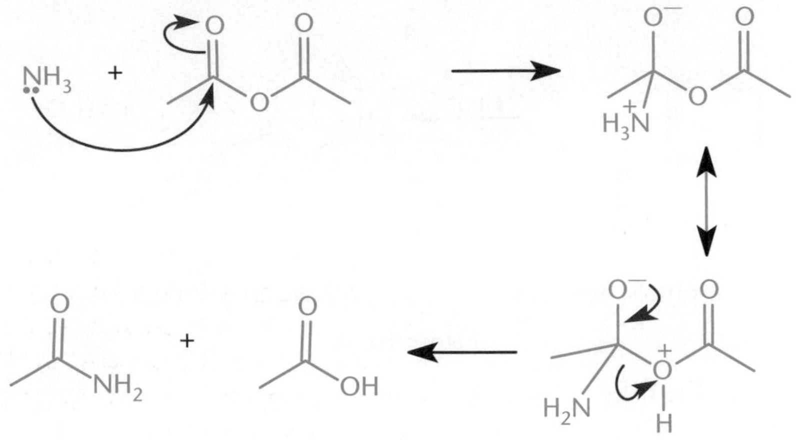

Then:

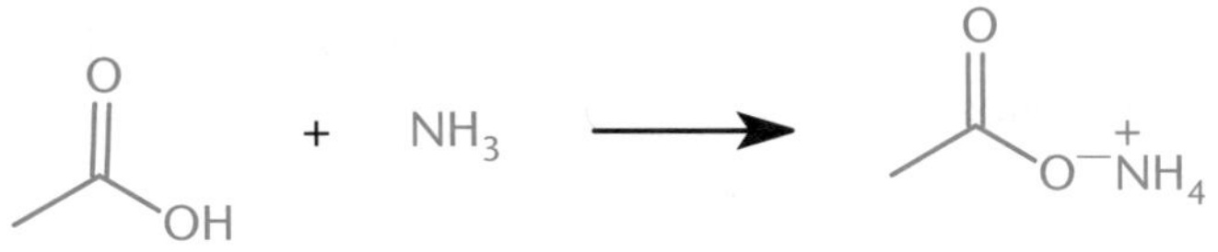

Figure 10.13

3. Conversion into Esters and Carboxylic Acids

Anhydrides react with alcohols to form esters and carboxylic acids.

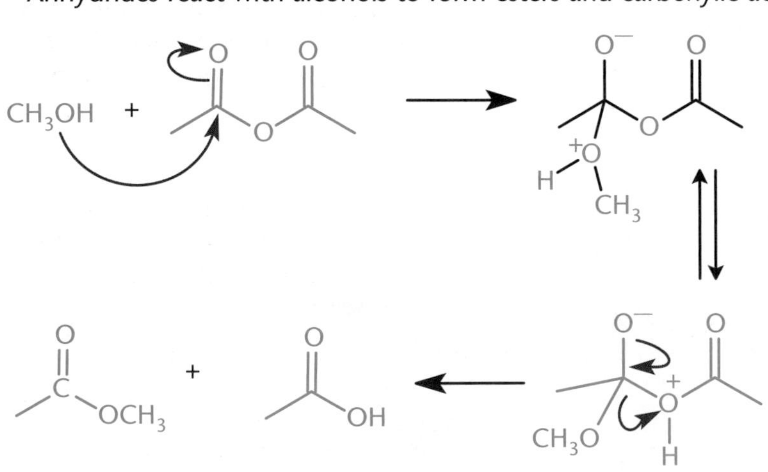

Figure 10.14

4. **Acylation**

Friedel-Crafts acylation occurs readily with AlCl$_3$ or other Lewis acid catalysts.

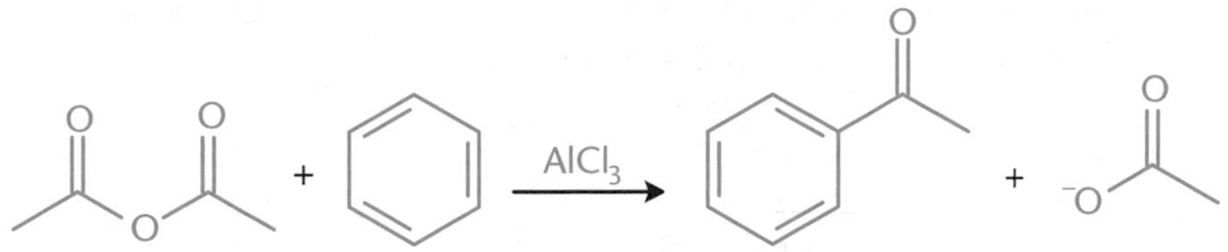

DAT Synopsis

This reaction proceeds via electrophilic aromatic substitution.

Figure 10.15

AMIDES

A. NOMENCLATURE

Amides are compounds with the general formula RCONR$_2$. They are named by replacing the *-oic* acid ending with **-amide**. Alkyl substituents on the nitrogen atom are listed as prefixes, and their location is specified with the letter *N*, as in the example in Figure 10.16.

Bridge

The peptide bond is actually an amide linkage.

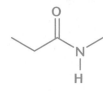

N-methylpropanamide

Figure 10.16

B. SYNTHESIS

Amides are generally synthesized by the reaction of acid chlorides with amines or by the reaction of acid anhydrides with ammonia (see above). Note that loss of hydrogen is required; thus, only primary and secondary amines will undergo this reaction.

DAT Synopsis

Only primary and secondary amines can be used to form amides.

C. REACTIONS

1. Hydrolysis

Amides can be hydrolyzed under acidic conditions, via nucleophilic substitution, to produce carboxylic acids or basic conditions to form carboxylates, as shown in Figure 10.17.

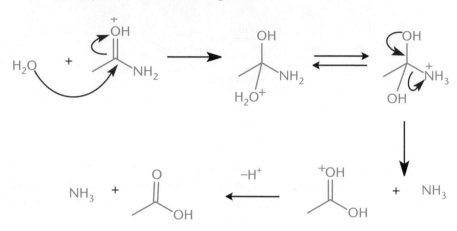

Figure 10.17

2. Hofmann Rearrangement

The **Hofmann rearrangement** converts amides to primary amines with the loss of the carbonyl carbon. The mechanism involves the formation of a **nitrene**, the nitrogen analog of a carbene. The nitrene is attached to the carbonyl group and rearranges to form an **isocyanate**, which under the reaction condition is hydrolyzed to the amine.

$$R-C(=O)-NH_2 \xrightarrow{BrO^-} R-C(=O)-\ddot{N}(H)-Br + OH^- \rightleftharpoons R-C(=O)-\ddot{N}^{-}-Br + H_2O$$

$$R-C(=O)-\ddot{N}-Br \longrightarrow O=C=\ddot{N}-R + Br^- \xrightarrow{H_2O} H_2\ddot{N}R + CO_2 + Br^-$$

nitrene   isocyanate

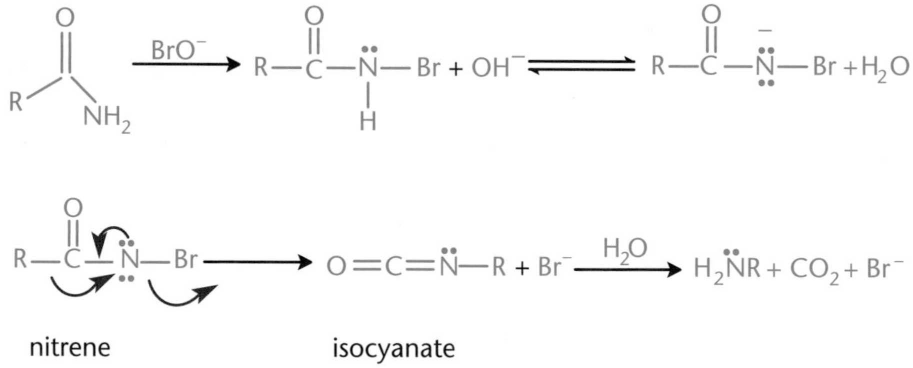

Figure 10.18

3. Reduction

Amides can be reduced with LAH to the corresponding amine. Notice in Figure 10.19 that this differs from the product of the Hofmann rearrangement in that no carbon atom is lost.

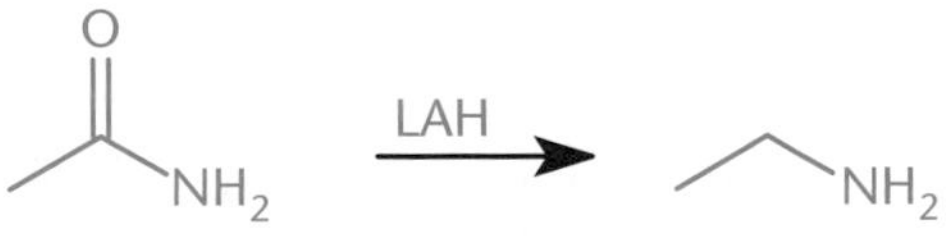

Figure 10.19

ESTERS

A. NOMENCLATURE

Esters are the dehydration products of carboxylic acids and alcohols. They are commonly found in many fruits and perfumes. They are named in the IUPAC system as **alkyl** or **aryl alkanoates**. For example, ethyl acetate, derived from the condensation of acetic acid and ethanol, is called ethyl ethanoate according to IUPAC nomenclature.

> **DAT Synopsis**
>
> An acid + an alcohol = an ester.

B. SYNTHESIS

Mixtures of carboxylic acids and alcohols will condense into esters, liberating water, under acidic conditions. Esters can also be obtained from reaction of acid chlorides or anhydrides with alcohols (see above). Phenolic (aromatic) esters are produced in the same way, although the aromatic acid chlorides are less reactive than aliphatic acid chlorides so that base must generally be added as a catalyst.

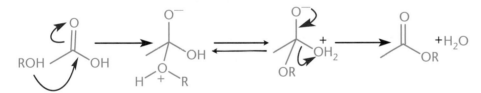

Figure 10.20

C. REACTIONS

1. Hydrolysis

Esters, like the other derivatives of carboxylic acids, can be hydrolyzed, yielding carboxylic acids and alcohols. Hydrolysis can take place under either acidic or basic conditions. Figure 10.21 shows this reaction under acidic conditions.

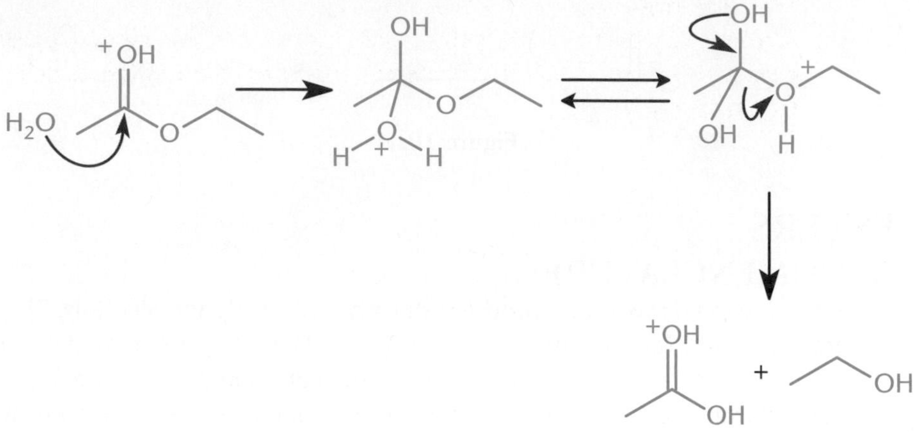

Figure 10.21

The reaction proceeds similarly under basic conditions, except that the oxygen on the C=O is not protonated, and the nucleophile is OH⁻.

Triacylglycerols, also called fats, are esters of long-chain carboxylic acids, often called fatty acids, and glycerol (1,2,3-propanetriol). **Saponification** is the process whereby fats are hydrolyzed under basic conditions to produce soaps. (Note: Acidification of the soap retrieves triacylglycerol.)

triacylglycerol   soap   glycerol

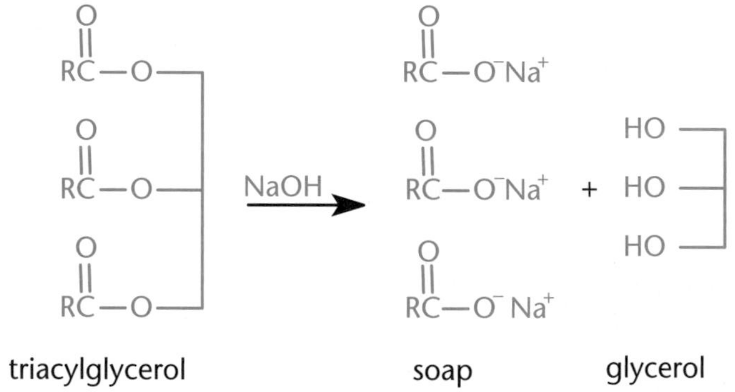

Figure 10.22

2. **Conversion into Amides**

Nitrogen bases, such as ammonia, will attack the electron-deficient carbonyl carbon atom, displacing alkoxide to yield an amide and an alcohol side-product. In Figure 10.23, ammonia is the nucleophile.

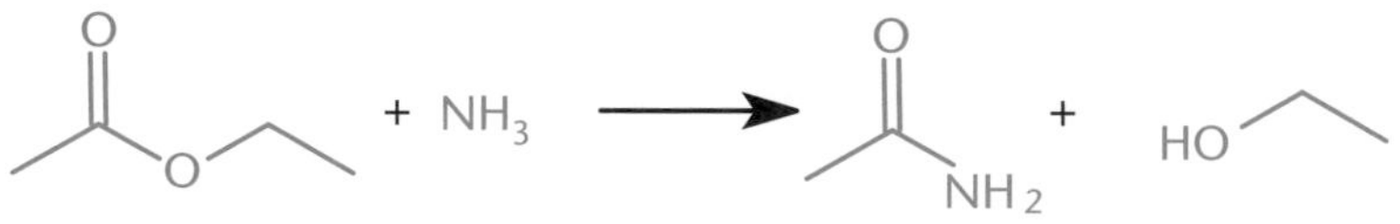

Figure 10.23

3. Transesterification

Alcohols can act as nucleophiles and displace the alkoxy groups on esters. This process, which transforms one ester into another, is called **transesterification**.

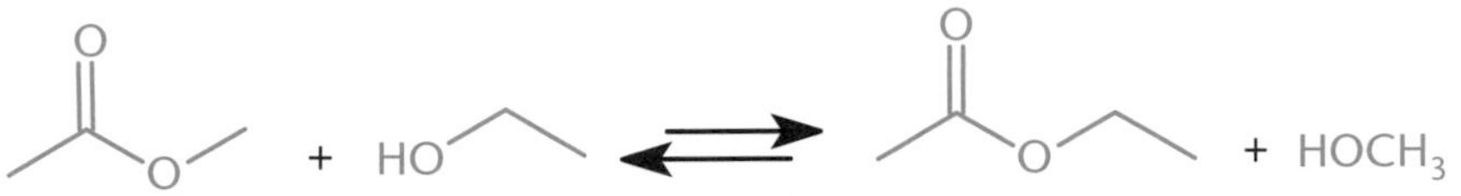

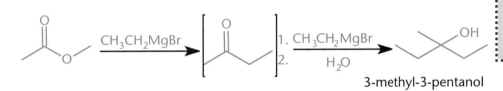

Figure 10.24

4. Grignard Addition

Grignard reagents add to the carbonyl groups of esters to form ketones; however, these ketones are more reactive than the initial esters and are readily attacked by more Grignard reagent. Two equivalents of Grignard reagent can thus be used to produce tertiary alcohols with good yield. (The intermediate ketone can be isolated only if the alkyl groups are sufficiently bulky to prevent further attack.) This reaction proceeds via nucleophilic substitution followed by nucleophilic addition.

3-methyl-3-pentanol

Figure 10.25

5. Condensation Reactions

An important reaction of esters is the **Claisen condensation**. In the simplest case, two moles of ethyl acetate react under basic conditions to produce a β-keto ester, ethyl 3-oxobutanoate, or acetoacetic ester by its common name. (The Claisen condensation is also called the **acetoacetic ester condensation**.) The reaction proceeds by addition of an enolate anion to the carbonyl group of another ester, followed by displacement of ethoxide ion. This mechanism is analogous to that of the aldol condensation.

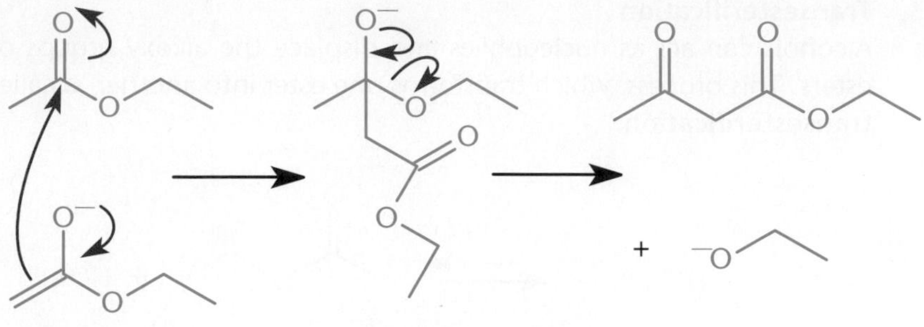

Figure 10.26

6. Reduction

Esters may be reduced to primary alcohols with LAH but not with NaBH₄. This allows for selective reduction in molecules with multiple functional groups.

> **DAT Synopsis**
>
> LAH is essentially equivalent to a H⁻ nucleophile.

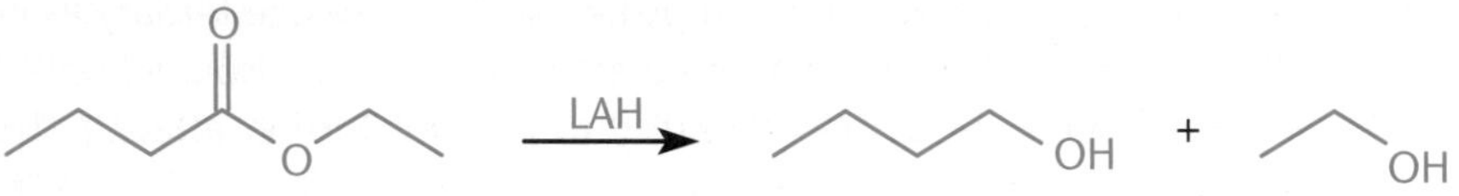

Figure 10.27

D. PHOSPHATE ESTERS

While phosphoric acid derivatives are not carboxylic acid derivatives, they form esters similar to those in the previous section.

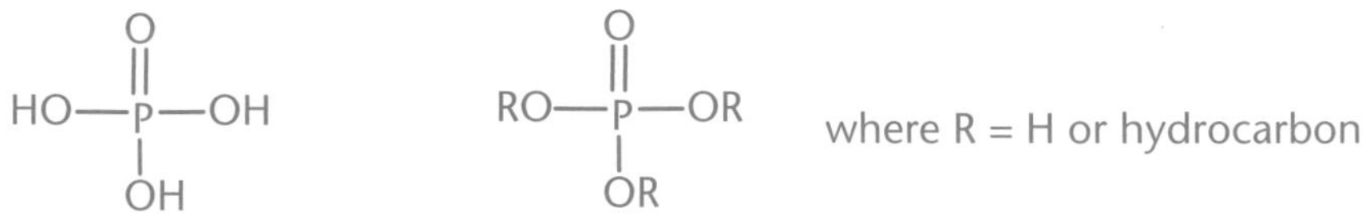

phosphoric acid   phosphoric ester   where R = H or hydrocarbon

Figure 10.28

Phosphoric acid and the mono- and diesters are acidic (more so than carboxylic acids) and usually exist as anions. Like all esters, under acidic conditions, they can be cleaved into the parent acid (in Figure 10.28, H_3PO_4) and alcohols.

Phosphate esters are found in living systems in the form of **phospholipids** (phosphoglycerides), in which glycerol is attached to two carboxylic acids and one phosphoric acid.

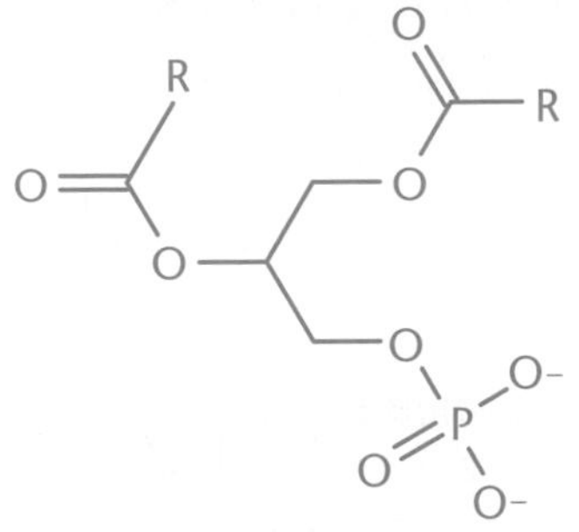

phosphatidic acid
diacylglycerol phosphate
(a phosphoglyceride)

Figure 10.29

Phospholipids are the main component of cell membranes, and phospholipid/carbohydrate polymers form the backbone of nucleic acids, the hereditary material of life (see chapter 15 and Biology chapter 3). The nucleic acid derivative **adenosine triphosphate (ATP)** can give up and regain one or more phosphate groups. ATP facilitates many biological reactions by releasing phosphate groups to other compounds, thereby increasing their reactivities.

Bridge

Remember phosphodiester bonds? They hold the backbone of DNA together, connecting nucleotides with covalent linkages.

SUMMARY OF REACTIONS

- The most important derivatives of carboxylic acid are acyl halides, anhydrides, esters, and amides. These are listed from most reactive (least stable) to least reactive (most stable).

ACYL HALIDES

- Can be formed by adding $RCOOH + SOCl_2$, PCl_3 or PCl_5, or PBr_3.
- Undergo many different nucleophilic substitutions; H_2O yields carboxylic acid, ROH yields an ester, and NH_3 yields an amide.
- Can participate in Friedel-Crafts acylation to form an alkyl aryl ketone.
- Can be reduced to alcohols or, selectively, to aldehydes.

ANHYDRIDES

- Can be formed by $RCOOH + RCOOH$ (condensation) or $RCOO^- + RCOCl$ (substitution).
- Undergo many nucleophilic substitution reactions, forming products that include carboxylic acids, amides, and esters.
- Can participate in Friedel-Crafts acylation.

ESTERS

- Formed by $RCOOH + ROH$ or, better, by acid chlorides or anhydrides + ROH.
- Hydrolyze to yield acids + alcohols; adding ammonia yields an amide.
- Reaction with Grignard reagent (2 moles) produces a tertiary alcohol.
- In Claisen condensation, analogous to the aldol, the ester acts both as nucleophile and target.
- Are very important in biological processes, particularly phosphate esters, which can be found in membranes, nucleic acids, and metabolic reactions.

AMIDES

- Can be formed by acid chlorides + amines or acid anhydrides + ammonia.
- Hydrolysis yields carboxylic acids or carboxylate anions.
- Can be transformed to primary amines via Hofmann rearrangement or reduction.

## 11

AMINES AND NITROGEN-CONTAINING COMPOUNDS

NOMENCLATURE

Amines are compounds of the general formula NR_3. They are classified according to the number of alkyl (or aryl) groups to which they are bound. A **primary (1°) amine** is attached to one alkyl group, a **secondary (2°)** amine to two, and a **tertiary (3°)** amine to three. A nitrogen atom attached to four alkyl groups is called a **quaternary ammonium compound**. The nitrogen carries a positive charge; thus, these compounds generally exist as salts.

In the common system, amines are generally named as alkylamines. The groups are designated individually or by using the prefixes di- or tri- if they are the same. In the IUPAC system, amines are named by substituting the suffix -**amine** for the final e of the name of the alkane to which the nitrogen is attached. N is used to label substituents attached to the nitrogen in secondary or tertiary amines. The prefix **amino-** is used for naming compounds containing an OH or a CO_2H group. Aromatic amines are named as derivatives of aniline ($C_6H_5NH_2$), the IUPAC name for which is benzenamine. Table 11.1 shows some examples.

Formula:	$CH_3CH_2NH_2$	$CH_3CH_2N(CH_3)_2$	$H_2NCH_2CH_2CH_2OH$
IUPAC:	ethanamine	N,N-dimethylethanamine	2-aminoethanol
Common:	ethylamine	dimethylethylamine	_____

Table 11.1

There are many other nitrogen-containing organic compounds. **Amides**, the condensation products of carboxylic acids and amines, have already been discussed in chapter 10. **Carbamates** are compounds with the general formula RNHC(O)OR'. They are also called **urethanes** and can form polymers called **polyurethanes**. Carbamates are derived from compounds called **isocyanates** (general formula RNCO) by the addition of an alcohol. **Enamines** are the nitrogen analogs of enols, with an amine group attached to one carbon of a double bond. **Imines** are nitrogen compounds that contain nitrogen-carbon double bonds. **Nitriles**, or **cyanides**, are compounds with a triple bond between a carbon atom and a nitrogen atom. They are named with either the prefix **cyano-** or the suffix **-nitrile**. **Nitro** compounds contain the nitro group, NO_2. **Diazo** compounds contain an N_2 functionality. They tend to lose N_2 to form carbenes. **Azides** are compounds with an N_3 functionality. When azides lose nitrogen (N_2), they form **nitrenes**, the nitrogen analogs of carbenes. Examples of these various compounds are shown in Figure 11.1.

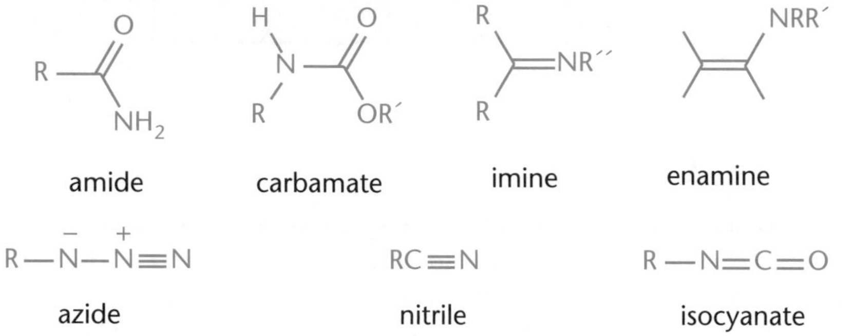

| amide | carbamate | imine | enamine |

| azide | nitrile | isocyanate |

Figure 11.1

PROPERTIES

The boiling points of amines are between those of alkanes and alcohols. For example, ammonia boils at −33°C, whereas methane boils at −161°C and methanol at 64.5°C. As molecular weight increases, so do boiling points. Primary and secondary amines can form hydrogen bonds, while tertiary amines cannot; therefore, tertiary amines have lower boiling points. Since nitrogen is not as electronegative as oxygen, the hydrogen bonds of amines are not as strong as those of alcohols.

The nitrogen atom in an amine is approximately sp^3 hybridized. Nitrogen must bond to only three substituents in order to complete its octet; a lone pair occupies the last sp^3 orbital. This lone pair is very important to the chemistry of amines; it is associated with their basic and nucleophilic properties.

Nitrogen atoms bonded to three different substituents are chiral because of the geometry of the orbitals. However, these enantiomers cannot be isolated, because they interconvert rapidly in a process called **nitrogen inversion**: an inversion of the sp^3 orbital occupied by the lone pair. The activation energy for this process is only 6 kcal/mol, and only at very low temperatures is it significantly slowed or stopped.

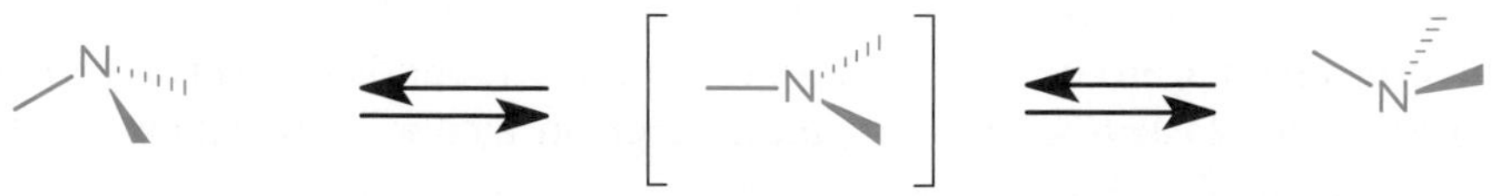

Figure 11.2

Amines are bases and readily accept protons to form ammonium ions. The pK_b values of alkyl amines are around 4, making them slightly more basic than ammonia (pK_b = 4.76) but less basic than hydroxide (pK_b = –1.7). Aromatic amines such as aniline (pK_b = 9.42) are far less basic than aliphatic amines, because the electron-withdrawing effect of the ring reduces the basicity of the amino group. The presence of other substituents on the ring alters the basicity of anilines: Electron-donating groups (such as –OH, $-CH_3$, and $-NH_2$) increase basicity, while electron-withdrawing groups (such as NO_2) reduce basicity.

Real-World Analogy

An interesting property of several nitrogen-containing compounds, such as nitroglycerin and nitrous oxide, is their ability to act as relaxants. Nitroglycerine is given sublingually to relieve coronary artery spasms in people with chest pain, and nitrous oxide (laughing gas) is a common dental anesthetic. Nitroglycerine has the additional property of rapidly decomposing to form gas and is thus fairly explosive.

Amines also function as very weak acids. The pK_a's of amines are around 35, and a very strong base is required for deprotonation. For example, the proton of diisopropylamine may be removed with butyllithium, forming the sterically hindered base lithium diisopropylamide, LDA.

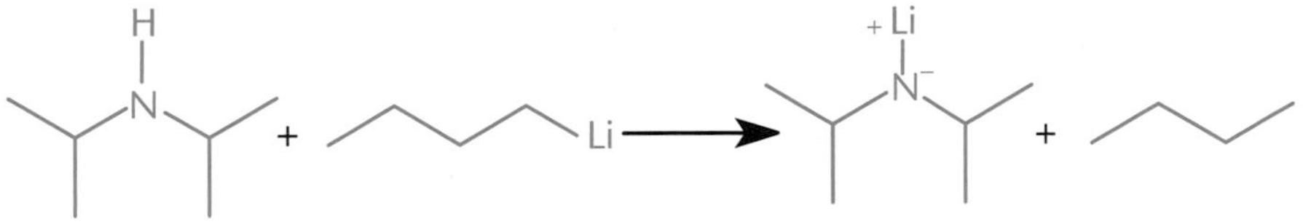

Figure 11.3

SYNTHESIS

A. ALKYLATION OF AMMONIA

1. Direct

Alkyl halides react with ammonia to produce alkylammonium halide salts. Ammonia functions as a nucleophile and displaces the halide atom. When the salt is treated with base, the alkylamine product is formed.

$$CH_3Br + NH_3 \longrightarrow CH_3\overset{+}{N}H_3Br^- \xrightarrow{NaOH} CH_3NH_2 + NaBr + H_2O$$

$$CH_3NH_2 + CH_3Br \longrightarrow CH_3{-}\underset{CH_3}{\underset{|}{NH}} + CH_3B \longrightarrow CH_3{-}\underset{CH_3}{\underset{|}{N}} \longrightarrow CH_3$$

$$\longrightarrow (CH_3)_4N^+$$

Figure 11.4

This reaction often leads to side products, because the alkylamine formed is nucleophilic and can react with the alkyl halide to form more complex products.

DAT Synopsis

Alkylation of ammonia proceeds to completion and forms of quaternary ammonium salts.

2. Gabriel Synthesis

The **Gabriel synthesis** converts a primary alkyl halide to a primary amine. The use of a disguised form of ammonia prevents side-product formation.

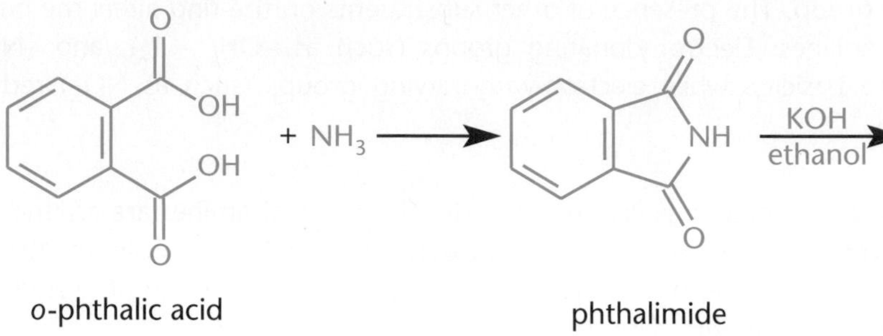

Flashback

Addition of ammonia to an alkyl halide and the Gabriel synthesis are both S_N2 reactions. With its unshared electron pair, ammonia is a very good nucleophile, while the halides are all good leaving groups (see chapter 4).

o-phthalic acid   phthalimide

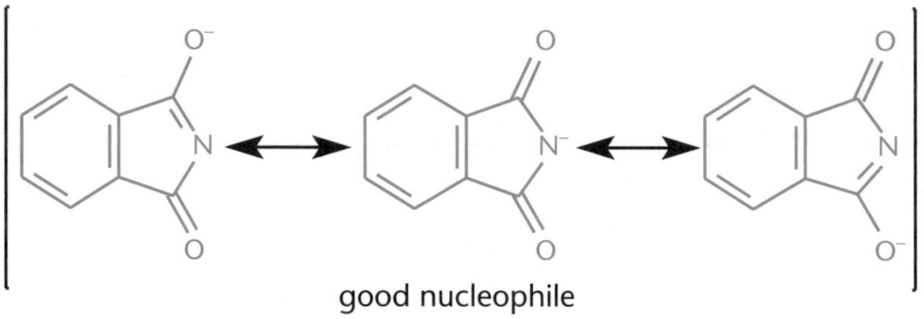

good nucleophile

Figure 11.5

Phthalimide, the condensation product of phthalic acid and ammonia, acts as a good nucleophile when deprotonated. It displaces halide ions, forming N-alkylphthalimides, which do not react with other alkyl halides. When the reaction is complete, the N-alkylphthalimide can be hydrolyzed with aqueous base to produce the alkylamine.

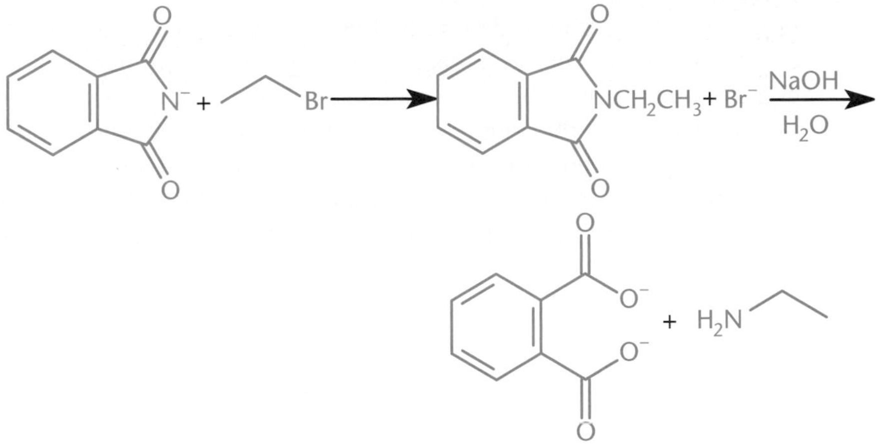

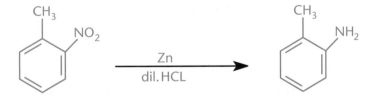

Figure 11.6

B. REDUCTION

Amines can be obtained from other nitrogen-containing functionalities via reduction reactions.

1. From Nitro Compounds

Nitro compounds are easily reduced to primary amines. The most common reducing agent is iron or zinc and dilute hydrochloric acid, although many other reagents can be used. This reaction is especially useful for aromatic compounds, because nitration of aromatic rings is facile.

Figure 11.7

2. From Nitriles

Nitriles can be reduced with hydrogen and a catalyst, or with lithium aluminum hydride (LAH), to produce primary amines.

$$CH_3CH_2C\equiv N \xrightarrow{\text{LAH}} CH_3CH_2CH_2NH_2$$

Figure 11.8

DAT Synopsis

Amines can be formed by
1) S_N2 reactions
   - ammonia reacting with alkyl halides
   - Gabriel synthesis

2) Reduction of
   - amides
   - aniline and its derivatives
   - nitriles
   - imines

Amines can be destroyed (converted to alkenes) by exhaustive methylation.

---

3. From Imines

Amines can be synthesized by **reductive amination**, a process whereby an aldehyde or ketone is reacted with ammonia, a primary amine, or a secondary amine to form a primary, secondary, or tertiary amine, respectively. When the amine reacts with the aldehyde or the ketone, an imine is produced. Consequently, it will undergo hydride reduction in much the same way that a carbonyl does. When the imine is reduced with hydrogen in the presence of a catalyst, an amine is produced.

DAT Synopsis

An imine is a nitrogen double-bonded to a carbon and has about the same polarity as a carbonyl functionality.

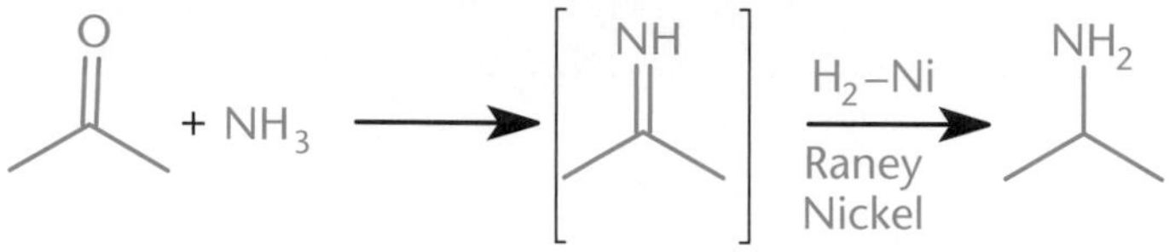

acetone   imine   amine
                       isopropylimine   isopropylamine
                                              (aminoisopropane)

Figure 11.9

4. From Amides

Amides can be reduced with LAH to form amines (see "Amides: Reaction" in chapter 10).

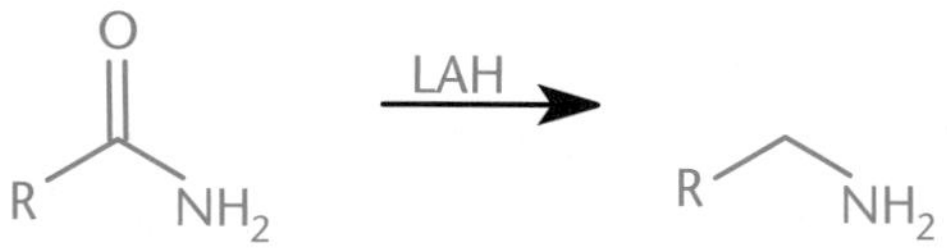

Figure 11.10

REACTIONS
A. EXHAUSTIVE METHYLATION

Exhaustive methylation is also known as **Hofmann elimination**. In this process, an amine is converted to a quaternary ammonium iodide by treatment with excess methyl iodide. Treatment with silver oxide and water converts this to the ammonium hydroxide, which, when heated, undergoes elimination to form an alkene and an amine. The predominant alkene formed is the least substituted, in contrast with normal elimination reactions where the predominant alkene product is the most substituted.

Flashback

Elimination reactions were discussed in chapter 5.

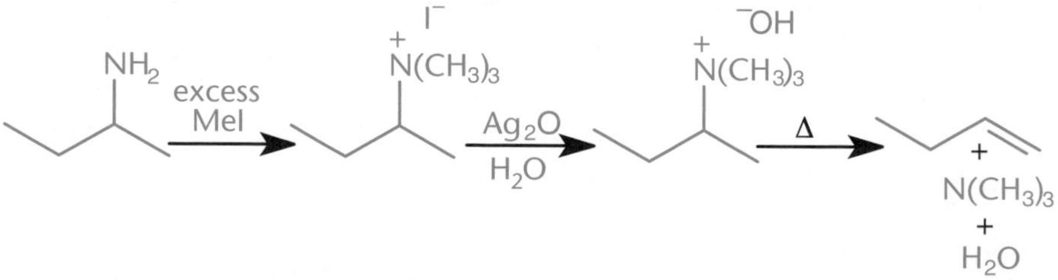

Figure 11.11

## 12

PURIFICATION AND SEPARATION

Much of organic chemistry is concerned with the isolation and purification of the desired reaction product. A reaction itself may be completed in a matter of minutes, but separating the product from the reaction mixture is often a difficult and time-consuming process. Many techniques have been developed to accomplish this objective: to obtain a pure compound separated from solvents, reagents, and other products.

BASIC TECHNIQUES
A. EXTRACTION

One way of separating out a desired product is through **extraction**, the transfer of a dissolved compound (here, the desired product) from one solvent into another in which it is more soluble. Most impurities will be left behind in the first solvent. The two solvents should be immiscible (form two layers that do not mix because of mutual insolubility). The two layers are temporarily mixed together so that solute can pass from one to the other. For example, a solution of isobutyric acid in diethyl ether can be extracted with water. Isobutyric acid is more soluble in water than in ether, so when the two solvents are placed together, isobutyric acid transfers to the water phase.

The water (aqueous) and ether (organic) phases are separated in a specialized piece of glassware called a separatory funnel (see Figure 12.1). Once separated, the isobutyric acid can be isolated from the aqueous phase in pure form. Some isobutyric acid will remain dissolved in the ether phase, so the extraction should be repeated several times with fresh solvent (water). More product can be obtained with successive extractions (i.e., it is more effective to perform three successive extractions of 10 mL each than to perform one extraction of 30 mL). Once the compound has been isolated in its purified form in a solvent, it can then be obtained by evaporation of the solvent.

> **DAT Synopsis**
>
> Think of the aqueous and organic layers as being like oil and water in salad dressing: You can shake the mixture to increase their interaction, but ultimately they will separate again.

Bridge

Extraction depends on the rules of solubility—"like dissolves like"! Remember the three intermolecular forces that affect solubility:

1. Hydrogen bonding: Compounds that can do this, such as alcohols or acids, will move most easily into the aqueous layer.
2. Dipole-dipole interactions: These compounds are less likely to move into the aqueous layer.
3. Van der Waals (London) forces: With only these interactions, compounds are least likely to move into the aqueous layer.

Bridge

You can use the properties of acids and bases to your advantage in extraction:

$$HA + base \longrightarrow A^- + Base: H^+$$

When the acid dissociates, the anion formed will be more soluble in the aqueous layer (because it is charged) than was the original form.

Thus, adding a *base* will help you extract an acid.

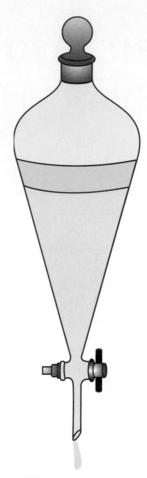

Figure 12.1. Separatory Funnel

An extraction carried out to remove unwanted impurities rather than to isolate a pure product is called a **wash**.

B. FILTRATION

Filtration is used to isolate a solid from a liquid. In this technique, a liquid/solid mixture is poured onto a paper filter that allows only the solvent to pass through. The result of this process is the separation of the solid (often referred to as the residue) from the liquid or **filtrate**. The two basic types of filtration are **gravity filtration** and **vacuum filtration**. In gravity filtration, the solvent's own weight pulls it through the filter. Frequently, however, the pores of the filter become clogged with solid, slowing the rate of filtration. For this reason, in gravity filtration it is generally desirable for the substance of interest to be in solution (dissolved in the solvent), while impurities remain undissolved and can be filtered out. This allows the desired product to flow more easily and rapidly through the apparatus. To ensure that the product remains dissolved, gravity filtration is usually carried out with hot solvent.

In vacuum filtration (see Figure 12.2), the solvent is forced through the filter by a vacuum on the other side. Vacuum filtration is used to isolate relatively large quantities of solid, usually when the solid is the desired product.

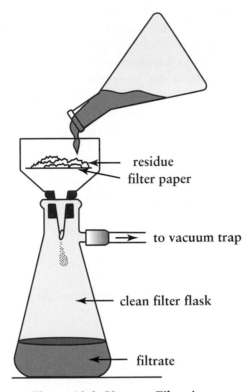

residue
filter paper

to vacuum trap

clean filter flask

filtrate

Figure 12.2. Vacuum Filtration

C. RECRYSTALLIZATION

Recrystallization is a process in which impure crystals are dissolved in a minimum amount of hot solvent. As the solvent is cooled, the crystals re-form, leaving the impurities in solution. For recrystallization to be effective, the solvent must be chosen carefully. It must dissolve the solid while it is hot, but not while it is cold. In addition, it must dissolve the impurities at both temperatures so that they remain in solution. Solvent choice is usually a matter of trial and error, although some generalizations can be made. An estimate of polarity is useful, since polar solvents dissolve polar compounds, while nonpolar solvents dissolve nonpolar compounds (see General Chemistry, chapter 9). A solvent with intermediate polarity is generally desirable in recrystallization. In addition, the solvent should have a low enough freezing point that the solution may be sufficiently cooled.

In some instances, a mixed solvent system may be used. Here the crude compound is dissolved in a solvent in which it is highly soluble. Another solvent, in which the compound is less soluble, is then added in drops, just until solid begins to precipitate. The solution is heated a bit more to redissolve the precipitate and then slowly cooled to induce crystal formation.

> ### DAT Synopsis
>
> Ideally, the desired product should have solubility that depends on temperature—it should be more soluble at high temperature, less so at low. In contrast, impurities should be equally soluble at various temperatures.

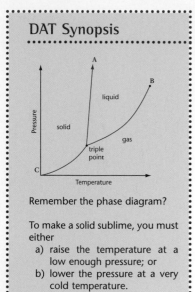
D. SUBLIMATION

Sublimation occurs when a heated solid turns directly into a gas without an intervening liquid stage. It is used as a method of purification because the impurities found in most reaction mixtures will not sublime easily. The vapors are made to condense on a **cold finger**, a piece of glassware packed with dry ice or with cold water running through it (see Figure 12.3). Most sublimations are performed under vacuum, because at higher pressures more compounds will pass through a liquid phase rather than subliming; low pressure also reduces the temperature required for sublimation and thus the danger that the compound will decompose. The optimal conditions depend on the compound to be purified, since each compound has a different phase diagram (see General Chemistry, chapter 8).

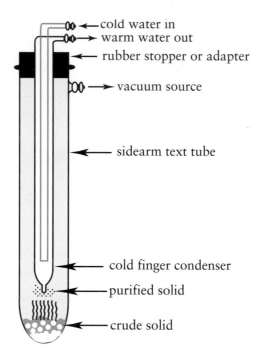

Figure 12.3. Sublimation

E. CENTRIFUGATION

Particles in a solution settle, or **sediment**, at different rates depending upon their mass, their density, and their shape. Sedimentation can be accelerated by **centrifuging** the solution. A centrifuge is an apparatus in which test tubes containing the solution are spun at high speed, which subjects them to centrifugal force (see Figure 12.4). Compounds of greater mass and density settle toward the bottom of the test tubes, while lighter compounds remain near the top. This method of separation is effective for many different types of compounds and is frequently used in biochemistry to separate cells, organelles, and biological macromolecules.

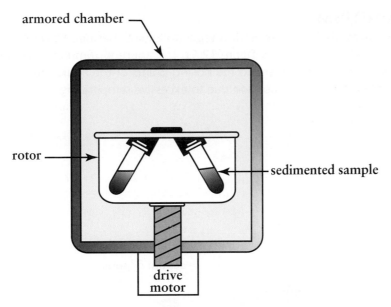

Figure 12.4. Centrifuge

DISTILLATION

Distillation is the separation of one liquid from another through vaporization and condensation. A mixture of two (or more) miscible liquids is slowly heated; the compound with the lowest boiling point is preferentially vaporized, condenses on a water-cooled distillation column, and is separated from the other, higher-boiling compound(s). (Immiscible liquids can be separated in a separatory funnel and thus do not require distillation.)

A. SIMPLE

Simple distillation is used to separate liquids that boil *below* 150°C and at least 25°C apart. The apparatus consists of a distilling flask containing the two liquids, a distillation column consisting of a thermometer and a condenser, and a receiving flask to collect the distillate.

DAT Synopsis

Boiling point is strongly affected by intermolecular forces:
- H bonds (this is why H_2O has such a high bp)
- Dipole-dipole interactions
- Van der Waals (London) forces (the reason that longer molecules tend to have higher bp than shorter ones)

B. VACUUM

Vacuum distillation is used to separate liquids that boil *above* 150°C and at least 25°C apart (see Figure 12.5). The entire system is operated under reduced pressure, lowering the boiling points of the liquids and thus preventing their decomposition due to excessive temperature.

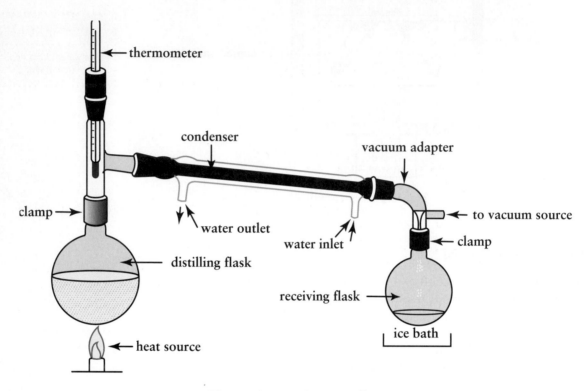

Figure 12.5. Vaccum Distillation

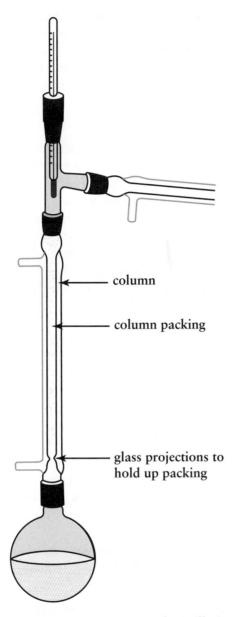

column

column packing

glass projections to
hold up packing

Figure 12.6. Fractional Distillation

C. FRACTIONAL

Fractional distillation is used to separate liquids that boil less than 25°C apart (see Figure 12.6). A fractionating column is used to connect the distilling flask to the distillation column. It is filled with inert objects, such as glass beads, which have a large surface area. The vapors condense on these surfaces, re-evaporate, and then condense further up the column.

> **DAT Synopsis**
>
> Fractional distillation can be thought of as repeated distillation: It's like distilling the compounds over and over again.

Each time the liquid evaporates, the vapors contain a greater proportion of the lower-boiling component. Eventually, near the top of the fractionating column, the vapor is composed solely of one component, which will condense on the distillation column and collect in the receiving flask.

CHROMATOGRAPHY

A. GENERAL PRINCIPLES

Chromatography is a technique that allows scientists to separate, identify, and isolate individual compounds from a complex mixture based on their differing chemical properties. First, the sample is placed, or loaded, onto a solid medium called the **stationary phase** or **adsorbant**. Then, the **mobile phase**, a liquid (or gas for gas chromatography), is run through the stationary phase, to displace (or **elute**) adhered substances. Different compounds will adhere to the stationary phase with different strengths and, therefore, migrate with different speeds. This causes separation of the compounds within the stationary phase, allowing each compound to be isolated.

Several forms of media are used as the stationary phase, which separate compounds based on different chemical properties. How quickly a compound travels through the stationary phase depends on a variety of factors. Commonly, the key is polarity. For instance, thin-layer chromatography often uses silica gel, which is highly polar. Thus, polar compounds bind tightly, eluting poorly into the less polar organic solvent. Size or charge may also play a role, as in column chromatography (described in detail below). Newer techniques, such as affinity chromatography, take advantage of unique properties of a substance (such as its strong binding to a specific antibody or to a known receptor or ligand) to bind it tightly to the stationary phase.

Compounds can be distinguished from each other because they travel across the stationary phase (adsorbant) at different rates. In practice, a substance can be identified based on

- how far it travels in a given amount of time (as in TLC); or
- how rapidly it travels a given distance (e.g., how quickly it elutes off the column, as in GC or column chromatography).

The four most commonly used types of chromatography are **thin-layer chromatography**, **column chromatography**, **gas chromatography**, and **high-pressure** (or **performance**) **liquid chromatography**.

B. THIN-LAYER CHROMATOGRAPHY

The adsorbant in thin-layer chromatography (TLC) is either a piece of paper or a thin layer of silica gel or alumina on a plastic or glass sheet (see Figure 12.7). The mixture to be separated is placed on the adsorbant; this is called **spotting**, because a small, well-defined spot is desirable. The TLC plate is then **developed**—placed upright in a developing chamber

---

DAT Synopsis

Key idea: Chromatography separates compounds based on how strongly they adhere to the *solid*, or *stationary*, phase (or, in other words, how easily they come off into the mobile phase).

(usually a beaker with a lid or a wide-mouthed jar), containing **eluant** (solvent) approximately 1/4-inch deep (this value depends on the size of the plate). It is imperative that the initial spots on the plate be above the level of the solvent, or else they will simply elute off the plate into the solvent rather than moving neatly up the plate itself. The solvent creeps up the plate by capillary action, moving different compounds at different rates. When the **solvent front** nears the top of the plate, the plate is removed from the chamber and allowed to dry.

Chromatography is often done with silica gel, which is very polar and hydrophilic. The mobile phase, usually an organic solvent of weak to moderate polarity, is then used to "run" the sample through the gel. Nonpolar compounds move very quickly, while polar molecules are stuck tightly to the gel. The more polar the solvent, the faster the sample will migrate. Reverse-phase chromatography is just the opposite. Here the stationary phase is very nonpolar, so polar molecules run very quickly, while nonpolar molecules stick more tightly.

The spots of individual compounds (usually white) are not usually visible on the white TLC plate. They are **visualized** by placing the TLC plate under UV light, which will show any compounds that are UV-sensitive (see chapter 13), or by allowing iodine, I_2, to stain the spots. Other chemical staining agents include phosphomolybdic acid and vanillin. Note that these compounds destroy the product (usually by oxidation), so it cannot be recovered for further study.

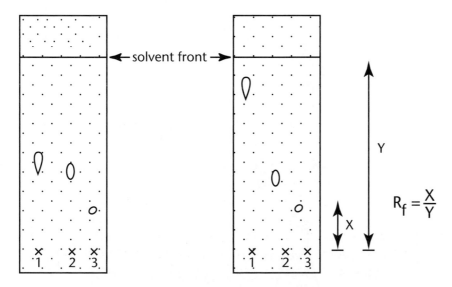

Figure 12.7. Thin-Layer Chromatograms

The distance a compound travels, divided by the distance the solvent travels, is called the **R_f value**. This value is relatively constant for a particular compound in a particular solvent and can, therefore, be used for identification.

TLC is most frequently used for qualitative identification (i.e., determining the identity of a compound). It can also be used on a larger scale as a means of purification. **Preparative** or **prep TLC** uses a large TLC plate upon which a sizeable streak of a mixture is placed. As the plate develops, the streak splits into bands of individual compounds, which can then be scraped off. Rinsing with a polar solvent will recover the pure compounds from the silica.

C. COLUMN CHROMATOGRAPHY

The principle behind column chromatography is the same as for TLC. Column chromatography, however, uses silica gel or alumina as an adsorbant (not paper), and this adsorbant is in the form of a column (not a layer), allowing much more separation (see Figure 12.8). In TLC, the solvent and compounds move up the plate (by capillary action), whereas in column chromatography, they move down the column (by gravity). Sometimes the solvent is forced through the column with nitrogen gas; this is called **flash column chromatography**.

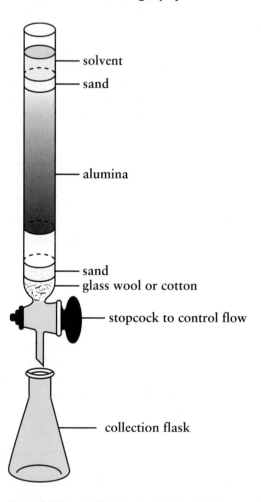

Figure 12.8. Column Chromatography

The solvent drips out the end of the column, and fractions are collected in flasks or test tubes. These fractions contain bands corresponding to the different compounds, and when the solvents are evaporated, the compounds can be isolated.

Column chromatography is particularly useful in biochemistry, because it can be used to separate macromolecules such as proteins or nucleic acids. Several techniques exist:

1) In *ion exchange chromatography*, the beads in the column are coated with charged substances, so they will attract or bind compounds with an opposing charge. For instance, a positively charged column will attract and hold negative substances while letting those with positive charge pass through.

2) In *size-exclusion chromatography*, the column contains beads with many tiny pores. Very small molecules can enter the beads, which slows down their progress, while large molecules move around/between the beads and thus travel through the column faster.

3) In *affinity chromotography*, columns can be "customized" to bind a substance of interest. For example, to purify substance A, a scientist might use a column of beads coated with something that binds A very tightly, such as a receptor for A, A's biological target, or even a specific antibody. Substance A will bind to the column very tightly. It can later be eluted by washing with free receptor (or target or antibody), which will compete with the bead-bound receptor and ultimately free substance A from the column.

D. GAS CHROMATOGRAPHY

Gas chromatography (GC) is another method of qualitative separation. In gas chromatography, also called **vapor-phase chromatography** (VPC), the eluant that passes through the adsorbant is a gas, usually helium or nitrogen. The adsorbant is inside a 30-foot column that is coiled and kept inside an oven to control its temperature (see Figure 12.9). The mixture to be separated is injected into the column and vaporized. The gaseous compounds travel through the column at different rates, because they adhere to the adsorbant to different degrees, and will separate by the time they reach the end of the column. At this point, they are registered by a detector, which records the presence of a compound as a peak.

> **DAT Synopsis**
>
> Again, note that there is a stationary phase (here, a 30-foot column) and a mobile phase or eluant (here, a gas).

> **DAT Synopsis**
>
> To identify a compound or distinguish two different compounds, look at their "retention times"—that is, how *long* it took for each to travel through the column.

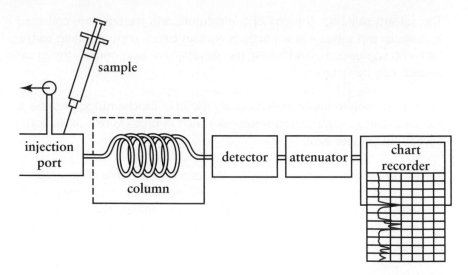

Figure 12.9. Gas Chromatography

GC can be used on a larger scale for quantitative separation; it is then called preparative or prep GC. This is, however, very tedious and difficult to perform.

E. HPLC

HPLC stands for either high-pressure or high-performance liquid chromatography. The eluant is a liquid that travels through a column similar to a GC column, but it is under pressure. In the past, very high pressures were used. Now they are much lower; hence, the change from high *pressure* to high *performance*.

In HPLC, a sample is injected into the column, and separation occurs as it flows through. The compounds pass through a detector and are collected as the solvent flows out the end of the apparatus. The eluant may vary, as in thin-layer or column chromatography.

ELECTROPHORESIS

When a molecule is placed in an electric field, it will move towards either the cathode or the anode, depending on its size and charge. **Electrophoresis** employs this phenomenon to separate macromolecules (usually biological macromolecules) such as proteins or DNA. The migration velocity, v, of a molecule is directly proportional to the electric field strength, E, and to the net charge on the molecule, z, and it is inversely proportional to a frictional coefficient, f, which depends on the mass and shape of the migrating molecules.

$$V = \frac{EZ}{f}$$

Therefore, in a constant electric field, highly charged molecules will move most rapidly, as will small molecules.

KAPLAN EXCLUSIVE

In electrophoresis:

Anions are attracted to the Anode while
Cations are attracted to the Cathode.

DAT Synopsis

In most forms of electrophoresis, the size of a macromolecule is usually the most important factor—small molecules move faster, while large ones move more slowly and may in fact take hours to leave the well.

A. AGAROSE GEL ELECTROPHORESIS

Agarose gel electrophoresis is used by molecular biologists to separate pieces of **nucleic acid** (usually **deoxyribonucleic acid**, DNA, but sometimes **ribonucleic acid**, RNA, as well; see chapter 15). Agarose is a plant gel, derived from seaweed, that is nontoxic and easy to manipulate (unlike SDS/polyacrylamide). Since every piece of nucleic acid is highly negatively charged, nucleic acids can be separated effectively on the basis of size even without the charge masking provided by SDS. Agarose gels are stained with a compound called ethidium bromide, which binds to nucleic acids and is visualized by its fluorescence under ultraviolet light.

Agarose gel electrophoresis can also be used preparatively by cutting the desired band out of the gel and eluting out the nucleic acid.

B. SDS-POLYACRYLAMIDE GEL ELECTROPHORESIS

SDS-polyacrylamide gel electrophoresis separates proteins on the basis of mass, not charge. Polyacrylamide gel is the standard medium for electrophoresis. SDS is sodium dodecyl sulfate, which disrupts noncovalent interactions. It binds to proteins and creates large negative net charges, neutralizing the protein's original net charge. As proteins move through the gel, the only variable affecting their velocity is f, the frictional coefficient, which is dependent on mass. After separation, the gel is stained so that the protein bands can be visualized.

C. ISOELECTRIC FOCUSING

A protein may be characterized by its **isoelectric point**, pI, which is the pH at which its net charge (the sum of the charges on all of its component amino acids; see chapter 15) is zero. If a mixture of proteins is placed in an electric field in a gel with a pH gradient, the proteins will move until they reach the point at which the pH is equal to their pI. At this location, the protein will be uncharged and will no longer move in the field. Molecules differing by as little as one charge can be separated in this manner, which is called **isoelectric focusing**.

Real–World Example

To make your gel run faster:
- Increase the voltage (∂E).
- Use a lower percent of agarose or acrylamide (f).

DAT Synopsis

SDS–PAGE and agarose gel electrophoresis separate molecules based on *size*.

DAT Synopsis

When pH = pI, a protein stops moving.

DAT Synopsis

Isoelectric focusing separates proteins based on *charge*.

SUMMARY OF PURIFICATION METHODS

Method	Use
Extraction	Separates dissolved substances based on differential solubility in aqueous versus organic solvents.
Filtration	Separates solids from liquids.
Recrystallization	Separates solids based on differential solubility; temperature is important here.
Sublimation	Separates solids based on their ability to sublime.
Centrifugation	Separates large things (like cells, organelles, and macromolecules) based on mass and density.
Distillation	Separates liquids based on boiling point, which in turn depends on intermolecular forces.
Chromatography	Uses a stationary phase and a mobile phase to separate compounds based on how tightly they adhere (generally due to polarity but sometimes size as well).
Electrophoresis	Used to separate biological macromolecules (such as proteins or nucleic acids) based on size and sometimes charge.

## 13

SPECTROSCOPY

Once an organic compound is isolated, it must be characterized and identified. If it is a known compound, identification can often be made from elemental analysis or determination of the melting point. With new or more complex compounds, other methods must be used. **Spectroscopy** is the process of measuring the energy differences between the possible states of a molecular system by determining the frequencies of electromagnetic radiation (light) absorbed by the molecules. The possible states are quantized energy levels associated with different types of molecular motion, including molecular rotation, vibration of bonds, and electron movement. Different types of spectroscopy measure these different types of molecular motion, identifying specific functional groups and how they are connected.

Spectroscopy is useful because only a very small quantity of sample is needed. In addition, the sample may be reused after an IR, NMR, or UV spectrum is obtained.

INFRARED
A. BASIC THEORY

Infrared (IR) spectroscopy measures molecular vibrations, which include bond **stretching**, **bending**, and **rotation**. The useful absorptions of infrared light occur in the 3,000–30,000 nm region, which corresponds to 3,500–300 cm^{-1} (called **wavenumbers**). When light of these wavelengths/wavenumbers is absorbed, the molecules enter higher (excited) vibrational states.

Bond stretching (which can be of two types: symmetric or asymmetric) involves the largest change in energy and is observed in the region 1,500–4,000 cm^{-1}. Bending vibrations are observed in the region 400–1500 cm^{-1}. Four types of vibration that can occur are shown in Figure 13.1.

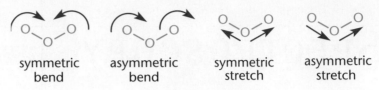

| symmetric bend | asymmetric bend | symmetric stretch | asymmetric stretch |

Figure 13.1

In addition to bending and stretching vibrations, more complex vibrations may occur. These can be combinations of bending, stretching, and rotation frequencies or complex frequency patterns caused by the motion of the whole molecule. Absorptions of these types are seen in the region 1,500–400 cm^{-1}. This region of the spectrum is known as the **fingerprint region** and is characteristic of a molecule; it is, therefore, frequently used to identify a substance.

For an absorption to be recorded, the motion must result in a change in a bond dipole moment. Molecules comprised of atoms with the same electronegativity, as well as symmetrical molecules, do not experience a changing dipole moment and, therefore, do not exhibit absorption. For example, O_2 and Br_2 do not absorb, but HCl and CO do.

A typical spectrum is obtained by passing infrared light (of frequencies from approximately 4,000–400 cm^{-1}) through a sample and recording the absorption pattern. Percent transmittance is plotted versus frequency, where percent transmittance = absorption^{-1} ($\%T = A^{-1}$); absorptions appear as valleys on the spectrum.

DAT Synopsis

Symmetric stretches do not show up in IR spectra since they involve no net change in dipole movement.

DAT Synopsis

Wavenumbers (cm^{-1}) are not the same as frequency.

$v = \dfrac{c}{\lambda}$ while wave number $= \dfrac{1}{\lambda}$.

B. CHARACTERISTIC ABSORPTIONS

Particular functional groups absorb at localized frequencies. For example, alcohols absorb around 3,300 cm^{-1}, carbonyl groups around 1,700 cm^{-1}, and ethers around 1,100 cm^{-1}. Table 13.1 lists the specific absorptions of key functional groups and the vibrations with which they are associated.

C. APPLICATION

A great deal of information can be obtained from an IR spectrum. Most of the useful functional group information is found between 1,400 and 4,000 cm^{-1}. Figure 13.2 shows the IR spectrum of an aliphatic alcohol. The large peak at 3,300 cm^{-1} is due to the presence of the hydroxyl group, while the peak at 3,000 cm^{-1} can be attributed to the alkane portion of the molecule.

Table 13.1. Common Infrared Absorption Peaks

Functional Group	Frequency (cm^{-1})	Vibration
Alkanes	2,800–3,000	C–H
	1,200	C–C
Alkenes	3,080–3,140	=C–H
	1,645	C=C
Alkynes	2,200	C≡C
	3,300	≡C–H
Aromatic	2,900–3,100	C–H
	1,475–1,625	C–C
Alcohols	3,100–3,500	O–H (broad)
Ethers	1,050–1,150	C–O
Aldehydes	2,700–2,900	(O)C–H
	1,725–1,750	C=O
Ketones	1,700–1,750	C=O
Carboxylic Acids	1,700–1,750	C=O
	2,900–3,300	O–H (broad)
Amines	3,100–3,500	N–H (sharp)

DAT Synopsis

IR spectroscopy is best used for identification of functional groups. The most important peaks to know are those for alcohols (don't forget this is a BROAD peak), acids (BROADEST peak), ketones, and amines (SHARP peak). If you know nothing else here, know these!

Frequency (cm^{-1})

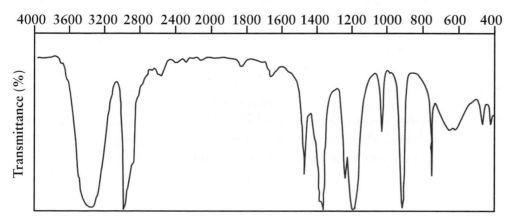

Figure 13.2

NUCLEAR MAGNETIC RESONANCE

A. BASIC THEORY

Nuclear magnetic resonance (NMR) spectroscopy is one of the most widely used spectroscopic tools in organic chemistry. NMR is based on the fact that certain nuclei have magnetic moments that are normally oriented at random. When such nuclei are placed in a magnetic field, their magnetic moments tend to align either with or against the direction of this applied field. Nuclei whose magnetic moments are aligned with the field are said to be in the α **state** (lower energy), while those whose moments are aligned against the field are said to be in the β **state** (higher energy). If the nuclei are then irradiated with electromagnetic radiation, some will be excited into the β state. The absorption corresponding to this excitation occurs at different frequencies depending on an atom's environment. The nuclear magnetic moments are affected by other nearby atoms that also possess magnetic moments. Hence, a compound may contain many nuclei that resonate at different frequencies, producing a very complex spectrum.

A typical NMR spectrum is a plot of frequency versus absorption of energy during resonance. Frequency *decreases* toward the right. Alternatively, varying magnetic field may be plotted on the *x*-axis, *increasing* towards the right. Because different NMR spectrometers operate at different magnetic field strengths, a standardized method of plotting the NMR spectrum has been adopted. An arbitrary variable, called **chemical shift** (represented by the symbol δ), with units of **parts per million (ppm)** of spectrometer frequency, is plotted on the *x*-axis.

NMR is most commonly used to study ^{1}H nuclei (protons) and ^{13}C nuclei, although any atom possessing a nuclear spin (any nucleus with an odd atomic number or odd mass number) can be studied, such as ^{19}F, ^{17}O, ^{14}N, ^{15}N, or ^{31}P.

B. ^{1}H-NMR

Most ^{1}H nuclei come into resonance between 0 and 10 δ downfield from TMS. Each distinct set of nuclei gives rise to a separate peak. The compound dichloromethyl methyl ether has two distinct sets of ^{1}H nuclei. The single proton attached to the dichloromethyl group is in a different magnetic environment than are the three protons on the methyl group, and the two classes resonate at different frequencies. The three protons on the methyl group are magnetically equivalent due to rotation about the oxygen-carbon single bond and resonate at the same frequency. Thus, two separate peaks are expected, as shown in Figure 13.3.

> ### DAT Synopsis
>
> TMS provides a reference peak. The signal for its H atoms is assigned a $\delta = 0$.

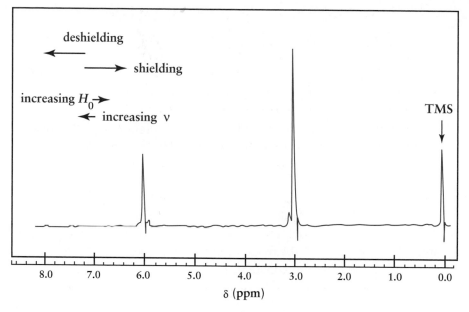

deshielding

shielding

increasing H_0

increasing ν

TMS

8.0 7.0 6.0 5.0 4.0 3.0 2.0 1.0 0.0

δ (ppm)

Figure 13.3

The left-hand peak corresponds to the single dichloromethyl proton and the middle peak to the three methyl protons (the one on the far right is the TMS reference peak). Notice that if the areas under the peaks are integrated, the ratio between them is 3:1, corresponding to the number of protons producing each peak.

The single proton comes into resonance downfield from the methyl protons. This phenomenon is due to the electron-withdrawing effect of the chlorine atoms. The electron cloud that surrounds the ^{1}H nucleus ordinarily screens the nucleus somewhat from the applied magnetic field. The chlorine atoms pull away the electron cloud and **deshield** the nucleus. Thus, the nucleus resonates in a lower field than it would otherwise. By the same rationale, electron-donating atoms, such as the silicon atoms in TMS, **shield** the ^{1}H nuclei, causing them to come into resonance at a higher field.

If two magnetically different protons are within three bonds of each other, a phenomenon known as **coupling,** or **splitting,** occurs. Consider two protons, H_a and H_b, on the molecule 1,1-dibromo-2,2-dichloroethane (Figure 13.4).

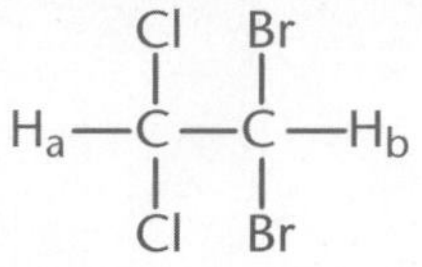

Figure 13.4

DAT Synopsis

The splitting of the peak represents the number of adjacent hydrogens. A peak will be split into $n + 1$ peaks, where n is the number of adjacent hydrogens.

At any given time, H_a can experience two different magnetic environments, since H_b can be in either the α or the β state. These different states of H_b influence nucleus H_a (if the two H atoms are within three bonds of each other), causing slight upfield and downfield shifts. Since there is approximately a 50 percent chance that H_b will be in either state, this results in a **doublet**, two peaks of equal intensity equally spaced around the true chemical shift of H_a. H_b experiences the two different states of H_a and is likewise coupled. The magnitude of the splitting, usually denoted in Hz, is called the **coupling constant, J**.

In 1,1-dibromo-2-chloroethane (Figure 13.5), the H_a nucleus is affected by two nearby H_b nuclei, and can experience four different states: $\alpha\alpha< \alpha\beta< \beta\alpha<$ or $\beta\beta$.

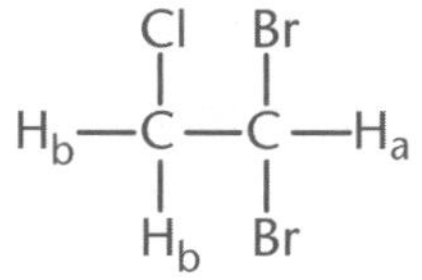

Figure 13.5

The α and α states have the same net effect on the H_a nucleus, and the resonances occur at the same frequency. The $\alpha\alpha$ and states resonate at frequencies different from each other and from the α / α frequency. The result is three peaks centered around the true chemical shift with an area ratio of 1:2:1. In general, n hydrogen atoms couple to give $n + 1$ peaks, whose area ratios are given by Pascal's triangle, shown in Table 13.2.

Table 13.2. Pascal's Triangle

Number of Adjacent Hydrogens	Total Number of Peaks	Area Ratios
0	1	1
1	2	1:1
2	3	1:2:1
3	4	1:3:3:1
4	5	1:4:6:4:1
5	6	1:5:10:10:5:1
6	7	1:6:15:20:15:6:1
7	8	1:7:21:35:35:21:7:1

Table 13.2 indicates the chemical shift ranges of several different types of protons:

Table 13.2. Chemical Shifts

Type of Proton	Approximate Chemical Shift δ (ppm) Downfield from TMS
RCH_3	0.9
RCH_2	1.25
R_3CH	1.5
–CH=CH	4.6–6.0
–C≡CH	2.0–3.0
Ar–**H**	6.0–8.5
–CHX	2.0–4.5
–CHOH/–CHOR	3.4–4.0
RCHO	9.0–10.0
RCHCO–	2.0–2.5
–CHCOOH/–CHCOOR	2.0–2.6
–CHOH–CH_2OH	1.0–5.5
ArOH	4.0–12.0
–COOH	10.5–12.0
$–NH_2$	1.0–5.0

DAT Synopsis

Proton MR is good for
1. determining the relative number of protons and their relative chemical environments.
2. showing how many adjacent protons there are by splitting patterns.
3. showing certain functional groups.

C. ^{13}C-NMR

^{13}C-NMR is very similar to ^{1}H-NMR. Most ^{13}C-NMR signals, however, occur 0–200 δ downfield from the carbon peak of TMS. Another significant difference is that only 1.1 percent of carbon atoms are ^{13}C atoms. This has two effects: First, a much larger sample is needed to run a ^{13}C spectrum (about 50 mg compared with 1 mg for ^{1}H-NMR), and second, coupling between carbon atoms is generally not observed.

Coupling *is* observed, however, between carbon atoms and the protons directly attached to them. This one-bond coupling is analogous to the three-bond coupling in ^{1}H-NMR. For example, if a carbon atom is attached to two protons, it can experience four different states of those protons (*αα*, *α* , *α*, and), and the carbon signal is split into a triplet with the area ratio 1:2:1.

An additional feature of ^{13}C-NMR is the ability to record a spectrum *without* the coupling of adjacent protons. This is called **spin decoupling**, and it produces a spectrum of **singlets**, each corresponding to a separate, magnetically equivalent carbon atom. For example, compare two spectra of 1,1,2-trichloropropane. One (Figure 13.6) is a typical **spin-decoupled spectrum**, and the other (Figure 13.7) is spin coupled.

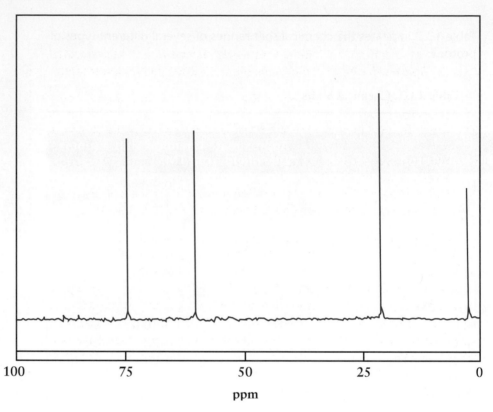

Figure 13.6 Spin-Decoupled Spectrum of 1,1,2-Trichloropropane

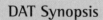

DAT Synopsis

Carbon NMR can show
1. the number of different carbons with their relative chemical environments.
2. their number of hydrogens (spin-coupled NMR only).

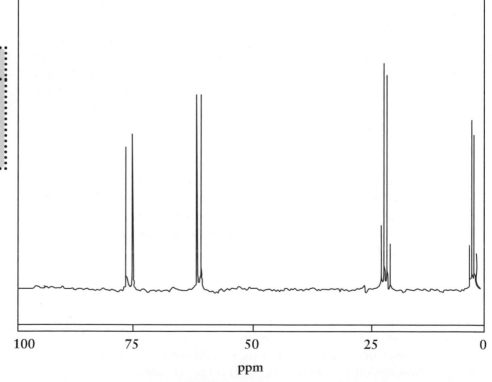

Figure 13.7 Spin-Coupled Spectrum of 1,1,2-Trichloropropane

In general, NMR spectroscopy provides information about the carbon skeleton of a compound, along with some suggestion of its functional groups. Specifically, NMR can provide the following types of information:

1. The number of nonequivalent nuclei, determined from the number of peaks
2. The magnetic environment of a nucleus, determined by the chemical shift
3. The relative numbers of nuclei, determined by integrating the peak areas
4. The number of neighboring nuclei, determined by the splitting pattern observed (except for ^{13}C in the spin-decoupled mode)

ULTRAVIOLET SPECTROSCOPY
A. BASIC THEORY

Ultraviolet spectra are obtained by passing ultraviolet light through a chemical sample (usually dissolved in an inert, nonabsorbing solvent) and plotting absorbance versus wavelength. The wavelength of maximum absorbance provides information on the extent of the conjugated system, as well as other structural and compositional information.

MASS SPECTROMETRY
A. BASIC THEORY

Mass spectrometry differs from the methods thus far discussed in that it is not true spectroscopy (i.e., no absorption of electromagnetic radiation is involved) and in that it is a destructive technique—mass spectrometry, does not allow for reuse of the sample once the analysis is complete. Most commonly used mass spectrometers utilize a high-speed beam of electrons to ionize the sample to be analyzed, a particle accelerator to put the charged particles in flight, a magnetic field to deflect the accelerated cationic fragments, and a detector that records the number of particles of each mass exiting the deflector area. The initially formed ion is the molecular cation-radical (M^+) resulting from a single electron being removed from a molecule of the sample. This unstable species usually decomposes rapidly into a cationic fragment and a radical fragment. Since there are many molecules in the sample and (usually) more than one way for the initially formed cation-radical to decompose into fragments, a typical mass spectrum is composed of many lines, each corresponding to a specific mass/charge ratio (m/e). The spectrum itself plots mass/charge on the horizontal axis and relative abundance of the various cationic fragments on the vertical axis (see Figure 13.8).

Flashback

Bonding and antibonding orbitals were discussed in chapter 3.

DAT Synopsis

UV spectroscopy is most useful for studying compounds containing double bonds and/or hetero atoms with lone pairs.

DAT Synopsis

UV spectroscopy can be applied quantitatively by using Beer's Law:

$$A = \epsilon bc$$

where A is absorbance (measured by UV spectroscopy), ϵ is a constant for the substance at a given wavelength, b is path length (usually equal to 1), and c is concentration.

B. CHARACTERISTICS

The tallest peak, belonging to the most common ion, is called the **base peak**, and it is assigned the relative abundance value of 100 percent. The peak with the highest m/e ratio (see Figure 13.8) is generally the **molecular ion peak (parent ion peak)**, **M⁺**, from which the molecular weight, M, can be obtained. The charge value is usually 1; hence, the m/e ratio can usually be read as the mass of the fragment.

C. APPLICATION

Fragmentation patterns often provide information that helps identify or distinguish certain compounds. In particular, the fragmentation pattern provides clues to the compound's structure. For example, while IR spectroscopy would be of little use in distinguishing between propionaldehyde and butyraldehyde, a mass spectrum would allow unambiguous identification.

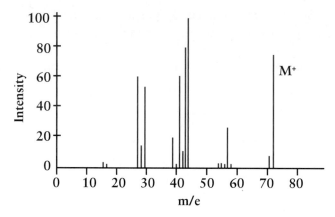

Figure 13.8

Figure 13.8 shows the mass spectrum of butyraldehyde. The peak at $m/e = 72$ corresponds to the molecular cation-radical, M⁺, while the base peak at $m/e = 44$ corresponds to the cationic fragment resulting from the loss of a C_2H_4 neutral fragment ($M - 28 = 44$). Other peaks of note include those at 57($M - 15$, loss of CH_3 radical), 43($M - 29$, loss of C_2H_5 radical), and at 29 ($M - 43$, loss of C_3H_7 radical). The small peak at $m/e = 15$ can be attributed to the unstable (and therefore not abundant) methyl cation.

## 14

CARBOHYDRATES

Carbohydrates are compounds containing carbon, hydrogen, and oxygen in the form of polyhydroxylated aldehydes or ketones. They have the general formula $C_n(H_2O)_n$ and serve many functions in biological systems, most notably as the chemical energy source for most organisms. A single carbohydrate unit is a **monosaccharide** (simple sugar), and a molecule with two sugars is a **disaccharide**. **Oligosaccharides** are short carbohydrate chains, while **polysaccharides** are long carbohydrate chains.

> **DAT Synopsis**
>
> Carbohydrates are aldehydes or ketones with many hydroxyl groups.

MONOSACCHARIDES

Monosaccharides are single sugar subunits. Examples of monosaccharides include fructose, glucose, galactose, and mannose. Monosacchaides are classified according to the number of carbons they possess.

> **DAT Synopsis**
>
> Monosaccharides are the simplest units and are classified by the number of carbons.

For example, **trioses**, **tetroses**, **pentoses**, and **hexoses** have 3, 4, 5, and 6 carbons, respectively. The basic structure of monosaccharides is exemplified by the simplest, glyceraldehyde.

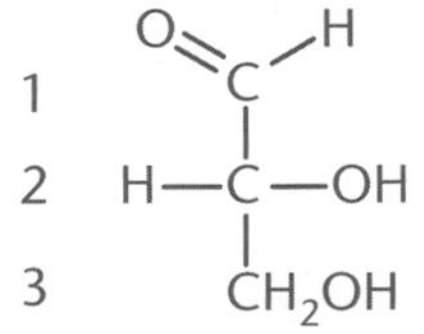

Figure 14.1. Glyceraldehyde

Glyceraldehyde is a polyhydroxylated aldehyde or **aldose** (aldehyde sugar). A polyhydroxylated ketone is called a **ketose** (ketone sugar). The numbering of the carbon atoms in a monosaccharide begins with the end closest to the carbonyl group.

> **DAT Synopsis**
>
> As usual, number the molecule from the end closest to the carbonyl.

A. STEREOCHEMISTRY

The stereochemistry of monosaccharides can be understood by studying the enantiomeric configurations of glyceraldehyde (see Figure 14.2).

DAT Synopsis

The *D* and *L* designations are based on the sterochemistry of glyceraldehyde. Further, they are enantimers.

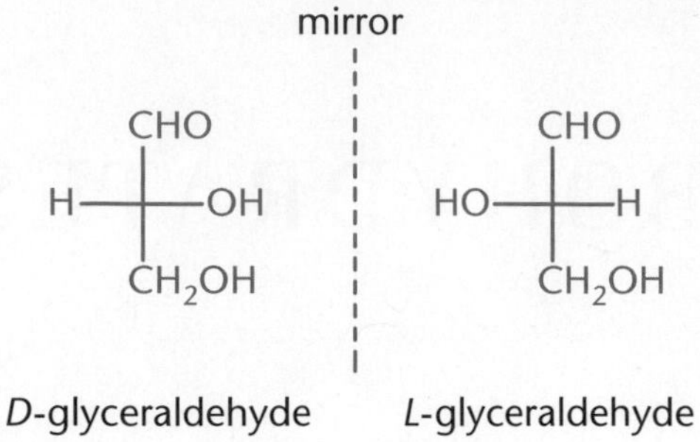
mirror
CHO
H
OH
CH_2OH
CHO
HO
H
CH_2OH
D-glyceraldehyde
L-glyceraldehyde

Figure 14.2

KAPLAN EXCLUSIVE

If Lowest –OH is on the Left, the molecule is L. If the –OH is on the Right, it's D (from the Latin root dextro, meaning "right").

The *D* and *L* configurations of glyceraldehyde were assigned early in this century (before the *R* and *S* configurations were used) to designate the optical rotation of each enantiomer. *D*-glyceraldehyde was later determined to exhibit a positive rotation (designated as *D*-(+)-glyceraldehyde), and *L*-glyceraldehyde a negative rotation (designated as *L*-(–)-glyceraldehyde. However, other monosaccharides are assigned the *D* or *L* configuration depending on their relationship to glyceraldehyde: A molecule whose highest-numbered chiral center (the chiral center farthest from the carbonyl) has the same configuration as *D*-(+)-glyceraldehyde is classed as a *D*-sugar. A molecule that has its highest-numbered chiral center in the same configuration as *L*-(–)-glyceraldehyde is classed as an *L*-sugar. This is illustrated Figure 14.3.

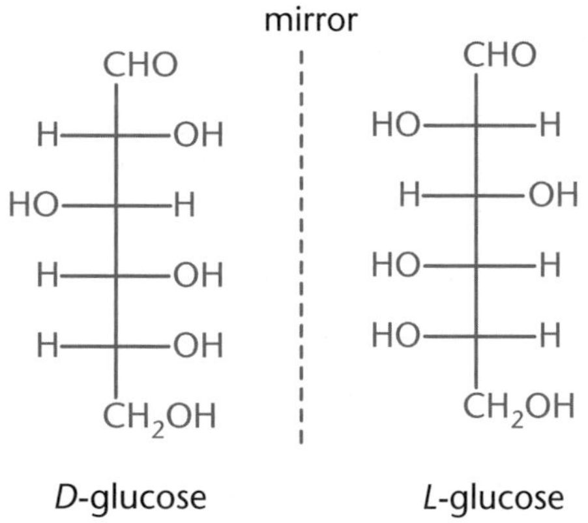
mirror
CHO
H
OH
HO
H
H
OH
H
OH
CH_2OH
CHO
HO
H
H
OH
HO
H
HO
H
CH_2OH
D-glucose
L-glucose

Figure 14.3

DAT Synopsis

Epimers differ in configuration at only one carbon.

Monosaccharide stereoisomers are divided into two optical families, *D* and *L*; the stereoisomers within one family are known as **diastereomers**. Aldose diastereomers that differ only about the configuration of one carbon are known as **epimers**. For instance, *D*-ribose and *D*-arabinose are pentose epimers. They differ in configuration only at C–2 (see Figure 14.4). Some important monosaccharides are shown in Figure 14.5.

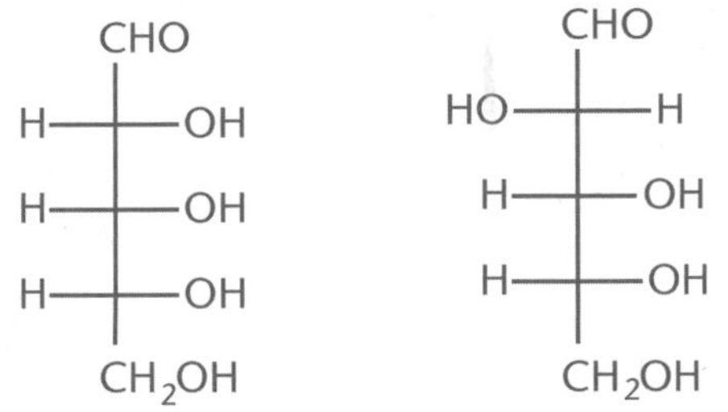

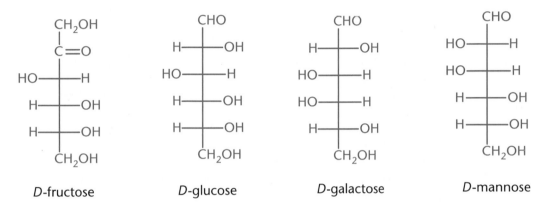

D-ribose *D*-arabinose

Figure 14.4

DAT Synopsis

Fructose is a ketose while glucose, galactose, and mannose are all aldoses.

D-fructose *D*-glucose *D*-galactose *D*-mannose

Figure 14.5

B. RING PROPERTIES

Because monosaccharides contain both a hydroxyl group and a carbonyl group, they can undergo intramolecular reactions to form cyclic hemiacetals (or hemiketals, in the case of ketoses). These cyclic molecules are stable in solution and may exist as six-membered **pyranose** rings (as in glucose) or five-membered **furanose** rings. Like cyclohexane, the pyranose rings adopt a chairlike configuration, and the substituents assume axial or equatorial positions so as to minimize steric hindrance. When converting the monosaccharide from its straight-chain Fischer projection to the Haworth projection (shown in Figure 14.6), it is important to remember that any group on the right of the Fischer projection will be pointing down, while any group on the left side of the Fischer projection will be pointing up. The following reaction scheme depicts the formation of a cyclic hemiacetal from *D*-glucose.

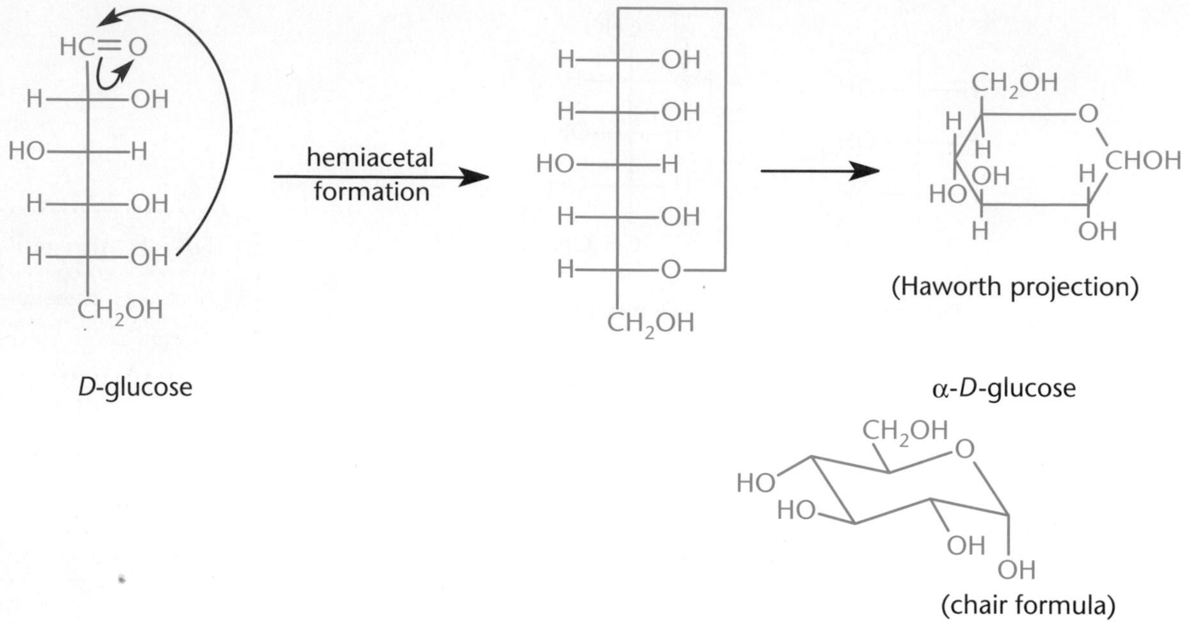

(Haworth projection)

α-D-glucose

(chair formula)

Figure 14.6

When a straight-chain monosaccharide is converted to its cyclic form, the carbonyl carbon (C–1 for glucose) becomes chiral. Cyclic stereoisomers differing about the new chiral carbon are known as **anomers**. In glucose, the alpha anomer has the –OH group of C–1 *trans* to the CH_2OH substituent (down), while the beta anomer has the –OH group of C–1 *cis* to the CH_2OH substituent (up).

When exposed to water, hemiacetal rings spontaneously open and then reform. Because of bond rotation between C–1 and C–2, either the alpha or beta anomer may be formed. The reaction is more rapid when catalyzed by an acid or a base. The spontaneous change of configuration about C–1 is known as **mutarotation**, and it results in a mixture containing both anomers in their equilibrium concentrations (for glucose, 36 percent alpha:64 percent beta). The alpha configuration is less favored because the hydroxyl group of C–1 is axial, making the molecule more sterically strained.

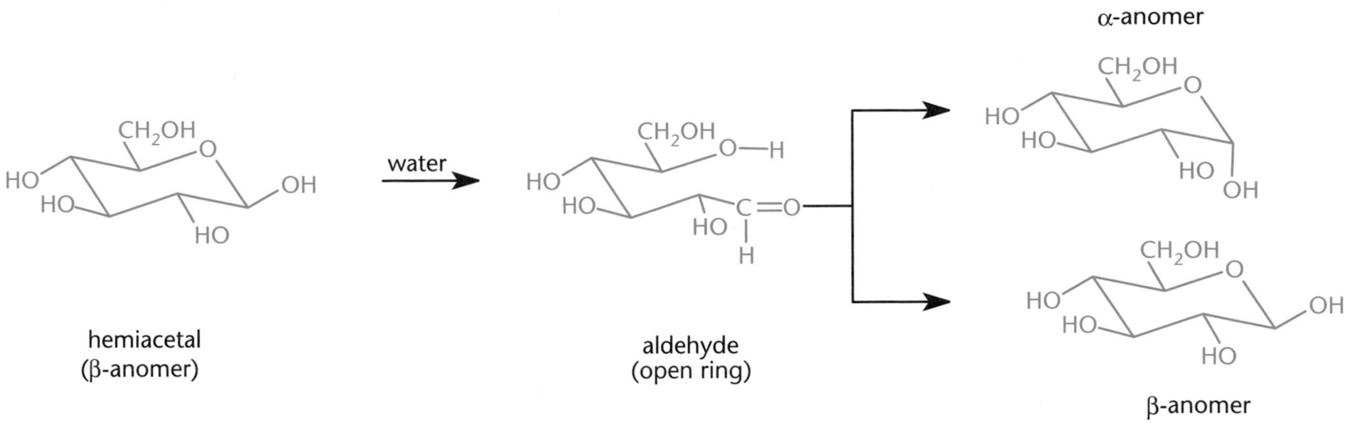

Figure 14.7

C. MONOSACCHARIDE REACTIONS

1. Ester Formation

Monosaccharides contain hydroxyl groups and can undergo many of the same reactions as simple alcohols. Therefore, they may be converted to either esters or ethers. In the presence of acid anhydride and base, all of the hydroxyl groups will be esterified. The reaction shown in Figure 14.8 is an example of glucose esterification.

> **DAT Synopsis**
>
> Reaction types are determined by the functional groups that are present. Think of alcohols and carbonyls.

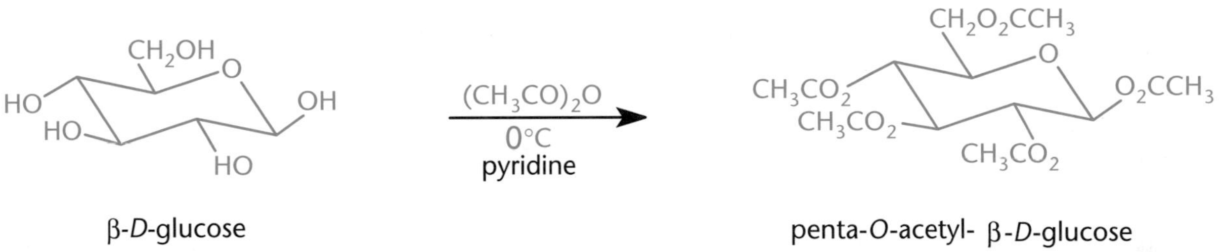

Figure 14.8

2. Oxidation of Monosaccharides

As they switch between anomeric configurations, the hemiacetal rings spend a short time in the open-chain aldehyde form. Like all aldehydes, these can be oxidized to carboxylic acids called **aldonic acids**. Thus, the aldoses are reducing agents. Any monosaccharide with a hemiacetal ring (–OH on C–1) is considered a **reducing sugar** and can be oxidized. Both Tollens' reagent and Benedict's reagent can be used to detect the presence of reducing sugars. A positive Tollens' test involves the reduction of Ag^+ to form metallic silver. When Benedict's reagent is used, a red precipitate of Cu_2O indicates the presence of a reducing sugar. Ketose sugars are also reducing sugars and give positive Tollen's and Benedict's tests, because they can isomerize to aldoses via keto-enol shifts.

> **DAT Synopsis**
>
> Key reactions of monosaccharides include
> - ester formation;
> - oxidation; and
> - glycosidic reactions.

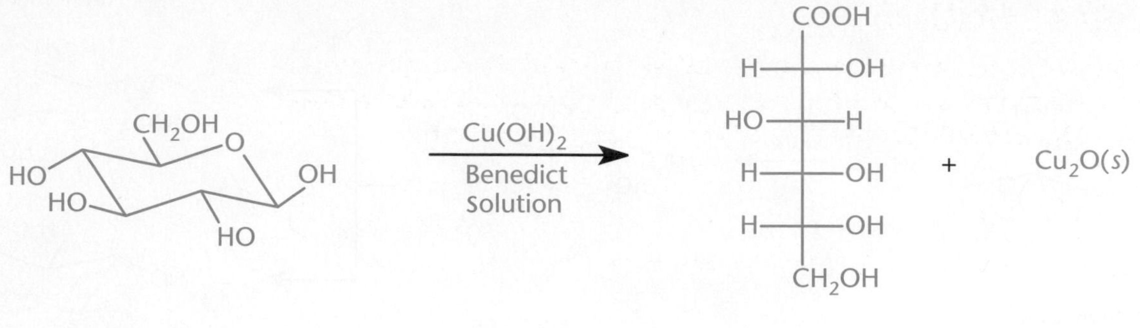

β-*D*-glucose

D-gluconic acid
(an aldonic acid)

(red solid)

Figure 14.9

3. **Glycosidic Reactions**

Hemiacetal monosaccharides will react with alcohols under acidic conditions. The anomeric hydroxyl group is transformed into an alkoxy group, yielding a mixture of the alpha and beta acetals. The resulting bond is called a **glycosidic linkage**, and the acetal is known as a **glycoside**. An example is the reaction of glucose with ethanol (see Figure 14.1). Glycosides do not mutarotate and are stable in water.

ethyl-α-*D*-glucoside
(an acetal)

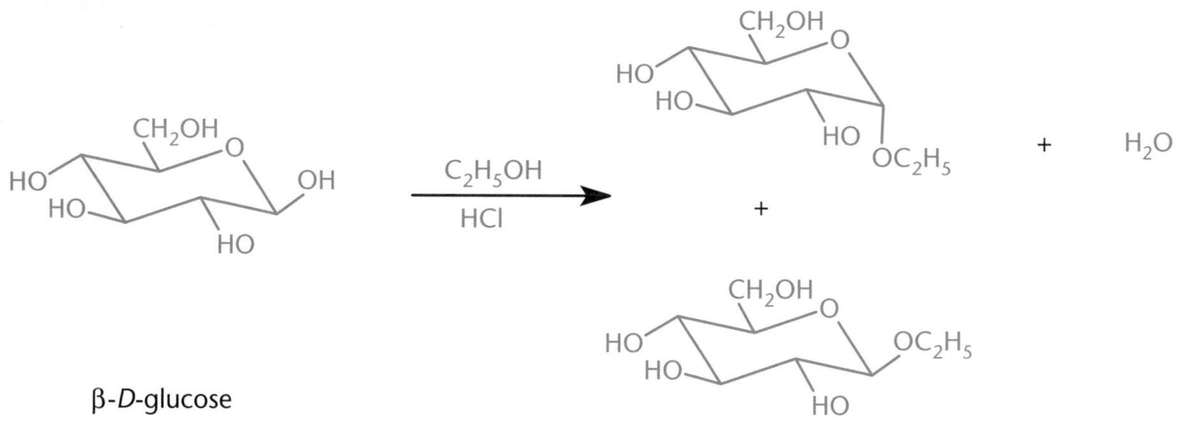

β-*D*-glucose

ethyl-β-*D*-glucoside
(an acetal)

Figure 14.10

> **DAT Synopsis**
>
> Glycosidic reactions:
>
> hemiacetal + alcohol acetal.

DISACCHARIDES

As discussed above, a monosaccharide may react with alcohols to give acetals. When that alcohol is another monosaccharide, the product is called a **disaccharide**. The formation of a disaccharide is shown in Figure 14.11.

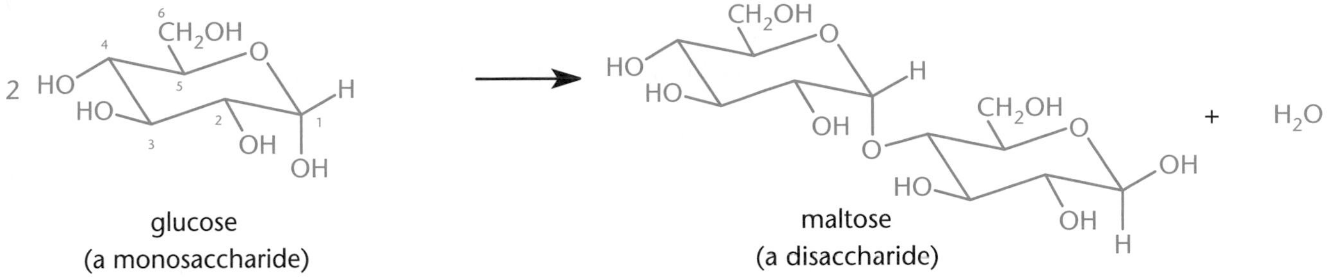

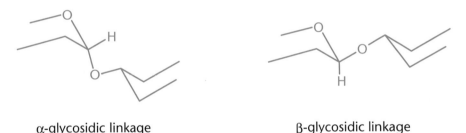

Figure 14.11

The most common glycosidic linkage occurs between C–1 of the first sugar and C–4 of the second, and it is designated as a 1,4' link; 1,6' and 1,2' bonds are also observed. The glycosidic bonds may be either alpha or beta, depending on the orientation of the hydroxyl group on the anomeric carbon.

> **DAT Synopsis**
>
> In the body, enzymes are needed to ensure that the correct glycosidic linkages form. Without enzymes, the reactions are non-specific and tend to keep going, never stopping at the disaccharide level.

α-glycosidic linkage   β-glycosidic linkage

Figure 14.12

These glycosidic linkages can often be cleaved in the presence of aqueous acid. For example, the glycosidic linkage of maltose, a disaccharide, can be cleaved to yield two molecules of glucose.

POLYSACCHARIDES

Polysaccharides are formed via linkage of monosaccharide units with glycosidic bonds. The three most important biological polysaccharides are **cellulose**, **starch**, and **glycogen**. Cellulose is comprised of *D*-glucose linked by 1,4'-beta-glycosidic bonds. Cellulose is the structural component of plants. Starch stores energy in plants, and glycogen stores energy in animals; both are formed by linking glucose units in 1,4'-alpha-glycosidic bonds, with occasional 1,6'-alpha-glycosidic bonds creating branches. While all three are composed of glucose subunits, the orientation about the anomeric carbon gives them biological differences. Cellulose cannot be digested by humans, while starch and glycogen can and are important energy sources for living organisms.

> **DAT Synopsis**
>
> Key biological polysaccharides:
> • Cellulose (1,4' beta)
> • Starch and glycogen (mostly 1,4' alpha; some 1,6' alpha)

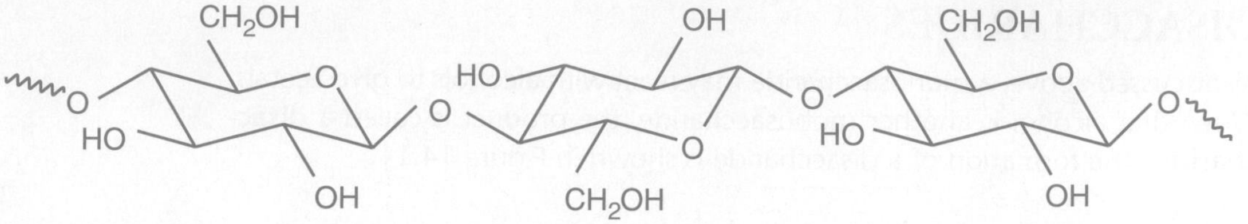

cellulose, a 1,4′,-β-*D*-glucose polymer

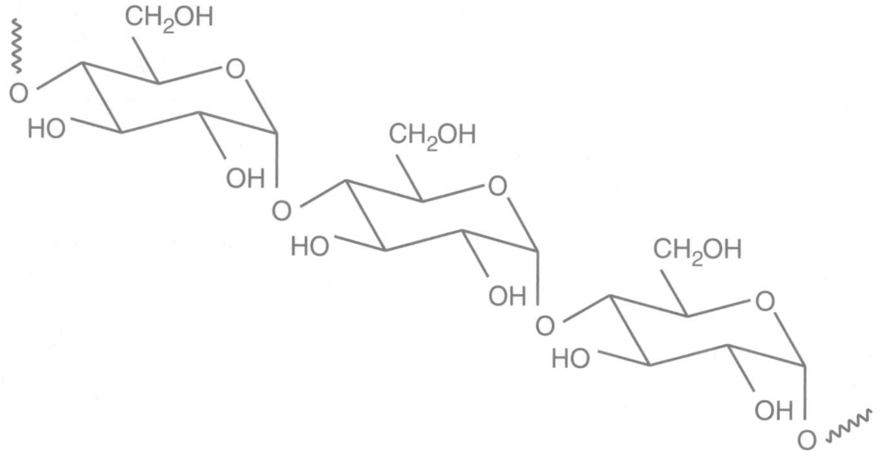

starch, a 1,4′,-α-*D*-glucose polymer

Figure 14.13

## 15

Amino Acids, Peptides, and Proteins

Proteins are large polymers composed of many amino acid subunits. Proteins have diverse biological roles; for example, they provide structure (keratin, collagen), regulate body metabolism via hormonal control (insulin), and serve as catalysts (enzymes).

AMINO ACIDS

Amino acids contain an amine group and a carboxyl group attached to a single carbon atom (the alpha carbon atom). The other two substituents of the alpha carbon are usually a hydrogen atom and a variable side chain referred to as the **R-group**.

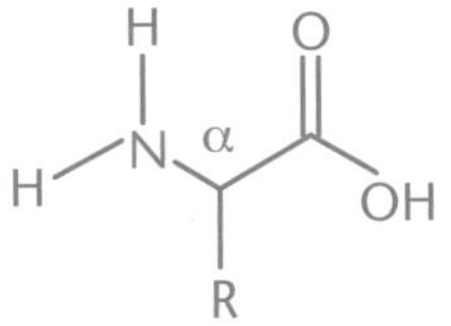

Figure 15.1

The alpha carbon is a chiral center (except in glycine, the simplest amino acid, where R=H), and thus all amino acids (except for glycine) are optically active. Naturally occurring amino acids (of which there are 20) are *L*-enantiomers (see chapters 2 and 14).

> **DAT Synopsis**
>
> Except for glycine, all amino acids are chiral.

By convention, the Fischer projection for an amino acid is drawn with the amino group on the left (see Figure 15.2).

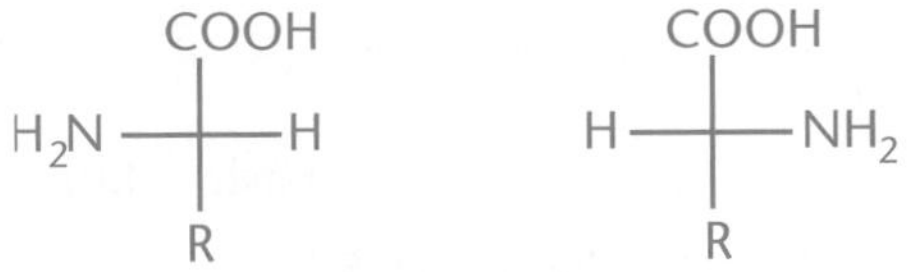

L-amino acid *D*-amino acid

Figure 15.2

A. ACID-BASE CHARACTERISTICS

Amino acids have an acidic carboxyl group and a basic amino group on the same molecule (see General Chemistry chapter 10 for a discussion of acids and bases). As a result, when they are in solution, amino acids sometimes take the form of dipolar ions, or **zwitterions** (from German *zwitter*, hybrid). The two halves of the molecules neutralize each other so that at neutral pH, they exist in the form of internal salts.

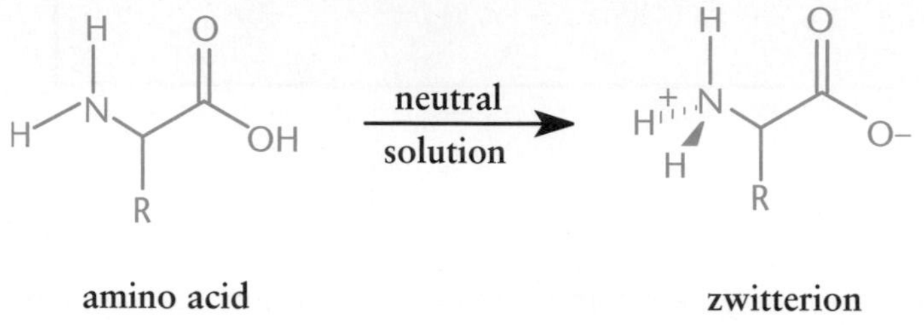

amino acid   zwitterion

Figure 15.3

Amino acids are **amphoteric** (i.e., they may act as either acids or bases, depending on their environment). Amino acids in acidic solution (see Figure 15.4) are fully protonated. Since they have two protons that can dissociate—one from the carboxyl group and one from the amino group—amino acids have at least two dissociation constants, K_{a1} and K_{a2}.

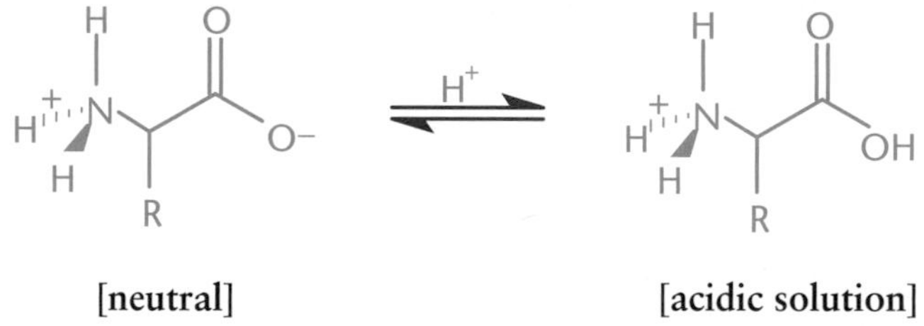

[neutral]   [acidic solution]

Figure 15.4

Amino acids in basic solution (see Figure 15.5) are deprotonated. They have two proton-accepting groups and, therefore, at least two dissociation constants, K_{b1} and K_{b2}.

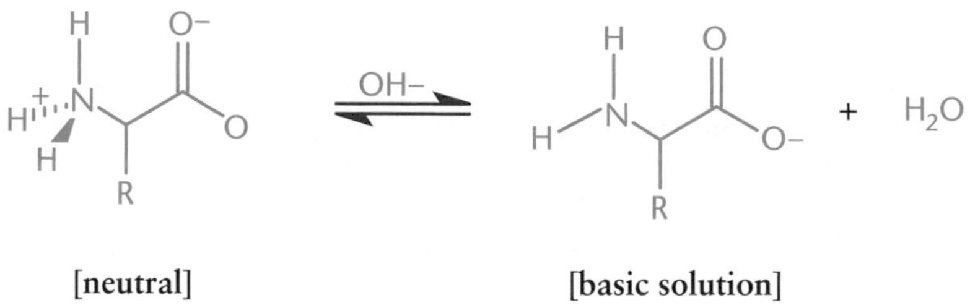

[neutral]   [basic solution]

Figure 15.5

At low pH, the amino acid carries an excess positive charge, and at high pH, the amino acid carries an excess negative charge. The intermediate pH, at which the amino acid is electrically neutral and exists as a zwitter-ion, is the **isoelectric point (pI)**, or **isoelectric pH**, of the amino acid.

The isoelectric pH lies between pK_{a1} and pK_{a2}.

B. TITRATION OF AMINO ACIDS

Because of their acidic and basic properties, amino acids can be titrated. The titration of each proton occurs as a distinct step resembling that of a simple monoprotic acid. The titration curve of glycine is shown in Figure 15.6.

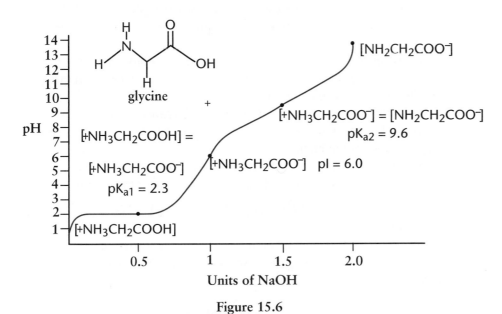

Figure 15.6

A 1M glycine solution is acidic; the glycine exists predominantly as $^+NH_3CH_2COOH$. The amino acid is fully protonated and carries a positive charge. As the solution is titrated with NaOH, carboxyl groups lose a proton. During this stage, the amino acid acts as a buffer, and the pH changes very slowly. When 0.5 mol of base has been added to the amino acid solution, the concentrations of $^+NH_3CH_2COOH$ and $^+NH_3CH_2COO^-$ (its zwitterion) are equimolar. At this point, the pH is equal to the pK_{a1}, and the solution is buffered against pH changes.

As more base is added, all of the carboxyl groups are deprotonated. The amino acid loses buffering capacity, and thus the pH rises more rapidly. When 1 mol of base has been added, glycine exists predominantly as $^+NH_3CH_2COO^-$. The amino acid is now electrically neutral; the pH is equal to glycine's pI.

Glycine passes through a second buffering stage during which pH change is slow because continued titration deprotonates amino groups. When 1.5 mol of base have been added, the concentrations of $^+NH_3CH_2COO^-$ and $NH_2CH_2COO^-$ are equimolar, and the pH is equal to pK_{a2}.

As another 0.5 mol of base is added, all of the amino groups are deprotonated to $NH_2CH_2COO^-$; glycine is now completely deprotonated.

Certain things should be noted about the titration of amino acids:

1. When adding base, the carboxyl group loses its proton first; after all of the carboxyl groups are fully deprotonated, the amino group loses its acidic proton.
2. Two moles of base must be added in order to deprotonate one mole of most amino acids. The first mole deprotonates the carboxyl group, while the second mole deprotonates the amino group.
3. The buffering capacity of the amino acid is greatest at or near the two dissociation constants, K_{a1} and K_{a2}. At the isoelectric point, its buffering capacity is minimal.
4. It is possible to perform the titration in reverse, from alkaline pH to acidic pH, with the addition of acid; the sequence of events is reversed.

C. HENDERSON-HASSELBALCH EQUATION

The ratio of an amino acid's ions are dependent on pH. The **Henderson-Hasselbalch equation** defines the relationship between pH and the ratio of conjugate acid to conjugate base, and it provides a mathematical expression for the dissociation constants of amino acids.

$$pH = pK_a + log \frac{[conjugate\ base]}{[conjugate\ acid]}$$

When the pK_{a1} of glycine is known, the ratio of conjugate acid to conjugate base for a particular pH can be determined. For example, at pH 3.3, glycine, which has a pK_a of 2.3, will have these ratios:

$$3.3 = 2.3 + log \frac{[H_3N^+CH_2COO^-]}{[H_3N^+CH_2COOH]}$$

By subtraction: $log \frac{[H_3N^+CH_2COO^-]}{[H_3N^+CH_2COOH]} = 1$

The antilog of 1 = 10. Thus: $\frac{[H_3N^+CH_2COO^-]}{[H_3N^+CH_2COOH]} = \frac{10}{1}$

So, in this example, there are ten times as many zwitterions as there are of the fully protonated form.

The Henderson-Hasselbalch equation can be used experimentally to prepare buffer solutions of amino acids. The best buffering regions of amino acids occur within one pH unit of the pK_a or pK_b. For example, the carboxyl group of glycine, which has a pK_a of 2.3, shows high buffering capacity between pH 1.3 and 3.3.

D. AMINO ACID SIDE CHAINS

Amino acid side chains (R-groups) give chemical diversity to the backbone of the amino acid molecule. They also give proteins some distinguishing features. The 20 amino acids are classified according to whether their side chains are **nonpolar, polar** (but uncharged), **acidic,** or **basic.**

1. **Nonpolar Amino Acids**

   Nonpolar amino acids (see Figure 15.7) have R-groups that are saturated hydrocarbons. The R-groups are hydrophobic and decrease the solubility of the amino acid in water. Amino acids with nonpolar side chains are usually found buried within protein molecules, away from the aqueous cellular environment.

alanine

valine

leucine

isoleucine

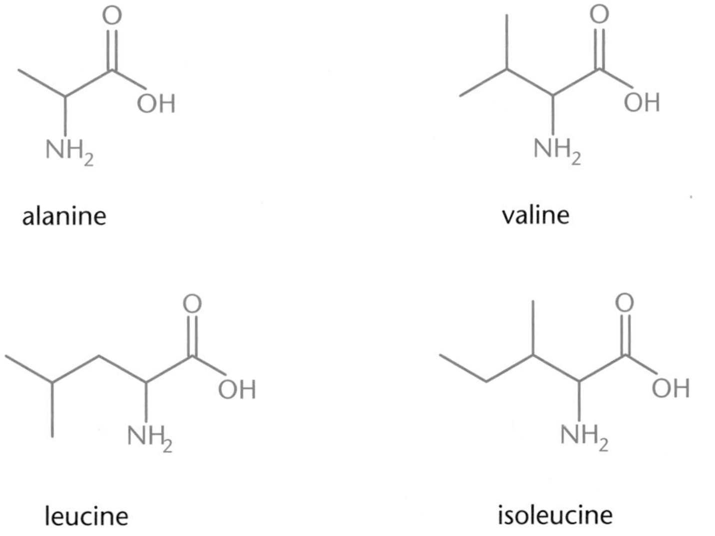

Figure 15.7a

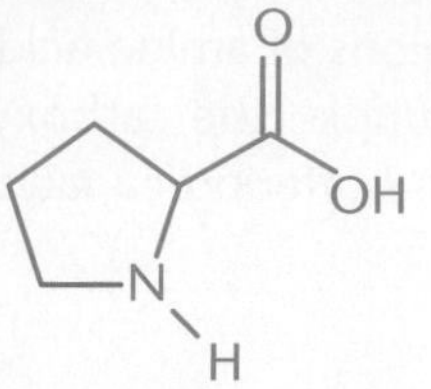

proline

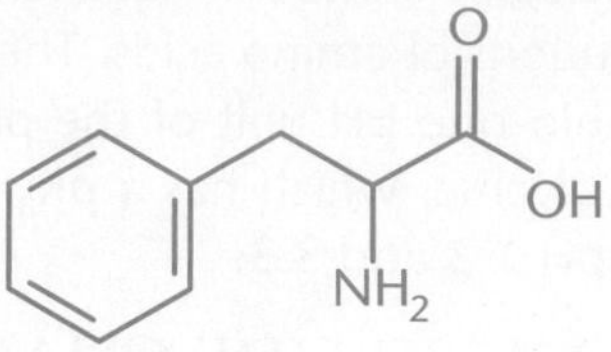

phenylalanine

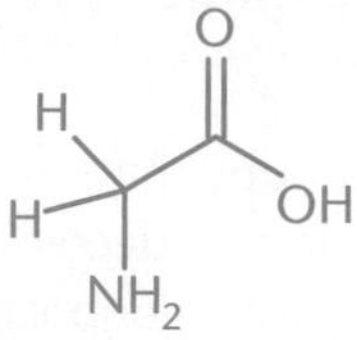

glycine

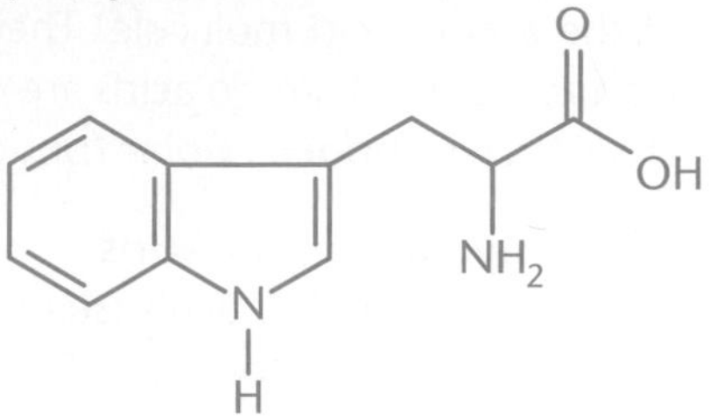

tryptophan

Figure 15.7b

2. **Polar Amino Acids**

Polar amino acids (see Figure 15.8) have polar, uncharged R-groups that are hydrophilic, increasing the solubility of the amino acid in water. They are usually found on protein surfaces.

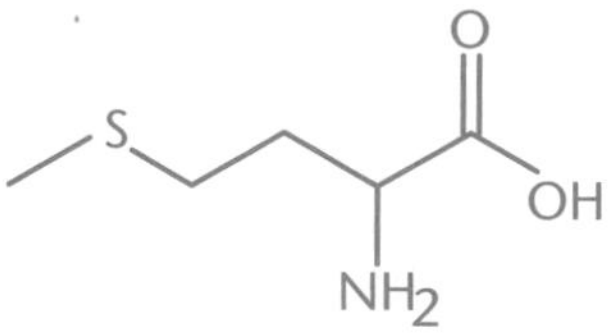

methionine

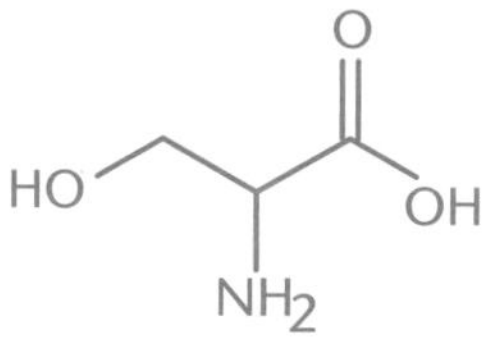

serine

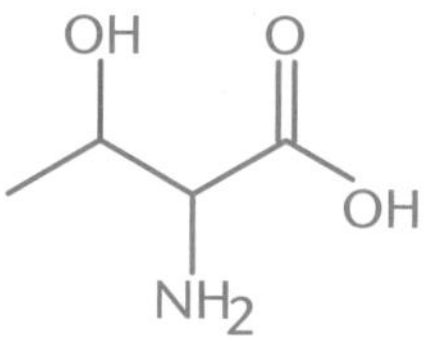

threonine

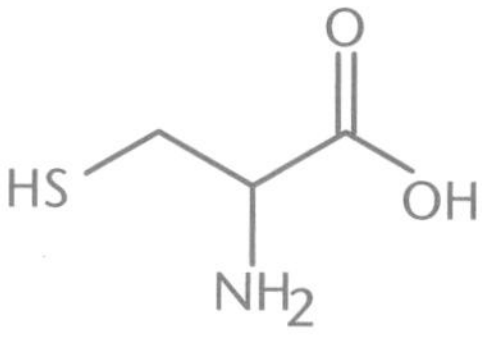

cysteine

Figure 15.8a

> ### DAT Synopsis
>
> The other types of amino acids (polar, acidic, and basic) are found in regions of proteins that are exposed to the aqueous, polar environment.

tyrosine

asparagine

glutamine

Figure 15.8b

3. **Acidic Amino Acids**
    Amino acids whose R-group contains a carboxyl group are called acidic amino acids (see Figure 15.9). They have a net negative charge at physiological pH (pH 7.4) and exist in salt form in the body. They often play important roles in the substrate-binding sites of enzymes.

> **DAT Synopsis**
>
> Acidic amino acids have a negative charge at physiological pH (pH 7.4).

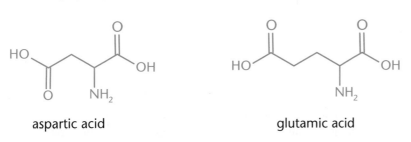

aspartic acid

glutamic acid

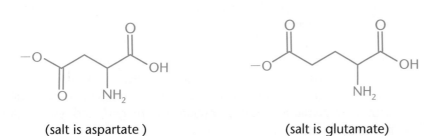

(salt is aspartate)

(salt is glutamate)

Figure 15.9

> **DAT Synopsis**
>
> Acidic amino acids have three distinct pK_a's.

Aspartic acid and glutamic acid each have three groups that must be neutralized during titration (two –COOH and one $-NH_3^+$). Therefore, their titration curve is different from the standard curve for amino acids (exemplified by glycine). The molecule has three distinct dissociation constants—pK_{a1}, pK_{a2}, and pK_{a3}—although the neutralization curves of the two carboxyl groups overlap to a certain extent. Because of the additional carboxyl group, the isoelectric point is shifted towards an acidic pH. Three moles of base are needed to deprotonate one mole of an acidic amino acid.

4. **Basic Amino Acids**

   Amino acids whose R-group contains an amino group are called basic amino acids and carry a net positive charge at physiological pH (see Figure 15.10).

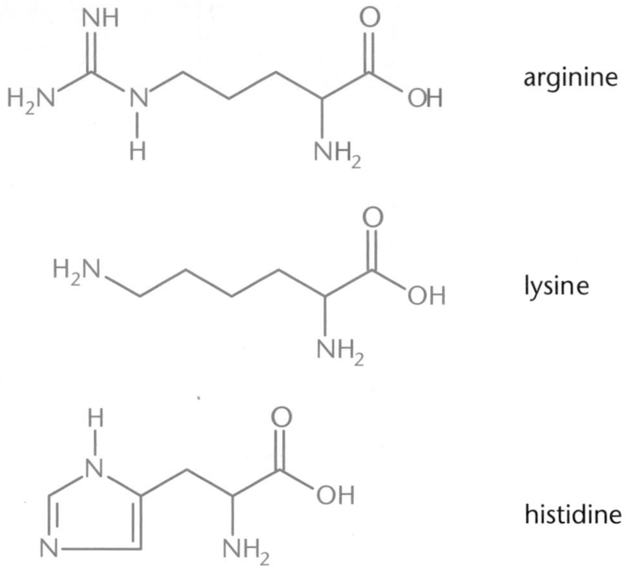

arginine

lysine

histidine

Figure 15.10

The titration curve of amino acids with basic R-groups is modified by the additional amino group that must be neutralized. Although basic amino acids have three dissociation constants, the neutralization curves for the two amino groups overlap. The isoelectric point is shifted toward an alkaline pH. Three moles of acid are needed to neutralize one mole of a basic amino acid.

Understanding titration curves and isoelectric points helps predict the charge of particular amino acids at a given pH. For example, in a mixture of glycine, glutamic acid, and lysine at pH 6.0, glycine will be neutral, glutamic acid will be negatively charged, and lysine will be positively charged.

PEPTIDES

Peptides are composed of amino acid subunits, sometimes called **residues**, linked by **peptide bonds**. Peptides are small proteins (the distinction between a peptide and protein is vague). Two amino acids joined together form a **dipeptide**, three form a **tripeptide**, and many amino acids linked together form a **polypeptide**.

> **DAT Synopsis**
>
> A peptide bond is an amide bond.

A. REACTIONS

Amino acids are joined by **peptide bonds** (amide bonds) between the carboxyl group of one amino acid and the amino group of another. This bond is formed via a condensation reaction (a reaction in which water is lost). The reverse reaction, hydrolysis (cleavage with the addition of water) of the peptide bond, is catalyzed by an acid or base.

> **Bridge**
>
> Refer to chapter 11 for the reactions concerning nitrogen-containing compounds.

Certain enzymes digest the chain at specific peptide linkages. For example, **trypsin** cleaves at the carboxyl end of arginine and lysine; chymotrypsin cleaves at the carboxyl end of phenylalanine, tyrosine, and tryptophan.

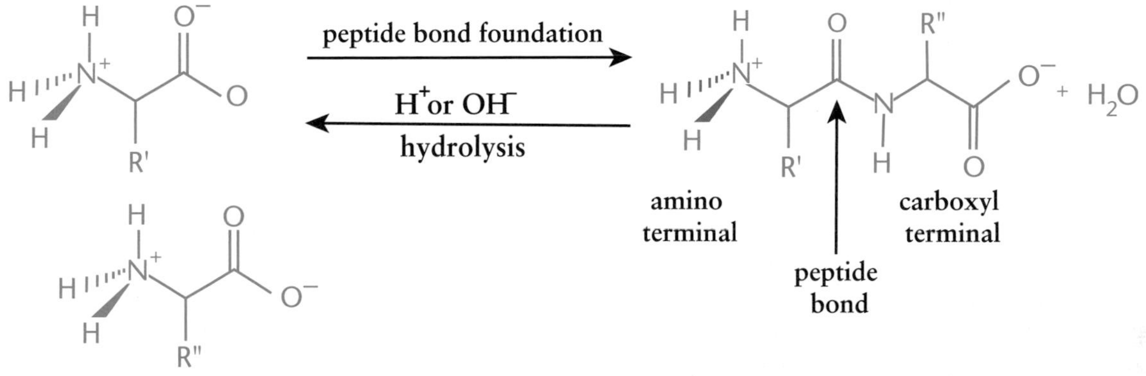

Figure 15.11

B. PROPERTIES

The terminal amino acid with a free alpha-amino group is known as the **amino-terminal** or **N-terminal** residue, while the terminal residue with a free carboxyl group is called the **carboxy-terminal** or **C-terminal** residue. By convention, peptides are drawn with the N-terminal end on the left and the C-terminal end on the right.

> **DAT Synopsis**
>
> Rotation is limited around the peptide bond because resonance gives the C–N bond partial double-bond character.

Amides have two resonance structures, and the true structure is a hybrid with partial double-bond character. As a result, rotation about the C–N bond is restricted. The bonds on either side of the peptide unit, however, have a great deal of rotational freedom.

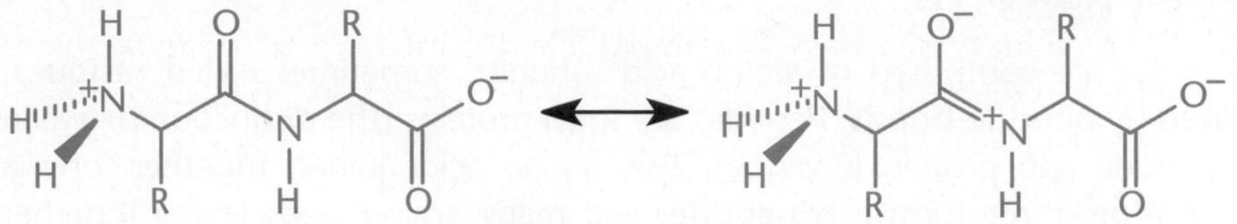

Figure 15.12

PROTEINS

Proteins are polypeptides that can range from only a few up to more than a thousand amino acids in length. Proteins serve many diverse functions in biological systems, acting as enzymes, hormones, membrane pores, receptors, and elements of cell structure. Four structural levels of protein structure—**primary**, **secondary**, **tertiary**, and **quaternary**—are described below.

A. PRIMARY STRUCTURE

The primary structure of the protein refers to the sequence of amino acids, listed from the N-terminus to the C-terminus, linked by covalent bonds between neighboring residues in the chain.

The higher-level structures of a protein are dependent on the primary sequence; in other words, a protein will assume whatever secondary, tertiary, and quaternary structures are most energetically favorable given its primary structure and environment. The primary structure of a protein can be determined using a laboratory procedure called **sequencing**.

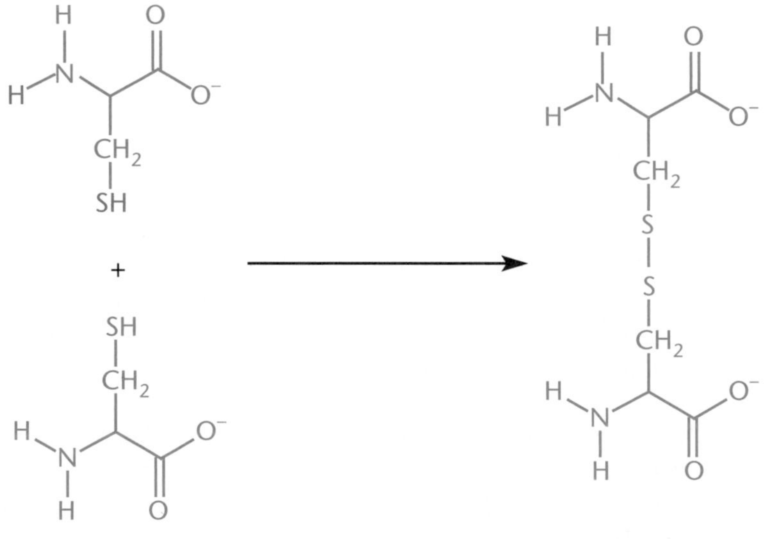

cysteine

cystine

Figure 15.13

B. SECONDARY STRUCTURE

The secondary structure of a protein refers to the local structure of neighboring amino acids, governed mostly by hydrogen bond interactions within and between peptide chains. The two most common types of secondary structures are the α-**helix** and the β-**pleated sheet**.

> **DAT Synopsis**
>
> Secondary structure describes hydrogen bonding. Common secondary structures include the α-helix and the β-pleated sheets.

1. α-Helix

The α-helix is a rod like structure in which the peptide chain coils clockwise about a central axis. The helix is stabilized by intramolecular hydrogen bonds between carbonyl oxygen atoms and amine hydrogen atoms four residues away. The side chains point away from the structure's core and interact with the cellular environment. A typical protein with this structure is **keratin**, which is found in feathers and hair.

2. β-Pleated Sheet

In β-pleated sheets, the peptide chains lie alongside each other in rows. The chains are held together by intramolecular hydrogen bonds between carbonyl oxygen atoms on one peptide chain and amine hydrogen atoms on another. To accommodate the maximum number of hydrogen bonds, the β-pleated sheet assumes a rippled, or pleated, shape (see Figure 15.14). The R-groups of the amino residues point above and below the plane of the β-pleated sheet. Silk fibers are composed of β-pleated sheets.

> **DAT Synopsis**
>
> - Primary structure consists of the amino acid sequence.
> - Secondary structure refers to the local structure of a protein, largely determined by hydrogen bond interactions within and between neighboring amino acids.
> - Tertiary structure is the three-dimensional shape of the protein.
> - Quaternary structure is the arrangement of polypeptide subunits.
> - Conjugated proteins have prosthetic groups.

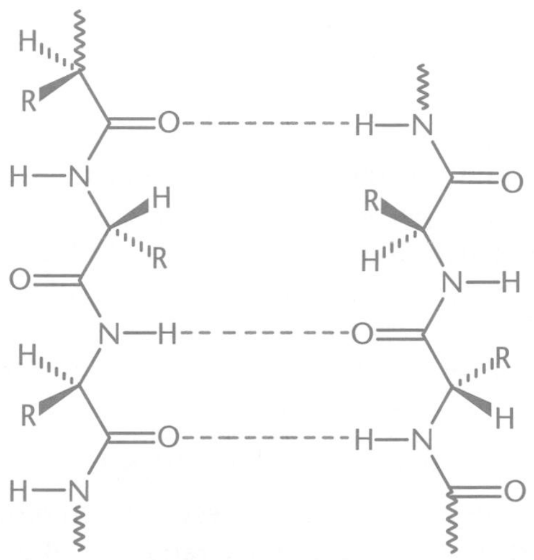

β-pleated sheet

Figure 15.14

C. TERTIARY STRUCTURE

Tertiary structure refers to the three-dimensional shape of the protein, as determined by hydrophilic and hydrophobic interactions between the R-groups of amino acids that are far apart on the chain and by the distribution of disulfide bonds. In a disulfide bond, two **cysteine** molecules become oxidized to form **cystine**. Disulfide bonds create loops in the protein chain.

Other amino acids have significant effects on tertiary structures as well. For instance, proline, because of its shape, cannot fit into an α-helix, thereby causing a kink in the chain.

Amino acids with hydrophilic (polar and charged) R-groups tend to arrange themselves toward the outside of the protein, where they interact with the aqueous cellular environment. Amino acids with hydrophobic R-groups tend to be found close together, protected from the aqueous environment by polar amino and carboxyl groups.

Proteins are divided into two major classifications on the basis of tertiary structure. **Fibrous proteins**, such as **collagen**, are found as sheets or long strands, while **globular proteins**, such as **myoglobin**, are spherical in shape.

D. QUATERNARY STRUCTURE

Some proteins contain more than one polypeptide subunit. The quaternary structure refers to the way in which these subunits arrange themselves to yield a functional protein molecule. **Hemoglobin**, which is composed of four polypeptide chains, possesses quaternary structure.

E. CONJUGATED PROTEINS

Certain proteins, known as **conjugated proteins**, derive part of their function from covalently attached molecules called **prosthetic groups**. Prosthetic groups may be organic molecules or metal ions. Many vitamins are prosthetic groups. Proteins with lipid, carbohydrate, and nucleic acid prosthetic groups are referred to as **lipoproteins**, **glycoproteins**, and **nucleoproteins**, respectively. Prosthetic groups play major roles in determining the function of the proteins with which they are associated. For example, the **heme group** carries oxygen in both myoglobin and hemoglobin. The heme is composed of an organic porphyrin ring with an iron atom bound in the center. Hemoglobin is inactive without the heme group.

F. DENATURATION OF PROTEINS

Denaturation, or **melting**, is a process in which proteins lose their three-dimensional structure and revert to a **random-coil** state. Denaturation can be caused by detergent or by changes in pH, temperature, or solute concentration. The weak intermolecular forces keeping the protein stable and functional are disrupted. When a protein denatures, the damage is usually permanent. However, certain gentle denaturing agents do not permanently disrupt the protein; removing the reagent might allow the protein to **renature** (regain its structure and function).

G. LIPIDS (FATS AND OILS)

Like carbohydrates, lipids are also composed of C,H, and O, but their H:O ratio is much greater than 2:1 as they have much more H than O. A lipid consists of **three fatty acid** molecules bonded to a single **glycerol** backbone. Fatty acids have long carbon chains that give them their hydrophobic (fatty) character and carboxylic acid groups that make them acidic. Three dehydration reactions are needed to form one fat molecule. Lipids do not form polymers.

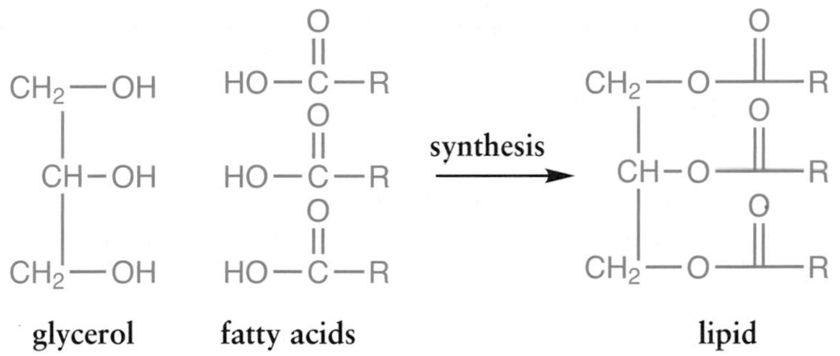

glycerol   fatty acids   →   lipid

1. **Lipid Derivatives**

   Lipids are the chief means of food storage in animals. They release more energy per gram weight than any other class of biological compounds. They also provide insulation and protection against injury since they are a major component of fatty **(adipose)** tissue. Lipid derivatives are the following:

   a. **Phospholipids**

      Phospholipids contain glycerol, two fatty acids, a phosphate group, and nitrogen-containing alcohol. Examples are lecithin (a major constituent of cell membranes) and cephalin (found in the brain, nerves, and neural tissue).

   b. **Waxes**

      Waxes are esters of fatty acids and monohydroxylic alcohols. They are found as protective coatings on skin, fur, leaves of higher plants, and the exoskeleton of many insects. An example is lanolin.

   c. **Steroids**

      All steroids have three fused cyclohexane rings and one fused cyclopentane ring. They include **cholesterol**, the **sex hormones** testosterone and estrogen, and **corticosteroids**.

d. **Carotenoids**

These are fatty, acidlike carbon chains containing conjugated double bonds and carrying six-membered carbon rings at each end. These compounds are the **pigments** that produce red, yellow, orange, and brown colors in plants and animals. Two subgroups are the **carotenes** and the **xanthophylls**.

e. **Porphyrins**

Porphyrins, also called tetrapyrroles, contain four joined **pyrrole** rings. They are often complexed with a metal. For example, the porphyrin **heme** complexes with Fe in hemoglobin. Chlorphyll is complexed with Mg.

C. PROTEINS

Proteins are composed primarily of the elements C, H, O, and N but may also contain phosphorus (P) and sulfur (S). They are polymers of **amino acids**.

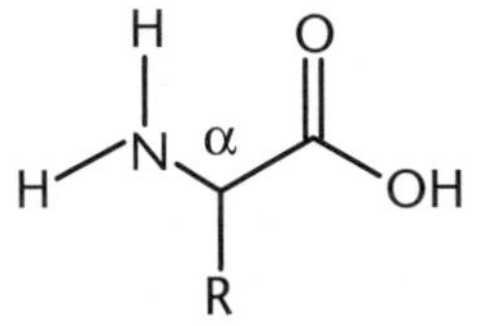

Amino acids are joined by **peptide bonds** through dehydration reactions. Chains of such bonds produce a polymer called a **polypeptide** or simply peptide. The sequence of amino acids in a protein is referred to as the 1° (primary) structure. Proteins can also coil or fold to form helices and β-pleated sheets. These are considered part of the protein's 2° (secondary) structure.

PERCEPTUAL ABILITY

INTRODUCTION TO THE PAT

The Perceptual Ability Test (PAT) is a section in the DAT that tests your spatial visualization skills, especially your ability to interpret two-dimensional representations of three-dimensional objects. These skills will be useful to you as a dentist as you construct a mental image of teeth from X-rays, deal with casts and fillings, etc.

The PAT contains a total of 90 questions, which you need to complete within 60 minutes. The 90 questions are divided into six categories, each consisting of 15 questions: Keyholes (Aperture Passing), Top-Front-End (Orthographic Procedures), Angle Ranking, Hole Punching, Cube Counting, and Pattern Folding. Some question types are more challenging than others—it is important that you pace yourself accordingly. For example, you should definitely spend less time on the Angle Ranking problems than on the Pattern Folding questions.

A description of each of the six categories (or question types) follows.

KEYHOLES

In each of the questions making up this subsection, you are presented with a three-dimensional object, and you must determine through which of five openings this object can pass. The object can pass through the opening in any orientation, but it cannot be rotated while it is passing through. The external outline of the object is the EXACT shape of the opening. In the example below, the cube could fit through any of the apertures. But on the PAT, there is only one correct answer: the projection of the cube.

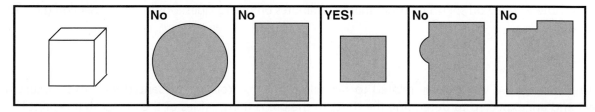

The object and the opening are drawn to the same scale.

The correct opening *must* be one of the three projections that can be drawn for the object: the top-bottom projection, the front-back projection, or the side projection. The most efficient way to arrive at the correct answer, therefore, is to determine the three projections of the object and pick the choice that matches one of these. (Since there is only one correct answer, only one of the projections will be found.) The following example illustrates this technique:

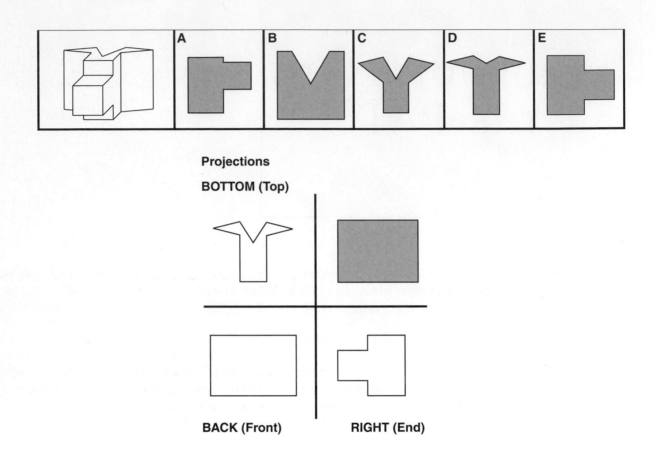

Projections

BOTTOM (Top)

BACK (Front)   **RIGHT (End)**

The correct choice is (E). Note how choice (D) is a "distractor" choice, designed to trap students who go for the "obvious" features of the object without paying attention to the finer aspects. This is a favorite DAT trap. Note also that in the projections we have drawn, we have omitted such details as solid and dashed lines within the projection, details that are very important in the next type of questions on the DAT, Top-Front-End (see below). For the purpose of this subsection, the overall shape of the projection suffices.

We recommend that you spend no more than ten minutes on the 15 questions in this subsection (i.e., 40 seconds per question).

TOP-FRONT-END

These questions are very closely related to Keyhole problems. You are presented with two projections of an object and are expected to determine the third. In the projections, edges of the object that cannot be seen are represented by dotted lines, while edges that can be seen are represented by solid lines. The following scenario illustrates this convention:

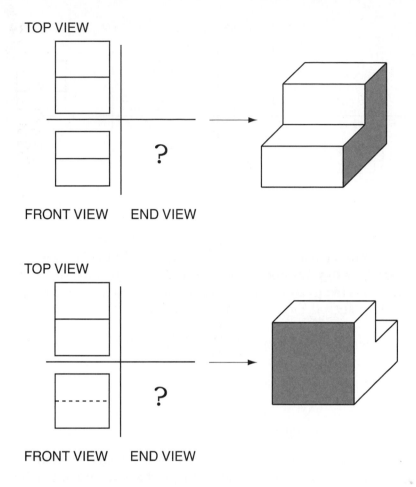

TOP VIEW

FRONT VIEW   END VIEW

TOP VIEW

FRONT VIEW   END VIEW

(On the DAT, you will not be given the three-dimensional object on the right—this is what you are expected to construct mentally.)

The top views of both objects are the same: They tell us that the object possesses some kind of "step," although we do not know which half is higher. This information is conveyed in the front views. In the first case, since we see a solid line, we know that the lower step is in front. In the second case, however, the higher step is in front, hiding the lower step from our view. Hence, a dotted line is used to indicate the presence of the step. The three-dimensional object that we construct is similar in either case, but the orientation is different. This is important because the end view is a lateral *from the right*. Hence, in the first case, the end view is an L-shape pointing from right to left, while in the second case the L-shape points from left to right. In short, unlike in Keyhole problems, orientation does matter here.

The correct interpretation of solid and dashed lines can be very helpful in the more challenging problems. Sometimes, it is very difficult to construct a three-dimensional image of the object from the two projections given. In these situations, it may be much easier to focus on some finer features and determine whether we expect solid or dotted lines in certain regions. The following example illustrates this point:

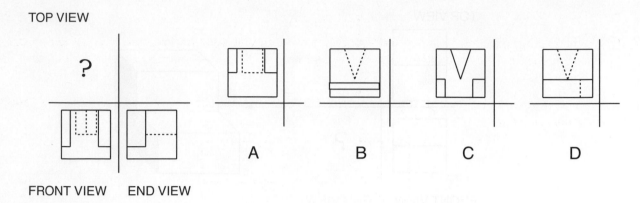

TOP VIEW

?

FRONT VIEW   END VIEW

A   B   C   D

In this question, we are asked to select the correct top view. The three-dimensional appearance of the object is not immediately obvious from the two given projections. However, in the front view, we see a substructure represented in dotted lines. Since this substructure is at the top, we expect to see it in solid lines in the top view. The substructure is also expected to be not in front (otherwise, the lines would be solid and not dotted in the front view). Only choice (C) fits.

It is recommended that you spend 15 minutes on the Top-Front-End section (1 minute per question).

ANGLE RANKING

In an Angle Ranking question, you are given four angles, labeled 1–4, which you need to rank in increasing order.

Some of the angles may be so close in size that it is almost impossible to assign the order unambiguously. However, it is not always necessary to do so to select the correct answer; use the answer choices to help you, at least in eliminating certain answer choices. This strategy is illustrated in the following example:

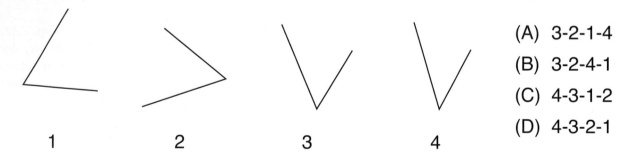

1   2   3   4

(A) 3-2-1-4

(B) 3-2-4-1

(C) 4-3-1-2

(D) 4-3-2-1

It is difficult to ascertain which angle is larger: 2 or 3. However, if we can see that 4 is the smallest angle and 1 is the largest, only one choice can be correct: choice (D).

It is important to move through this part of the PAT quickly. Try to spend no more than five minutes on the 15 Angle Ranking questions.

HOLE PUNCHING

In a Hole Punching question, a square piece of paper is folded one, two, or three times, and then one or more holes are punched at specific locations. You are asked to unfold the paper mentally and determine the locations of the holes.

The paper is always folded towards the front. The folds are also not arbitrary—in fact, there are only four possible first folds, as follows:

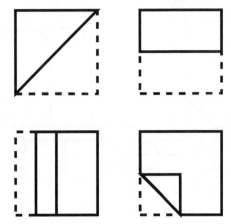

Each of these four first folds can be rotated 90, 180, or 270 degrees to give a seemingly larger variety of first folds.

After the first fold, the paper may be folded one or more times. In the following example, we see the paper folded diagonally in the first fold, then folded halfway down before a hole is punched.

We can mentally unfold the paper as follows:

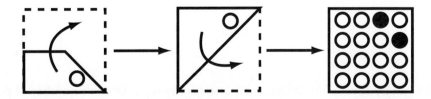

Note that in the answer, the holes are indicated by filled circles.

We recommend that you spend five minutes on the Hole Punching section.

CUBE COUNTING

In this part of the PAT, you will be presented with several stacks of cubes. Each stack is constructed by cementing together identical cubes. You are asked to imagine that the stack as a whole is painted (or "varnished") on all sides except for the bottom (on which the stack rests). You are then asked to determine how many cubes have a particular number of sides varnished. The following example makes the description more concrete:

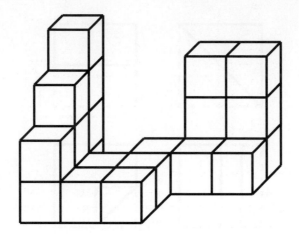

In the figure, how many cubes have two of their sides painted?

   A.   5 cubes

   B.   6 cubes

   C.   7 cubes

   D.   8 cubes

   E.   9 cubes

In the figure, how many cubes have three of their sides painted?

   A.   5 cubes

   B.   6 cubes

   C.   7 cubes

   D.   8 cubes

   E.   9 cubes

(Each structure is followed by several questions, each one specifying a different number of painted sides.)

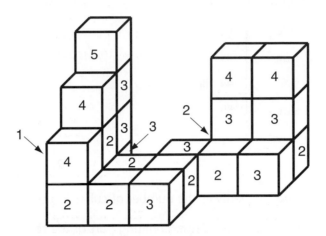

The complete assignation of the cubes is as follows.

As the diagram illustrates, it is important not to neglect cubes that are not clearly visible. The general rule as devised by the test makers is that the only hidden cubes are the ones necessary to support other cubes. In the diagram, we infer the presence of a hidden cube with one side painted on the left, because without such a cube, the four-sided and the two-sided cubes would not be supported.

Sometimes cubes can be totally hidden within the stack and have no sides painted, as shown below.

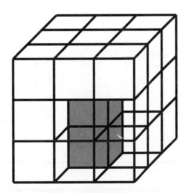

One strategy that you may find useful is to make a tally of all the cubes in the object. In other words, rather than going over each cube in the stack for each question, which duplicates your efforts, spend some time up front with the object. Make a table on your scratch paper with entries of "0 sides painted" to "5 sides painted." Then, methodically go over the stack and, for each cube, check off the appropriate column. After you have constructed the table, add up the entries to make sure you haven't omitted any cubes. Now, as you look at the questions, it is easy to obtain the answer from your table. The table for the example shown above would look something like this:

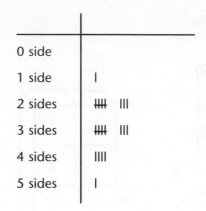

0 side	
1 side	I
2 sides	⽢⽢ III
3 sides	⽢⽢ III
4 sides	IIII
5 sides	I

The entries add up to 22, which we can verify as the number of cubes in the object.

Try to spend no more than ten minutes on the Cube Counting part of the test.

PATTERN FOLDING

In Pattern Folding questions, a flat pattern is presented, and you are asked to select the three-dimensional figure into which it folds. Some questions require only that you identify the structure, while others also present shading that you need to identify, as shown in the following examples:

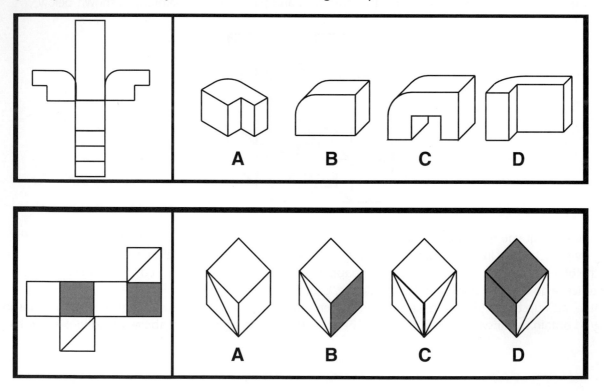

In questions such as the first one, a very effective strategy—in case the three-dimensional structure does not suggest itself immediately—is to eliminate answer choices that require faces obviously lacking in the flat pattern. For example, choice (B) requires that there be a face that is a rectangle with one rounded corner. (Actually, *two* such faces are required, since a similar face appears at the back.) This is clearly not satisfied by the pattern. The front and back faces of choice (C) also correspond to a shape not present in the flat pattern. The only choices left are (A) and (D). We can eliminate choice (D) because the faces with the rounded corner do not have the same proportions as shown in the flat pattern.

For questions of the second type, where shading is a factor, we need to work out which faces will be adjacent to which. Again, elimination of answer choices is a very powerful technique. In the second example shown above, the blank faces will be opposite each other, as will the shaded faces. We can therefore eliminate choices (A) and (D). A striped face will be adjacent to both blank and shaded faces, as those "wrap around" the edges of a striped face. However, the two striped faces are also opposite each other. Choice (C) can therefore also be eliminated.

Pattern Folding questions are some of the more challenging ones in the PAT. We recommend that you spend about 15 minutes on this section: 1 minute per question.

The remainder of this section provides you with six comprehensive practice sets on each of the PAT question types.

Keyholes Practice Set

15 questions—10 minutes

DIRECTIONS: For each question, a three-dimensional object is displayed at left. This figure is followed by outlines of five openings or apertures.

The assignment is the same for each question. Imagine how the object at left looks from all directions, not just the one shown. Choose one of the five openings presented which would allow the object to pass through if the proper side were inserted first.

Basic Rules:

1. The irregular object at left may be rotated in any manner. It may be inserted through the aperture starting with a side not shown.

2. Once the irregular object has started through the aperture, it may not be rotated or turned in any way. The object must pass completely through the aperture. The aperture is always the exact shape of the external outline of the object.

3. Both the irregular object and openings are drawn to the same scale.

4. There are no irregularities in any hidden part of the object. If a figure has symmetric indentations, hidden portions are symmetric with visible parts.

5. There is only one correct answer choice for each object.

Try the following example problem:

Example

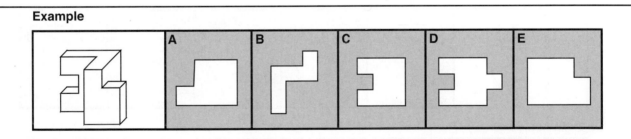

The correct answer is choice (B), since the object would pass through this aperture if the top were inserted first.

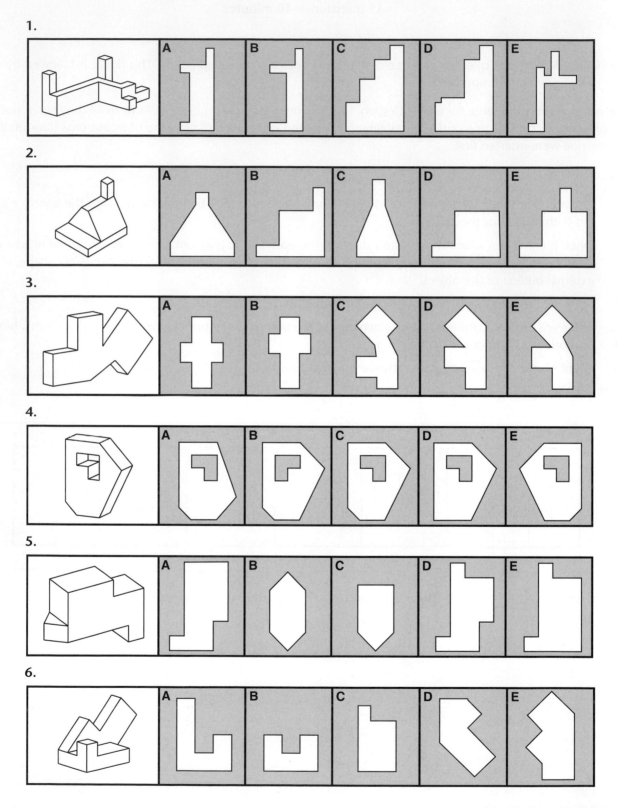

GO TO THE NEXT PAGE.

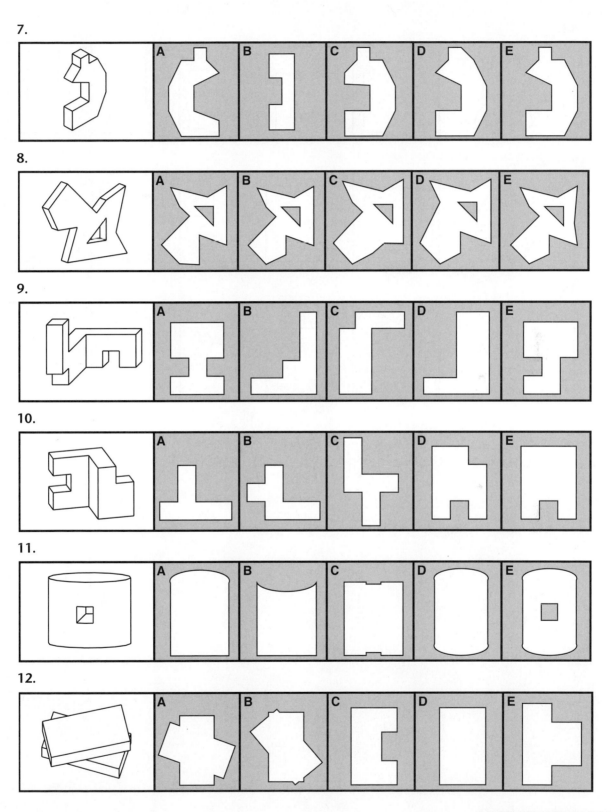

GO TO THE NEXT PAGE.

13.

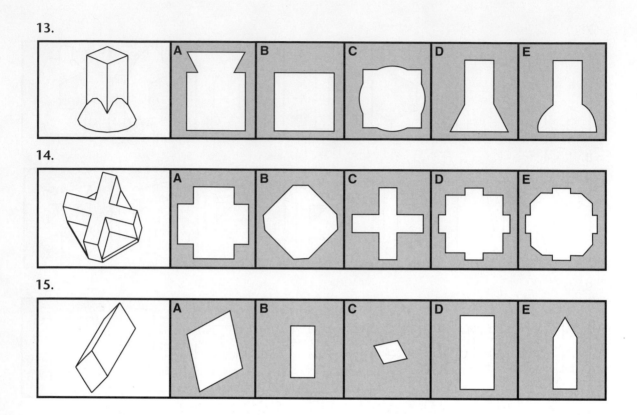

14.

15.

STOP! END OF TEST

The Answer Key Appears on the Following Page.

Keyholes Practice Set Answer Key

1. B
2. B
3. E
4. C
5. D
6. A
7. E
8. B
9. C
10. D
11. C
12. E
13. D
14. B
15. D

Keyholes Practice Set Explanations

1. B

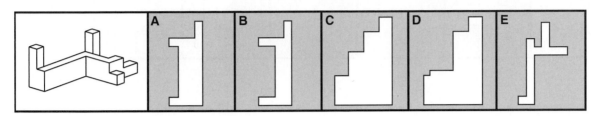

Projections

BOTTOM (Top)

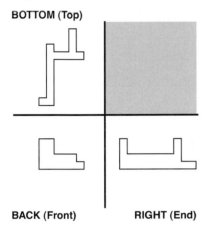

BACK (Front)   **RIGHT (End)**

2. B

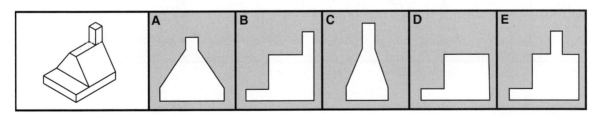

Projections

BOTTOM (Top)

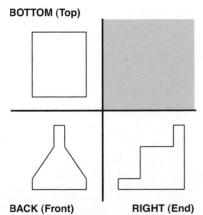

BACK (Front)   **RIGHT (End)**

485

3. E

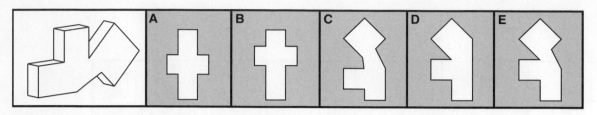

Projections

BOTTOM (Top)

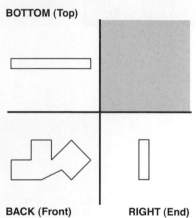

BACK (Front)   **RIGHT (End)**

4. C

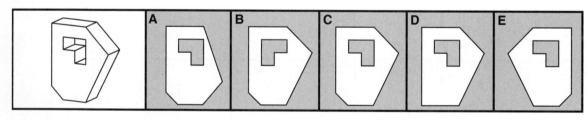

Projections

BOTTOM (Top)

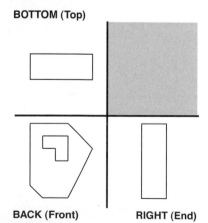

BACK (Front)   **RIGHT (End)**

5. D

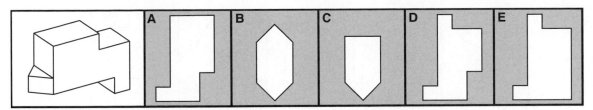

Projections

BOTTOM (Top)

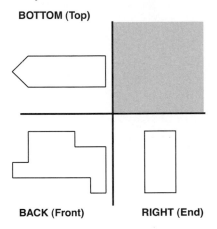

BACK (Front)   **RIGHT (End)**

6. A

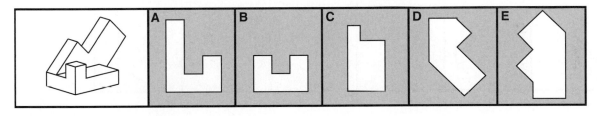

Projections

BOTTOM (Top)

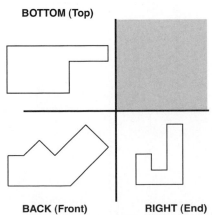

BACK (Front)   **RIGHT (End)**

7. E

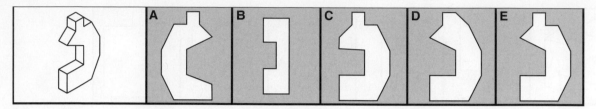

Projections

BOTTOM (Top)

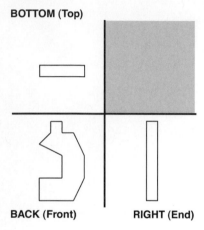

BACK (Front)   **RIGHT (End)**

8. B

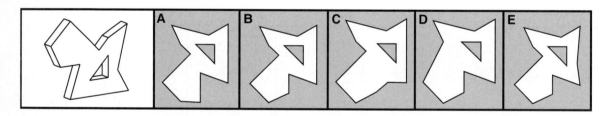

Projections

BOTTOM (Top)

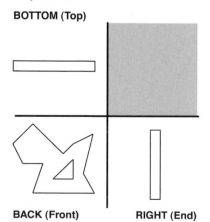

BACK (Front)   **RIGHT (End)**

9. C

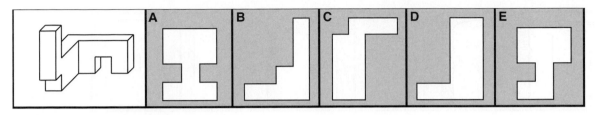

Projections

BOTTOM (Top)

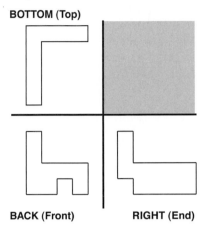

BACK (Front)   **RIGHT (End)**

10. D

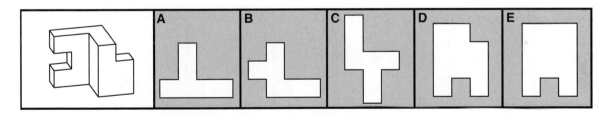

Projections

BOTTOM (Top)

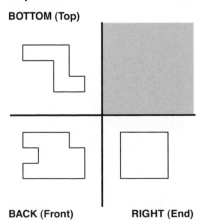

BACK (Front)   **RIGHT (End)**

11. C

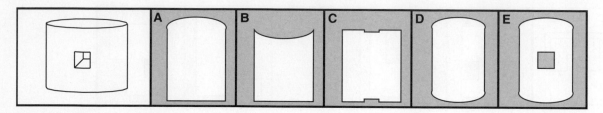

Projections

BOTTOM (Top)

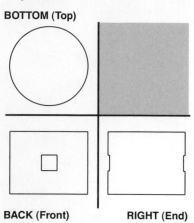

BACK (Front)   **RIGHT (End)**

12. E

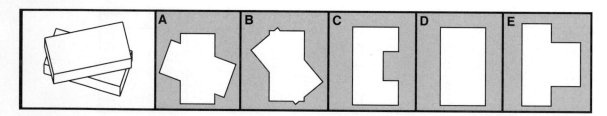

Projections

BOTTOM (Top)

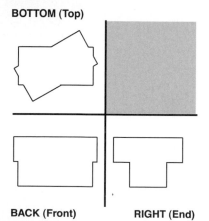

BACK (Front)   **RIGHT (End)**

13. D

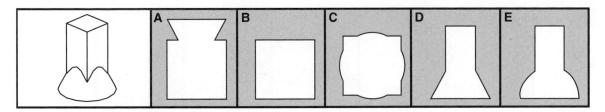

Projections

BOTTOM (Top)

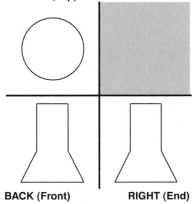

BACK (Front)   **RIGHT (End)**

14. B

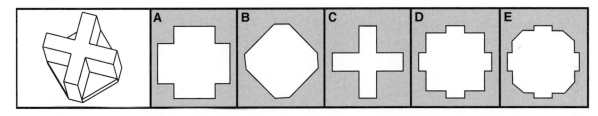

Projections

BOTTOM (Top)

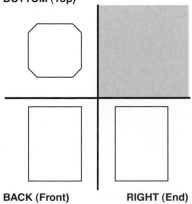

BACK (Front)   **RIGHT (End)**

15. D

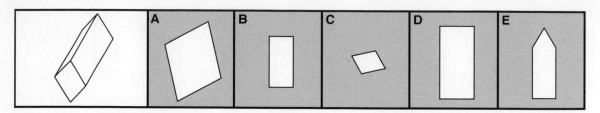

Projections

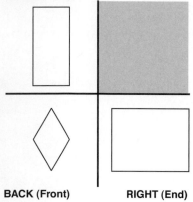

Top-Front-End Practice Set
15 questions—15 minutes

DIRECTIONS:

In each of the following questions, top, front, and end views of various solid objects are presented. All views are presented without perspective. Points in the viewed surface are presented along parallel lines of sight.

The TOP VIEW image of the object presents the projection of looking down on the object. The FRONT VIEW image presents a view of the object from the front. The END VIEW illustrates a lateral view of the object from the right. These views are always in the same position.

Lines that cannot be seen in some perspectives are represented by DOTTED lines.

The problems that follow present two views of a particular object. Four alternatives are shown to complete the set. You will need to select the correct alternative. Try the following example:

Example: Choose the correct **END VIEW**

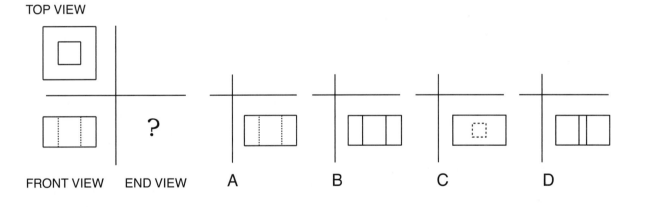

The correct answer is choice A. The following views are shown:

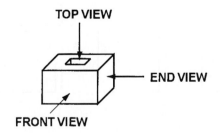

---

1. Choose the correct **END VIEW.**

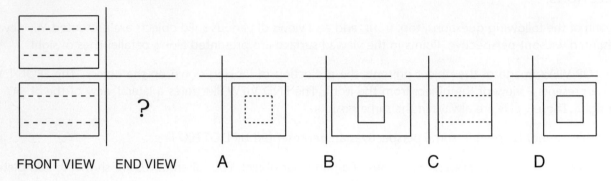

TOP VIEW

FRONT VIEW   END VIEW   A   B   C   D

2. Choose the correct **END VIEW.**

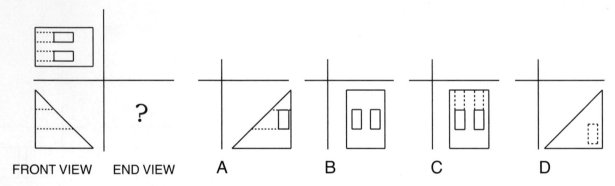

TOP VIEW

FRONT VIEW   END VIEW   A   B   C   D

3. Choose the correct **END VIEW.**

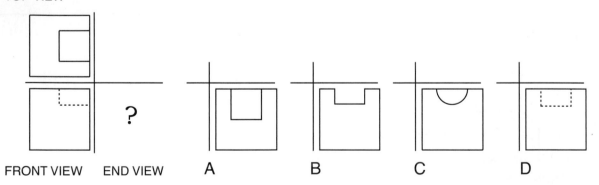

TOP VIEW

FRONT VIEW   END VIEW   A   B   C   D

GO TO THE NEXT PAGE.

4. Choose the correct **END VIEW**.

TOP VIEW

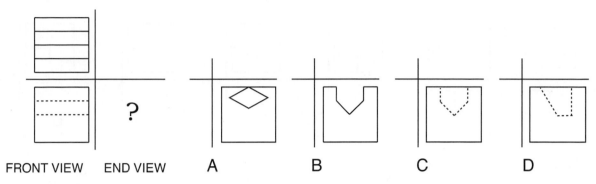

FRONT VIEW   END VIEW   A   B   C   D

5. Choose the correct **END VIEW**.

TOP VIEW

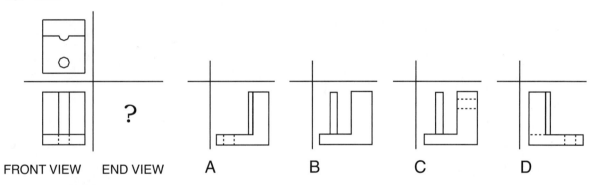

FRONT VIEW   END VIEW   A   B   C   D

6. Choose the correct **END VIEW**.

TOP VIEW

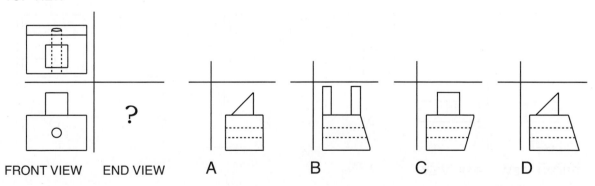

FRONT VIEW   END VIEW   A   B   C   D

GO TO THE NEXT PAGE.

7. Choose the correct **TOP VIEW.**

TOP VIEW

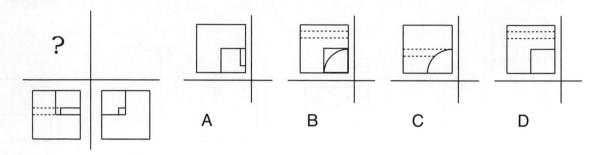

FRONT VIEW   END VIEW

8. Choose the correct **TOP VIEW.**

TOP VIEW

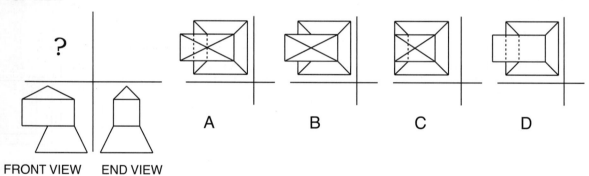

FRONT VIEW   END VIEW

9. Choose the correct **TOP VIEW.**

TOP VIEW

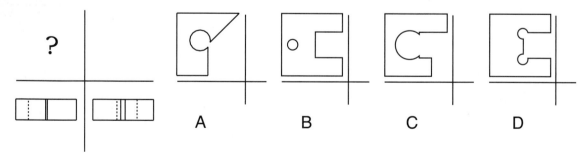

FRONT VIEW   END VIEW

GO TO THE NEXT PAGE.

10. Choose the correct **TOP VIEW.**

TOP VIEW

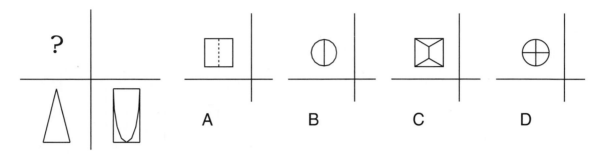

FRONT VIEW   END VIEW

11. Choose the correct **TOP VIEW.**

TOP VIEW

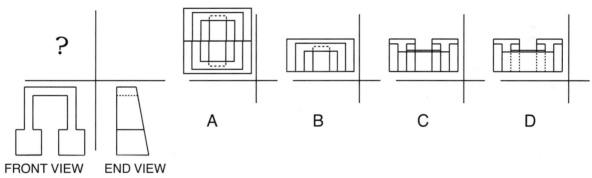

FRONT VIEW   END VIEW

12. Choose the correct **TOP VIEW.**

TOP VIEW

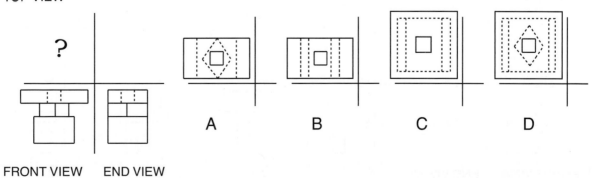

FRONT VIEW   END VIEW

GO TO THE NEXT PAGE.

13. Choose the correct **END VIEW.**

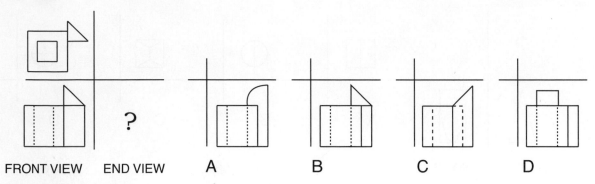

14. Choose the correct **END VIEW.**

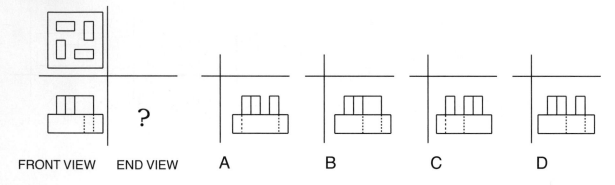

15. Choose the correct **END VIEW.**

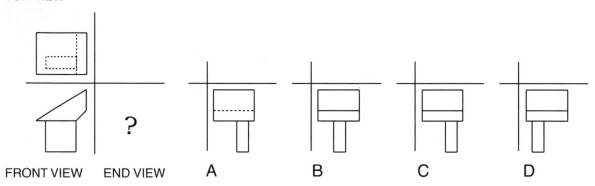

STOP! END OF TEST

The Answer Key Appears on the Following Page.

Top-Front-End Practice Set Answer Key

1. D
2. B
3. C
4. B
5. A
6. D
7. C
8. A
9. A
10. B
11. D
12. A
13. C
14. D
15. D

Top-Front-End Practice Set Explanations

1. Choose the correct END VIEW.

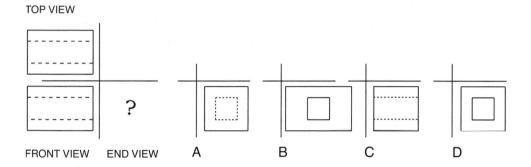

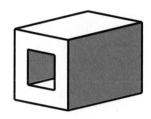

Answer: D

2. Choose the correct END VIEW.

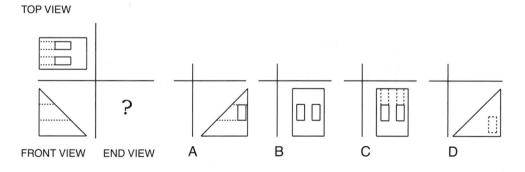

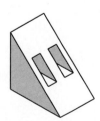

Answer: B

3. Choose the correct END VIEW.

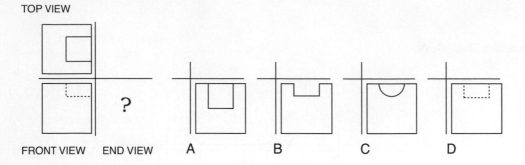

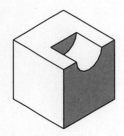

Answer: C

4. Choose the correct END VIEW.

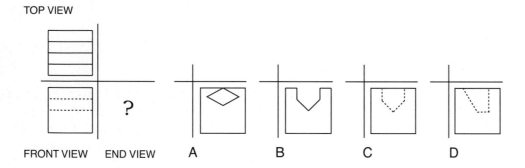

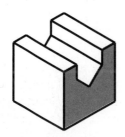

Answer: B

5. Choose the correct END VIEW.

TOP VIEW

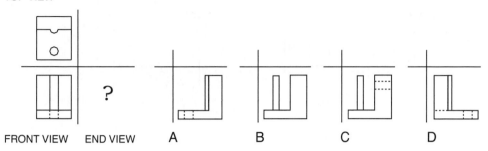

FRONT VIEW   END VIEW   A   B   C   D

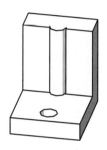

Answer: A

6. Choose the correct END VIEW.

TOP VIEW

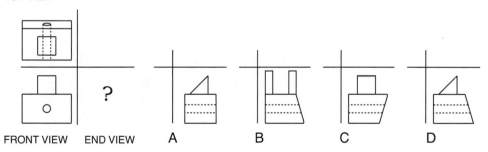

FRONT VIEW   END VIEW   A   B   C   D

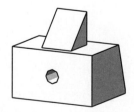

Answer: D

7. Choose the correct TOP VIEW.

TOP VIEW

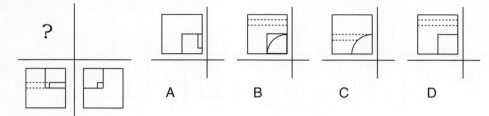

FRONT VIEW   END VIEW

A   B   C   D

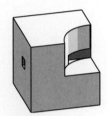

Answer: C

8. Choose the correct TOP VIEW.

TOP VIEW

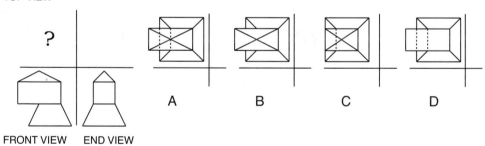

FRONT VIEW   END VIEW

A   B   C   D

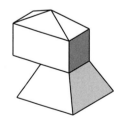

Answer: A

9. Choose the correct TOP VIEW.

TOP VIEW

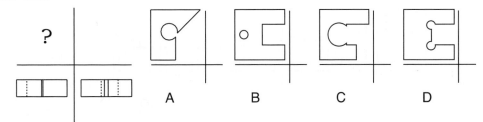

A   B   C   D

FRONT VIEW   END VIEW

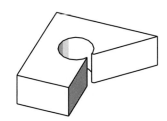

Answer: A

10. Choose the correct TOP VIEW.

TOP VIEW

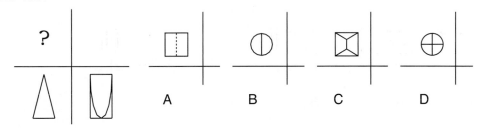

A   B   C   D

FRONT VIEW   END VIEW

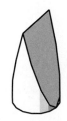

Answer: B

11. Choose the correct TOP VIEW.

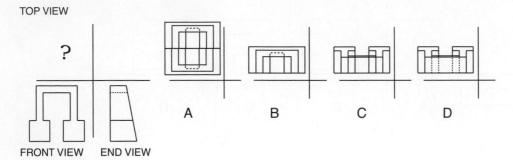

TOP VIEW

?

FRONT VIEW   END VIEW

A   B   C   D

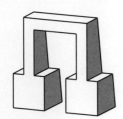

Answer: D

12. Choose the correct TOP VIEW.

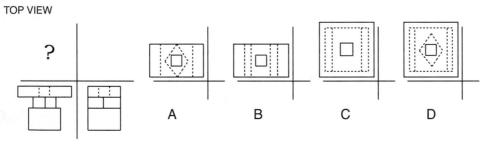

TOP VIEW

?

FRONT VIEW   END VIEW

A   B   C   D

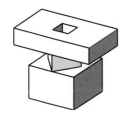

Answer: A

13. Choose the correct END VIEW.

TOP VIEW

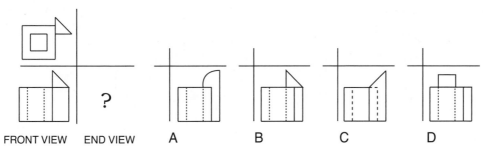

FRONT VIEW   END VIEW   A   B   C   D

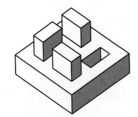

Answer: C

14. Choose the correct END VIEW.

TOP VIEW

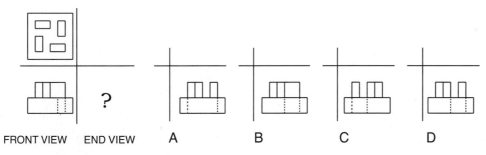

FRONT VIEW   END VIEW   A   B   C   D

Answer: D

15. Choose the correct END VIEW.

TOP VIEW

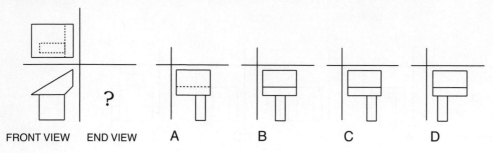

FRONT VIEW   END VIEW   A   B   C   D

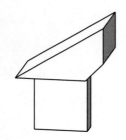

Answer: D

Angle Ranking Practice Set

15 questions—5 minutes

DIRECTIONS:

Each question in this section presents four INTERIOR angles, labeled 1 through 4. Examine the four interior angles presented in each question.

Rank each question's angles in order from smallest to largest. You will need to select the answer choice that represents the correct ranking. Try the following example problem.

Example:

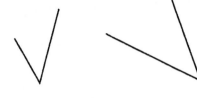

   1   2   3   4

(A) 4-1-2-3

(B) 2-1-4-3

(C) 1-4-2-3

(D) 3-2-1-4

The correct ranking of the angles from small to large is 4-1-2-3. Therefore, the correct answer is choice (A).

1.

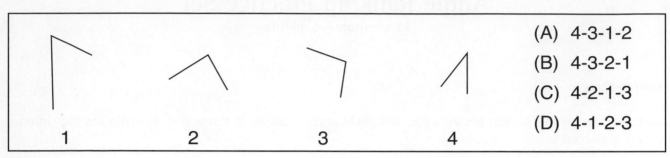

(A) 4-3-1-2
(B) 4-3-2-1
(C) 4-2-1-3
(D) 4-1-2-3

2.

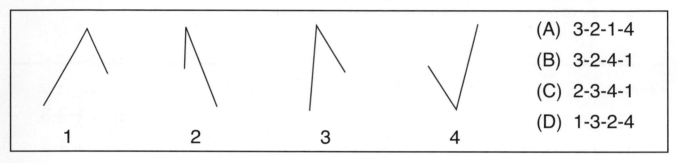

(A) 3-2-1-4
(B) 3-2-4-1
(C) 2-3-4-1
(D) 1-3-2-4

3.

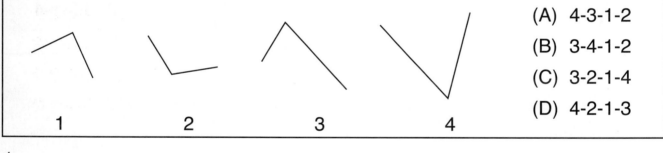

(A) 4-3-1-2
(B) 3-4-1-2
(C) 3-2-1-4
(D) 4-2-1-3

4.

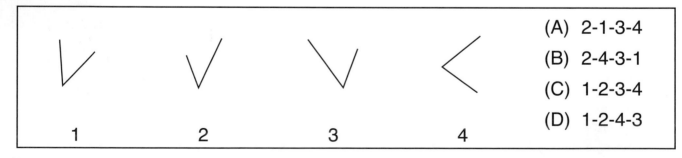

(A) 2-1-3-4
(B) 2-4-3-1
(C) 1-2-3-4
(D) 1-2-4-3

GO TO THE NEXT PAGE.

5.

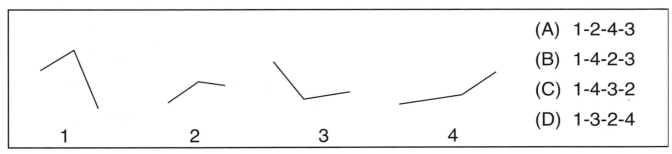

(A) 1-2-4-3

(B) 1-4-2-3

(C) 1-4-3-2

(D) 1-3-2-4

6.

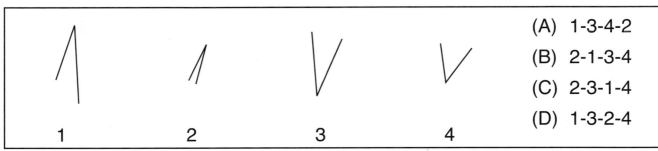

(A) 1-3-4-2

(B) 2-1-3-4

(C) 2-3-1-4

(D) 1-3-2-4

7.

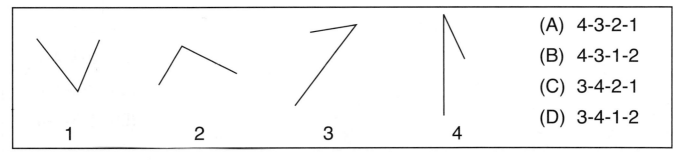

(A) 4-3-2-1

(B) 4-3-1-2

(C) 3-4-2-1

(D) 3-4-1-2

8.

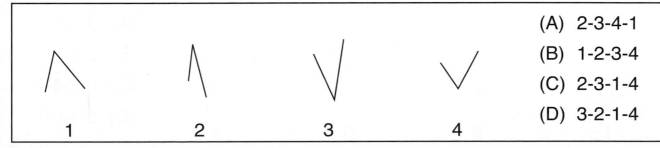

(A) 2-3-4-1

(B) 1-2-3-4

(C) 2-3-1-4

(D) 3-2-1-4

GO TO THE NEXT PAGE.

9.

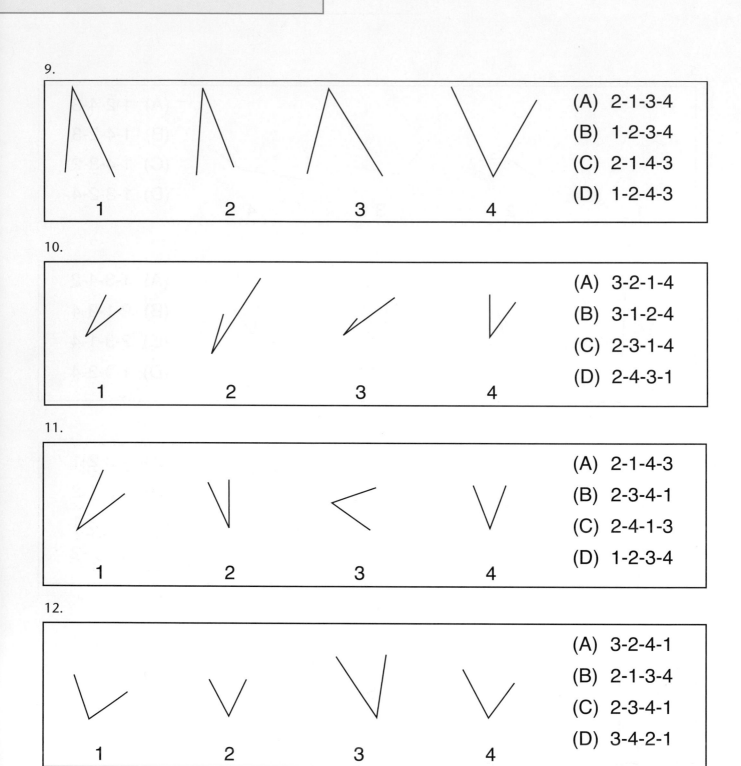

(A) 2-1-3-4
(B) 1-2-3-4
(C) 2-1-4-3
(D) 1-2-4-3

10.

(A) 3-2-1-4
(B) 3-1-2-4
(C) 2-3-1-4
(D) 2-4-3-1

11.

(A) 2-1-4-3
(B) 2-3-4-1
(C) 2-4-1-3
(D) 1-2-3-4

12.

(A) 3-2-4-1
(B) 2-1-3-4
(C) 2-3-4-1
(D) 3-4-2-1

GO TO THE NEXT PAGE.

13.

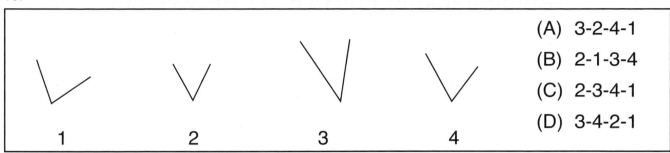

(A) 3-2-4-1

(B) 2-1-3-4

(C) 2-3-4-1

(D) 3-4-2-1

14.

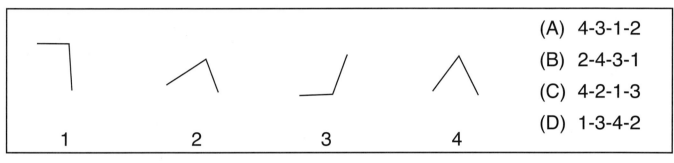

(A) 4-3-1-2

(B) 2-4-3-1

(C) 4-2-1-3

(D) 1-3-4-2

15.

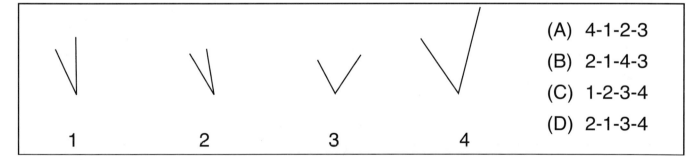

(A) 4-1-2-3

(B) 2-1-4-3

(C) 1-2-3-4

(D) 2-1-3-4

STOP! END OF TEST

Angle Ranking Practice Set Answer Key

1. D
2. C
3. A
4. A
5. D
6. B
7. B
8. C
9. A
10. A
11. A
12. A
13. A
14. C
15. B

Hole Punching Practice Set
15 questions—5 minutes

DIRECTIONS:

In these questions, a flat, square piece of paper is folded one or more times. Broken lines indicate the original position of the paper, and solid lines indicate the position of the folded paper. The folded paper remains within the boundaries of the original, flat sheet. The paper is not turned or twisted. There are one, two, or three folds per question.

Once the final fold is performed, one or more holes are punched in the paper. Once the hole(s) is/are punched, mentally unfold the paper and ascertain the position(s) of the hole(s) on the original flat sheet.

Select the answer choice that represents the same pattern of dark circles that would reflect the position of holes on the unfolded sheet. There is only one correct pattern for each question. Try the following example:

Example:

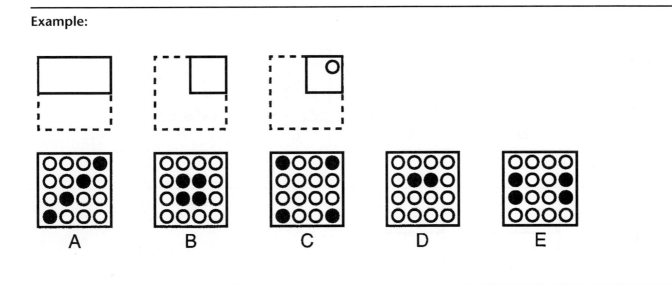

The correct answer is choice (C).

1.

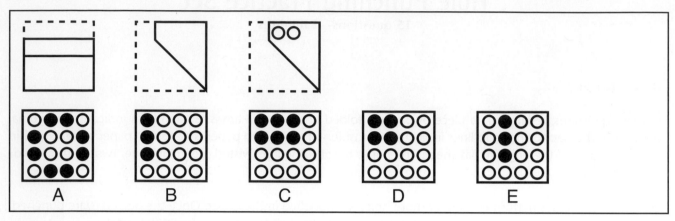

2.

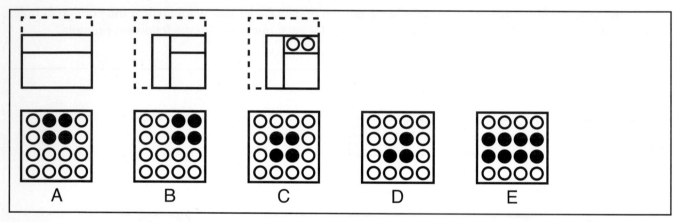

3.

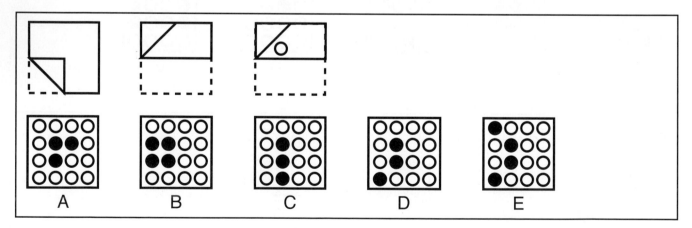

GO TO THE NEXT PAGE.

4.

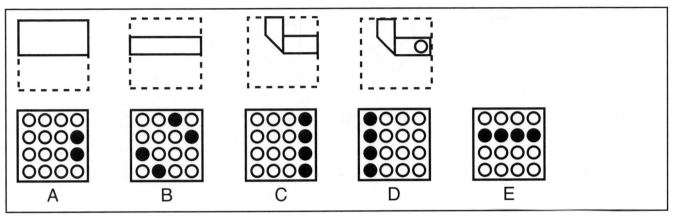

5.

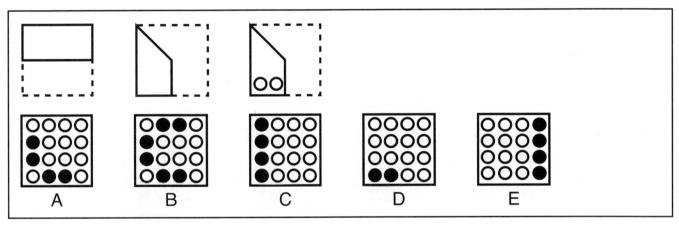

6.

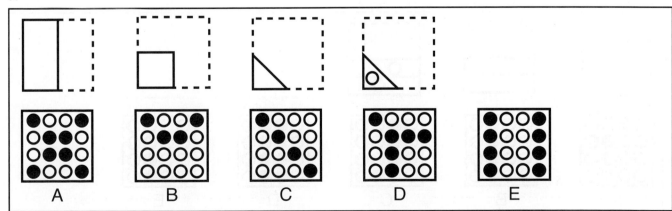

GO TO THE NEXT PAGE.

7.

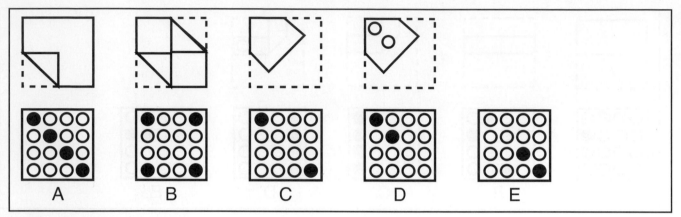

8.

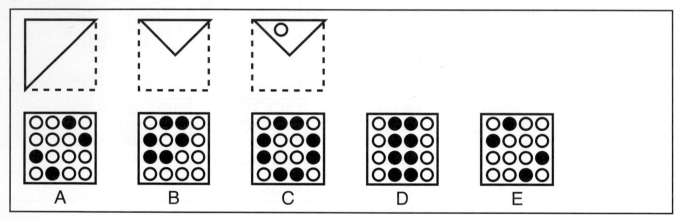

9.

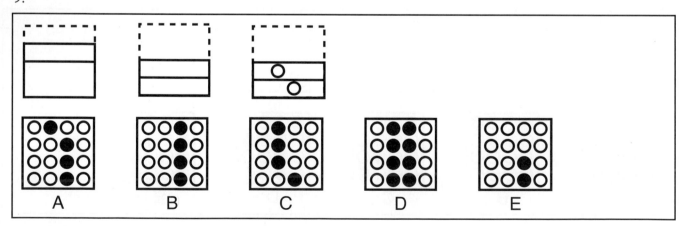

GO TO THE NEXT PAGE.

10.

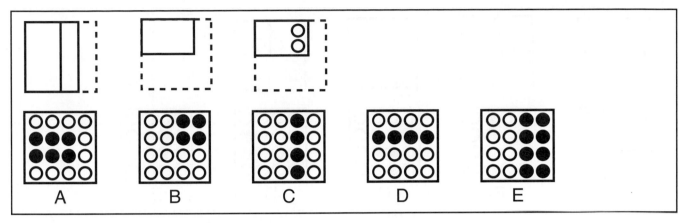

11.

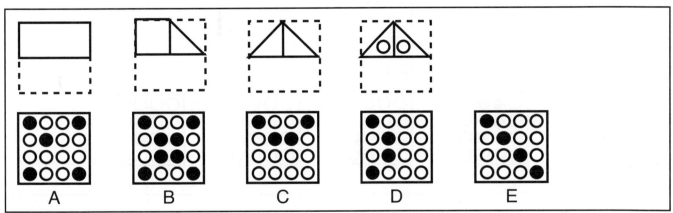

12.

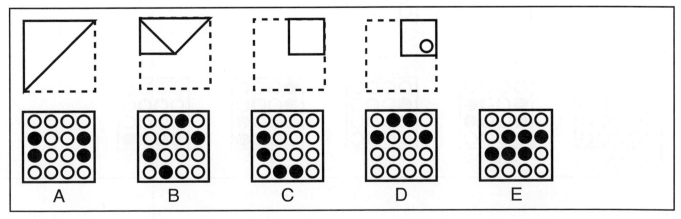

GO TO THE NEXT PAGE.

13.

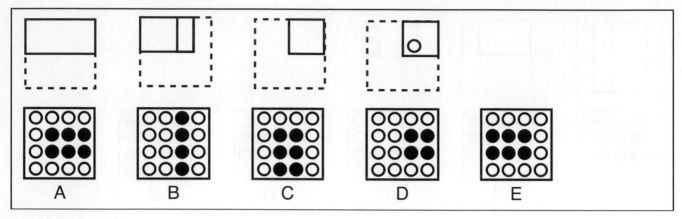

14.

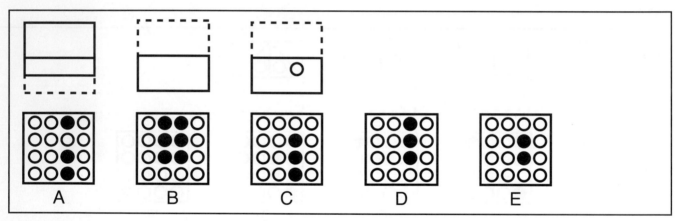

15.

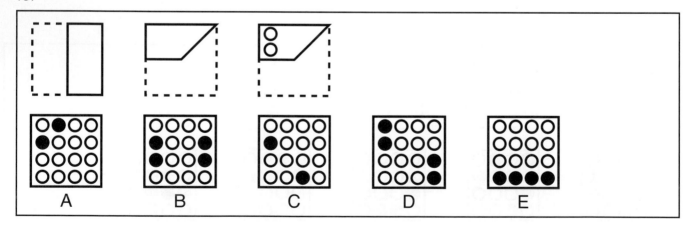

STOP! END OF TEST

The Answer Key Appears on the Following Page.

Hole Punching Practice Set Answer Key

1. B
2. B
3. D
4. C
5. E
6. A
7. A
8. E
9. C
10. E
11. B
12. C
13. A
14. C
15. E

Hole Punching Practice Set Explanations

1. B

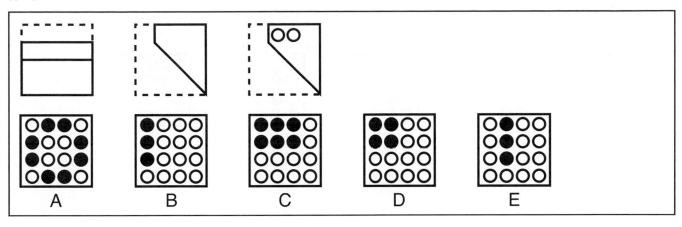

Always make sure to eliminate answer choices by looking at the symmetry of the first fold.

Eliminate (A).

2. B

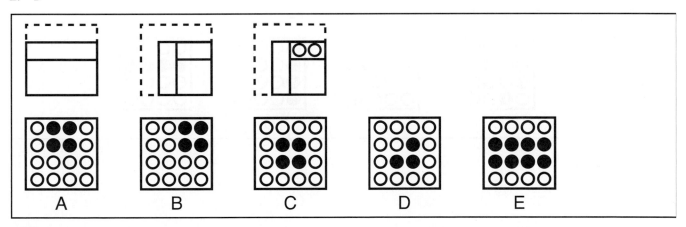

Eliminate (C), (D), and (E).

3. D

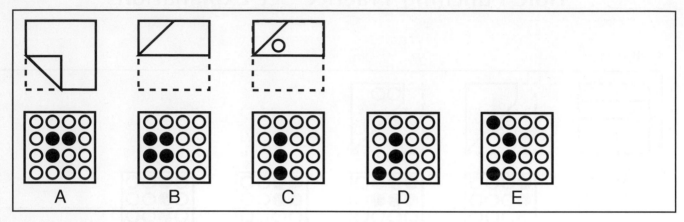

Eliminate (A), (B), and (C).

4. C

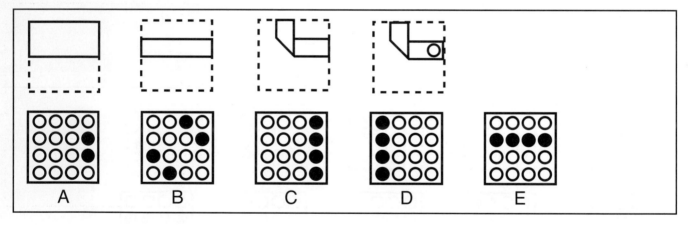

Eliminate (B) and (E).

5. E

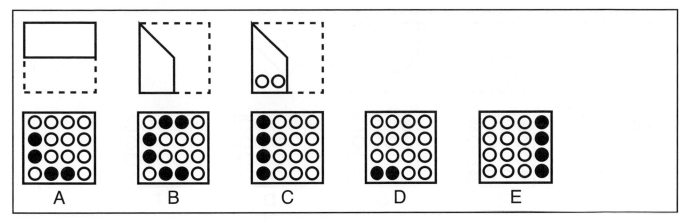

Eliminate (A) and (D).

6. A

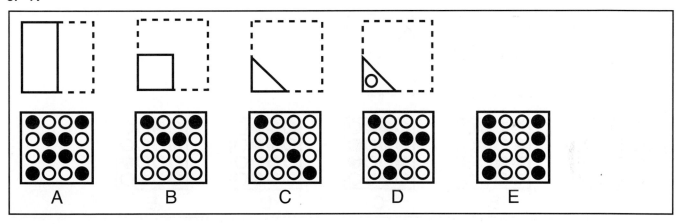

Eliminate (C) and (D).

7. A

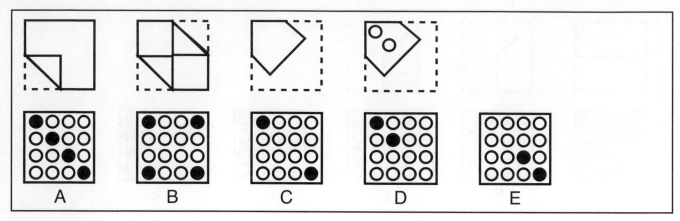

Eliminate (B).

8. E

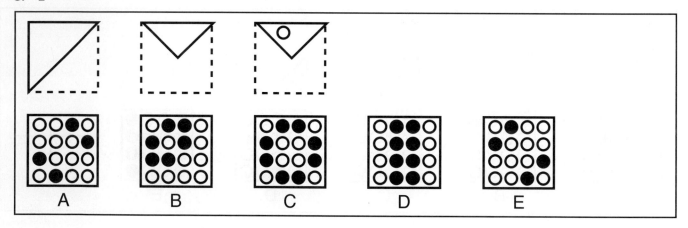

Eliminate (B) and (D).

9. C

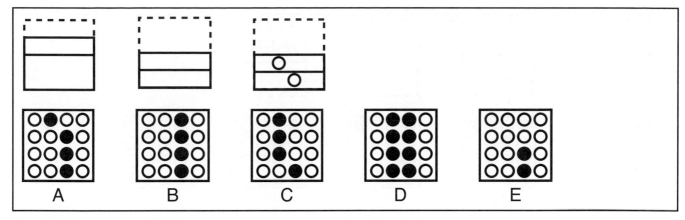

Eliminate (A).

10. E

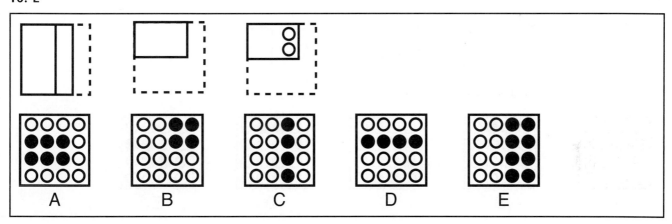

Eliminate (A) and (C).

11. B

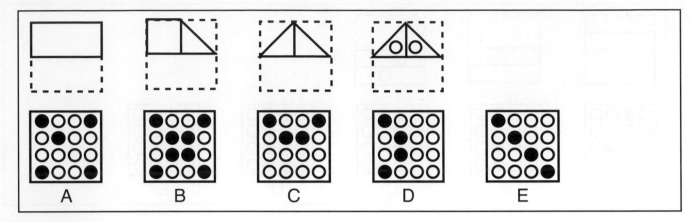

Eliminate (A), (C), and (D).

12. C

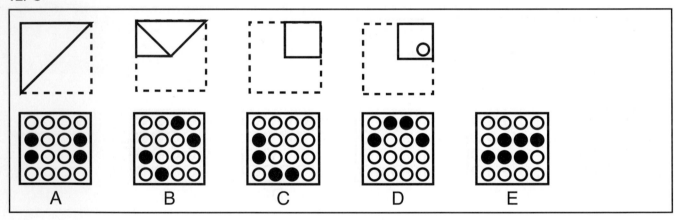

Eliminate (A), (D), and (E).

13. A

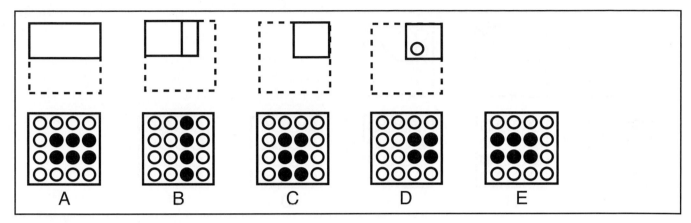

Eliminate (C).

14. C

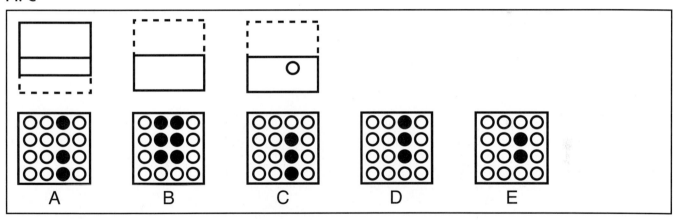

Eliminate (B), (D), and (E).

15. E

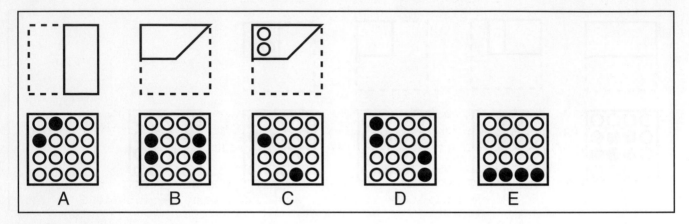

Eliminate (A), (C), and (D).

Cube Counting Practice Set
15 questions—10 minutes

DIRECTIONS:

Each figure presented in this section has been constructed by cementing together identical cubes. After being cemented, each figure was varnished on all sides EXCEPT for the bottom (the side on which the figure rests). The only hidden cubes are the ones necessary to support other cubes in the figure.

Examine each figure carefully regarding the number of sides on each cube that have been varnished. The following questions ask for this information. Select the correct answer choice from the ones provided.

Note: Zero (0) is not the correct answer for any question.

Example:

    In the Example Figure, how many cubes have two of their exposed sides painted?

    A. 1 cube

    B. 2 cubes

    C. 3 cubes

    D. 4 cubes

    E. 5 cubes

Example Figure

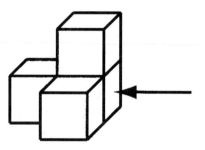

The correct answer is choice (A). The cube is indicated with an arrow.

Problem A

Figure A

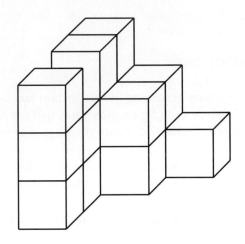

1. In Figure A, how many cubes have one of their exposed sides painted?

   A. 1 cube

   B. 2 cubes

   C. 3 cubes

   D. 4 cubes

   E. 5 cubes

2. In Figure A, how many cubes have two of their exposed sides painted?

   A. 1 cube

   B. 2 cubes

   C. 3 cubes

   D. 4 cubes

   E. 5 cubes

3. In Figure A, how many cubes have three of their exposed sides painted?

   A. 1 cube

   B. 2 cubes

   C. 3 cubes

   D. 4 cubes

   E. 5 cubes

4. In Figure A, how many cubes have four of their exposed sides painted?

   A. 1 cube

   B. 2 cubes

   C. 3 cubes

   D. 4 cubes

   E. 5 cubes

GO TO THE NEXT PAGE.

Problem B

Figure B

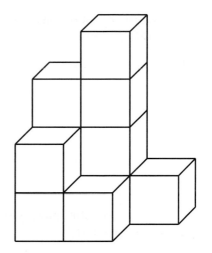

5. In Figure B, how many cubes have one of their exposed sides painted?

    A. 1 cube

    B. 2 cubes

    C. 3 cubes

    D. 4 cubes

    E. 5 cubes

6. In Figure B, how many cubes have two of their exposed sides painted?

    A. 1 cube

    B. 2 cubes

    C. 3 cubes

    D. 4 cubes

    E. 5 cubes

7. In Figure B, how many cubes have three of their exposed sides painted?

    A. 1 cube

    B. 2 cubes

    C. 3 cubes

    D. 4 cubes

    E. 5 cubes

8. In Figure B, how many cubes have five of their exposed sides painted?

    A. 1 cube

    B. 2 cubes

    C. 3 cubes

    D. 4 cubes

    E. 5 cubes

GO TO THE NEXT PAGE.

Problem C

9. In Figure C, how many cubes have one of their exposed sides painted?

   A. 1 cube

   B. 2 cubes

   C. 3 cubes

   D. 4 cubes

   E. 5 cubes

10. In Figure C, how many cubes have two of their exposed sides painted?

   A. 1 cube

   B. 2 cubes

   C. 3 cubes

   D. 4 cubes

   E. 5 cubes

11. In Figure C, how many cubes have four of their exposed sides painted?

   A. 1 cube

   B. 2 cubes

   C. 3 cubes

   D. 4 cubes

   E. 5 cubes

Figure C

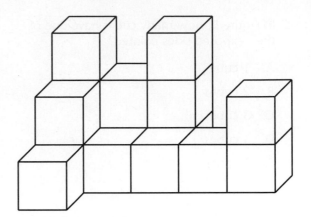

GO TO THE NEXT PAGE.

Problem D

Figure D

12. In Figure D, how many cubes have four of their exposed sides painted?

    A. 1 cube

    B. 2 cubes

    C. 3 cubes

    D. 4 cubes

    E. 5 cubes

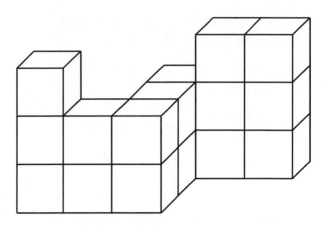

13. In Figure D, how many cubes have five of their sides painted?

    A. 1 cube

    B. 2 cubes

    C. 3 cubes

    D. 4 cubes

    E. 5 cubes

GO TO THE NEXT PAGE.

Problem E

Figure E

14. In Figure E, how many cubes have three of their exposed sides painted?

    A. 1 cube

    B. 2 cubes

    C. 3 cubes

    D. 4 cubes

    E. 5 cubes

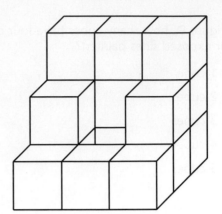

15. In Figure E, how many cubes have four of their sides painted?

    A. 1 cube

    B. 2 cubes

    C. 3 cubes

    D. 4 cubes

    E. 5 cubes

STOP! END OF TEST

The Answer Key Appears on the Following Page.

Cube Counting Practice Set Answer Key

1. C
2. D
3. E
4. C
5. A
6. C
7. C
8. A
9. B
10. E
11. B
12. B
13. A
14. D
15. D

Cube Counting Practice Set Explanations

Problem A

Figure A

1. In Figure A, how many cubes have one of their exposed sides painted?

   A. 1 cube

   B. 2 cubes

   C. 3 cubes

   D. 4 cubes

   E. 5 cubes

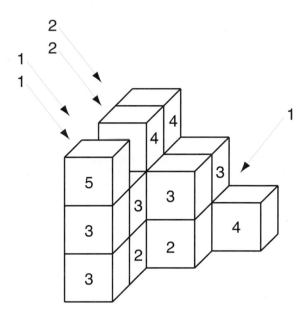

2. In Figure A, how many cubes have two of their exposed sides painted?

   A. 1 cube

   B. 2 cubes

   C. 3 cubes

   D. 4 cubes

   E. 5 cubes

3. In Figure A, how many cubes have three of their exposed sides painted?

   A. 1 cube

   B. 2 cubes

   C. 3 cubes

   D. 4 cubes

   E. 5 cubes

4. In Figure A, how many cubes have four of their exposed sides painted?

   A. 1 cube

   B. 2 cubes

   C. 3 cubes

   D. 4 cubes

   E. 5 cubes

Problem B

Figure B

5. In Figure B, how many cubes have one of their exposed sides painted?

    A. 1 cube

    B. 2 cubes

    C. 3 cubes

    D. 4 cubes

    E. 5 cubes

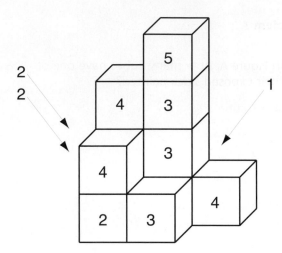

6. In Figure B, how many cubes have two of their exposed sides painted?

    A. 1 cube

    B. 2 cubes

    C. 3 cubes

    D. 4 cubes

    E. 5 cubes

7. In Figure B, how many cubes have three of their exposed sides painted?

    A. 1 cube

    B. 2 cubes

    C. 3 cubes

    D. 4 cubes

    E. 5 cubes

8. In Figure B, how many cubes have five of their exposed sides painted?

    A. 1 cube

    B. 2 cubes

    C. 3 cubes

    D. 4 cubes

    E. 5 cubes

Problem C

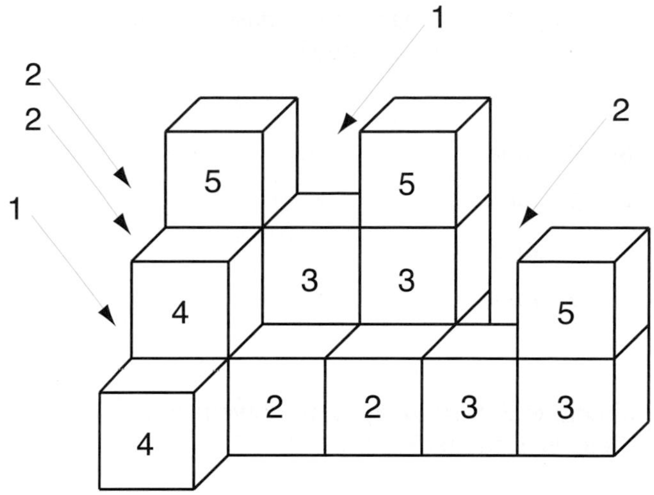

9. In Figure C, how many cubes have one of their exposed sides painted?

   A. 1 cube

   B. 2 cubes

   C. 3 cubes

   D. 4 cubes

   E. 5 cubes

10. In Figure C, how many cubes have two of their exposed sides painted?

   A. 1 cube

   B. 2 cubes

   C. 3 cubes

   D. 4 cubes

   E. 5 cubes

11. In Figure C, how many cubes have four of their exposed sides painted?

   A. 1 cube

   B. 2 cubes

   C. 3 cubes

   D. 4 cubes

   E. 5 cubes

Figure C

Problem D

12. In Figure D, how many cubes have four of their exposed sides painted?

    A. 1 cube

    B. 2 cubes

    C. 3 cubes

    D. 4 cubes

    E. 5 cubes

13. In Figure D, how many cubes have five of their sides painted?

    A. 1 cube

    B. 2 cubes

    C. 3 cubes

    D. 4 cubes

    E. 5 cubes

Figure D

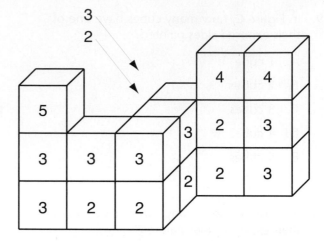

Problem E

14. In Figure E, how many cubes have three of their exposed sides painted?

    A. 1 cube

    B. 2 cubes

    C. 3 cubes

    D. 4 cubes

    E. 5 cubes

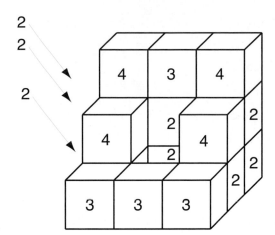

15. In Figure E, how many cubes have four of their sides painted?

    A. 1 cube

    B. 2 cubes

    C. 3 cubes

    D. 4 cubes

    E. 5 cubes

Pattern Folding Practice Set
15 questions—15 minutes

DIRECTIONS:

In these questions, a flat pattern is presented. This pattern will be folded into a three-dimensional figure, and the correct three-dimensional figure is one of the four answer choices illustrated at the right of the pattern. There is only one correct three-dimensional figure for each question. The pattern at the left represents the outside of the figure.

Select the three-dimensional figure that directly corresponds to the pattern at the left. Mark the appropriate answer choice on your answer grid that represents the correct figure. Try the following example:

Example:

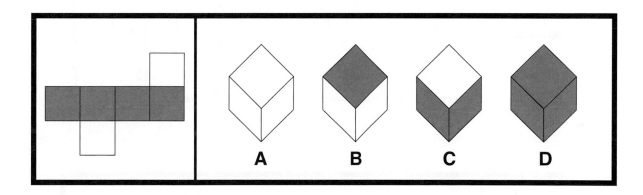

The correct answer is choice (C).

1.

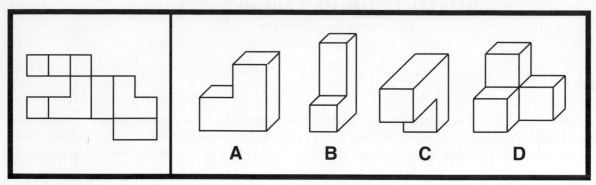

2.

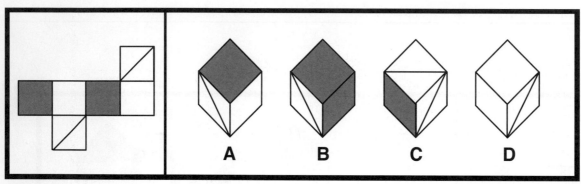

3.

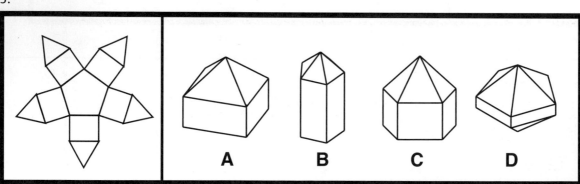

GO TO THE NEXT PAGE.

4.

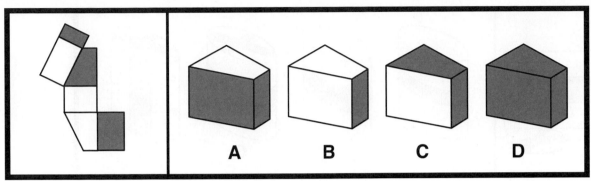

5.

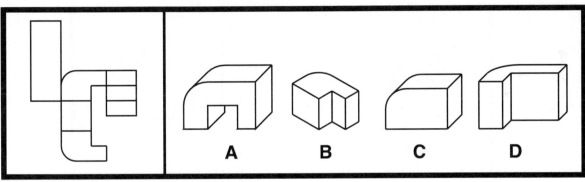

6.

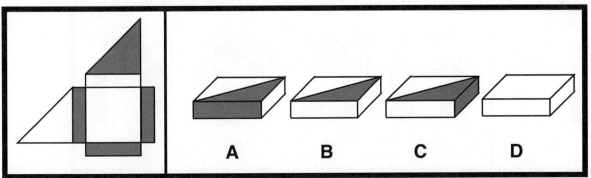

GO TO THE NEXT PAGE.

7.

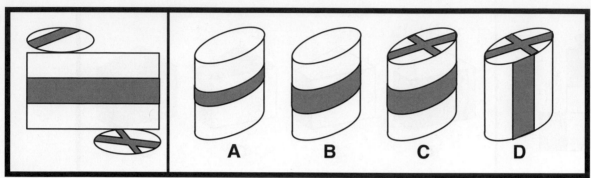

8.

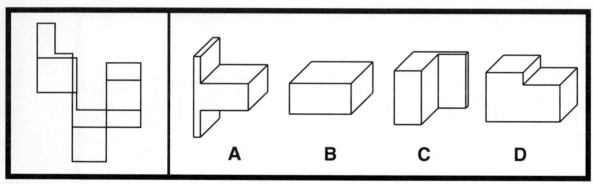

9.

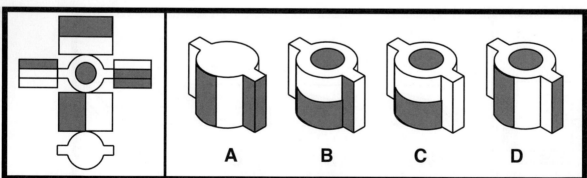

GO TO THE NEXT PAGE.

10.

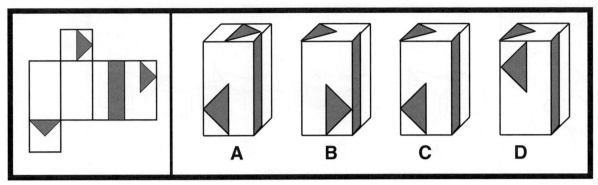

11.

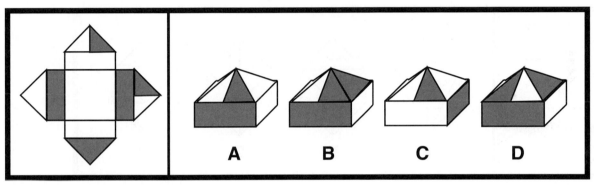

12.

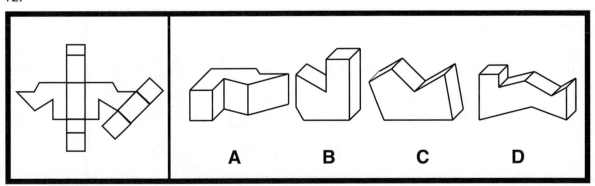

GO TO THE NEXT PAGE.

13.

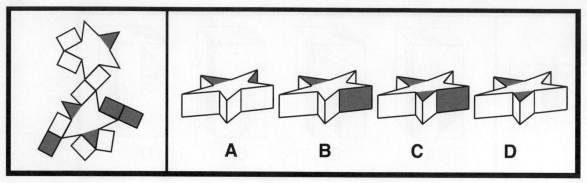

14.

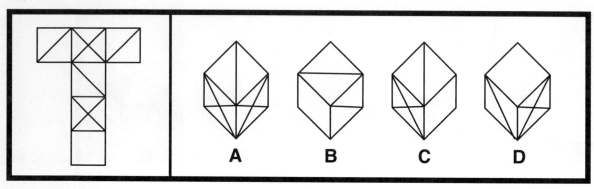

15.

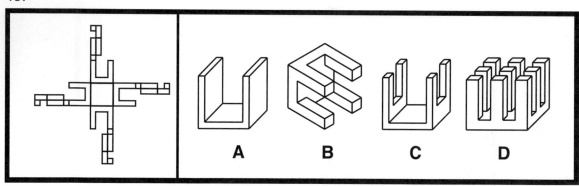

STOP! END OF TEST

The Answer Key Appears on the Following Page.

Pattern Folding Practice Set Answer Key

1. A
2. A
3. C
4. D
5. B
6. C
7. C
8. C
9. B
10. C
11. D
12. A
13. A
14. C
15. B

READING COMPREHENSION

Reading Comprehension Practice Test

50 minutes—50 questions

DIRECTIONS: The following test consists of several reading passages and questions that test your comprehension of the passages. Read each passage carefully, and when you believe you have sufficient comprehension of the passage, go on to the questions. You may look back at a passage as often as you wish. Each question item consists of a question or an unfinished sentence followed by possible answers or completions. After reading a question, decide which choice is best and mark your answer.

The growth and development of mammalian teeth is the result of a complex series of tissue interactions that occurs during the embryonic and post-natal periods. The permanent tooth and its associated structures are composed of a wide variety of tissue types, including bone, epithelium, connective tissue, nerves, and blood vessels. Its anatomic structure is based upon a central pulp cavity containing the neural and vascular supply. This is surrounded by a layer of dentin, a yellowish material that is somewhat harder than bone. Finally, the dentin is covered by a layer of mineralized enamel, the hardest substance in the body. The dentin and enamel are each produced by highly specialized cells known as odontoblasts and ameloblasts, respectively.

The nerves responsible for pain sensation in the teeth are the superior and inferior alveolar nerves, which are derived from the fifth cranial (trigeminal) nerve. These are the sole sensory nerves for the teeth. The autonomic nervous system also innervates the teeth through the parasympathetic vasodilator fibers of the otic ganglion of the ninth cranial (glossopharyngeal) nerve and the fibers of the cervical sympathetic chain.

The blood supply to the upper jaw is provided by the superior alveolar arteries, which arise from the infraorbital and maxillary arteries. Blood to the lower jaw is carried by the inferior alveolar artery, another branch of the maxillary artery. These arteries are controlled by the vasoconstrictor fibers of the cervical sympathetic system, which stimulates contraction of the arterial smooth muscle fibers. All of the blood to the teeth comes originally from the right and left common carotid arteries, which supply the entire head and face.

The rate of tooth eruption in mammals has been studied for over 150 years. Early observations in 1823 led Oudet to conclude that rat incisors were capable of persistent growth, even in mature animals. Although it was long suspected that innervation might be responsible for control of this growth, it was not until 1919 that Moral and Hosemann were the first to measure tooth growth after cutting the inferior alveolar nerve. In 1927, Leist reported increased growth of guinea pig incisors after cutting the inferior alveolar nerve and the cervical sympathetic chain. However, he believed that the observed increase may have been due to secondary hyperemia of the pulp following the cervical sympathectomy.

This belief shifted attention, at least temporarily, away from the nervous system and toward the circulatory system. Despite the wide range of possible explanations for the control of tooth growth, the most commonly accepted theory was that first proposed by Leist—that blood supply was the important regulatory influence. it was not until the work of Butcher and Taylor in 1951 that any significant change in thought evolved.

The two investigators, working at New York University, studied five factors—blood supply, innervation, the shape of the tooth, physical stress, and the consistency of the diet—and their influence upon tooth growth rates. They explained that rat incisors were capable of two processes, eruption and attrition. The former refers to extrusion of a tooth into the oral cavity, while the latter results in a shortening of the tooth due to breakage or grinding, usually the result of normal feeding activity. Changes in tooth length were measured by initially cutting a notch in the tooth at the gingival crest. Eruption was quantified by measuring the distance between the notch and the gingival crest after a period of a few days, during which the tooth was allowed to grow. Attrition was measured as the decrease in distance from the notch to the incisal edge after breaking or grinding had occurred.

Studying the blood supply, Butcher and Taylor found that unilateral ligation of the common carotid artery decreased blood supply to teeth on the corresponding side but also produced bilateral fluctuation in eruption rate, although there was no clear decrease in tooth growth. Further, they showed that ligation of the inferior alveolar artery, while decreasing blood flow considerably, had no effect on rate of eruption. However, when all blood flow to a tooth was stopped by applying retroactive tension to the tooth, eruption ceased. Thus, the demonstration that only complete ischemia, or total lack of blood, would drastically reduce tooth growth led Butcher and Taylor to conclude that circulation was not the most important regulatory factor.

Considering innervation, they discovered that cutting the inferior alveolar nerve resulted in an average increase in growth rate of 26 to 30 percent. Teeth so denervated appeared microscopically normal, except for a decrease in nerve fibers in the periodontal tissue and pulp cavity. Sympathetic denervation in the rats had no effect on tooth growth, despite contrary results observed in guinea pigs. Likewise, removal of the rat's otic ganglion had no effect upon the rate of growth. Thus, Butcher and Taylor surmised that the role of the inferior alveolar nerve was due to is sensory fibers, since the autonomic system had no apparent influence. They hypothesized that the phenomenon was due to sensory impulses conducted from the tooth by the inferior alveolar nerve whenever the tooth met its antagonist in occlusion. This suggested the presence of a feedback system where lack of sensory impulse served as a stimulus to additional growth and presence of sensory impulse served to inhibit additional growth. A loss of the sensory nerve, then, would render the animal unable to detect normal occlusion of the tooth or injury to the tooth.

This hypothesis was tested by artificially altering the physical stress upon a tooth by adjusting its shape. When all occlusal stress was relieved by repeated fracture of the incisor, eruption rate was accelerated. Extrusion rate was increased in every case of relieved functional pressure, and the increase reached a maximum of 200 percent above normal with prolonged repeated fracture. This was considered to be the maximum growth potential of the tooth. When the tooth was allowed to resume normal contact with its antagonist, there was an immediate return of growth rate to the normal levels. Rapidly erupting teeth were found to be abnormal in cross-sectional appearance, with decreased content of dentin and enamel and a widely dilated pulp cavity. Individual odontoblasts and ameloblasts, however, were found to be normal.

Finally, the consistency of the diet and its relation to functional stress were considered, and the results further supported the sensory feedback hypothesis. The standard consistency diet of all experiments was Purina Dog Chow. To prevent fracture and grinding, a soft consistency diet of cornmeal was used; to promote fracture and grinding, a hard consistency diet of whole kernel corn was used. When animals were placed on the soft consistency diet, eruption rate decreased 20 percent from the normal value of 0.5 mm/day. The rate gradually returned to normal when the animals were returned to the dog chow.

Similarly, eruption rate increased when the rats were fed whole kernel corn, a food that caused increased fracture and grinding. The overall difference in eruption rate from the hard to soft consistency diets was 35 percent.

Thus, the work of Butcher and Taylor shifted the focus of attention from the circulatory system to the nervous system and was largely responsible for the direction and emphasis of future research. To date, no major evidence in opposition to the theory of Butcher and Taylor has been found.

1. Vasodilator nerve fibers that innervate teeth in mammals are found in

   A. the trigeminal nerve.
   B. the otic ganglion.
   C. the cervical sympathetic chain.
   D. the inferior alveolar nerve.
   E. the superior alveolar nerves.

2. Since the work of Butcher and Taylor, the accepted theory for control of tooth eruption rate has been based upon

   A. sensory nerve feedback.
   B. blood supply.
   C. the role of odontoblasts.
   D. the role of ameloblasts.
   E. None of the above

3. In the experiment described in the passage, when a rat on a soft diet was returned to the standard consistency diet, its tooth growth rate

   A. remained depressed.
   B. immediately returned to normal.
   C. gradually returned to normal.
   D. remained elevated.
   E. decreased even further.

4. Which of the following statements correctly summarizes the sensory feedback hypothesis of Butcher and Taylor?

   A. Lack of sensory impulse causes increased blood flow to the tooth.
   B. Lack of sensory impulse causes decreased tooth growth rate.
   C. Lack of sensory impulse causes gradual pulp ischemia.
   D. Lack of sensory impulse causes increased tooth growth rate.
   E. The absence of a feedback system allows for an increased tooth growth rate.

5. Teeth that are denervated by cutting the inferior alveolar nerve show

   A. an average decrease in growth rate of 30 percent.
   B. no change in normal growth rate.
   C. an average increase in growth rate of 45 percent.
   D. no change in microscopic appearance except for a proliferation of capillaries.
   E. no change in microscopic appearance except for a decrease in nerve fibers.

6. Removal of the otic ganglion in rats

   A. caused an immediate increase in growth rate.
   B. caused an immediate decrease in growth rate.
   C. caused a delayed decrease in growth rate.
   D. caused a delayed increase in growth rate.
   E. had no effect on growth rate.

7. Before 1951, tooth growth was commonly thought to be regulated by

   A. diet.
   B. physical stress.
   C. blood supply.
   D. innervation.
   E. both (C) and (D).

8. Which of the following would be most likely to cause the greatest increase in blood supply to the teeth in mammals?

   A. A cervical sympathectomy
   B. Ligation of the common carotid artery
   C. Cutting the inferior alveolar nerve
   D. Removal of the otic ganglion
   E. Ligation of the inferior alveolar nerve

9. Based on information in the passage, which of the following statements best defines the term *antagonistic teeth?*

   A. Two adjacent teeth on the upper jaw
   B. Two adjacent teeth on the lower jaw
   C. Two teeth with opposite functional properties
   D. One tooth on the upper jaw, one on the lower
   E. Upper and lower teeth that meet in normal biting

10. According to the author, odontoblasts are responsible for the production of

    A. enamel.
    B. dentin.
    C. pulp.
    D. gingival tissue.
    E. dentin and enamel.

11. In the experiments on normal adult rats, significant incisor growth could be measured within

    A. 24 hours.
    B. 48 hours.
    C. 72 hours.
    D. 1 week.
    E. 2 weeks.

12. The greatest increase in eruption rate was achieved by

    A. altering the consistency of the diet.
    B. relieving the tooth of all functional stress.
    C. ligating the common carotid artery.
    D. removing the otic ganglion.
    E. returning the tooth to normal contact with its antagonist.

13. The central structure of the adult tooth is composed of

    A. epithelium.
    B. mineralized enamel.
    C. cementum.
    D. nerves and blood vessels.
    E. bone.

14. To destroy pain sensation in the teeth, which of the following nerves must be cut?

    A. The ninth cranial nerve
    B. The cervical sympathetic fibers
    C. The otic ganglion
    D. The glossopharyngeal nerve
    E. The inferior alveolar nerve

15. What observation was made about rat teeth that were permitted to grow at their maximum potential rate?
    A. They were more prone to fracture.
    B. They were lacking in nerve fibers.
    C. They had decreased amounts of dentin and enamel.
    D. They had unusually small pulp cavities.
    E. They appeared normal at the microscopic level.

16. Which of the following may be concluded from the observation of Butcher and Taylor?

    A. Teeth are more likely to fracture in older mammals.
    B. Occlusal stress may account for suppression of the maximum tooth growth rate.
    C. Mammals fed a "soft" diet will exhibit an increased number of ameloblasts.
    D. Occlusion involves only antagonistic teeth.
    E. Circulation plays a critical role in the regulation of tooth growth.

17. Butcher and Taylor's findings on the effects of dietary consistency upon tooth growth rate

    A. are inconsistent with the hypothesis of a sensory feedback system.
    B. show that consistency of the diet has little effect on rate of tooth eruption in rats, even if the diet consists solely of Purina Dog Chow.
    C. suggest that a mechanism other than sensory feedback affects tooth growth rate.
    D. are irrelevant, since rats would never duplicate the experimental diet under normal circumstances.
    E. indicate that tooth growth rate is affected by more than one factor.

Since estimates of future population growth are based on projections regarding complex and changeable social factors, it is not surprising to find that the estimates are often markedly inaccurate. For several decades following World War II, unprecedented population growth in the United States exceeded all projections. A 1947 Census Bureau prediction of the U.S. population in 1970, for example, underestimated the actual 1970 population by 65 million, falling far short of the count of 205 million that year. Today, predicting population growth is still an inexact science, but discrepancies often stem from overestimation rather than underestimation. Only a few years ago, demographers projected that our national population would reach the 300 million mark in the year 2000, but even after the turn of the century, the nation's population has not reached that mark. Such discrepancies stem from the fact that population predictions involve a certain amount of guesswork. The complexity and variability of social and economic factors involved in predicting population make the enterprise one of educated speculation.

Population predictions are based primarily upon studies of the "total fertility rate" of a country, defined as the average number of births a woman is expected to have over the course of her reproductive life. This rate is related to the "replacement level," a constant that describes the fertility rate at which a population neither grows nor declines. Today, the U.S. fertility rate is 1.7, considerably less than the replacement level of 2.1, so our population is expected to decrease. While demographers differ on exactly why and to what extent this diminution will occur, many agree that the decline in fertility is related to changes in the status and expectations of women.

Radical and rapid changes in attitudes toward marriage and family partly explain recent unanticipated declines in the rate of U.S. population growth. In the past few decades, there has been a considerable decline in the number of women who marry young. In 1960, only 29 percent of women under 24 had never married; by 1978, that percentage had jumped to 48 percent. This seems related to the tendency for unmarried couples to postpone marriage and live together, an arrangement that has become increasingly popular in recent years. Whether cohabitation is a likely prelude to marriage or an indication of a basic change in attitudes toward that institution, it is clear that cohabitation results in lower fertility than does marriage. Growing instability of marital relationships also affects fertility rates: As marriage rates have declined, divorce rates have increased, with half of all American marriages ending in divorce.

The shifting economic role that women play in society also effects childbearing. The relationship between fertility and the growing participation of women in the workplace is complex. A few demographers actually suggest that there is a positive correlation between women's working and fertility; this school of thought speculates that because increased prosperity positively affects fertility, women's economic gains will result in boosted fertility rates. But most demographers agree that work and fertility are negatively correlated in women. Some believe that women will have fewer children in order to facilitate their ability to join the workforce and gain financial stability. Others claim that, at the same time as increasingly effective methods of contraception have given women greater control over their own childbearing, the growing financial independence of women has weakened the economic rationale for marriage. This theory suggests that marriage offers women financial security in return for their childbearing and housekeeping services. Thus, if women no longer need to "barter" for economic support, childbearing becomes less of an automatic and expected social response.

In addition to the changing attitudes and status of women, even larger, more sweeping processes are at work in declining birthrates. Broad societal trends, including increasing urbanization and decreasing religiosity, are playing a significant role in lowering fertility rates. Migration to urban areas, for instance, has stripped away a powerful economic incentive for childbearing. In agrarian economies, there is a need for large families, as children play an important role in agricultural production. But in industrial economies, children are—in an economic

sense—burdens, as they consume limited resources without producing much in return.

Similarly, declining subscription to traditional religious values weakens the emphasis formerly placed upon and reduces attachment to family and childbearing. Some demographers have argued that the spread of evangelical religious movements, with their strong emphasis on traditional values, may eventually reverse this trend, but this seems doubtful. While these movements are certainly attracting an increasing number of adherents, they appeal mainly to rural elements of the population. Put differently, evangelical movements tend to attract people who are already very religious, so it is unlikely that their ultimate impact on demographic trends will be significant.

Hence, most demographers now agree that a declining birthrate is a long-term feature of U.S. society, especially since there does not appear to be any sense of urgency about altering the status quo. Indeed, the general belief about desirable population levels in this country was best summed up by the Commission on Population Growth and the American Future, which concluded that declining fertility was a positive development, since it may—in sheer terms of numbers—help to alleviate many of our most pressing social and economic problems.

Consequently, the United States has expressed no interest in pronatalist policies. In contrast, many nations in both Eastern and Western Europe have instituted a wide variety of pronatalist measures. In most instances, national security was cited as the reason for their introduction—demographic projections for many of these nations predicted rapid falls in population by the 21st century. Whatever the case, pronatalist polices led to an almost immediate rise in European birthrates. In former East Germany, for example, the birthrate went from 10.6 per 1,000 inhabitants in 1975 to 13.3 in 1977. Most of these countries have thus far restricted themselves mainly to liberal economic measures, such as family cash allowances, generous tax relief, subsidized child care services, and improved housing.

Should the U.S. government ever decide that the declining birthrate has become a threat to the nation's well-being, it may very well take steps to encourage population growth similar to those adopted by European countries. If that were to occur, once again demographers would have to revise drastically today's population predictions.

18. According to the passage, in 1947 the Census Bureau estimated that the 1970 U.S. population would be

    A. 205 million.
    B. 65 million.
    C. 283 million.
    D. 140 million.
    E. 270 million.

19. Which of the following statements best expresses the author's opinion about the relationship between marriage and the economic status of women?

    A. Lower economic status generally results in reduced fertility.
    B. Working women give birth to fewer children than do nonworking women.
    C. The effect of women's economic position on fertility has not yet been determined.
    D. Women who receive economic support tend to exhibit lower fertility rates.
    E. Urban women of lower economic status have higher birth rates than do rural women of lower economic status.

20. The "replacement level" is defined as

    A. the number of births the average woman has over her lifetime.
    B. the difference between a nation's birth and death rates.
    C. the birthrate necessary to ensure population growth.
    D. the number of deaths that must occur in order to keep the population from increasing.
    E. the birthrate at which a nation's population will remain stable.

21. Which of the following "total fertility rates" would most probably signal an increase in U.S. population?

    A. 2.0
    B. 1.7
    C. 1.8
    D. 2.1
    E. 2.4

22. The author mentions the increasingly popular trend of cohabitation in order to

    A. make a generalization about shifting moral values.
    B. support the claim that marriage is losing its economic rationale.
    C. provide an example of a social factor that contributes to lower fertility rates.
    D. underscore the relationship between cohabitation and increased divorce rates.
    E. recommend it as a guarantor of increased fertility.

23. Which of the following would most demographers probably NOT consider a factor in decreasing fertility rates?

   A. Increasingly effective methods of birth control
   B. Greater societal acceptance of childless marriages
   C. Growing demand for women in the workplace
   D. Liberalized attitudes toward unwed motherhood
   E. An increasing divorce rate

24. It can be inferred from the author's discussion of the economic rationale for marriage that

   A. the institution of marriage has generally lost its romantic veneer.
   B. women seek financial security when choosing husbands.
   C. romantic illusions often mask exploitive financial relationships.
   D. marriage is an idyllic state of shared responsibility.
   E. some demographers consider marriage primarily an economic relationship.

25. Which of the following is the most appropriate title for the passage?

   A. Decline in Birthrate Illustrates New Social Realities
   B. Growth Rate Falls as Women's Economic Status Improves
   C. Demographers Admit Futility of Population Prediction
   D. Shifting Social Values Lessen Nation's Social and Economic Ills
   E. New Women's Attitudes and National Birthrate Trends

26. According to the passage, the Commission on Population Growth and the American Future concluded that declining fertility will

   A. harm our national security.
   B. improve our quality of life.
   C. make our political problems more severe.
   D. convince our government to adopt pronatalist policies.
   E. escalate the divorce rate.

27. Which of the following is NOT mentioned in the passage as a pronatalist measure?

   A. Tax relief
   B. Cash allowances
   C. Subsidized child care
   D. Land grants
   E. Improved housing

28. According to most demographers, the U.S. birthrate will

   A. decline for a few more years but then increase.
   B. decline steadily for the indefinite future.
   C. increase over the next decade but then decline.
   D. increase drastically over the next couple of centuries.
   E. remain stable, without decline or increase.

29. The primary purpose of the first paragraph is to

   A. suggest that demographers are poor statisticians.
   B. argue that predicting population is difficult.
   C. prove that Census Bureau figures are highly accurate.
   D. discuss the social and economic factors that affect population estimates.
   E. analyze the Census Bureau's prediction of the U.S. population in 1970.

30. Many European nations have adopted pronatalist measures because

    A. their immigrant populations are expanding at alarming rates.
    B. they want to encourage long-term economic growth.
    C. they wish to reflect American pronatalist policies.
    D. their populations are heavily influenced by traditional religious values.
    E. they believe that population levels affect national security.

31. Rural families tend to be larger than their urban counterparts. The passage implies that this is because

    A. children are important as productive members of agrarian economies.
    B. rural couples are more likely to be traditional and religious.
    C. women are less likely to pursue careers in an agrarian environment.
    D. rural couples experience less difficulty conceiving than urban couples.
    E. urban couples are better educated about the use of contraception.

32. The author believes that the growth of evangelical religious movements will

    A. eventually lead to an upswing in the U.S. birthrate.
    B. cause an immediate drop in the U.S. birthrate.
    C. have no real impact on the U.S. birthrate.
    D. cause an upswing in the U.S. birthrate initially but a drop in the long run.
    E. cause an eventual decline in the U.S. birthrate.

33. The passage suggests that, in the future, young women will become

    A. more interested in marrying at a young age.
    B. less likely to give birth out of wedlock.
    C. more interested in pursuing a career.
    D. less interested in being financially independent.
    E. uninterested in maintaining a long-term career.

34. The author suggests that current population predictions

    A. are extremely accurate.
    B. overestimate the actual population.
    C. underestimate the actual population.
    D. ignore the growth of illegal immigrant populations.
    E. are anomalous in their inaccuracy.

Adequate nutrition is essential to the development, growth, and sustenance of the human organism. A good diet must supply the body with sufficient energy to power all life support activities. Amino acids play an important role in this dietary process.

The amino acid molecule is composed of an amino group ($-NH_2$), a carboxyl group (-COOH), a hydrogen atom (-H), and a unique R group (or side chain), all bonded to a central alpha carbon atom (C). Although amino acids occur in two stereoisomeric forms, D- (dextrorotary) and L- (levorotary), only the L-form is nutritionally active in the human body. There are twenty L-amino acids in total, each identifiable by its side chains, which differ in terms of size, shape, charge, hydrogen-bonding capacity, and chemical reactivity.

The primary role of L-amino acids is to provide the biologically active building blocks for proteins. Proteins are formed when groups of amino acids become linked in polypeptide chains. Peptide bonds are formed between the alpha-carboxyl group of one amino acid and the alpha-amino group of the next. These polypeptide chains link in turn to become proteins—in certain cells, they become the precursors of neurotransmitters, skin pigments, or hormones. All twenty amino acids must be present for the complete range of body proteins to be synthesized. The human body is capable of synthesizing several amino acids, such as alanine, glutamate, and proline, and these are classified as nonessential in dietary terms. Others, however, designated essential amino acids, must be supplied in the diet. The absence of any single amino acid disrupts protein synthesis and can result in a negative nitrogen balance within the body. When this occurs, protein degradation exceeds protein synthesis, and the body excretes a greater quantity of nitrogen than it ingests to replace it.

The body obtains essential amino acids by extracting them from food proteins in the digestive process, which begins in the stomach. Firstly, the oxyntic (parietal) cells of the fundic gastric glands lower the pH level of the stomach by secreting 0.15m HCl into the stomach. Zymogenic (chief) cells secrete quantities of pepsin, the first proteolytic enzyme to break down the ingested proteins, as well as rennin, an enzyme that curdles milk. The pepsin is secreted in an inactive form (pepsinogen) and is converted to the active enzymatic form by the HCl acid. In this state, it catalyzes the hydrolysis of the peptide bonds between amino acids within the proteins.

The majority of protein degradation and absorption occurs in the small intestine. The two primary proteolytic enzymes of the small intestine are trypsin and chymotrypsin. Trypsin breaks polypeptide chains on the carboxyl side of arginine and lysine residues. Chymotrypsin, on the other hand, cleaves preferentially on the carboxyl side of aromatic and other bulky nonpolar amino acids.

The major end products of digestion are L-amino acids, which are absorbed by the intestinal mucosa cells through a complex transport mechanism. First, a basolateral membrane Na^+-K^+-ATPase pump (powered by cellular ATP) sets up a favorable concentration gradient, where the concentration of sodium ions is greater outside the cell than inside. Then, as sodium ions diffuse into the cell, L-amino acids are transported simultaneously with sodium ions across the cell membrane.

The intestinal mucosal cells are also capable of absorbing dipeptides and tripeptides; their microvillus membranes contain enzymes that specifically split off dipeptides from the amino terminal end of protein polypeptide chains prior to absorption. All of the amino acids absorbed from the lumen of the intestine are then transported by the mucosal cells into the blood, where they proceed to the liver via the hepatic portal system. Any excess of absorbed amino acids, above that required for protein synthesis, is not stored in the body is much too valuable to be excreted. Instead, surplus amino acids are degraded in the liver and utilized as metabolic fuel.

Amino acid degradation primarily involves conversion of the alpha-amino group to urea. This group is transferred to the molecule alpha-ketoglutarate to form glutamate, which is subsequently oxidatively deaminated to the ammonium ion (NH_4^+) by the enzyme glutamate dehydrogenase, then converted via the enzymes of the urea cycle into the excretion product.

A special class of enzymes called transaminases catalyzes the transfer of the amino group from an alpha-amino acid to an alpha-keto acid, such as alpha-ketoglutarate. These transaminases require a prosthetic group (or coenzyme) called pyridoxal phosphate, which is derived from pyridoxine (vitamin B_6) to become active. The transaminase enzyme has a terminal lysine residue at its active site that combines with the aldehyde group of pyridoxal phosphate in a covalent Schiff-base linkage prior to the binding of the amino acid substrate. The transaminases form a new covalent Schiff-base intermediate with the alpha-amino group of the amino acid, which displaces an epsilon-amino group of the enzyme's active site lysine. As a result of this reaction, the pyridoxal phosphate is converted to pyridoxamine phosphate, and the alpha-amino becomes an alpha-keto acid. The pyridoxamine phosphate-enzyme complex subsequently combines with alpha-ketoglutarate to yield glutamates and a regenerated pyridoxal phosphate enzyme. Other pyridoxal phosphate enzymes can catalyze decarboxylations, deaminations, racemizations, and aldol cleavages of amino acid substrates.

The main benefits of the transamination process are that it enables the glutamate formed to be oxidatively deaminated by glutamate dehydrogenase to regenerate alpha-ketoglutarate and thus form ammonium ions for the urea cycle. In this particular process, either NAD^+ or $NADP^+$ are energized with electrons to form NADH or NADPH respectively, and both can be used as electron carriers. NADH is an active electron carrier in the oxidative phosphorylation, which generates cellular ATP, whereas NADPH is more active in reductive biosynthesis.

The process of energy production is controlled by the enzyme glutamate dehydrogenase and the pre-existing cellular energy levels. It is an allosterically regulated enzyme (i.e., it is only active when low-energy precursors are present, such as ADP and GDP). Conversely, it is inhibited when high-energy molecules are in abundance, such as ATP and GTP. Thus, under low-energy states, surplus amino acids can generate high-energy molecules and raise the caloric content in the body. In contrast, amino acid carbon skeletons are transformed into acetyl-CoA, pyruvate, or one of the intermediates of the citric acid cycle. The citric acid cycle is the final common route of oxidation of fuel molecules such as carbohydrates, fatty acids, and amino acids. The reactions of this cycle occur within the cells' mitochondria, and most fuel molecules enter as acetyl-CoA. However, some amino acids enter the cycle in the form of intermediates. Phenylalanine (derived from phenylpyruvate) is degraded to tyrosine by phenylalanine hydroxylase, and tyrosine is further transaminated back to p-hydroxyphenylpyruvate (the precursor of tyrosine), which is in turn oxidized to homogentisate. Homogentisate oxidase then converts homogentisate to 4-maleylacetoacetate, which is subsequently isomerized and hydrolyzed to become acetoacetate and fumarate, a cycle intermediate.

Those amino acids that are degraded to acetyl-CoA or acetoacetyl-CoA are called ketogenic and ultimately may also give rise to the ketone bodies acetone, d-3-hydroxybutyrate, and acetoacetate, which is a preferred fuel of heart muscle and renal cortex cells. Other amino acids are called glucogenic because they are degraded to pyruvate and fumarate or oxaloacetate. Of all the twenty acids, only leucine is purely ketogenic, while isoleucine, lysine, phenylalanine, tryptophan, and tyrosine are both ketogenic and glucogenic. The remaining fourteen amino acids are purely glucogenic.

35. Negative nitrogen balance is a state in the body in which

    A. essential amino acids are absent.
    B. protein synthesis exceeds protein degradation.
    C. protein degradation exceeds protein synthesis.
    D. the body ingests too much nitrogen.
    E. Both (A) and (C) are correct.

36. When the alpha-carboxyl group of one amino acid is bonded to the alpha-amino group of the subsequent amino acid, this is called

    A. a hydrogen bond.
    B. a polar covalent.
    C. a nonpolar covalent bond.
    D. a peptide bond.
    E. an ionic bond.

37. The low pH of the stomach is provided by the

    A. secretion of 0.25M HCl by chief cells.
    B. secretion of 0.15M HCl by parietal cells.
    C. secretion of 0.15M phosphoric acid by oxyntic cells.
    D. secretion of 10M HCl by oxyntic cells.
    E. secretion of 0.15M HCl by zymogenic cells.

38. In the process of absorption, an *L*-amino acid is cotransported with

    A. a K^+ ion.
    B. a Cl^- ion.
    C. a Na^+ ion.
    D. a Na^+ and a Cl^- ion simultaneously.
    E. a glucose molecule.

39. Transamination is the enzymatic process

    A. of transferring the alpha-amino group of an alpha-amino acid to an alpha-keto acid.
    B. of transferring the alpha-amino group of an alpha-keto acid to an alpha-amino acid.
    C. of transferring the carboxyl group of an alpha-amino acid to a lysine residue.
    D. used to split and transfer a carboxyl group from an alpha-amino acid to an alpha-keto acid.
    E. used to create pyridoxine.

40. Which of the following amino acids is purely ketogenic?

    A. Tyrosine
    B. Phenylalanine
    C. Leucine
    D. Isoleucine
    E. Tryptophan

41. Ketone bodies are

    A. *d*-3-hydroxybutyrate molecules.
    B. acetone molecules.
    C. used by renal and heart cells as fuel.
    D. products of degradation.
    E. All of the above

42. Pyridoxal phosphate enzymes

    A. can only catalyze transaminations.
    B. catalyze aldol cleavages of amino acids.
    C. catalyze carboxylations of amino acids.
    D. All of the above
    E. None of the above

43. The bond formed by a transaminase and its coenzyme
    A. is a covalent Schiff-base reaction.
    B. is a noncovalent Schiff-base reaction.
    C. occurs between a lysine residue of the enzyme and an aldehyde group of the coenzyme.
    D. occurs between a tyrosine residue of the enzyme and a carboxyl group of the coenzyme.
    E. Both (A) and (C) are correct.

44. The main benefit of transamination is
    A. conversion of coenzyme to NH_4^+.
    B. decrease in the caloric content of the body.
    C. generation of GDP and ADP.
    D. generation of NADH to participate in oxidative phosphorylation.
    E. the catabolism of ammonium ions.

45. The main site of amino acid degradation in the body is
    A. the pancreas.
    B. the stomach.
    C. the small intestine.
    D. the liver.
    E. the gall bladder.

46. Side chains of amino acids differ in regard to which of the following?
    A. Size
    B. Hydrogen-binding capacity
    C. Shape
    D. Charge
    E. All of the above

47. The enzyme glutamate dehydrogenase is allosterically regulated, such that
    A. an increase in GTP and ATP levels activates the enzyme.
    B. an increase in YUTP and GTP levels activates the enzyme.
    C. an increase in GDP and ADP levels activates the enzyme.
    D. only an increase in UTP activates the enzyme.
    E. only a decrease in UTP activates the enzyme.

48. Trypsin and chymotrypsin cleave protein polypeptide chains at or between
    A. the same site.
    B. different sites.
    C. arginine and lysine residues for trypsin and aromatic residues for chymotrypsin.
    D. (A), (B), and (C) are correct.
    E. Both (B) and (C) are correct.

49. Amino acid degradation involves
    A. transamination.
    B. change of amino acids to acetyl-CoA and acetoacetyl-CoA.
    C. change of amino acids to pyruvate and fumarate.
    D. conversion of the alpha-amino group to urea.
    E. All of the above

50. Which of the following compounds can act as electron carriers in oxidative phosphorylation?
    A. $NADP^+$
    B. NAD^+
    C. Both $NADP^+$ and NAD^+
    D. ATP
    E. None of the above

STOP! END OF TEST.

Reading Comprehension Practice Test: Answers and Explanations

ANSWER KEY

1.	B	26.	B
2.	A	27.	D
3.	C	28.	B
4.	D	29.	B
5.	E	30.	E
6.	E	31.	A
7.	C	32.	C
8.	A	33.	C
9.	E	34.	B
10.	B	35.	E
11.	C	36.	D
12.	B	37.	B
13.	D	38.	C
14.	E	39.	A
15.	C	40.	C
16.	B	41.	E
17.	E	42.	B
18.	D	43.	E
19.	B	44.	D
20.	E	45.	D
21.	E	46.	E
22.	C	47.	C
23.	D	48.	E
24.	E	49.	E
25.	A	50.	C

EXPLANATIONS

1. B The passage states that the vasodilator nerve fibers are parasympathetic fibers found in the otic ganglion of the glossopharyngeal nerve, making choice (B) correct. They are not found in the inferior alveolar nerve, the superior alveolar nerve, a branch of the trigeminal nerve, or the cervical sympathetic chain. Thus, answer choices (A), (C), (D), and (E) are all incorrect.

2. A Each of the five factors (blood supply, innervation, shape of the tooth, physical stress, and the consistency of the diet) that Butcher and Taylor examined pointed to sensory nerve feedback, choice (A), as the predominant controller of

the rate of tooth growth. While the blood supply was thought at one point in time to be important in tooth eruption, Taylor and Butcher concluded that it was not the most important regulatory factor. In addition, the accepted theory for control of tooth eruption rate since Butcher and Taylor has not been based in the roles of odontoblasts or of ameloblasts.

3. C Although animals who were placed on a soft consistency diet experienced decreases of tooth eruption rate of up to 20 percent from the normal value of 0.5 mm/day, the passage states that the animals' eruption rates gradually returned to normal when the animals returned to the dog chow (the standard consistency diet).

4. D The passage states that Butcher and Taylor surmised that the sensory fibers of the inferior alveolar nerve would provide a feedback system where a lack of sensory impulse would serve as a stimulus for a tooth to grow—choice (D) and, conversely, the presence of a sensory impulse would serve to inhibit a tooth's growth. The sensory feedback hypothesis did not address the lack of sensory impulses and their relation to blood flow or ischemia.

5. E After cutting the inferior alveolar nerve, Butcher and Taylor discovered that teeth demonstrated an average increase in growth rate of 26–30 percent, not 45 percent as in choice (C). When examined microscopically, these teeth were normal except for a decrease in nerve fibers. Therefore, choice (D) is incorrect.

6. E In contrast to the question above, denervation of the otic ganglion had no effect on growth rate. Butcher and Taylor surmised that this was due to the presence of sensory fibers in the inferior alveolar nerve that were not present in the autonomic nerves.

7. C The passage states that prior to 1951 and subsequent to 1927, the most commonly accepted theory of tooth growth was the one proposed by Leist—that blood supply was the important regulatory influence. Although innervation was considered at one time, it is not the optimal answer because in the years pursuant to 1951, blood supply was more highly considered. Physical stress and diet were never thought to be extremely important regulators of tooth growth.

8. A The passage states that following cervical sympathectomy, a secondary hyperemia (increase in blood flow to the site of innervation) occurs. Therefore, choice (A) would be most correct. Ligation of the common carotid artery would decrease the amount of blood flow to teeth, and the denervation of the inferior alveolar nerve would have little to do with blood supply. Finally, the removal of the otic ganglion may actually decrease the amount of blood to the teeth due to the presence of parasympathetic autonomic nerve fibers.

9. E The use of the word *antagonist* in the passage refers to a tooth that makes normal contact with another. Therefore, answer choice (E) is most correct. While the word *antagonists* might conjure up images of teeth with opposite functional properties—choice (C), it was not used in this context in the passage. Clearly, answer choices (A) and (B) are incorrect; they are not mentioned as valid choices in the passage. Finally, answer choice (D) is too vague—choice (E) is far more accurate.

10. B The author states that odontoblasts are responsible for the production of dentin and that ameloblasts are responsible for the production of enamel. The pulp is littered with neural and vascular supply, and the author does not mention the origin of gingival tissue.

11. C The passage states that eruption (the extrusion of a tooth into the oral cavity) was measured by examining the distance between the notch (cut initially at the gingival crest) and the gingival crest after a period of a few days (during which time the tooth was allowed to grow). Three days, or 72 hours, is the best choice.

12. B The passage states that ligating the common carotid artery or removing the otic ganglion did nothing to affect the eruption rate. Altering the consistency of the diet, while affecting the eruption rate slightly, could not compare to relieving the tooth of all functional stress (which was shown to increase eruption by 200 percent). Finally, returning the tooth to normal contact with its antagonist reinstituted normal growth rates.

13. D The passage specifically states that the central pulp cavity of a tooth contains the neural and vascular supply. The mineralized enamel is a layer that covers the dentin, which in turn surrounds the central pulp cavity. No mention is made of cementum or bone in the composition of the central structure of the adult tooth.

14. E The inferior alveolar nerve carries sensory nerve fibers that the cervical sympathetic fibers and the otic ganglion do not. While the glossopharyngeal nerve does have sensory fibers, this nerve does not innervate the teeth. Therefore, the inferior alveolar nerve is the most correct answer.

15. C The passage states that Butcher and Taylor found that rapidly erupting teeth were abnormal in cross-sectional appearance (thus, answer choice (E) is not correct). They possessed decreased contents of dentin and enamel—choice (C)—and a widely dilated pulp cavity (therefore, choice (D) is not correct). No mention was made of their propensity for fracture or their abundance of nerve fibers; therefore, these answers—choices (A) and (B)—are incorrect.

16. B According to the sensory feedback hypothesis proposed by Butcher and Taylor, it is the absence of sensory influences that causes an increase in the growth rate of teeth. No mention is made of tooth fracture and older mammals or of the occlusive ability of nonantagonistic teeth. Mammals fed on a "soft" diet exhibit a decrease in the eruption rate, indicating—if anything—a decrease in the number of ameloblasts.

17. E Butcher and Taylor's experiments revealed that both occlusal stress and diet consistency affected tooth eruption. This corresponds to many other findings in science, namely that they are multifactorial. The fact that dietary consistency affected tooth growth rate does not obviate the hypothesis of a sensory feedback system, nor does it suggest that a sole mechanism other than sensory feedback affects tooth growth rate. These diet consistency experiment results are relevant and should be examined from a multifactorial perspective.

18. D The passage states the census count for the year 1970 was 205 million people and that the 1947 Census Bureau prediction was 65 million short of that. Therefore, 140 million was the predicted number.

19. B Although the author concedes that some demographers believe that there is a positive correlation between women's working and fertility, he argues that most demographers agree that work and fertility are negatively correlated in women. He also believes that higher economic status of women generally results in reduced fertility and that women who receive economic support (i.e., are dependent upon it) tend to exhibit higher fertility rates. Finally, although the author states that higher economic status is associated with lower fertility, he never compares the fertility rates of women of lower economic status in rural and urban areas. One factor that immediately undermines this supposition is the indication that urbanization provides fewer incentives for childbearing and has thus played a role in lowering fertility rates.

20. E The passage defines "replacement level" as a birthrate at which a nation's population will remain stable (will neither decline nor grow). Note that the question stem refers to "replacement," which implies a need for production to fill a void (or births to fill the population void caused by deaths). Thus, one could automatically eliminate choice (D), which only focuses on deaths, and choice (C), which refers to actual growth, not just replacement. Choice (A) is incorrect, as well, as it refers to "total fertility rate" as defined in the passage, and choice (B) is incorrect as it refers to a measurement of a status quo, not of a determined "level."

21. E The total fertility rate of a country is defined as the average number of births a woman is expected to have over the course of her reproductive life. This rate is related to the replacement level (the fertility rate at which population remains stable), which is defined as 2.1 in the passage. As the total fertility rate must exceed the replacement rate for population growth to occur, the answer choice must be greater than 2.1. Choice (E) satisfies this requirement.

22. C The author cites cohabitation as an example of a social factor that contributes to lower fertility rates. She makes little judgment about shifting moral values; she does not support the claim that marriage is losing its economic rationale. In addition, the author never correlates cohabitation with increased divorce rates. Finally, cohabitation is anything but a guarantor of fertility, as the author indicates that it is more clearly associated with lower fertility rates than is marriage.

23. D The author cites several factors that demographers believe to be important in decreasing fertility rates. They include contraception, more women working, increased societal acceptance of one-parent families, and increased divorce rates. However, the author does not address the role of liberalized attitudes toward unwed motherhood, implying that it is not a factor.

24. E The passage discusses the rationale behind marriage in strictly economic terms and indicates that many demographers regard marriage in this way. While it might be argued that choice (B) is also correct, it is not, since it makes an assumption about all women's reasons for marriage—an inference that is too drastic. Note that choice (E) makes a less inclusive conclusion by referring to "some demographers." Finally, answers (A), (C), and (D) are poor choices because they are not addressed in the passage.

25. A Whether the author talks about urbanization, contraception, or cohabitation, it is clear that she is referring to the relationship of new social realities and decline in birthrate. While answer choice (B) is factually correct, it is a limited title because it does not include other causes of declining birthrates. The author does not deem population prediction futile; she only admits that it is an "enterprise of educated speculation." In addition, the author never correlates shifting social values with a lessening of the nation's social and economic ills. Finally, national birthrate trends are related not just to women's new attitudes but to other issues such as divorce, cohabitation, and contraception (all of which might or do involve men's attitudes, as well).

26. B   The passage states that the Commission on Population Growth and the American Future concluded that declining fertility was a positive development because it may help to alleviate many of our most pressing social and economic problems.

27. D   The passage mentions that European pronatalist policies included family cash allowances, generous tax relief, subsidized childcare services, and improved housing. There is no mention in the passage of land grants, choice (D).

28. B   The passage states that most demographers now agree that the present declining birthrate is a long-term feature of U.S. society, especially since there does not appear to be any sense of urgency about altering the status quo.

29. B   The purpose of the first paragraph can be identified in its last sentence, which states, "The complexity and variability of social and economic factors involved in predicting population make the enterprise one of educated speculation." In other words, it is difficult. The paragraph never states that demographers are poor statisticians. Rather, it says population growth prediction is an inexact science. And, on the contrary, it reveals the inaccuracy of Census Bureau figures. Finally, while the paragraph mentions social and economic factors, as well as the Census Bureau's prediction of the 1970 U.S. population, it does not focus on any of these points as its central purpose.

30. E   The passage states that in most instances, European pronatalist policies have been introduced for reasons of national security. Thus, choice (E) is the most directly applicable choice.

31. A   The author states that rural families have higher fertility rates than urban families. This is, she argues, because in agrarian (i.e., more rural) economies, children play an important role in agricultural production and are thus necessities of life. While it may be that rural couples are more likely to be traditional and religious, this cannot be argued from the passage. Further, the passage provides no indication that women are less likely to pursue careers in rural areas, that rural couples experience less difficulty conceiving than urban couples, or that urban couples are better educated about contraception.

32. C   The author does correlate a decline in subscription to religious values with a reduced attachment to childbearing, which would imply that an extension of religious values through evangelism would potentially increase birthrates. However, the author specifically indicates that "evangelical movements tend to attract people who are already very religious," or who already embrace values of family and childbearing. Thus, evangelism, according to the passage, causes neither an increase nor decline in the birthrate.

33. C   The author claims that there is a growing financial independence of women owing to an increased number of women in the workplace. Therefore, it follows that women will be less interested in marrying at a young age, more likely to give birth out of wedlock, more interested in remaining financially independent, and more interested in maintaining a long-term career. These are the opposite responses seen in choice (A), (B), (D), and (E), respectively.

34. B   The first paragraph of the passage states that discrepancies in current population predictions for the year 2000 reflect an overestimation rather than an underestimation. Thus, choices (A) and (C) are automatically eliminated as possibilities. In terms of choice (D), the author never indicates that current population predictions fail to account for the growth of illegal immigrant populations. Finally, the author's description of the 1947 overestimation of the population for 1970 indicates that present overestimations in prediction are not anomalous.

35. E The passage defines nitrogen balance as a process in which protein degradation exceeds protein synthesis, so the body excretes a greater quantity of nitrogen than it ingests to replace it. In this state, essential amino acids are absent, making choice (E) the most correct one.

36. D The passage states that peptide bonds are formed between the alpha-carboxyl group of one amino acid and the alpha-amino group of another. Therefore, choice (D) is most correct.

37. B The passage states that the first process in gastric digestion of food is the secretion of 0.15 M HCl from the oxyntic, or parietal, cells of the fundic stomach. Therefore, choice (B) is most correct.

38. C The passage states that end products of digestion—L-amino acids—are absorbed by the intestinal mucosal cells via a complex transport mechanism that involves cotransport of sodium ion. It makes no mention of the simultaneous transport of chloride ions, making choice (C) optimal.

39. A Transamination, mediated by enzymes called transaminases, catalyzes the transfer of amino groups from alpha amino acids to alpha-keto acids (e.g., alpha-ketoglutarate).

40. C The last few sentences of the passage categorize amino acids, which are either gluconeogenic, ketogenic, or both. Leucine is the only ketogenic amino acid; therefore, choice (C) is the correct answer.

41. E All of the answer choices work. Amino acids that are degraded to acetyl-CoA or acetoacetyl-CoA are considered ketogenic. They may give rise to D-3-hydroxybutyrate, acetone molecules, and acetoacetate. They are the preferred fuel of cardiac muscle and renal cortical cells; thus, choice (E) is correct.

42. B Pyridoxal phosphate enzymes may cause transamination, decarboxylation deamination, racemization, and aldol cleavage of amino acids. Therefore, choice (B) is correct.

43. E The bond between pyridoxal phosphate and a transaminase occurs at a terminal lysine residue. The bond is a Schiff-base linkage, which is covalent in property. Therefore, choice (E) correct.

44. D According to the passage, the main benefit of the transamination process is that it enables the glutamate formed to be oxidatively deaminated (by glutamate dehydrogenase) to regenerate alpha-ketoglutarate. This results in the formation of ammonium ions (from the glutamate, not the coenzyme pyridoxal phosphate) for the urea cycle and the regeneration of NADH and NADPH (involved in oxidative phosphorylation and reductive biosynthesis, respectively). Therefore, answer choice (D) is correct.

45. D The passage states that the main degradation site of amino acids is in the liver, although the main absorption site is the small intestine. Therefore, choice (D) is correct.

46. E The passage states the differences in amino acids are in their side chains, which themselves differ in size, shape, charge, hydrogen bonding capacity, and chemical reactivity. The passage does not indicate that side chains differ in carbon-binding capacity or number. Therefore, choice (E) is correct.

47. C The passage states that glutamate dehydrogenase is an allosterically regulated enzyme that is active only when low-energy precursors are present, such as ADP and GDP. In contrast, the activity of glutamate dehydrogenase is low when ATP and GTP are present. Therefore, choice (C) is correct.

48. E The passage states that trypsin breaks polypeptide chains on the carboxyl side of arginine and lysine residues, while chymotrypsin cleaves preferentially on the carboxyl side of aromatic and other bulky, nonpolar amino acids. Therefore, choice (E) is correct.

49. E The passage states that amino acid degradation involves primarily the conversion of an alpha-amino group to urea. The alpha-amino group is initially transferred to the molecule alpha-ketoglutarate to form glutamate, which is oxidatively deaminated to form NH_4^+. The ammonium ion is then converted to an excretion product and launched into the urea cycle. Amino acid skeletons may be converted to acetyl-CoA, pyruvate, or one of the intermediates of the citric acid cycle (e.g., fumarate). Alternatively, for ketogenic amino acids, degradation may involve the formation of acetyl-CoA or acetoacetyl-Coa and may give rise to ketone bodies, such as acetone, 3-hydroxybutyrate, and acetoacetate. Therefore, choice (E) is correct.

50. C The passage states that while NADH is an active electron carrier in the oxidative phosphorylation that generates cellular ATP, NADPH is more active in reductive biosynthesis. However, this implies that NADPH has some activity in oxidative phosphorylation. Therefore, choice (C) is correct.

QUANTITATIVE REASONING

ARITHMETIC

FRACTIONS

A. FAST FRACTIONS OVERVIEW

$$\frac{7}{8} \quad \begin{array}{l}\leftarrow \text{Numerator}\\ \leftarrow \text{Denominator}\end{array}$$

Multiplying fractions: Multiply numerators by each other and denominators by each other.

$$\frac{3}{4} \times \frac{9}{7} = \frac{3 \times 9}{4 \times 7} = \frac{27}{28}$$

Dividing fractions: Flip the numerator and denominator of the fraction that you're dividing by, then multiply.

$$\frac{1}{5} \div \frac{4}{11} = \frac{1}{5} \times \frac{11}{4} = \frac{1 \times 11}{5 \times 4} = \frac{11}{20}$$

Adding fractions: You can add fractions only when they have the same denominator. When you add, add only the numerators, NOT the denominators.

$$\frac{2}{3} + \frac{5}{3} = \frac{2 + 5}{3} = \frac{7}{3}$$

If you don't have a common denominator, you have to find one. The fastest way to get a common denominator is to multiply each fraction by a fraction whose numerator and denominator are the same as the denominator of the other fraction. (You can do this because any fraction with the same numerator and denominator is equal to 1, and multiplying any number by 1 doesn't change the value of the number.)

$$\frac{1}{3} + \frac{2}{5} = \left(\frac{1}{3} \times \frac{5}{5}\right) + \left(\frac{2}{5} \times \frac{3}{3}\right) = \frac{5}{15} + \frac{6}{15} = \frac{11}{15}$$

Subtracting fractions: This works the same way as adding fractions, except you subtract the numerators instead of adding them.

$$\frac{6}{7} - \frac{1}{2} = \left(\frac{6}{7}\right)\left(\frac{2}{2}\right) - \left(\frac{1}{2}\right)\left(\frac{7}{7}\right) = \frac{12}{14} - \frac{7}{14} = \frac{5}{14}$$

Remember, parentheses can be used to indicate multiplication instead of the "×" sign.

Reducing fractions: Whenever there is a common factor in the numerator and denominator, you can reduce the fraction by removing the factor from both parts of the fraction. You can do this because dividing the numerator and denominator by the same number doesn't change the value of the fraction as a whole. This will often make working with the fraction much easier, because you'll be using smaller numbers.

$$\frac{4}{12} = \frac{1 \times 4}{3 \times 4} = \frac{1}{3} \times \frac{4}{4} = \frac{1}{3} \times 1 = \frac{1}{3}$$

Obviously, you don't have to write out all this math. We're just doing it to show you exactly what's going on. On the test, you should do easy fractions like these in one step like in the next example.

You can reduce $\dfrac{42}{28}$ by canceling like this:
$$\frac{\overset{6}{\cancel{42}}}{\underset{4}{\cancel{28}}} = \frac{\overset{3}{\cancel{6}}}{\underset{2}{\cancel{4}}} = \frac{3}{2}$$

Let's look more closely at how we reduced $\dfrac{42}{28}$. Since both 42 and 28 are divisible by 7, we can divide both the numerator (42) and the denominator (28) by 7. Thus $\dfrac{42}{28}$ was reduced to $\dfrac{6}{4}$. Since both 6 and 4 are divisible by 2, we can divide both the numerator (6) and the denominator (4) by 2. Thus $\dfrac{6}{4}$ was reduced to $\dfrac{3}{2}$.

Canceling: Whenever you have to multiply two or more fractions, you should cancel common factors before you multiply. This is a lot like reducing and has the same advantages. $\dfrac{1}{7} \times \dfrac{7}{3}$ can be cancelled like this:

$$\frac{1}{\cancel{7}} \times \frac{\overset{1}{\cancel{7}}}{3} = \frac{1}{1} \times \frac{1}{3} = \frac{1}{3}$$

$\dfrac{4}{5} \times \dfrac{15}{12}$ can be cancelled like this:

$$\frac{\overset{1}{\cancel{4}}}{\underset{1}{\cancel{5}}} \times \frac{\overset{3}{\cancel{15}}}{\underset{3}{\cancel{12}}} = \frac{1}{1} \times \frac{3}{3} = 1$$

Notice that we divided both the 5 in the denominator of the first fraction and the 15 in the numerator of the second fraction by 5. We also divided the 4 in the numerator of the first fraction and the 12 in the denominator of the second fraction by 4.

B. COMPARING FRACTIONS

One way to compare fractions is to re-express them with a **common denominator**: $\frac{3}{4} = \frac{21}{28}$ and $\frac{5}{7} = \frac{20}{28}$ because $\frac{21}{28}$ is greater than $\frac{20}{28}$, $\frac{3}{4}$ is greater than $\frac{5}{7}$. Another way to compare fractions is to convert them both to decimals: $\frac{3}{4}$ converts to 0.75, and $\frac{5}{7}$ converts to approximately 0.714.

C. MIXED NUMBERS AND IMPROPER FRACTIONS

A mixed number consists of an integer and a fraction. For example, $3\frac{1}{4}$, $12\frac{2}{5}$, and $5\frac{7}{8}$ are all mixed numbers.

To convert an improper fraction (a fraction whose numerator is greater than its denominator) to a mixed number, divide the numerator by the denominator. The number of "whole" times that the denominator goes into the numerator will be the integer portion of the improper fraction; the remainder will be the numerator of the fractional portion.

Example: Convert $\frac{23}{4}$ to a mixed number.

Dividing 23 by 4 gives you 5 with a remainder of 3, so $\frac{23}{4} = 5\frac{3}{4}$.

To change a mixed number to a fraction, keep the denominator of the fraction. To figure out the numerator, multiply the integer portion of the mixed number by the number in the denominator. Then add this result to the numerator of the mixed number.

Example: Convert $2\frac{3}{7}$ to a fraction.

$$2\frac{3}{7} = \frac{(2 \times 7) + 3}{7} = \frac{17}{7}$$

Example: Convert $5\frac{8}{9}$ to a fraction.

$$5\frac{8}{9} = \frac{(5 \times 9) + 8}{9} = \frac{53}{9}$$

D. ADDING AND SUBTRACTING MIXED NUMBERS

Adding or subtracting mixed numbers whose fractional parts have the same denominator will probably be on the test.

Example: $3\dfrac{12}{17} + 4\dfrac{10}{17} = ?$

First, add the integer parts: $3 + 4 = 7$.

Next, add the fractional parts: $\dfrac{12}{17} + \dfrac{10}{17} = \dfrac{22}{17}$.

Now, $\dfrac{22}{17} = 1\dfrac{5}{17}$.

Therefore, $3\dfrac{12}{17} + 4\dfrac{10}{17} = 7 + 1\dfrac{5}{17} = 8\dfrac{5}{17}$.

Example: $4\dfrac{5}{8} - 2\dfrac{7}{8} = ?$

The wrinkle here is that the fractional part of the first number is smaller than the fractional part of the second number (i.e., $\dfrac{5}{8}$ is smaller then $\dfrac{7}{8}$). What we need to do, therefore, is to borrow from the integer part of the first number to make the fractional part of the first number bigger. We'll borrow 1 from the integer part and add it to the fractional part (remembering that 1 can be rewritten as $\dfrac{8}{8}$).

So $4\dfrac{5}{8} = 3 + \dfrac{8}{8} + \dfrac{5}{8} = 3\dfrac{13}{8}$. So the problem of finding $4\dfrac{5}{8} - 2\dfrac{7}{8}$ has been replaced with the problem of finding $3\dfrac{13}{8} - 2\dfrac{7}{8}$, which is easier, because the fractional part of the first number is greater than the fractional part of the second number.

Notice that all we've done is replace $4\dfrac{5}{8}$ with $3\dfrac{13}{8}$, which is equal to $4\dfrac{5}{8}$. To find $3\dfrac{13}{8} - 2\dfrac{7}{8}$, first subtract the integer parts: $3 - 2 = 1$. Next subtract the fractional parts: $\dfrac{13}{8} - \dfrac{7}{8} = \dfrac{6}{8} = \dfrac{3}{4}$. So $4\dfrac{5}{8} - 2\dfrac{7}{8} = 1\dfrac{3}{4}$.

Example: $5\dfrac{1}{4} - 1\dfrac{3}{4} = ?$

$$5\dfrac{1}{4} - 1\dfrac{3}{4} = 5 + \dfrac{1}{4} - 1\dfrac{3}{4} = \left(4 + \dfrac{4}{4}\right) + \dfrac{1}{4} - 1\dfrac{3}{4} = 4\dfrac{5}{4} - 1\dfrac{3}{4} = 3\dfrac{2}{4} = 3\dfrac{1}{2}$$

When you gain experience with this, you'll be able to skip some of the steps and do this type of problem more quickly.

Example: $8\frac{3}{25} - 4\frac{12}{25} = ?$

$$8\frac{3}{25} - 4\frac{12}{25} = 7 + \frac{25}{25} + \frac{3}{25} - 4\frac{12}{25} = 7\frac{28}{25} - 4\frac{12}{25} = 3\frac{16}{25}$$

RATIOS

A. SETTING UP A RATIO

To find a ratio, put the number associated with the word *of* **on top** and the quantity associated with the word *to* **on the bottom** and reduce. The ratio of 20 oranges to 12 apples is $\frac{20}{12}$, which reduces to $\frac{5}{3}$.

B. PART-TO-PART RATIOS AND PART-TO-WHOLE RATIOS

If the parts add up to the whole, a part-to-part ratio can be turned into two part-to-whole ratios by putting each number in the original ratio over the sum of the numbers. If the ratio of males to females is 1 to 2, then the males-to-people ratio is $\frac{1}{1+2} = \frac{1}{3}$ and the females-to-people ratio is $\frac{2}{1+2} = \frac{2}{3}$. In other words, $\frac{2}{3}$ of all the people are female.

C. SOLVING A PROPORTION

To solve a proportion, **cross multiply:**

$$\frac{x}{5} = \frac{3}{4}$$
$$4x = 5 \times 3$$
$$x = \frac{15}{4} = 3.75$$

DECIMALS

There are two different ways to express numbers that are not integers: as fractions and as decimals. Fractions we've already discussed; now it's time to talk about decimals.

A. CHANGING FRACTIONS TO DECIMALS

It's easy to change a fraction into a decimal—all you do is divide the denominator of the fraction into the numerator.

Example: Change $\dfrac{415}{3,220}$ into a decimal.

First write the fraction as long division.

$$3,220\overline{)415}$$

Since 3,220 is much bigger than 415, what we do is add a zero to the 415 to make the division work out. The only way we can do this without changing the value of 415 is if we add a decimal point after the 5. Then we're just changing 415 to 415.00—and those zeros don't change the value of anything. We divide normally, but we put a decimal point in the quotient (the answer) directly above the decimal point in 415.

$$
\begin{array}{r}
.12 \\
3,220\overline{)415.000} \\
4150 \\
\underline{3220} \\
9330 \\
\underline{6440} \\
28600
\end{array}
$$

How far we should go depends on how much accuracy we need, but at this point, we can tell that the answer is going to be close to 0.13.

B. CHANGING DECIMALS TO FRACTIONS

How do you express 0.5 as a fraction? Well, 0.1 represents $\dfrac{1}{10}$, and 0.5 is five times as much as 0.1, so 0.5 must represent 5 times $\dfrac{1}{10}$ or $\dfrac{5}{10}$. Of course, we can reduce $\dfrac{5}{10}$ to $\dfrac{1}{2}$.

How do you express 0.55 as a fraction? Well—let's think of it in terms of dollars and cents. We know that $0.01 is one cent, and that's $\dfrac{1}{100}$ of a dollar. Then $0.55 is 55 cents, and that's 55 times as much, so $0.55 must be $\dfrac{55}{100}$ of a dollar. We can reduce this by dividing the top and bottom by 5, giving us $\dfrac{11}{20}$. That's the fractional equivalent of 0.55.

Hopefully by this point you recognize a pattern:

$$0.1 = 1 \times \frac{1}{10} \text{ or } \frac{1}{10}$$

$$0.11 = 11 \times \frac{1}{100} \text{ or } \frac{11}{100}$$

$$0.111 = 111 \times \frac{1}{1,000} \text{ or } \frac{111}{1,000}$$

$$0.1111 = 1,111 \times \frac{1}{10,000} \text{ or } \frac{1,111}{10,000}$$

and so on.

What we did on the previous page to change these decimals to fractions was to put the digits to the right of the decimal point in the numerator. To figure out the denominator, we put a 1 in the denominator and followed it with as many zeros as there were digits to the right of the decimal point.

Example: Change 0.564 to a fraction.

There are three digits to the right of the decimal point, so the denominator of our fraction will be 1,000 (a 1 followed by three zeros). The numerator of the fraction is 564.

$$0.564 = \frac{564}{1,000}$$

But notice that $\frac{564}{1,000}$ can be reduced. Since both 564 and 1,000 are divisible by 4, we can divide both the numerator and the denominator by 4; therefore, $\frac{564}{1,000} = \frac{564 \div 4}{1,000 \div 4} = \frac{141}{250}$.

C. ADDITION AND SUBTRACTION OF DECIMALS

You add and subtract decimals the same way you add and subtract whole numbers. Just make sure the decimal points are lined up, then add. In the answer, put the decimal point directly below the other decimal points.

$$0.456 + 1.234 = \begin{array}{r} 0.456 \\ + 1.234 \\ \hline 1.690 \end{array} = 1.69$$

If one of the terms you are adding or subtracting is longer than another (has more digits to the right of the decimal), it helps to add zeros to the shorter number.

$$6.97 - 3.567 = \begin{array}{r} 6.970 \\ - 3.567 \\ \hline 3.403 \end{array}$$

D. MULTIPLICATION OF DECIMALS

As with addition and subtraction, you multiply decimals as if they were whole numbers and worry about the decimal points later. You don't need to add zeros to make the numbers the same length when you multiply, however.

$$
\begin{array}{r}
4.5 \times 3.2 = 4.5 \\
\times\ 3.2 \\
\hline
9\,0 \\
1\,3\,5 \\
\hline
14.40
\end{array}
$$

To place the decimal point in the answer, count the number of digits to the right of the decimal point in each number. Here we have one decimal place in 4.5 and one in 3.2 for a total of 1 + 1 or 2 places. Put the decimal point two places from the right in the answer: 14.40.

It's a good idea when you get the answer to check that you put the decimal point in the right place by seeing if the answer makes sense. Here the answer should be a little bigger than 4×3, or 12. So 14.40 should be about right. If you had placed the decimal point incorrectly and ended up with 144, you would know that was wrong.

E. DIVISION OF DECIMALS

It's easiest to discuss division of decimals if we express the division in fractional form.

Example: $4.15 \div 32.2 = \dfrac{4.15}{32.2}$

Make both the numerator and the denominator of the fraction whole numbers; to do this, multiply both top and bottom by a sufficient power of 10. In our example, we need to multiply by 100; this will make the denominator 3,220 and the numerator 415. We're left with

$$
\frac{4.15}{32.2} = \frac{415}{3,220}
$$

Now divide 3,220 into 415.

F. ROUNDING DECIMALS TO THE NEAREST PLACE

To round a decimal to the nearest place, look at the digit immediately to the right of that place. If that digit is 5, 6, 7, 8, or 9, then round up the place you are rounding to. If the digit immediately to the right of the place you are rounding to is 0, 1, 2, 3, or 4, then don't change the digit at the place you are rounding to. In either case, in the rounded-off number, there will be no digits to the right of the place you are rounding off to.

Example: Round 0.12763 to the nearest thousandth.

The digit in the thousandths place is 7. The digit immediately to the right of the 7 is a 6. Since 6 is among the digits that are 5 or more, we round up the thousandths digits from 7 to 8. So 0.12763 rounded to the nearest thousandth is 0.128.

Example: Round 0.5827 to the nearest hundredth.

The digit in the hundredths place is 8. Immediately to the right of the 8 is a 2. Since 2 is among the digits 0 through 4, we keep the digit in the hundredths place the same. So 0.5827 rounded to the nearest hundredth is 0.58.

Example: Round $\frac{5}{37}$ to the nearest hundredth.

$$\begin{array}{r} 0.135 \\ 37\overline{)5.000} \\ 50 \\ \underline{37} \\ 130 \\ \underline{111} \\ 190 \\ \underline{185} \\ 5 \end{array}$$

Since the digit in the thousandths place is a 5, which is among the digits 5 through 9, the hundredths digit is rounded up from 3 to 4. So $\frac{5}{37}$ rounded to the nearest hundredth is 0.14.

PERCENTS

Percents are a special kind of ratio. Any percent can be expressed as a fraction with a denominator of 100 (*cent* means "one hundred," so *percent* means "*per one hundred*"). Because of this, it is very easy to convert percents into decimals as well as fractions.

To convert a percent to a fraction or decimal, just drop the percent symbol and divide the number by 100. (To convert to decimals, the shortcut is simply to drop the percent symbol and move the decimal point two places to the left.)

Percent to fraction: $78\% = \frac{78}{100}$

Percent to decimal: $78\% = 0.78$

$\frac{78}{100} = 0.78$

To convert any fraction or decimal to a percent, just multiply by 100 and add a percent sign. (For decimals, just move the decimal point two places to the right and add a percent sign. For fractions, remember to reduce if you can before you multiply.)

Decimal to percent: $0.29 = 29\%$

$$0.3 = 30\%$$

$$1.45 = 145\%$$

Fraction to percent: $\dfrac{3}{5} = \dfrac{3}{5} \times 100\% = \dfrac{3(100)}{5}\% = 3(20)\% = 60\%$

Know these common conversions. They come up frequently on the test, and you can avoid errors and save time by memorizing them instead of having to calculate them on the test.

In general, a digit with a bar over it means that the digit repeats indefinitely. In the table below, $0.3\overline{3}$ means that the 3 with the bar over it repeats indefinitely. Thus, $0.3\overline{3} = 0.3333....$

Fraction	Decimal	Percent
$\dfrac{1}{1}$	1.0	100%
$\dfrac{3}{4}$	0.75	75%
$\dfrac{2}{3}$	$0.6\overline{6}$	$66\dfrac{2}{3}\%$
$\dfrac{1}{2}$	0.5	50%
$\dfrac{1}{3}$	$0.3\overline{3}$	$33\dfrac{1}{3}\%$
$\dfrac{1}{4}$	0.25	25%
$\dfrac{1}{5}$	0.2	20%
$\dfrac{1}{8}$	0.125	$12\dfrac{1}{2}\%$
$\dfrac{1}{10}$	0.1	10%
$\dfrac{1}{20}$	0.05	5%

A. THE PERCENT FORMULA

The percent formula is commonly expressed in two different ways that are mathematically identical. Memorize and use whichever version of the formula you prefer. Notice how easy it is to get from one formula to the other—just multiply or divide both sides of the equation by the Whole.

$$\text{Percent} = \frac{\text{Part}}{\text{Whole}}$$

or

$$\text{Percent} \times \text{Whole} = \text{Part}$$

If the Part is 3 and the Whole is 4, then the Percent $= \dfrac{3}{4} = 0.75 = 75\%$.

If the Percent is 20% and the Whole is 8, then the Part $= 20\%(8) = (0.2)(8) = 1.6$

If the Percent is 60% and the Part is 12, then 60% (Whole) = 12. Thus,

$$\text{Whole} = \frac{12}{60\%} = \frac{12}{\left(\dfrac{6}{10}\right)} = 12\left(\frac{10}{6}\right) = 20.$$

B. PERCENT INCREASE/DECREASE

Once you understand percents, calculating percent increase and decrease is not as difficult as it may seem.

$$\%\text{ increase} = \frac{\text{Amount of increase}}{\text{Original whole}}(100\%)$$

$$\%\text{ decrease} = \frac{\text{Amount of decrease}}{\text{Original whole}}(100\%)$$

New Whole = Original whole ± Amount of change

Look at the first equation above. To find a percent increase, divide the amount of increase by the original whole. Then multiply this fraction by 100%.

Example: If a number increases from 50 to 70, what is the percent increase?

The amount of increase is 70 – 50, or 20. The original whole is 50. So the percent increase is $\frac{20}{50} \times 100\% = \frac{2}{5} \times 100\%$. What you learned reducing fractions can help here.

$$\frac{2}{5} \times 100\% = 2 \times 20\% = 40\%$$

If the new price of an item is 130% of its previous price, then it has increased in price by 30%. If an item goes on sale at 60% of its previous price, then it has decreased in price by 40%.

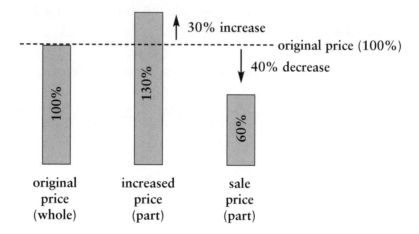

The percent increase or decrease is just the difference in percent from the whole (which is always equal to 100%).

When you come across the following phrases, use the percent increase/decrease formula:

If *X* is 10% greater than *Y*, then *X* is 110% of *Y*.

If *X* is 70% less than *Y*, then *X* is 30% of *Y*.

Example: If the value of a certain piece of property now is 350% of its original value when Kim purchased it, by what percent has the value of the property increased since Kim purchased it?

The percent increase is the difference from 100%. So 350% – 100% = 250% increase.

AVERAGES
A. FORMULA FOR COMPUTING AVERAGES

To find the average of a set of numbers, add them up and divide by the number of terms (the number of numbers).

$$\text{Average} = \frac{\text{Sum of the terms}}{\text{Number of terms}}$$

To find the average of the five numbers 12, 15, 23, 40, and 40, first add them: 12 + 15 + 23 + 40 + 40 = 130. Then divide the sum by 5: 130 ÷ 5 = 26.

B. USING THE AVERAGE TO FIND THE SUM

Sum = (Average) × (Number of terms)

If the average of 10 numbers is 50, then they add up to 10 × 50, or 500.

C. FINDING THE MISSING NUMBER

To find a missing number when you're given the average, **use the sum.** If the average of four numbers is 7, then the sum of those four numbers is 4 × 7, or 28. Suppose that three of the numbers are 3, 5, and 8. These three numbers add up to 16 of that 28, which leaves 12 for the fourth number.

PROBABILITY

The probability of an event is the possible number of desired outcomes divided by the total number of possible outcomes. Its numerical value is always less than or equal to 1. The probability of two independent events both occurring is the product of the individual probabilities.

Example: If we rolled two dice, what is the probability that we would make a total of 4?

There are six possible outcomes for each roll of a die, so with two dice, there are 6 × 6 = 36 possible outcomes. There are three outcomes that will lead to a total of 4: rolling 1 and 3, 3 and 1, or 2 and 2. The probability is therefore $\frac{3}{36} = \frac{1}{12}$.

## 2

ALGEBRA

EXPONENTS—KEY OPERATIONS

You can't be adept at algebra unless you're completely at ease with exponents. Here's what you need to know.

Multiplying powers with the same base: To multiply powers with the same base, keep the base and add the exponents:

$$x^3 \times x^4 = x^{3+4} = x^7$$

Dividing powers with the same base: To divide powers with the same base, keep the base and subtract the exponents:

$$y^{13} \div y^8 = y^{13-8} = y^5$$

Raising a power to an exponent: To raise a power to an exponent, keep the base and multiply the exponents:

$$(x^3)^4 = x^{3 \times 4} = x^{12}$$

Multiplying powers with the same exponent: To multiply powers with the same exponent, multiply the bases and keep the exponent:

$$(3^x)(4^x) = 12^x$$

Dividing powers with the same exponent: To divide powers with the same exponent, divide the bases and keep the exponent:

$$\frac{6^x}{2^x} = 3^x$$

> **DAT Synopsis**
>
> 1. $(x^m)(x^n) = x^{m+n}$.
>
> 2. $\dfrac{x^m}{x^n} = x^{m-n}$.
>
> 3. $(x^m)^n = x^{mn}$.
>
> 4. $(x^n)(y^n) = (xy)^n$.
>
> 5. $\dfrac{x^n}{y^n} = \left(\dfrac{x}{y}\right)^n$.

Example: For all $xyz \neq 0$, $\dfrac{6x^2y^{12}z^6}{(2x^2yz)^3} =$

There's nothing tricky about this question if you know how to work with exponents. The first step is to eliminate the parentheses. Everything inside gets cubed:

$$\frac{6x^2y^{12}z^6}{(2x^2yz)^3} = \frac{6x^2y^{12}z^6}{8x^6y^3z^3}$$

The next step is to look for factors common to the numerator and denominator. The 6 on top and the 8 on bottom reduce to 3 over 4. The x^2 on top cancels with the x^6 on bottom, leaving x^4 on bottom.

You're actually subtracting the exponents: $2 - 6 = -4$, since x^{-4} is the same as $\dfrac{1}{x^4}$. The y^{12} on top cancels with the y^3 on bottom, leaving y^9 on top. And the z^6 on top cancels with the z^3 on bottom, leaving z^3 on top:

$$\frac{6x^2y^{12}z^6}{8x^6y^3z^3} = \frac{3y^9z^3}{4x^4}$$

ADDING, SUBTRACTING, AND MULTIPLYING POLYNOMIALS

Algebra is the basic language of mathematics, and you will want to be fluent in that language. You might not get a whole lot of questions that ask explicitly about such basic algebra procedures as combining like terms, multiplying binomials, or factoring algebraic expressions, but you will do all of those things in the course of working out the answers to more advanced questions. So it's essential that you be at ease with the mechanics of algebraic manipulations.

Combining like terms: To combine like terms, keep the variable part unchanged while adding or subtracting the coefficients:

$$2a + 3a = (2 + 3)a = 5a$$

Adding or subtracting polynomials: To add or subtract polynomials, combine like terms:

$$(3x^2 + 5x - 7) - (x^2 + 12) =$$

$$(3x^2 - x^2) + 5x + (-7 - 12) =$$

$$2x^2 + 5x - 19$$

Multiplying monomials: To multiply monomials, multiply the coefficients and the variables separately:

$$2x \times 3x = (2 \times 3)(x \times x) = 6x^2$$

Multiplying binomials: To multiply binomials, use FOIL. To multiply $(x + 3)$ by $(x + 4)$, first multiply the **First** terms: $x \times x = x^2$. Next the **Outer** terms: $x \times 4 = 4x$. Then the **Inner** terms: $3 \times x = 3x$. And finally the **Last** terms: $3 \times 4 = 12$. Then add and combine like terms:

$$x^2 + 4x + 3x + 12 = x^2 + 7x + 12$$

Multiplying polynomials: To multiply polynomials with more than two terms, make sure you multiply each term in the first polynomial by each term in the second. (FOIL works only when you want to multiply two binomials.)

$$(x^2 + 3x + 4)(x + 5) = x^2(x + 5) + 3x(x + 5) + 4(x + 5)$$

$$= x^3 + 5x^2 + 3x^2 + 15x + 4x + 20$$

$$= x^3 + 8x^2 + 19x + 20$$

After multiplying two polynomials together, the number of terms in your expression before simplifying should equal the number of terms in one polynomial multiplied by the number of terms in the second. In the example above, you should have $3 \times 2 = 6$ terms in the product before you simplify like terms.

DIVIDING POLYNOMIALS

To divide polynomials, you can use long division. For example, divide $2x^3 + 13x^2 + 11x - 16$ by $x + 5$:

$$x + 5 \,\overline{)\,2x^3 + 13x^2 + 11x - 16}$$

The first term of the quotient is $2x^2$, because that's what will give you a $2x^3$ as a first term when you multiply it by $x + 5$:

$$
\begin{array}{r}
2x^2 \\
x + 5 \,\overline{)\,2x^3 + 13x^2 + 11x - 16} \\
\underline{2x^3 + 10x^2}
\end{array}
$$

Subtract and continue in the same way as when dividing numbers:

$$
\begin{array}{r}
2x^2 + 3x - 4 \\
x + 5 \,\overline{)\,2x^3 + 13x^2 + 11x - 16} \\
\underline{2x^3 + 10x^2} \\
3x^2 + 11x \\
\underline{3x^2 + 15x} \\
-4x - 16 \\
\underline{-4x - 20} \\
4
\end{array}
$$

The result is $2x^2 + 3x - 4$ with a remainder of 4.

DAT Synopsis

$(a + b)(c + d) = ?$

First $= ac$

Outer $= ad$

Inner $= bc$

Last $= bd$

Product $= ac + ad + bc + bd$

Long division is the way to do the following:

Example: When $2x^3 + 3x^2 - 4x + k$ is divided by $x + 2$, the remainder is 3. What is the value of k?

To answer this question, start by cranking out the long division:

$$
\require{enclose}
\begin{array}{r}
2x^2 - x - 2 \\
x + 2 \enclose{longdiv}{2x^3 + 3x^2 - 4x + k} \\
\underline{2x^3 + 4x^2} \\
-x^2 - 4x \\
\underline{-x^2 - 2x} \\
-2x + k \\
\underline{-2x - 4}
\end{array}
$$

The question says that the remainder is 3, so, whatever k is, when you subtract -4 from it, you get 3:

$$k - (-4) = 3$$

$$k + 4 = 3$$

$$k = -1$$

FACTORING

Performing operations on polynomials is largely a matter of cranking it out. Once you know the rules, adding, subtracting, multiplying, and even dividing is automatic. Factoring algebraic expressions is a different matter. To factor successfully you have to do more thinking and less cranking. You have to try to figure out what expressions multiplied will give you the polynomial you're looking at. Sometimes that means having a good eye for the test makers' favorite factorables:

- Factor common to all terms

- Difference of squares

- Square of a binomial

A. FACTOR COMMON TO ALL TERMS

A factor common to all the terms of a polynomial can be factored out. This is essentially the distributive property in reverse. For example, all three terms in the polynomial $3x^3 + 12x^2 - 6x$ contain a factor of $3x$. Pulling out the common factor yields $3x(x^2 + 4x - 2)$.

B. DIFFERENCE OF SQUARES

You will want to be especially keen at spotting polynomials in the form of the difference of squares. Whenever you have two identifiable squares with a minus sign between them, you can factor the expression like this:

$$a^2 - b^2 = (a + b)(a - b)$$

$4x^2 - 9$, for example, factors to $(2x + 3)(2x - 3)$.

C. SQUARES OF BINOMIALS

Learn to recognize polynomials that are squares of binomials:

$$a^2 + 2ab + b^2 = (a + b)^2$$
$$a^2 - 2ab + b^2 = (a - b)^2$$

For example, $4x^2 + 12x + 9$ factors to $(2x + 3)^2$, and $a^2 - 10a + 25$ factors to $(a - 5)^2$.

D. FACTORING OTHER EXPRESSIONS

Sometimes you'll want to factor a polynomial that's not in any of these classic factorable forms. When that happens, factoring becomes a kind of logic exercise, with some trial and error thrown in. To factor a quadratic expression, think about what binomials you could use FOIL to get that quadratic expression. For example, to factor $x^2 - 5x + 6$, think about what **First** terms will produce x^2, what **Last** terms will produce $+6$, and what **Outer** and **Inner** terms will produce $-5x$. Some common sense—and a little trial and error—will lead you to $(x - 2)(x - 3)$.

Example:　For all $x \neq \pm3$, $\dfrac{3x^2 - 11x + 6}{9 - x^2} =$

(A) $\dfrac{2 - 3x}{x - 3}$　　(B) $\dfrac{2 - 3x}{x + 3}$　　(C) $\dfrac{2x - 3}{x - 3}$　　(D) $\dfrac{3x - 2}{x + 3}$　　(E) $\dfrac{3x - 2}{x - 3}$

To reduce a fraction, you eliminate factors common to the top and bottom. So the first step in reducing an algebraic fraction is to factor the numerator and denominator. Here the denominator is easy since it's the difference of squares: $9 - x^2 = (3 - x)(3 + x)$. The numerator takes some thought and some trial and error. For the first term to be $3x^2$, the first terms of the factors must be $3x$ and x. For the last term to be $+6$, the last terms must be either $+2$ and $+3$, or -2 and -3, or $+1$ and $+6$, or -1 and -6. After a few tries, you should come up with $3x^2 - 11x + 6 = (3x - 2)(x - 3)$. Now the fraction looks like this:

$$\frac{3x^2 - 11x + 6}{9 - x^2} = \frac{(3x - 2)(x - 3)}{(3 - x)(3 + x)}$$

In this form, there are no precisely common factors, but there is a factor in the numerator that's the opposite (negative) of a factor in the denominator: $x - 3$ and $3 - x$ are opposites. Factor -1 out of the numerator and get this:

$$\frac{(3x - 2)(x - 3)}{(3 - x)(3 + x)} = \frac{(-1)(3x - 2)(3 - x)}{(3 - x)(3 + x)}$$

Now $(3 - x)$ can be eliminated from both the top and the bottom:

$$\frac{(-1)(3x - 2)(3 - x)}{(3 - x)(3 + x)} = \frac{-(3x - 2)}{3 + x} = \frac{-3x + 2}{3 + x}$$

That's the same as choice (B):

$$\frac{-3x + 2}{3 + x} = \frac{2 - 3x}{x + 3}$$

Alternative method: Here's another way to answer this question. *Pick a number for x and see what happens.* One of the answer choices will give you the same value as the original fraction will, no matter what you plug in for *x*. Pick a number that's easy to work with—like 0.

When you plug $x = 0$ into the original expression, any term with an *x* drops out, and you end up with $\frac{6}{9}$, or $\frac{2}{3}$. Plug $x = 0$ into each answer choice to see which ones equal $\frac{2}{3}$.

When you get to (B), it works, but you can't stop there. It might be just a coincidence. When you pick numbers, *look at every answer choice*. Choice (E) also works for $x = 0$. At least you know one of those is the correct answer, and you can decide between them by picking another value for *x*.

This is not a sophisticated approach, but who cares? You don't get points for elegance. You get points for right answers.

DAT Synopsis

When the answer choices are algebraic expressions, it often works to pick numbers for the unknowns, plug those numbers into the stem and see what you get, and then plug those same numbers into the answer choices to find matches.

Warning: When you pick numbers, you have to check all the answer choices. Sometimes more than one works with the number(s) you pick, in which case you have to pick numbers again.

THE GOLDEN RULE OF EQUATIONS

You probably remember the basic procedure for solving algebraic equations: *Do the same thing to both sides.* You can do almost anything you want to one side of an equation as long as you preserve the equality by doing the same thing to the other side. Your aim in whatever you do to both sides is to get the variable (or expression) you're solving for all by itself on one side.

Example: If $\sqrt[3]{8x + 6} = -3$, what is the value of *x* ?

To solve this equation for *x* means to do whatever is needed to both sides of the equation to get *x* all by itself on one side. Layer by layer, you want to peel away all those extra symbols and numbers around the *x*. First you want to get rid of that cube-root symbol. The way to undo a cube root is to cube both sides:

$$\sqrt[3]{8x + 6} = -3$$

$$\left(\sqrt[3]{8x + 6}\right)^3 = (-3)^3$$

$$8x + 6 = -27$$

The rest is easy. Subtract 6 from both sides and divide both sides by 8:

$$8x + 6 = -27$$

$$8x = -27 - 6$$

$$8x = -33$$

$$x = -\frac{33}{8} = -4.125$$

The test makers have a couple of favorite equation types that you should be prepared to solve. Solving linear equations is usually pretty straightforward. Generally it's obvious what to do to isolate the unknown. But when the unknown is in a denominator or an exponent, it might not be so obvious how to proceed.

UNKNOWN IN A DENOMINATOR

The basic procedure for solving an equation is the same even when the unknown is in a denominator: Do the same thing to both sides. In this case you multiply in order to undo division.

If you wanted to solve $1 + \dfrac{1}{x} = 2 - \dfrac{1}{x}$, you would multiply both sides by x:

$$1 + \frac{1}{x} = 2 - \frac{1}{x}$$

$$x\left(1 + \frac{1}{x}\right) = x\left(2 - \frac{1}{x}\right)$$

$$x + 1 = 2x - 1$$

Now you have an equation with no denominators, which is easy to solve:

$$x + 1 = 2x - 1$$

$$x - 2x = -1 - 1$$

$$-x = -2$$

$$x = 2$$

Another good way to solve an equation with the unknown in the denominator is to *cross multiply*. That's the best way to do the following example.

Example: If $\dfrac{5}{x + 3} = \dfrac{1}{x} + \dfrac{1}{2x}$, what is the value of x?

Before you can cross multiply, you need to re-express the right side of the equation as a single fraction. That means giving the two fractions a common denominator and adding them. The common denominator is $2x$:

$$\frac{5}{x+3} = \frac{1}{x} + \frac{1}{2x}$$

$$\frac{5}{x+3} = \frac{2}{2x} + \frac{1}{2x}$$

$$\frac{5}{x+3} = \frac{3}{2x}$$

Now you can cross multiply:

$$\frac{5}{x+3} = \frac{3}{2x}$$
$$(5)(2x) = (x+3)(3)$$
$$10x = 3x + 9$$
$$10x - 3x = 9$$
$$7x = 9$$
$$x = \frac{9}{7}$$

UNKNOWN IN AN EXPONENT

The procedure for solving an equation when the unknown is in an exponent is a little different. What you want to do in this situation is to re-express one or both sides of the equation so that the two sides have the same base.

Example: If $8^x = 16^{x-1}$, then $x =$

(A) $\frac{1}{8}$ (B) $\frac{1}{2}$ (C) 2   (D) 4   (E) 8

In this case, the base on the left is 8 and the base on the right is 16. They're both powers of 2, so you can reexpress both sides as powers of 2:

$$(2^3)^x = (2^4)^{x-1}$$
$$2^{3x} = 2^{4x-4}$$

Now that both sides have the same base, you can simply set the exponent expressions equal and solve for x:

$$3x = 4x - 4$$
$$3x - 4x = -4$$
$$-x = -4$$
$$x = 4$$

Alternative method: Here's another way to answer this question. Nobody says you have to figure out the answer to the question and then look for your solution among the answer choices. If you don't see how to do it the front way, *try working backwards*. Try plugging the answer choices back into the problem until you find the one that works. Here, if you start with (C) and

$x = 2$, you get $8^x = 8^2 = 64$ on the left side of the equation and $16^{x-1} = 16^1 = 16$ on the right side. It's not clear whether (C) was too small or too large, so you should probably try (D) next—it's easier to work with than (B), which is a fraction. If $x = 4$, then $8^x = 8^4 = 4,096$ on the left, and $16^{x-1} = 16^3 = 4,096$. No need to do any more. (D) works, so it's the answer.

Don't depend on backsolving too much. There are lots of math questions that can't be backsolved at all. And most that *can* be backsolved are almost certainly more *quickly* solved by a more direct approach.

QUADRATIC EQUATIONS

To solve a quadratic equation, put it in the $ax^2 + bx + c = 0$ form, factor the left side (if you can), and set each factor equal to 0 separately to get the two solutions. For example, to solve $x^2 + 12 = 7x$, first rewrite it as $x^2 - 7x + 12 = 0$. Then factor the left side:

$$x^2 - 7x + 12 = 0$$
$$(x - 3)(x - 4) = 0$$
$$x - 3 = 0 \text{ or } x - 4 = 0$$
$$x = 3 \text{ or } 4$$

Sometimes the left side may not be obviously factorable. You can always use the *quadratic formula.* Just plug in the coefficients a, b, and c from $ax^2 + bx + c = 0$ into the formula:

$$x = \frac{-b \pm \sqrt{b^2 - 4ac}}{2a}$$

For example, to solve $x + 4x + 2 = 0$, plug $a = 1$, $b = 4$, and $c = 2$ into the formula:

$$x = \frac{-4 \pm \sqrt{4^2 - 4 \times 1 \times 2}}{2 \times 1}$$
$$= \frac{-4 \pm \sqrt{8}}{2} = -2 \pm \sqrt{2}$$

"IN TERMS OF"

So far in this chapter, solving an equation has meant finding a numerical value for the unknown. When there's more than one variable, it's generally impossible to get numerical solutions. Instead, what you do is solve for the unknown *in terms of* the other variables.

To solve an equation for one variable in terms of another means to isolate the one variable on one side of the equation, leaving an expression containing the other variable on the other side of the equation.

For example, to solve the equation $3x - 10y = -5x + 6y$ for x in terms of y, isolate x:

$$3x - 10y = -5x + 6y$$
$$3x + 5x = 6y + 10y$$
$$8x = 16y$$
$$x = 2y$$

Example: If $a = \dfrac{b + x}{c + x}$, what is the value of x in terms of a, b, and c?

You want to get x on one side by itself. First thing to do is eliminate the denominator by multiplying both sides by $c + x$:

$$a = \frac{b + x}{c + x}$$

$$a(c + x) = \left(\frac{b + x}{c + x}\right)(c + x)$$

$$ac + ax = b + x$$

Next move all terms with x to one side and all terms without to the other:

$$ac + ax = b + x$$
$$ax - x = b - ac$$

Now factor x out of the left side and divide both sides by the other factor to isolate x:

$$ax - x = b - ac$$
$$x(a - 1) = b - ac$$
$$x = \frac{b - ac}{a - 1}$$

SIMULTANEOUS EQUATIONS

DAT Synopsis

You don't always have to find the value of each variable to answer a simultaneous equations question.

You can get numerical solutions for more than one unknown if you are given more than one equation. Simultaneous equations questions take a little thought to answer. Solving simultaneous equations almost always involves combining equations, but you have to figure out what's the best way to combine the equations.

You can solve for two variables only if you have two distinct equations. Two forms of the same equation will not be adequate. Combine the equations in such a way that one of the variables cancels out. For example, to solve the two equations $4x + 3y = 8$ and $x + y = 3$, multiply both sides of the second equation by -3 to get $-3x - 3y = -9$. Now add the two equations; the $3y$ and the $-3y$ cancel out, leaving $x = -1$. Plug that back into either one of the original equations, and you'll find that $y = 4$.

Example: If $2x - 9y = 11$ and $x + 12y = -8$, what is the value of $x + y$?

If you just plow ahead without thinking, you might try to answer this question by solving for one variable at a time. That would work, but it would take a lot more time than this question needs. As usual, the key to this simultaneous equations question is to combine the equations, but combining the equations doesn't necessarily mean losing a variable. Look what happens here if you just add the equations as presented:

$$2x - 9y = 11$$
$$+[x + 12y = -8]$$
$$\overline{3x + 3y = 3}$$

Suddenly you're almost there! Just divide both sides by 3, and you get $x + y = 1$.

ABSOLUTE VALUE AND INEQUALITIES

To solve an equation that includes absolute value signs, think about the two different cases. For example, to solve the equation $|x - 12| = 3$, think of it as two equations:

$$x - 12 = 3 \text{ or } x - 12 = -3$$
$$x = 15 \text{ or } 9$$

To solve an inequality, do whatever is necessary to both sides to isolate the variable. Just remember that when you multiply or divide both sides by a negative number, you must reverse the sign. To solve $-5x + 7 < -3$, subtract 7 from both sides to get $-5x < -10$. Now divide both sides by -5, remembering to reverse the sign: $x > 2$.

Example: What is the solution set of $|2x - 3| < 7$?

(A) $\{x: -5 < x < 2\}$
(B) $\{x: -5 < x < 5\}$
(C) $\{x: -2 < x < 5\}$
(D) $\{x: x < -5 \text{ or } x > 2\}$
(E) $\{x: x < -2 \text{ or } x > 5\}$

What does it mean if $|2x - 3| < 7$? It means that if the expression between the absolute value bars is positive, it's less than +7, or if the expression between the bars is negative, it's greater than −7. In other words, $2x - 3$ is between −7 and +7:

$$-7 < 2x - 3 < 7$$
$$-4 < 2x < 10$$
$$-2 < x < 5$$

> **DAT Synopsis**
>
> If $n > 0$,
>
> $|whatever| < n$
> ⇓
> $-n < whatever < n$
>
> $|whatever| > n$
> ⇓
> $whatever < -n \text{ OR } whatever > n$

In fact, there's a general rule that applies here: To solve an inequality in the form $|\text{whatever}| < p$, where $p > 0$, just put that "whatever" inside the range $-p$ to p:

$$|\text{whatever}| < p \text{ means } -p < \text{whatever} < p$$

For example, $|x - 5| < 14$ becomes $-14 < x - 5 < 14$.

And here's another general rule: To solve an inequality in the form $|\text{whatever}| > p$, where $p > 0$, just put that "whatever" outside the range $-p$ to p :

$$|\text{whatever}| > p \text{ means whatever} < -p \text{ OR whatever} > p$$

For example, $\left|\dfrac{3x + 9}{2}\right| > 7$ becomes $\dfrac{3x + 9}{2} < -7$ OR $\dfrac{3x + 9}{2} > 7$.

## 3

PLANE GEOMETRY

ADDING AND SUBTRACTING SEGMENT LENGTHS

Example:

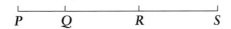

$$P \quad Q \quad R \quad S$$

In the figure above, the length of segment *PS* is 2x + 12, and the length of segment *PQ* is 6x – 10. If *R* is the midpoint of segment *QS*, what is the length of segment *PR*?

Usually the best thing to do to start on a plane geometry question is to mark up the figure. Put as much of the information into the figure as you can. That's a good way to organize your thoughts. And that way, you don't have to go back and forth between the figure and the question.

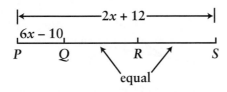

DAT Synopsis

Try to put all the given information into the figure so that you can see everything at a glance and don't have to keep going back and forth between the question stem and the figure.

Now you can plan your attack. First subtract *PQ* from the whole length *PS* to get *QS*:

$$QS = PS - PQ = (2x + 12) - (6x - 10) = 2x + 12 - 6x + 10 = -4x + 22$$

Then, because *R* is the midpoint of *QS*, you can divide *QS* by 2 to get *QR* and *RS*:

$$QR = RS = \frac{QS}{2} = \frac{-4x + 22}{2} = -2x + 11$$

What you're looking for is *PR*, so you have to add:

$$PR = PQ + QR = (6x - 10) + (-2x + 11) = 4x + 1$$

BASIC TRAITS OF TRIANGLES

Most plane geometry questions are about closed figures: polygons and circles. And the test makers' favorite closed figure by far is the three-sided polygon; that is, the triangle. All three-sided polygons are interesting because they share so many characteristics, and certain special three-sided polygons—equilateral, isosceles, and right triangles—are interesting because of their special characteristics.

Let's look at the traits that all triangles share.

Sum of the interior angles: The three interior angles of any triangle add up to 180°.

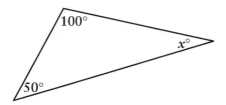

In the figure above, $x + 50 + 100 = 180$, so $x = 30$.

Measure of an exterior angle: The measure of an exterior angle of a triangle is equal to the sum of the measures of the remote interior angles.

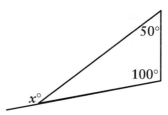

In the figure above, the measure of the exterior angle labeled $x°$ is equal to the sum of the measures of the remote interior angles: $x = 50 + 100 = 150$.

Sum of the exterior angles: The measures of the three exterior angles of any triangle add up to 360°.

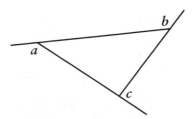

In the figure above, $a + b + c = 360°$. (Note: In fact, the measures of the exterior angles of any polygon add up to 360°.)

Area formula: The general formula for the area of a triangle is always the same:

$$\text{Area of Triangle} = \frac{1}{2}(\text{base})(\text{height})$$

The height is the perpendicular distance between the side that's chosen as the base and the opposite vertex.

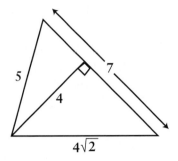

In the triangle above, 4 is the height when the 7 side is chosen as the base.

$$\text{Area of Triangle} = \frac{1}{2}(\text{base})(\text{height})$$

$$= \frac{1}{2}(7)(4) = 14$$

Triangle inequality theorem: The length of any one side of a triangle must be greater than the positive difference and less than the sum of the lengths of the other two sides. For example, if it is given that the length of one side is 3 and the length of another side is 7, then the length of the third side must be greater than $7 - 3 = 4$ and less than $7 + 3 = 10$.

SIMILAR TRIANGLES

Example:

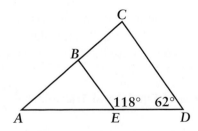

In the figure above, $AB = BC$. If the area of $\triangle ABE$ is x, what is the area of $\triangle ACD$?

You might wonder here how you're supposed to find the area of $\triangle ACD$ when you're given no lengths you can use for a base or an altitude. The only numbers you have are the angle measures. They must be there for some reason—the test makers rarely provide superfluous information. In fact, because the two angle measures provided add up to 180°, they tell you that BE and CD are parallel. And that, in turn, tells you that $\triangle ABE$ is similar to $\triangle ACD$—because they have the same three angles.

Similar triangles are triangles that have the same shape: Corresponding angles are equal, and corresponding sides are proportional. In this case, because it's given that $AB = BC$, you know that AC is twice AB and that corresponding sides are in a ratio of 2:1. Each side of the larger triangle is twice the length of the corresponding side of the smaller triangle. That doesn't mean, however, that the ratio of the areas is also 2:1. In fact, the area ratio is the square of the side ratio, and the larger triangle has four times the area of the smaller triangle, so the answer is $4x$.

THREE SPECIAL TRIANGLE TYPES

Three special triangle types deserve extra attention:

- Isosceles triangles

- Equilateral triangles

- Right triangles

Be sure you know not just the definitions of these triangle types but, more importantly, their special characteristics: side relationships, angle relationships, and area formulas.

Isosceles triangle: An isosceles triangle is a triangle that has two equal sides. Not only are two sides equal, but the angles opposite the equal sides, called base angles, are also equal.

Equilateral triangle: An equilateral triangle is a triangle that has three equal sides. Since all the sides are equal, all the angles are also equal. All three angles in an equilateral triangle measure 60 degrees, regardless of the lengths of the sides. You can find the area of an equilateral triangle by dividing it into two 30°-60°-90° triangles, or you can use this formula in terms of the length of one side s:

$$\text{Area of Equilateral Triangle} = \frac{s^2\sqrt{3}}{4}$$

Right triangle: A right triangle is a triangle with a right angle. The two sides that form the right angle are called *legs*, and you can use them as the base and height to find the area of a right triangle.

$$\text{Area of Right Triangle} = \frac{1}{2}(\text{leg}_1)(\text{leg}_2)$$

Pythagorean theorem: If you know any two sides of a right triangle, you can find the third side by using the Pythagorean theorem:

$$(\text{leg}_1)^2 + (\text{leg}_2)^2 = (\text{hypotenuse})^2$$

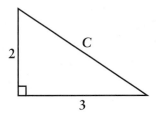

For example, if one leg is 2 and the other leg is 3, then

$$2^2 + 3^2 = c^2$$

$$c^2 = 4 + 9$$

$$c = \sqrt{13}$$

Pythagorean triplet: A Pythagorean triplet is a set of integers that fits the Pythagorean theorem. The simplest Pythagorean triplet is (3, 4, 5). In fact, any integers in a 3:4:5 ratio make up a Pythagorean triplet. And there are many other Pythagorean triplets: (5, 12, 13); (7, 24, 25); (8, 15, 17); (9, 40, 41); all their multiples; and infinitely many more.

3-4-5 triangle: If a right triangle's leg-to-leg ratio is 3:4, or if the leg-to-hypotenuse ratio is 3:5 or 4:5, then it's a 3-4-5 triangle, and you don't need to use the Pythagorean theorem to find the third side. Just figure out what multiple of 3-4-5 it is.

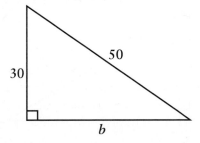

In the right triangle shown, one leg is 30 and the hypotenuse is 50. This is 10 times 3-4-5. The other leg is 40.

5-12-13 triangles: If a right triangle's leg-to-leg ratio is 5:12, or if the leg-to-hypotenuse ratio is 5:13 or 12:13, then it's a 5-12-13 triangle and you don't need to use the Pythagorean theorem to find the third side. Just figure out what multiple of 5-12-13 it is.

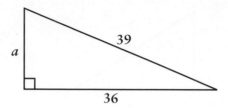

Here one leg is 36 and the hypotenuse is 39. This is 3 times 5-12-13. The other leg is 3×5 or 15.

45°-45°-90° triangles: The sides of a 45°-45°-90° triangle are in a ratio of $1:1:\sqrt{2}$

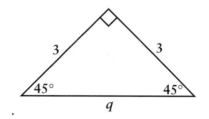

If one leg is 3, then the other leg is also 3, and the hypotenuse is equal to a leg times $\sqrt{2}$, or $3\sqrt{2}$.

30°-60°-90° triangles: The sides of a 30°-60°-90° triangle are in a ratio of $1:\sqrt{3}:2$. You don't need to use the Pythagorean theorem.

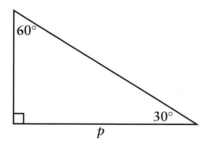

If the hypotenuse is 6, then the shorter leg is half that, or 3; and then the longer leg is equal to the short leg times $\sqrt{3}$, or $3\sqrt{3}$.

Example:

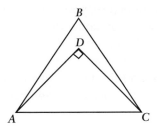

In the above figure, $\triangle ABC$ is equilateral and $\triangle ADC$ is isosceles. If $AC = 1$, what is the distance from B to D?

To get the answer to this question, you need to know about equilateral, 45°-45°-90°, and 30°-60°-90° triangles. If you drop an altitude from B through D, you will divide the equilateral triangle into two 30°-60°-90° triangles, and you will divide the right isosceles (or 45°-45°-90°) triangle into two smaller right isosceles triangles:

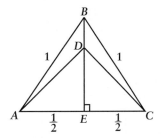

Using the side ratios for 30°-60°-90° and 45°-45°-90° triangles, you know that

$BE = \dfrac{\sqrt{3}}{2}$ and that $DE = \dfrac{1}{2}$.

Therefore, $BD = BE - DE = \dfrac{\sqrt{3}}{2} - \dfrac{1}{2} = \dfrac{\sqrt{3} - 1}{2}$.

HIDDEN SPECIAL TRIANGLES

It happens a lot that the key to solving a geometry problem is to add a line segment or two to the figure. Often what results is one or more special triangles.

Example:

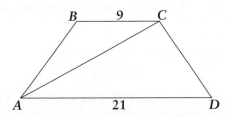

In the above figure, the perimeter of isosceles trapezoid $ABCD$ is 50. If $BC = 9$ and $AD = 21$, what is the length of diagonal AC?

DAT Synopsis

Often the breakthrough on a plane geometry problem comes when you add a line segment or two to the figure. Perpendiculars can be especially useful. They can function as rectangle sides or triangle altitudes or right triangle legs.

As you read the stem, you might wonder what an *isosceles trapezoid* is. If you'd never heard the term before, you still might have been able to extrapolate its meaning from what you know of isosceles triangles. *Isosceles* means "having two equal sides." When applied to a trapezoid, it tells you that the two nonparallel sides—the legs—are equal. In this case, that's *AB* and *CD*. If the total perimeter is 50, and the two marked sides add up to 21 + 9 = 30, then the two unmarked sides split the difference of 50 − 30 = 20. In other words, *AB* = *CD* = 10.

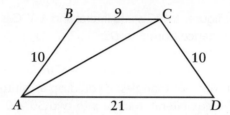

There aren't any special triangles yet. As so often happens, though, you can get some by constructing altitudes. Drop perpendiculars from points *B* and *C*, and you make two right triangles. The length 21 of side *AD* then gets split into 6, 9, and 6.

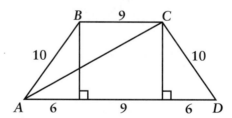

Now you can see that those right triangles are 3-4-5s (times 2) and that the height of the trapezoid is 8. Now look at the right triangle of which *AC* is the hypotenuse.

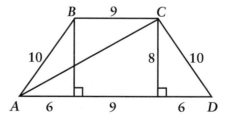

One leg is 6 + 9 = 15, and the other leg is 8; therefore, the hypotenuse *AC* is as follows:

$$\text{hypotenuse} = \sqrt{(\text{leg}_1)^2 + (\text{leg}_2)^2}$$
$$= \sqrt{15^2 + 8^2}$$
$$= \sqrt{225 + 64} = \sqrt{289} = 17$$

SPECIAL QUADRILATERALS

The trapezoid is just one of five special quadrilaterals you need to be familiar with. As with triangles, there is some overlap among these categories, and some figures fit into none of these categories. Just as a 45°-45°-90° triangle is both right and isosceles, a quadrilateral with four equal sides and four right angles is not only a square but also a rhombus, a rectangle, and a parallelogram. It is wise to have a solid grasp of the definitions and special characteristics of these five quadrilateral types.

A. TRAPEZOIDS

A trapezoid is a four-sided figure with one pair of parallel sides and one pair of nonparallel sides.

$$\text{Area of Trapezoid} = \left(\frac{\text{base}_1 + \text{base}_2}{2}\right) \times \text{height}$$

Think of this formula as the average of the bases (the two parallel sides) times the height (the length of the perpendicular altitude).

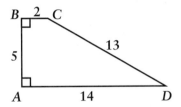

In the trapezoid *ABCD* above, you can use side *AB* for the height. The average of the bases is $\frac{2 + 14}{2} = 8$, so the area is 8×5, or 40.

B. PARALLELOGRAMS

A parallelogram is a four-sided figure with two pairs of parallel sides. Opposite sides are equal. Opposite angles are equal. Consecutive angles add up to 180°.

$$\text{Area of Parallelogram} = \text{base} \times \text{height}$$

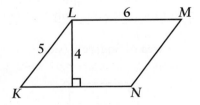

In parallelogram *KLMN* above, 4 is the height when *LM* or *KN* is used as the base. Base × height = $6 \times 4 = 24$.

Remember that to find the area of a parallelogram you need the height, which is the perpendicular distance from the base to the opposite side. You can use a side of a parallelogram for the height only when the side is perpendicular to the base, in which case you have a rectangle.

C. RECTANGLES

A rectangle is a four-sided figure with four right angles. Opposite sides are equal. Diagonals are equal. The perimeter of a rectangle is equal to the sum of the lengths of the four sides, which is equal to 2(length + width).

Area of Rectangle = length × width

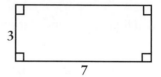

The area of a 7-by-3 rectangle is $7 \times 3 = 21$.

D. RHOMBUS

A rhombus is a four-sided figure with four equal sides.

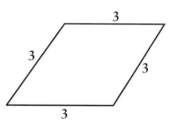

All four sides of the quadrilateral above have the same length, so it's a rhombus. A rhombus is also a parallelogram, so to find the area of a rhombus, you need its height. The more a rhombus "leans over," the smaller the height and, therefore, the smaller the area. The maximum area for a rhombus of a certain perimeter is a rhombus that has each pair of adjacent sides perpendicular, in which case you have a square.

E. SQUARE

A square is a four-sided figure with four right angles and four equal sides. A square is also a rectangle, a parallelogram, and a rhombus. The perimeter of a square is equal to 4 times the length of one side.

Area of Square = (side)^2

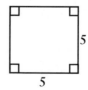

The square above, with sides of length 5, has an area of $5^2 = 25$.

POLYGONS—PERIMETER AND AREA

The test makers like to write problems that combine the concepts of perimeter and area. What you need to remember is that perimeter and area are not directly related. In the following example, for instance, you have two figures with the same perimeter, but that doesn't mean they have the same area.

Example: A square and a regular hexagon have the same perimeter. If the area of the square is 2.25, what is the area of the hexagon?

The way to get started with this question is to sketch what's described in the question. A square of area 2.25 has sides each of length $\sqrt{2.25} = 1.5$. So the perimeter of the square is $4(1.5) = 6$. Since that's also the perimeter of the regular hexagon, and a regular hexagon has six equal sides, the length of each side of the hexagon is 1.

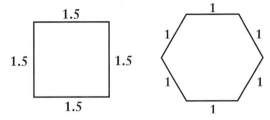

Now the problem is one of finding the area of a regular hexagon of side length 1. The fastest way to do that would be to use the formula, if you know it. If the length of one side is s,

$$\textbf{Area of Hexagon} = \frac{3s^2\sqrt{3}}{2}$$

This formula is not one the test makers expect you to know—there's always a way around it—but if you like formulas and you're good at memorizing them, it can only help. Let's proceed, however, as if we didn't know the formula. Another way to go about finding this area is to add a line segment or two to the figure and divide it up into more familiar shapes. You could, for example, draw in three diagonals and turn the hexagon into six equilateral triangles of side 1:

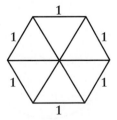

Each of those six triangles has base 1 and height $\frac{\sqrt{3}}{2}$, and therefore,

$$\textbf{Area of one triangle} = \frac{1}{2}(\text{base})(\text{height}) = \frac{1}{2}(1)\left(\frac{\sqrt{3}}{2}\right) = \frac{\sqrt{3}}{4}$$

The area of the hexagon is 6 times that.

$$\text{Area of Hexagon} = 6\left(\frac{\sqrt{3}}{4}\right) = \frac{3\sqrt{3}}{2}$$

CIRCLES—FOUR FORMULAS

After the triangle, the test makers' favorite plane geometry figure is the circle. Circles don't come in as many varieties as triangles do. In fact, all circles are similar—they're all the same shape. The only difference among them is size. So you don't have to learn to recognize types or remember names. All you have to know about circles is how to find four things:

- Circumference

- Length of an arc

- Area

- Area of a sector

You could think of the task as one of memorizing four formulas, but you'll be better off in the end if you have some idea of where the arc and sector formulas come from and how they are related to the circumference and area formulas.

A. CIRCUMFERENCE

Circumference is a measurement of length. You could think of it as the perimeter: It's the total distance around the circle. If the radius of the circle is r,

$$\textbf{Circumference} = 2\pi r$$

Since the diameter is twice the radius, you can easily express the formula in terms of the diameter d:

$$\text{Circumference} = \pi d$$

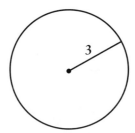

In the circle above, the radius is 3, so the circumference is $2\pi(3) = 6\pi$.

B. LENGTH OF AN ARC

An arc is a piece of the circumference. If n is the degree measure of the arc's central angle, then the formula is

$$\text{Length of an Arc} = \left(\frac{n}{360}\right)(2\pi r)$$

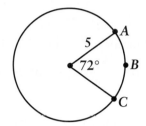

In the figure above, the radius is 5 and the measure of the central angle is 72°. The arc length is $\frac{72}{360}$ or $\frac{1}{5}$ of the circumference:

$$\left(\frac{72}{360}\right)(2\pi)(5) = \left(\frac{1}{5}\right)(10\pi) = 2\pi$$

C. AREA

The area of a circle is usually found using this formula in terms of the radius r:

$$\text{Area of a Circle} = \pi r^2$$

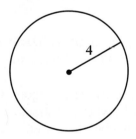

The area of the circle above is $\pi(4)^2 = 16\pi$.

D. AREA OF A SECTOR

A sector is a piece of the area of a circle. If n is the degree measure of the sector's central angle, then the area formula is

$$\text{Area of a Sector} = \left(\frac{n}{360}\right)(\pi r^2)$$

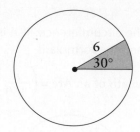

In the figure above, the radius is 6 and the measure of the sector's central angle is 30°. The sector has $\frac{30}{360}$ or $\frac{1}{12}$ of the area of the circle:

$$\left(\frac{30}{360}\right)(\pi)(6^2) = \left(\frac{1}{12}\right)(36\pi) = 3\pi$$

CIRCLES COMBINED WITH OTHER FIGURES

Some of the most challenging plane geometry questions are those that combine circles with other figures.

Example:

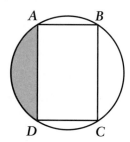

In the figure above, rectangle *ABCD* is inscribed in a circle. If the radius of the circle is 1 and *AB* = 1, what is the area of the shaded region?

Once again, the key here is to add to the figure. And in this case, as is so often the case when there's a circle, what you should add is radii. The equilateral triangles tell you that the central angles are 60° and 120°.

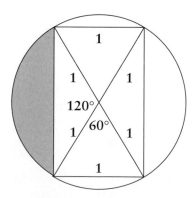

The shaded region is what's left of the 120° sector after you subtract the triangle with the 120° vertex angle.

To find the area of the shaded region, you want to find the areas of the sector and triangle, then subtract. The sector is exactly one-third of the circle (because 120° is one-third of 360°), so

$$\text{Area of sector} = \frac{1}{3}\pi r^2 = \frac{1}{3}\pi(1)^2 = \frac{\pi}{3}$$

You can divide the triangle into two 30°-60°-90° triangles:

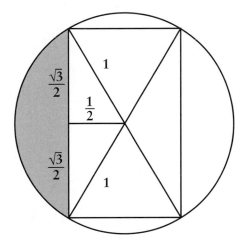

The area of each 30°-60°-90° triangle is $\frac{1}{2}\left(\frac{1}{2}\right)\left(\frac{\sqrt{3}}{2}\right) = \frac{\sqrt{3}}{8}$, so the area of

the triangle with the 120° vertex is twice that, or $\frac{\sqrt{3}}{4}$.

The area of the shaded region is, therefore,

$$\frac{\pi}{3} - \frac{\sqrt{3}}{4}$$

## 4

SOLID GEOMETRY

FIVE FORMULAS

A. LATERAL AREA OF A CONE

Given base circumference c and slant height ℓ,

$$\text{Lateral Area of Cone} = \frac{1}{2}c\ell$$

The lateral area of a cone is the area of the part that extends from the vertex to the circular base. It does not include the circular base.

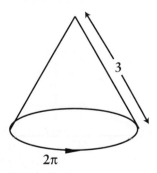

Flashback to Chapter 2

You can't escape algebra! Even a lot of the geometry questions are partly algebra questions as well. Make sure your algebra skills are in peak condition by test day.

For example, in the figure above, $c = 2\pi$ and $\ell = 3$, so
$$\text{Lateral Area} = \frac{1}{2}(2\pi)(3) = 3\pi$$

B. VOLUME OF A CONE

Given base radius r and height h,

$$\text{Volume of Cone} = \frac{1}{3}\pi r^2 h$$

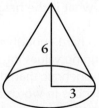

For example, in the figure on the previous page, $r = 3$ and $h = 6$, so

$$\text{Volume} = \frac{1}{3}\pi(3^2)(6) = 18\pi$$

C. SURFACE AREA OF A SPHERE

Given radius r,

Surface Area of Sphere = $4\pi r^2$

For example, if the radius of a sphere is 2, then

$$\text{Surface Area} = 4\pi(2^2) = 16\pi$$

D. VOLUME OF A SPHERE

Given radius r,

Volume of Sphere $= \frac{4}{3}\pi r^3$

For example, if the radius of a sphere is 2, then

$$\text{Volume} = \frac{4}{3}\pi(2)^3 = \frac{32\pi}{3}$$

E. VOLUME OF A PYRAMID

Given base area B and height h,

Volume of Pyramid $= \frac{1}{3}Bh$

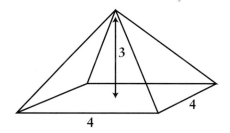

For example, in the figure above, $h = 3$, and if the base is a square, $B = 16$. Thus,

$$\text{Volume} = \frac{1}{3}(16)(3) = 16$$

Here's a question that uses some of these formulas.

Example: A right circular cone and a sphere have equal volumes. If the radius of the base of the cone is 2x and the radius of the sphere is 3x, what is the height of the cone in terms of x?

As you can see, this question is hard enough even with the formulas provided. This is no mere matter of plugging values into a formula and cranking out the answer. This question is more algebraic than that and takes a little thought. It's really a word problem. It describes in words a mathematical situation (in this case, geometric) that can be translated into algebra. The pivot in this situation is that the cone and sphere have equal volumes. You're looking for the height *h* in terms of *x*, and fortunately you can express both volumes in terms of those two variables. Be careful. Both formulas include *r*, but they're not the same *r*'s. In the case of the cone, *r* = 2*x* , but in the case of the sphere, *r* = 3*x*:

$$\text{Volume of cone} = \frac{1}{3}\pi r^2 h = \frac{1}{3}\pi(2x)^2 h = \frac{4}{3}\pi x^2 h$$

$$\text{Volume of sphere} = \frac{4}{3}\pi r^3 = \frac{4}{3}\pi(3x)^3 = 36\pi x^3$$

Now write an equation that says that the expressions for the two volumes are equal to each other and solve for *h*:

$$\frac{4}{3}\pi x^2 h = 36\pi x^3$$

$$\pi x^2 h = \frac{3}{4}(36\pi x^3)$$

$$\pi x^2 h = 27\pi x^3$$

$$h = \frac{27\pi x^3}{\pi x^2}$$

$$h = 27x$$

THE RECTANGULAR SOLID

The rectangular solid is the official geometric term for a box, which has 6 rectangular faces and 12 edges that meet at right angles at 8 vertices.

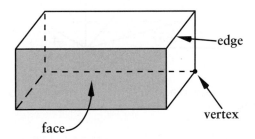

The surface area of a rectangular solid is simply the sum of the areas of the faces. That's what the formula Surface Area = 2ℓ*w* + 2*wh* + 2ℓ*h* says. If the length is ℓ, the width is *w*, and the height is *h*, then two rectangular faces have area ℓ*w*, two have area *wh*, and two have area ℓ*h*. The total surface area is the sum of those three pairs of areas.

Instead of the surface area, you may be asked to find the distance between opposite vertices of a rectangular solid.

Example:

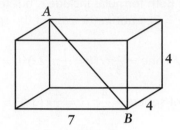

In the rectangular solid in the above figure, what is the distance from vertex *A* to vertex *B*?

One way to find this distance is to apply the Pythagorean theorem twice. First plug the dimensions of the base into the Pythagorean theorem to find the diagonal of the base:

$$\text{Diagonal of base} = \sqrt{4^2 + 7^2} = \sqrt{16 + 49} = \sqrt{65}$$

Notice that the base diagonal combines with an edge and with the segment *AB* you're looking for to form a right triangle:

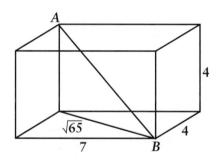

So you can plug the base diagonal and the height into the Pythagorean theorem to find *AB*:

$$AB = \sqrt{(\sqrt{65})^2 + 4^2} = \sqrt{65 + 16} = \sqrt{81} = 9$$

Another way to find this distance is to use the formula, which you could say is just the Pythagorean theorem taken to another dimension. If the length is ℓ, the width is w, and the height is h, the formula is

$$\text{Distance} = \sqrt{\ell^2 + w^2 + h^2}$$

UNIFORM SOLIDS

A rectangular solid is one type of *uniform solid*. A uniform solid is what you get when you take a plane and move it, without tilting it, through space. Here are some uniform solids.

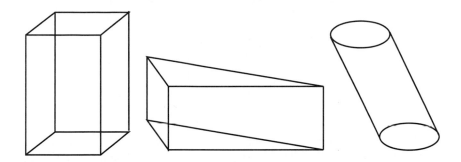

The way these solids are drawn, the top and bottom faces are parallel and congruent. These faces are called the *bases*. You can think of each of these solids as the result of sliding the base through space. The perpendicular distance through which the base slides is called the *height*.

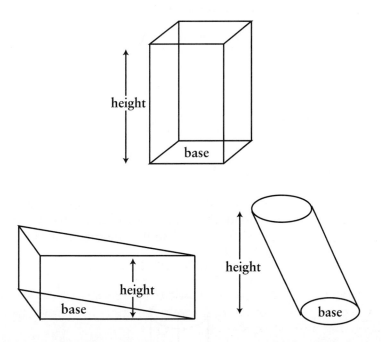

In every one of the above cases—indeed, in the case of *any* uniform solid—the volume is equal to the area of the base times the height. So you can say that for any uniform solid, given the area of the base B and the height h,

Volume of a Uniform Solid = Bh

A. VOLUME OF A RECTANGULAR SOLID

A rectangular solid is a uniform solid whose base is a rectangle and whose height is perpendicular to its base. Given the length ℓ, width w, and height h, the area of the base is ℓw, so the volume formula is

Volume of a Rectangular Solid = ℓwh

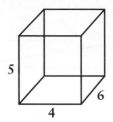

The volume of a 4-by-5-by-6 box is

$$4 \times 5 \times 6 = 120$$

B. VOLUME OF A CUBE

A cube is a rectangular solid with length, width, and height all equal. If e is the length of an edge of a cube, the volume formula is

Volume of a Cube = e^3

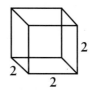

The volume of this cube is $2^3 = 8$.

C. VOLUME OF A CYLINDER

A cylinder is a uniform solid whose base is a circle. Given base radius r and height h, the area of the base is πr^2, so the volume formula is

Volume of a Cylinder = $\pi r^2 h$

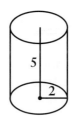

In the cylinder above, $r = 2$ and $h = 5$, so

$$\text{Volume} = \pi(2^2)(5) = 20\pi$$

Example:

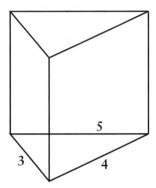

In the figure above, the bases of the right uniform solid are triangles with sides of lengths 3, 4, and 5. If the volume of the solid is 30, what is the total surface area?

The surface area is the sum of the areas of the faces. To find the areas of the faces, you need to figure out what kinds of polygons they are so that you'll know what formulas to use. Start with the bases, which are said to be "triangles with sides of lengths 3, 4, and 5." If side lengths don't ring a bell in your head, then you'd better go back and bone up on your special triangles. This is a 3-4-5 triangle, which means that it's a right triangle, which means that you can use the legs as the base and height to find the area:

$$\text{Area of Right Triangle} = \frac{1}{2}(\text{leg}_1)(\text{leg}_2) = \frac{1}{2}(3)(4) = 6$$

That's the area of each of the bases. The other three faces are rectangles. To find their areas, you need first to determine the height of the solid. If the area of the base is 6, and the volume is 30, then

$$\text{Volume} = Bh$$

$$30 = 6h$$

$$h = 5$$

So the areas of the three rectangular faces are $3 \times 5 = 15$, $4 \times 5 = 20$, and $5 \times 5 = 25$. The total surface area, then, is $6 + 6 + 15 + 20 + 25 = 72$.

## 5

COORDINATE GEOMETRY

MIDPOINTS AND DISTANCES

Some of the more basic coordinate geometry questions concern themselves with the layout of the grid, the location of points, distances between them, midpoints, and so on.

Example:

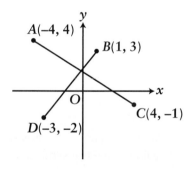

In the above figure, what is the distance from the midpoint of segment *AC* to the midpoint of segment *BD*?

To find the midpoint of a segment, average the *x*-coordinates and average the *y*-coordinates of the endpoints:

$$\text{midpoint of } AC = \left(\frac{-4 + 4}{2}, \frac{4 - 1}{2}\right) = (0, 1.5)$$

$$\text{midpoint of } BD = \left(\frac{-3 + 1}{2}, \frac{-2 + 3}{2}\right) = (-1, 0.5)$$

To find the distance between two points, use the distance formula:

$$\text{Distance} = \sqrt{(x_1 - x_2)^2 + (y_1 - y_2)^2}$$

The distance from (0, 1.5) to (–1, 0.5) is calculated as follows:

$$\text{Distance} = \sqrt{(-1-0)^2 + (0.5-1.5)^2}$$
$$= \sqrt{1+1}$$
$$= \sqrt{2}$$

SLOPE-INTERCEPT EQUATION FORM

DAT Synopsis

For any equation in the form $y = mx + b$:
m = slope
b = y-intercept

Slopes and intercepts are descriptions of lines and points on the grid, but the processes of finding and/or using slopes and/or intercepts are generally algebraic processes.

Example: Which of the following lines has no point of intersection with the line $y = 4x + 5$?

(A) $y = \frac{1}{4}x - 5$

(B) $y = -\frac{1}{4}x - 5$

(C) $y = 4x + \frac{1}{5}$

(D) $y = -4x + \frac{1}{5}$

(E) $y = -4x - \frac{1}{5}$

What does *has no intersection with* mean? It means that the lines are parallel, which in turn means that the lines have the same slope. If you know the slope-intercept equation form, you're able to spot the correct answer instantly.

When an equation is in the form $y = mx + b$, the letter m represents the slope, and the letter b represents the y-intercept. The equation in the stem is $y = 4x + 5$. That's in slope-intercept form, so the coefficient of x is the slope.

$$y = \textcircled{4}x + 5$$
slope = 4

Now look for the answer choice with the same slope. Conveniently, all the answer choices are presented in slope-intercept form, so spotting the one with $m = 4$ is a snap. It's (C):

$$y = \textcircled{4}x + \frac{1}{5}$$
slope = 4

People who are good at memorizing methods and formulas are not necessarily the ones who get the best scores; instead it's the people who have a deeper understanding of mathematics. If you really want to ace coordinate geometry questions, it's not enough to memorize the midpoint formula, the distance formula, the slope definition, the slope-intercept equation form, and so on. What you want is to have a real grasp of what slope is and what perpendicular, parallel, positive, negative, zero, and undefined slopes tell you.

Slope is a description of the "steepness" of a line. Lines that go uphill (from left to right) have positive slopes:

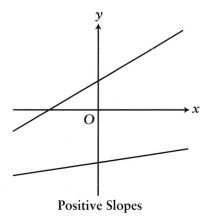

Positive Slopes

Lines that go downhill have negative slopes:

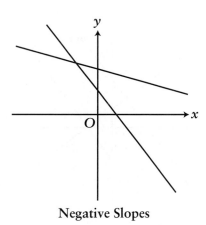

Negative Slopes

Lines parallel to the *x*-axis have slope = 0, and lines parallel to the *y*-axis have undefined slope.

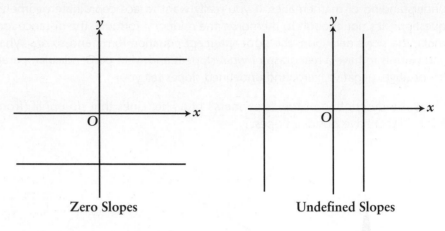

Zero Slopes   Undefined Slopes

Lines that are parallel to each other have the same slope, and lines that are perpendicular to each other have negative-reciprocal slopes.

In the figure below, the two parallel lines both have slope = 2, and the line that's perpendicular to them has slope = $-\frac{1}{2}$:

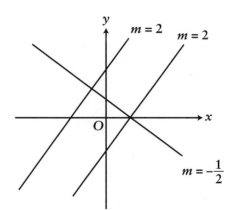

Parallel and Perpendicular Lines

ABSOLUTE VALUE AND INEQUALITIES

Example: Which of the following shaded regions shows the graph of the inequality $y \leq |x + 2|$?

(A)
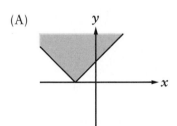

(B)
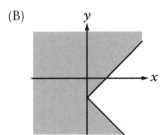

(C)
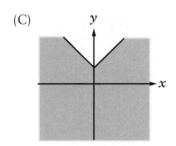

(D)
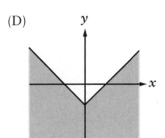

(E)
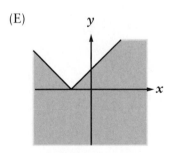

The way to handle an inequality is to think of it as an equation first, plot the line, and then figure out which side of the line to shade. This inequality is extra complicated because of the absolute value. When you graph an equation with absolute value, you generally get a line with a bend, as in all of the answer choices above. To find the graph of an absolute value equation, figure out where that bend is. In this case, $|x + 2|$ has a turning-point value of 0, which happens when $x = -2$. So the bend is at the point $(-2, 0)$. That narrows the choices down to (A) and (E).

Next, figure out which side gets shaded. Pick a convenient point on either side and see if that point's coordinates fit the given inequality. The point (0, 0) is an easy one to work with. Do those coordinates satisfy the inequality?

$$y \leq x + 2$$

$$0 \overset{?}{\leq} 0 + 2$$

$$0 \overset{?}{\leq} 2 \quad \text{Yes.}$$

The point (0, 0) must be on the shady side of the bent line. The answer is (E).

TRIGONOMETRY

RIGHT TRIANGLES AND SOH-CAH-TOA

Trigonometry is really all about right triangles—and we're concerned not with the right angle, per se, but with one of the other angles, denoted by the θ in the figure below. The sine of angle θ is simply the length of the side opposite the angle divided by the length of the hypotenuse (the hypotenuse is the side opposite the right angle). The mathematical abbreviation for sine is "sin," and in mathematics, the sine of the angle θ is written sin θ. The cosine is simply the length of the side adjacent to angle θ (actually, there will be two sides adjacent to the angle, but one of those sides will be the hypotenuse, so by *adjacent*, we really mean the side adjacent to angle that is NOT the hypotenuse) divided by the length of the hypotenuse. The mathematical abbreviation for cosine is "cos," and in mathematics, the cosine of the angle θ is written cos θ. Finally, the tangent of angle is the length of the opposite side over the length of the adjacent side. The mathematical abbreviation for tangent is "tan," and in mathematics, the tangent of the angle is written tan θ.

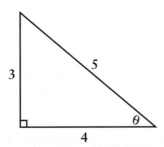

So for instance, in the figure above, the sine of angle θ, sin θ, is the length of the side opposite angle θ (3) divided by the length of the hypotenuse (5). So the sine is 0.60. That is, sin θ = 0.60. The cosine of angle θ is the length of the side adjacent to angle θ (4) divided by the length of the hypotenuse (5). So the cosine of angle θ is 0.80, or cos θ = 0.80. Finally, the tangent is the length of the side opposite angle θ (3) divided by the length of the side adjacent to angle θ (4). So the tangent of angle θ is 0.75, or tan θ = 0.75. To help you remember the definitions of sine, cosine, and tangent as they apply to right triangles, use the mnemonic SOHCAHTOA (the first letters of each of the words below).

$$\text{Sine} = \frac{\text{Opposite}}{\text{Hypotenuse}} \qquad \text{Cosine} = \frac{\text{Adjacent}}{\text{Hypotenuse}} \qquad \text{Tangent} = \frac{\text{Opposite}}{\text{Adjacent}}$$

We can also use this information to help us figure out the lengths of sides of triangles.

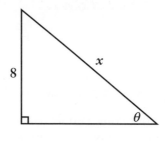

Figure 1

Example: In the right triangle in Figure 1, if the sine of angle $\theta = 0.5$, what is the value of x?

The angle is opposite the given 8, and the side you're looking for is the hypotenuse, so you can use the sine formula to find x:

$$\sin \theta = \frac{\text{Opposite}}{\text{Hypotenuse}}$$

$$0.5 = \frac{8}{x}$$

$$x = \frac{8}{0.5}$$

$$x = 16$$

There are three other trig functions you should be aware of—and each is the reciprocal of one of the trig functions introduced above. They are called cotangent, secant, and cosecant.

$$\text{Cotangent} = \frac{\text{Adjacent}}{\text{Opposite}} \qquad \text{Secant} = \frac{\text{Hypotenuse}}{\text{Adjacent}} \qquad \text{Cosecant} = \frac{\text{Hypotenuse}}{\text{Opposite}}$$

The mathematical abbreviation for cotangent is "cot," and in mathematics, the cotangent of the angle θ is written cot θ. The mathematical abbreviation for secant is "sec," and in math, the secant of the angle θ is written sec θ. The mathematical abbreviation for cosecant is "csc," and in math, the cosecant of the angle θ is written csc θ.

There are also three identities that you should probably be aware of:

$$\sin^2 x + \cos^2 x = 1$$
$$\tan^2 x + 1 = \sec^2 x$$
$$1 + \cot^2 x = \csc^2 x$$

So for any angle x, you could take the sine and cosine, square them both, and the squares will add up to 1. These relationships are really just restatements of the Pythagorean theorem. To make it easier for you to remember them, the proof of the first identity is presented below, but you certainly don't need to know the proof.

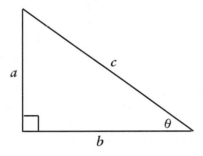

The Pythagorean theorem says that in a right triangle, the square of the hypotenuse is equal to the sum of the squares of the legs. In the right triangle in the figure above, $c^2 = a^2 + b^2$. Let's write this as $a^2 + b^2 = c^2$. Now divide both sides of this equation by c^2. Then $\dfrac{a^2 + b^2}{c^2} = \dfrac{c^2}{c^2}$, $\dfrac{a^2}{c^2} + \dfrac{b^2}{c^2} = 1$, and $\left(\dfrac{a}{c}\right)^2 + \left(\dfrac{b}{c}\right)^2 = 1$. Now $\dfrac{a}{c} = \sin\theta$ and $\dfrac{b}{c} = \cos\theta$. So $\sin^2\theta + \cos^2\theta = 1$.

The identity $\tan^2 x + 1 = \sec^2 x$ is proved by dividing both sides of the equation $a^2 + b^2 = c^2$ by b^2, and the identity $1 + \cot^2 x = \csc^2 x$ is proved by dividing both sides of the equation $a^2 + b^2 = c^2$ by a^2.

Example: Simplify $5\sin^2 x + 5\cos^2 x$.

When you spot a trigonometric expression where quantities are being squared, as in $5\sin^2 x + 5\cos^2 x$, you should think immediately about how to extract $\sin^2 x + \cos^2 x$ from it. You do that by factoring out a 5:

$$5\sin^2 x + 5\cos^2 x = 5(\sin^2 x + \cos x)$$
$$= 5(1)$$
$$= 5$$

DEGREE MEASURE AND RADIAN MEASURE

By definition, if you go all the way around a circle, you have traveled 360 degrees. The degree is a unit of measure for describing angles. An angle that is 1 degree is $\frac{1}{360}$ of a complete circle.

The radian is another measure used to describe an angle and is often used in trigonometry.

The word *radian* is related to the word *radius*. Before we define *radian*, let's repeat the definition of a central angle of a circle. In a circle, a central angle is the angle formed by two radii of the circle.

If a central angle of a circle intercepts an arc of a circle with length ℓ, then the number of radians in the central angle that contains this arc is $\frac{\ell}{r}$.

If a central angle in a circle intercepts an arc equal in length to 1 radius of a circle, that central angle has a radian measure of 1. So an angle can be described by its degree measure or by its radian measure. The circumference C of a circle is related to its radius r by the formula $C = 2\pi r$. So the number of radians in the circumference of any circle is 2π because there are precisely 2π radii in the length of the circumference of any circle. However, there are also 360 degrees in any full circle, so 2π radians is equal to 360 degrees.

Therefore 1 radian is equal to $\frac{360}{2\pi} = \frac{180}{\pi}$ degrees. $\frac{180}{\pi}$ is approximately 57.3.

So 1 radian is approximately 57.3 degrees. You are probably best off if you remember that 2π radians is equal to 360 degrees. Then you can work with this to convert from some other given number of degrees to the corresponding number of radians, or you can convert from the number of radians to the corresponding number of degrees. (You may also remember that π radians is equal to 180 degrees and do your converting based on this, if you are more comfortable doing so.)

Example: How many degrees are there in $\frac{5\pi}{6}$ radians?

Let x be the number of degrees. Then $\dfrac{x}{\left(\dfrac{5\pi}{6}\right)} = \dfrac{360}{2\pi}$.

So $x = \dfrac{5\pi}{6} \times \dfrac{360}{2\pi} = \dfrac{5}{6} \times \dfrac{360}{2} = \dfrac{5}{1} \times \dfrac{60}{2} = 5 \times 30 = 150.$

So there are 150 degrees in $\frac{5\pi}{6}$ radians.

Example: How many radians are there in 270 degrees?

Let y be the number of radians. Then $\dfrac{y}{270} = \dfrac{2\pi}{360}$. So $y = 270 \times \dfrac{2\pi}{360} = 3 \times \dfrac{\pi}{2} = \dfrac{3\pi}{2}.$

There are $\frac{3\pi}{2}$ radians in 270 degrees.

Notice that in the first example, we set up our equation so that we had the number of degrees in the numerator and the number of radians in the denominator, while in the second example, our equation had the number of radians in the numerator and the number of degrees in the denominator. This is just a matter of setting up an equation so that might be a little easier to work with. It seemed easier to begin with the unknown in the numerator in each case. What's really important is that you set up your equation correctly. Then if you can, try to work with an equation that's a little easier.

TRIGONOMETRIC FUNCTIONS OF OTHER ANGLES

To find a trigonometric function of an angle greater than or equal to 90°, sketch a circle of radius r and centered at the origin of the coordinate grid. Start from the point $(r, 0)$ and rotate the appropriate number of degrees counterclockwise.

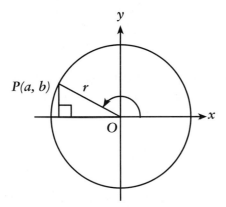

In this "circle setup," the basic trigonometric functions are defined in terms of the coordinates a and b:

$$\sin \theta = \frac{b}{r}$$

$$\cos \theta = \frac{a}{r}$$

$$\tan \theta = \frac{b}{a}$$

$$\cot \theta = \frac{a}{b}$$

$$\sec \theta = \frac{r}{a}$$

$$\csc \theta = \frac{r}{b}$$

Notice that tan and sec are undefined if $a = 0$ and cot and csc are undefined if $b = 0$. Notice also that you are working with a right triangle whose hypotenuse is a radius of the circle. One of the legs of this right triangle is on the part of the x-axis that is closest to the hypotenuse (which is the rotated radius).

Example: sin 210° = ?

Setup: Sketch a 210° angle in the coordinate plane:

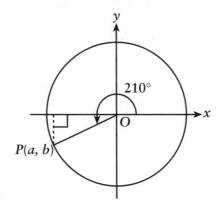

Because the triangle shown in the figure above is a 30°-60°-90° right triangle whose side lengths are in the ratio of $1:\sqrt{3}:2$, it is convenient to use a radius of 2. The coordinates of point P are $(-\sqrt{3}, -1)$.

Therefore $b = -1$, $r = 2$, and sin 210° $= \dfrac{b}{r} = \dfrac{-1}{2} = -\dfrac{1}{2}$.

THE GRAPHS OF $Y = \text{SIN } X$, $Y = \text{COS } X$, AND $Y = \text{TAN } X$

The graph of $y = \sin x$ repeats itself every interval of length 360 degrees (or 2π radians). When $0 \leq x \leq 90°$, sin x increases from 0 (when $x = 0°$) to 1 (when $x = 90°$). When $90 \leq x \leq 180°$, sin x decreases from 1 (when $x = 90°$) to 0 (when $x = 180°$). When $180 \leq x \leq 270°$, sin x decreases from 0 (when $x = 180°$) to –1 (when $x = 270°$). When $270 \leq x \leq 360°$, sin x increases from –1 (when $x = 270°$) to 0 (when $x = 360°$). Right after 360°, sin x begins another cycle. Sin x increases from 0 to 1 (in the interval $360° \leq x \leq 450°$), then decreases from 1 to 0 (in the interval $450° \leq x \leq 540°$), then continues to decrease from 0 to –1 (interval $540° \leq x \leq 630°$), and then increases from –1 to 0 (in the interval $630° \leq x \leq 720°$). This graph also repeats its cycle for values of x less than 0°.

This is the graph of $y = \sin x$.

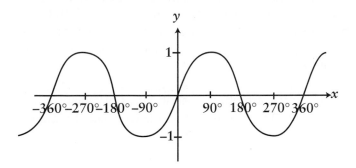

The graph of $y = \cos x$ also repeats itself every 360 degrees or 2π radians. It begins at 1 when $x = 0°$, and in the interval $0 \leq x \leq 90°$, it decreases from 1 to 0. When $90° \leq x \leq 180°$, cos x continues its decrease from 0 when $x = 90°$ to –1 when $x = 180°$. When $180 \leq x \leq 270°$, cos x increases from –1 when $x = 180°$ to 0 when $x = 270°$. When $270 \leq x \leq 360°$, cos x increases from 0 when $x = 270°$ to 1 when $x = 360°$. Then, for $360° \leq x \leq 720°$, the graph repeats itself again with one more complete cycle in the interval $360° \leq x \leq 720°$.

This is the graph of $y = \cos x$.

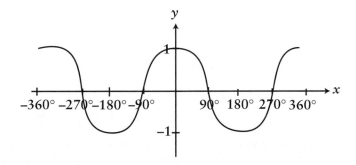

The graph of $y = \tan x$ repeats itself every 180°, which is unlike the graphs of $y = \sin x$ and $y = \cos x$, which repeat themselves every 360°. This is because tan x is positive for $0° < x < 90°$, tan x is negative for $90° < x < 180°$, tan x is positive again for $180° < x < 270°$, and tan x is negative again for $270° < x < 360°$.

Notice that tan x is undefined for every odd multiple of 90° or $\frac{\pi}{2}$. Thus, tan x is undefined when x is any of . . . , –630°, –450°, –270°, –90°, 90°, 270°, 450°, 630°, . . . , or in terms of radians, tan x is undefined when x is any of . . . , $-\frac{7\pi}{2}$, $-\frac{5\pi}{2}$, $\frac{-3\pi}{2}$, $\frac{-\pi}{2}$, $\frac{\pi}{2}$, $\frac{3\pi}{2}$, $\frac{5\pi}{2}$, $\frac{7\pi}{2}$, ...

When $-90° < x < 0°$, tan x is negative, and tan x increases from negative numbers with very large absolute values when x is near but greater than –90° to negative values with small absolute values when x is near but less than 0°. So in the interval $-90° < x < 0°$, tan x is increasing. When $x = 0°$, tan $x = 0$. When $0 < x < 90°$, tan x continues to increase from positive values that have a small absolute value for values of x that are near but greater than 0° to positive values that have a large absolute value for values of x that are close to but less than 90°. The graph of $y =$ tan x in the interval $-90° < x < 90°$ is repeated in the interval $90° < x < 270°$.

In trigonometry, scales are often given in terms of radians. The x-axis of the graph of $y =$ tan x will be labeled with radians, unlike the graphs of $y =$ sin x and $y =$ cos x, which had their x-axes labeled with degrees.

This is the graph of $y =$ tan x.

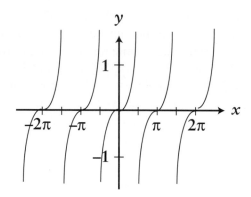

It can be seen from the graph above that when x approaches $\frac{\pi}{2}$ through values of x that are greater than $\frac{\pi}{2}$, $y =$ tan x approaches negative infinity. When x approaches $\frac{\pi}{2}$ through values of x that are less than $\frac{\pi}{2}$, $y =$ tan x approaches positive infinity. This can be seen on the graph of $y =$ tan x above.

PERIODIC FUNCTIONS

A function f is a set of instructions that associates with each number of a set A (which is called the domain) and a number in a set B (which is called the range). Often the domain and/or the range are not specified. What is important is that you just follow the instructions: For each given number, use the function to find the number associated with it.

If x is a point of the domain, then $f(x)$ is the number associated with x by the function f. Notice the difference between f and $f(x)$. f refers to the entire process of using the instructions to associate numbers with other numbers, while $f(x)$ means the exact number that the function f associates with the number x. So $f(x)$ is a number for any specified x. (While f is probably the most common, other letters such as g, h, and r may all be used to denote functions.)

The trigonometric function sin x repeats itself every 360°. For example, sin30° equals sin390°; both of these equal $\frac{1}{2}$.

Let R be a positive constant. If f is a function such that $f(x) = f(x + R)$ for all x, and R is the smallest positive number for which this is true, then the function is said to be periodic with period R. Notice that for the function f defined by $f(x) = \sin x$, $\sin (x + 2\pi) = \sin x$ for all x. Because 2π is the smallest possible positive value for R for which $\sin (x + R) = \sin x$ for all x, 2π is the period of sin x. While it is also true that $\sin (x + 4\pi) = \sin x$ for all x, 4π is not the smallest possible positive value for R such that $\sin (x + R) = \sin x$ for all x. So even though for any x, sin x does have the same value at $x + 4\pi$ that is has at x, we would not say that the period of $f(x) = \sin x$ is 4π. Again, the period of sin x is 2π.

THE INVERSE SINE FUNCTION AND THE INVERSE TANGENT FUNCTION

By the inverse sine function of x, that is denoted by arcsin x, or $\sin^{-1} x$, it is meant that angle y that is such that $\sin y = x$ and $-90° \leq y \leq 90°$. Because $-1 \leq \sin y \leq 1$, the inverse sine function cannot be defined for values of x such that $x < -1$ or $x > 1$. Therefore, the inverse sine function of x is defined only for x such that $-1 \leq x \leq 1$.

For example, $\arcsin\left(\frac{1}{2}\right) = \sin^{-1}\left(\frac{1}{2}\right) = 30°$ because $\sin 30° = \frac{1}{2}$ and 30° is in the interval $-90° \leq y \leq 90°$.

The reason that for a given x, the value of $\sin^{-1} x$ is defined to be in the interval $-90° \leq y \leq 90°$ is that for a given x, there are infinitely many y such that $\sin y = x$, and a function must associate exactly one number with each number.

For example, look at $\sin^{-1}\left(\frac{1}{2}\right)$ again. It is true that . . . , $\sin(-570°) = \frac{1}{2}$, $\sin(-330°) = \frac{1}{2}$, $\sin(-210°) = \frac{1}{2}$, $\sin 30° = \frac{1}{2}$, $\sin 150° = \frac{1}{2}$, $\sin 390° = \frac{1}{2}$, $\sin 510° = \frac{1}{2}$, $\sin 750° = \frac{1}{2}$, ... To be able to assign a unique value to $\sin^{-1}\left(\frac{1}{2}\right)$, the requirement that the angle be in the interval $-90° \leq y \leq 90°$ is included.

By the inverse tangent function of x, which is denoted by arctan x, or $\tan^{-1} x$, it is meant that angle y that is such that $-90° < y < 90°$ and $\tan y = x$. The inverse tangent function is defined for all real x. For example, $\arctan(-1) = \tan^{-1}(-1) = -45°$ because $-45°$ is in the interval $-90° < y < 90°$ and $\tan(-45°) = -1$.

The reason that for a given x the value of $\tan^{-1} x$ is defined to be in the interval $-90° < y < 90°$ is that for any given real number x, there are infinitely many values of y such that $\tan y = x$ and a function must associate exactly one number with each number. For example, look at $\tan^{-1} (-1)$ again. It is true that $\tan (-765°) = -1$, $\tan (-585°) = -1$, $\tan (-405°) = -1$, $\tan (-225°) = -1$, $\tan (-45°) = -1$, $\tan (135°) = -1$, $\tan 315° = -1$, $\tan 495° = -1$, $\tan 675° = -1$,.... To be able to assign a unique value to $\tan^{-1} (-1)$, the requirement that the angle be in the interval $-90° < y < 90°$ is included.

Notice that the possible values of the inverse sine function are in the interval $-90° \le y \le 90°$, while the possible values of the inverse tangent function are in the interval $-90° < y < 90°$. The values of $-90°$ and $90°$ are not possible values of the inverse tangent function because $\tan 90°$ and $\tan (-90°)$ are both undefined.

Example: Which of the following is equal to $\tan\left(\sin^{-1}\left(\dfrac{7}{\sqrt{74}}\right)\right)$?

   (A) $\dfrac{\sqrt{74}}{7}$ (B) $\dfrac{5}{\sqrt{74}}$ (C) $\dfrac{5}{7}$ (D) $\dfrac{7}{\sqrt{74}}$ (E) $\dfrac{7}{5}$

We want to find the tangent of a certain angle. That angle is $\sin^{-1}\left(\dfrac{7}{\sqrt{74}}\right)$. Call $\sin^{-1}\left(\dfrac{7}{\sqrt{74}}\right)$ the angle y. Then $\sin y = \dfrac{7}{\sqrt{74}}$. Remember that in a right triangle, the sine of an angle is equal to the length of the leg opposite that angle divided by the length of the hypotenuse. So draw yourself a picture of a right triangle with an angle y whose sine is $\dfrac{7}{\sqrt{74}}$:

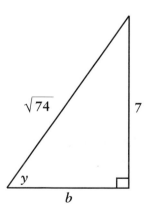

If we can find the length of b, we can find $\tan\left(\sin^{-1}\left(\dfrac{7}{\sqrt{74}}\right)\right) = \tan y$ by remembering that in a right triangle, the tangent of an angle is equal to the length of the leg opposite that angle divided by the length of the leg adjacent to that angle. The length b of the other leg can be found by using the Pythagorean theorem, which says that in a right triangle, the square of the hypotenuse is equal to the sum of the squares of the legs. Here,

$$7^2 + b^2 = (\sqrt{74})^2$$
$$49 + b^2 = 74$$
$$b^2 = 25$$
$$b = 5$$

(By the way, $b = -5$ is also a solution of the equation $b^2 = 25$, but here we're concerned with lengths and you can't have a negative length, so $b = -5$ is a solution of the equation $b^2 = 25$ that does not apply here.)

So $b = 5$, and now we can find tan y: $\tan y = \tan\left(\sin^{-1}\left(\dfrac{7}{\sqrt{74}}\right)\right) = \dfrac{7}{5}$, and choice (E) is correct.

FULL-LENGTH
PRACTICE DAT

Instructions for Taking the Practice Test

Before taking the practice test, find a quiet place where you can work uninterrupted. Make sure you have a comfortable desk and several No. 2 pencils.

Use the answer grid provided to record your answers. You'll find the answer key and score conversion chart following the test.

The test consists of four sections: Survey of the Natural Sciences (90 minutes), Perceptual Ability Test (60 minutes), Reading Comprehension (50 minutes), and Quantitative Reasoning (45 minutes). Remember, if you finish a section early, you may review any questions within that section, but you may not go back or forward a section.

Good luck.

MARK ONE AND ONLY ONE ANSWER TO EACH QUESTION. BE SURE TO FILL IN COMPLETELY THE SPACE FOR YOUR INTENDED ANSWER CHOICE. IF YOU ERASE, DO SO COMPLETELY. MAKE NO STRAY MARKS.

RIGHT MARK: ●   WRONG MARKS: ⊘ ✗ ●

Remove this answer sheet and use it to complete the full-length practice DAT.

Survey of the Natural Sciences

100 questions—90 minutes

DIRECTIONS: This examination is composed of 100 items: Biology (1–40), General Chemistry (41–70), and Organic Chemistry (71–100).

PERIODIC TABLE OF THE ELEMENTS

1 H 1.0																	2 He 4.0
3 Li 6.9	4 Be 9.0											5 B 10.8	6 C 12.0	7 N 14.0	8 O 16.0	9 F 19.0	10 Ne 20.2
11 Na 23.0	12 Mg 24.3											13 Al 27.0	14 Si 28.1	15 P 31.0	16 S 32.1	17 Cl 35.5	18 Ar 39.9
19 K 39.1	20 Ca 40.1	21 Sc 45.0	22 Ti 47.9	23 V 50.9	24 Cr 52.0	25 Mn 54.9	26 Fe 55.8	27 Co 58.9	28 Ni 58.7	29 Cu 63.5	30 Zn 65.4	31 Ga 69.7	32 Ge 72.6	33 As 74.9	34 Se 79.0	35 Br 79.9	36 Kr 83.8
37 Rb 85.5	38 Sr 87.6	39 Y 88.9	40 Zr 91.2	41 Nb 92.9	42 Mo 95.9	43 Tc (98)	44 Ru 101.1	45 Rh 102.9	46 Pd 106.4	47 Ag 107.9	48 Cd 112.4	49 In 114.8	50 Sn 118.7	51 Sb 121.8	52 Te 127.6	53 I 126.9	54 Xe 131.3
55 Cs 132.9	56 Ba 137.3	57 La* 138.9	72 Hf 178.5	73 Ta 180.9	74 W 183.9	75 Re 186.2	76 Os 190.2	77 Ir 192.2	78 Pt 195.1	79 Au 197.0	80 Hg 200.6	81 Tl 204.4	82 Pb 207.2	83 Bi 209.0	84 Po (209)	85 At (210)	86 Rn (222)
87 Fr (223)	88 Ra 226.0	89 Ac† 227.0	104 Unq (261)	105 Unp (262)	106 Unh (263)	107 Uns (262)	108 Uno (265)	109 Une (267)									

*	58 Ce 140.1	59 Pr 140.9	60 Nd 144.2	61 Pm (145)	62 Sm 150.4	63 Eu 152.0	64 Gd 157.3	65 Tb 158.9	66 Dy 162.5	67 Ho 164.9	68 Er 167.3	69 Tm 168.9	70 Yb 173.0	71 Lu 175.0
†	90 Th 232.0	91 Pa (231)	92 U 238.0	93 Np (237)	94 Pu (244)	95 Am (243)	96 Cm (247)	97 Bk (247)	98 Cf (251)	99 Es (252)	100 Fm (257)	101 Md (258)	102 No (259)	103 Lr (260)

GO TO THE NEXT PAGE.

1. Which of the following aspects of cellular respiration is correctly paired with the location in the cell where it occurs?

   A. Electron transport chain—inner mitochondrial membrane
   B. Glycolysis—inner mitochondrial membrane
   C. Krebs cycle—cytoplasm
   D. Fatty acid degradation—lysosomes
   E. ATP synthesis—outer mitochondrial membrane

2. If a strand of DNA underwent four rounds of replication, what percentage of the total DNA present would be comprised of the original DNA molecule?

   A. 0%
   B. 3.125%
   C. 6.25%
   D. 12.5%
   E. 25%

3. You discover an organism you believe to be a prokaryote. The presence of which of the following would support your hypothesis?

   A. Photosynthetic granules
   B. Cell wall made of peptidoglycans
   C. mRNA
   D. Cell wall made of cellulose
   E. Linear DNA

4. All of the following statements about the glycolytic pathway are true EXCEPT

   A. It occurs in the cytoplasm.
   B. Glycolysis is anaerobic.
   C. One molecule of glucose breaks down into one molecule of pyruvate.
   D. One molecule of glucose results in the formation of 2 net ATP and 2 reduced molecules of NAD^+.
   E. Glucose is partially oxidized.

5. Which of the following is NOT true regarding DNA?

   A. The basic unit is a nucleotide.
   B. Adenine and guanine are pyrimidines.
   C. The strands are antiparallel.
   D. Guanine always binds with cytosine with three hydrogen bonds.
   E. The sugar molecule is deoxyribose.

6. Fats differ from carbohydrates in that

   A. they have much more hydrogen than oxygen.
   B. they have much more oxygen than hydrogen.
   C. carbohydrates release more energy per gram than fats.
   D. they are more likely to form polymers.
   E. they contain nitrogen.

7. Which stage of embryonic development consists of a hollow ball of cells surrounding a fluid-filled center?

   A. Zygote
   B. Morula
   C. Blastula
   D. Two-layer gastrula
   E. Three-layer gastrula

8. You isolate a membrane-bound vesicle containing hydrolytic enzymes. It is most likely a

   A. chloroplast.
   B. microbody.
   C. phagosome.
   D. vacuole.
   E. lysosome.

GO TO THE NEXT PAGE.

9. In a population in Hardy–Weinberg equilibrium, the frequency of the dominant allele D is three times that of the recessive allele d. What is the frequency of heterozygotes in the population?

   A. 6.25%
   B. 25%
   C. 37.5%
   D. 56.25%
   E. 75%

10. Shortly after gastrulation, a teratogen affects the development of the endoderm. You will most likely see a deformity in the

    A. lens of the eye.
    B. gonads.
    C. nervous system.
    D. bladder lining.
    E. connective tissue.

11. Which of the following is involved in respiration and excretion and develops into the placenta in humans?

    A. Chorion
    B. Allantois
    C. Amnion
    D. Yolk sac
    E. Placenta

12. Which component of blood is involved in clot formation?

    A. Erythrocytes
    B. Macrophages
    C. T cells
    D. B cells
    E. Platelets

13. Ten turns of the Calvin cycle will produce

    A. 10 CO_2.
    B. 20 PGAL.
    C. 20 RBP.
    D. 36 ATP.
    E. 5 glucose.

14. Which of the following elements is not found in nucleic acids?

    A. Sulfur
    B. Carbon
    C. Oxygen
    D. Nitrogen
    E. Phosphorus

15. The next Mars probe brings back spores from an unknown plant. You discover that the spores have 18 chromosomes. Therefore,

    A. the haploid number is 9.
    B. the diploid number is 18.
    C. the haploid number is 36.
    D. the diploid number is 36.
    E. the diploid number is 9.

16. A color-blind male X_cY is crossed with a normal female who is a carrier of fragile X and color blindness (X_fX_c). What is the probability that a male child will be phenotypically normal?

    A. 0%
    B. 25%
    C. 50%
    D. 75%
    E. 100%

17. Which of the following is NOT true regarding the cytoskeleton?

    A. It is composed of microtubules and microfilaments.
    B. It gives the cell mechanical support.
    C. It maintains the cell's shape.
    D. It makes up the cell wall.
    E. It is functional in the cell's motility.

GO TO THE NEXT PAGE.

18. Someone turned the dial to 56°C from 37°C on the heat bath that you are using for an enzyme-catalyzed reaction you are studying. Your reaction will

    A. proceed more quickly, as the increased heat increases the energy level of the system.
    B. proceed more quickly, as the optimum temperature for most enzymes is 56°C.
    C. have a rapid drop in rate due to the heat denaturation of the proteins.
    D. have a rapid drop in rate due to too much energy in the system leading to ineffective collisions.
    E. None of the above

19. Cell division is different in plants than in animals. One difference is that

    A. plant cells have centrioles.
    B. plant cells divide via a cell plate.
    C. plant cells divide with a cleavage furrow.
    D. animal cells lack centrioles.
    E. plant cell divisions have unequal cytokinesis.

20. One molecule of glucose is catabolized via cellular respiration. How many molecules of ATP are produced by oxidative phosphorylation?

    A. 2
    B. 4
    C. 32
    D. 36
    E. 40

21. *Drosophila melanogaster* can have several eye colors. Red eyes are dominant over white eyes and sepia eyes. If a red-eyed fly that resulted from a mating of red-eyed and sepia-eyed parents is crossed with a sepia-eyed fly, what percentage of the offspring will have sepia eyes?

    A. 0%
    B. 25%
    C. 50%
    D. 75%
    E. 100%

22. The retina of the eye is a derivative of the

    A. endoderm.
    B. ectoderm.
    C. mesoderm.
    D. ectoderm and mesoderm.
    E. mesoderm and endoderm.

23. All of the following are characteristics of osmosis EXCEPT

    A. passive transport.
    B. it occurs with water.
    C. the solvent will spontaneously move from a hypertonic environment to a hypotonic environment.
    D. the solvent spontaneously moves from an area of high solvent concentration to low solvent concentration.
    E. it is a special form of diffusion.

24. Natural selection that favors variants of both phenotypic extremes over the intermediate phenotypes is known as

    A. stabilizing selection.
    B. genetic drift.
    C. disruptive selection.
    D. directional selection.
    E. gene flow.

25. Which of the following is a secondary consumer?

    A. Snake that eats mice
    B. Aphid that eats wheat
    C. Fungus that grows in dead tree trunks
    D. Photosynthetic bacterium
    E. Hawk that eats the snake from (A)

26. What region of the brain controls the breathing rate?

    A. Medulla oblongata
    B. Hypothalamus
    C. Cerebrum
    D. Cerebellum
    E. Pituitary gland

GO TO THE NEXT PAGE.

27. The lysogenic life cycle of a bacteriophage

    A. replicates with the host DNA.
    B. can remain dormant indefinitely.
    C. can exist as a prophage.
    D. None of the above
    E. All of the above

28. Which of the following hormones is released from the posterior pituitary?

    A. Oxytocin
    B. FSH
    C. Glucagon
    D. Estrogen
    E. Calcitonin

29. The tick bird feeds on parasites on the skin of a rhinoceros. This is an example of which of the following relationships?

    A. Parasitism
    B. Commensalism
    C. Predation
    D. Mutualism
    E. None of the above

30. In the Linnaen classification system, we are classified as *Homo sapiens*. The term *sapiens* refers to our

    A. class.
    B. family.
    C. order.
    D. genus.
    E. species.

31. Which of the following is TRUE about the role of LH in the menstrual cycle?

    A. LH inhibits the secretion of GnRH.
    B. LH is secreted by the ovary.
    C. LH induces the ruptured follicle to become the corpus luteum and secrete progesterone and estrogen.
    D. LH stimulates the development and maintenance of the endometrium in preparation for implantation of the embryo.
    E. LH stimulates milk production after birth.

32. Cardiac muscle

    A. is innervated by the somatic motor nervous system.
    B. is not striated.
    C. is multinucleated.
    D. has involuntary contraction.
    E. does not require Ca^{2+}.

33. Which of the following is an example of a fixed action pattern?

    A. Startle response
    B. Removing your hand from a hot stove
    C. Circadian rhythms
    D. Characteristic movement of herd animals
    E. None of the above

34. Which part of the flower produces the monoploid cells that develop into pollen grains?

    A. Style
    B. Petal
    C. Sepal
    D. Anther
    E. Stigma

35. Which of the following is an example of a pioneer organism?

    A. Lichens
    B. Mosses
    C. Ferns
    D. Annual grasses
    E. Birches

36. Which region of the kidney has the lowest solute concentration?

    A. Nephron
    B. Cortex
    C. Medulla
    D. Pelvis
    E. Epithelia

GO TO THE NEXT PAGE.

37. Two species occupying similar niches will

    A. both be driven to extinction.
    B. be nocturnal.
    C. evolve in a convergent direction.
    D. compete for at least one resource.
    E. Two species will never occupy similar niches.

38. Resting membrane potential depends on

    A. the differential distribution of ions across the axon membrane.
    B. active transport.
    C. selective permeability.
    D. the Na^+/K^+ pump.
    E. All of the above

39. A patient is diagnosed with a tumor located in the cerebellum. You might notice which of the following symptoms?

    A. Loss of temperature regulation
    B. Change in heart rate
    C. Loss of sense of smell
    D. Loss of hunger and thirst drives
    E. Loss of hand-eye coordination

40. Which metal is complexed to chlorophyll?

    A. Zinc
    B. Copper
    C. Iron
    D. Magnesium
    E. Manganese

41. Which one of the following correctly lists elements in order of decreasing electronegativity?

    A. N, P, As, Sb, Bi
    B. Ga, Ge, As, Se, Br
    C. Hg, In, Ge, P, O
    D. Ra, Ba, Sr, Ca, Mg
    E. Rn, Xe, Kr, Ar, Ne

42. Which one of the following elements has the largest second ionization energy?

    A. Mg
    B. Ca
    C. Sr
    D. Rb
    E. Cs

43. What is the molecular geometry of PH_2Cl?

    A. Square planar
    B. Trigonal planar
    C. Tetrahedral
    D. Trigonal bipyramid
    E. Trigonal pyramid

44. A rigid container holds 3.00 moles of an ideal gas at 298 K. How many moles of gas would need to be added to the container at constant temperature to increase the pressure from 1.00 atm to 1.80 atm?

    A. 73.4 moles
    B. 24.4 moles
    C. 22.4 moles
    D. 2.4 moles
    E. 0.80 moles

45. Determine the numerical value of the rate constant for the reaction $A + B \rightarrow C$ from the experimental rate data given below.

Experiment	$[A]_0$ (M)	$[B]_0$ (M)	$rate_0$ (Ms^{-1})
1	0.181	0.148	1.87
2	0.181	0.300	1.87
3	0.543	0.148	16.83

    A. $k = \dfrac{1.87}{(0.181)(0.148)}$

    B. $k = \dfrac{1.87}{(0.181)(0.148)^2}$

    C. $k = \dfrac{1.87}{(0.181)^2(0.323)}$

    D. $k = \dfrac{(0.181)(0.148)}{1.87}$

    E. $k = \dfrac{1.87}{(0.181)^2}$

GO TO THE NEXT PAGE.

46. The balanced equation below is for a nonspontaneous reaction ($\Delta H° = 131$ kJ/mol and $\Delta S° = 134$ J/mol·K). Assuming that ΔH and ΔS do not vary with temperature, at what temperature will the reaction become spontaneous?

$$C(s) + H_2O\ (\ell) \rightarrow CO(g) + H_2(g)$$

   A. 1250°C
   B. 1022°C
   C. 978°C
   D. 900°C
   E. 749°C

47. At 0°C, a mixture of neon and argon gases occupies a volume of 44.8 liters with a total pressure of 1 atm. If the mixture contains 1.5 moles of argon, how many moles of neon are present?

   A. 3.0
   B. 1.5
   C. 1.0
   D. 0.75
   E. 0.5

48. Which of the series of elements below correctly lists a halogen, an alkaline earth metal, and a transition metal, respectively?

   A. Cl, Na, Sr
   B. Br, Ca, Cr
   C. Se, Sr, Sn
   D. Rb, Ra, Rh
   E. I, Rb, Cu

49. What is the percentage of oxygen by mass in a 200 gram sample of $CuSO_4 \bullet 5H_2O$?

   A. 19.2%
   B. 30.1%
   C. 32.1%
   D. 36.1%
   E. 57.7%

50. Which of the following could be the correct electron configuration for the ground state neutral atom of a nonmetallic element?

   A. $1s^22s^22p^63s^2$
   B. $1s^22s^22p^63s^3$
   C. $1s^22s^22p^63s^24s^2$
   D. $1s^22s^22p^63s^23p^4$
   E. $1s^22s^22p^63s^23p^7$

51. Which of the following is a stable resonance structure of N_2O_4?

   A.

   B.

   C.

   D.

   E.

GO TO THE NEXT PAGE.

52. Which of the following is the most polar molecular compound?

   A. BF_3
   B. CF_4
   C. CBr_4
   D. CH_2Cl_2
   E. CH_2Br_2

53. What volume of hydrogen gas, in liters, at 40°C and 763 torr can be produced by the complete reaction of 5.05 grams of zinc with excess HCl (*aq*)?

   $Zn\ (s) + 2\ HCl\ (aq) \rightarrow ZnCl_2\ (aq) + H_2\ (g)$

   Note: R = 0.0821 L•atm/mol•K.

   A. $\left(\dfrac{5.05}{65.4}\right)\left(\dfrac{760}{763}\right)(0.0821)(313)$

   B. $\left(\dfrac{5.05}{65.4}\right)\left(\dfrac{763}{760}\right)(0.0821)(40)$

   C. $\left(\dfrac{5.05}{65.4}\right)\left(\dfrac{760}{763}\right)(0.0821)(40)$

   D. $\left(\dfrac{5.05}{65.4}\right)\left(\dfrac{763}{760}\right)(0.0821)(313)$

   E. $(2.0)\left(\dfrac{5.05}{65.4}\right)\left(\dfrac{760}{763}\right)(0.0821)(313)$

54. If one isotope of an element has a mass number of 208 and an atomic number of 82, then another isotope of this element could have

   A. 124 neutrons.
   B. 126 neutrons.
   C. a mass number of 208.
   D. an atomic number of 80.
   E. 84 protons.

55. A sample of a pure compound is analyzed and found to contain 0.537 moles of N, 1.074 moles of H, and 0.537 moles of Cl. What is the empirical formula of this compound?

   A. NH_4Cl
   B. NH_2Cl
   C. $NHCl_2$
   D. $N_2H_2Cl_2$
   E. N_2HCl

56. Given the reactions and thermodynamic data below, calculate the ΔH_f^0 for C_6H_5OH in kcal/mol.

reaction	$\Delta H°$(kcal)
$C_6H_5OH + 7\ O_2 \rightarrow 6\ CO_2 + 3\ H_2O$	729.8
$C + O_2 \rightarrow CO_2$	94.4
$2\ H_2 + O_2 \rightarrow 2\ H_2O$	136.8

   A. –247.0
   B. –41.7
   C. 0.00
   D. 41.7
   E. 247.0

57. What is the percent yield if 78 g of C_6H_6 reacts and 82 g of $C_6H_5NO_2$ is formed according to the reaction below?

   $C_6H_6 + HNO_3 \rightarrow C_6H_5NO_2 + H_2O$

   A. 17%
   B. 33%
   C. 50%
   D. 67%
   E. 100%

58. Hydrogen fluoride, HF, is a gas at room temperature, while water, H_2O, is a liquid. The best explanation for this observed difference in physical properties is that

   A. the difference in molecular weights indirectly accounts for the difference in boiling points because of van der Waals forces.
   B. the O–H bond dipoles of water are greater than the F–H bond dipoles of HF and account for the greater dipole-dipole interactions between water molecules.
   C. hydrogen bonding between water molecules is significantly greater than that between HF molecules.
   D. dispersion forces are significant between HF molecules but not between water molecules.
   E. water, as a universal solvent, is more likely than HF to be contaminated with impurities.

GO TO THE NEXT PAGE.

59. When 100 g of an unknown compound is dissolved in water to produce 1.00 liters of solution, the pH of the resulting solution is measured as 4.56. Which of the following statements is most likely true of the unknown compound?

    A. It is a strong base with a formula weight of less than 50 g/mol.
    B. It is a weak base with a pK_b of less than 5.
    C. It is a strong acid with a formula weight of less than 50 g/mol.
    D. It is a weak acid with a pK_a of more than 1.
    E. It is a weak acid with a formula weight of less than 10 g/mol.

60. 35 mL of 0.10 M KOH is required to neutralize 50 mL of a monoprotic acid solution. The molarity of the acid solution is

    A. (35)(50)(0.10).
    B. (35/0.10)(50).
    C. (50/35)(0.10).
    D. (35/50)(0.10).
    E. (50/0.10)(35).

61. When 22.2 g of a soluble ionic compound (formula weight = 111 g/mol) are added to 1.0 kg of water (K_f = 1.86°C/m), the freezing point of the resulting solution is –1.12°C. Which of the following could be the general formula of the ionic compound?

    A. MX
    B. MX_2
    C. M_2X_2
    D. MX_3
    E. M_2X_3

62. In which two compounds does sulfur have the same oxidation state?

    A. H_2S and $SOCl_2$
    B. H_2SO_4 and $SOCl_2$
    C. H_2SO_3 and $SOCl_2$
    D. H_2S and H_2SO_4
    E. H_2SO_3 and H_2SO_4

63. When carbon-14 undergoes beta decay, the daughter element is

    A. carbon-12.
    B. carbon-13.
    C. nitrogen-14.
    D. oxygen-15.
    E. silicon-28.

64. The balanced equation below is for a spontaneous oxidation-reduction reaction.

    $8\ Al\ (s) + 3\ NO_3^-\ (aq) + 5\ OH^-\ (aq) + 18\ H_2O\ (\ell) \rightarrow$
    $8\ Al\ (OH)_4^-\ (aq) + 3\ NH_3\ (g)$

    Which of the following is the best oxidizing agent?

    A. Al (s)
    B. NO_3^- (aq)
    C. NH_3 (g)
    D. Al $(OH)_4^-$ (aq)
    E. OH^- (aq)

65. What is the pH of a saturated aqueous solution of $Ca(OH)_2$? The K_{sp} of $Ca(OH)_2$ is 8.0×10^{-6}.

    A. 15.6
    B. 12.4
    C. 7.0
    D. 1.6
    E. 1.0

GO TO THE NEXT PAGE.

Questions 66–67 refer to the following diagram:

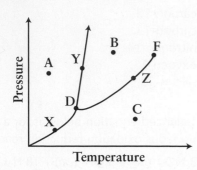

66. At which point(s) on the graph could ice, water, and water vapor exist at equilibrium together in a sealed beaker?

    A. D
    B. D and X
    C. D and Y
    D. D and Z
    E. Z

67. At which point(s) on the graph could condensation occur?

    A. D
    B. Y
    C. Z
    D. D and Y
    E. D and Z

68. Increasing the amount of liquid in a sealed container will cause the vapor pressure of the liquid to

    A. increase, regardless of the identity of the liquid.
    B. increase, if the liquid is sufficiently volatile.
    C. decrease, regardless of the identity of the liquid.
    D. remain the same, regardless of the identity of the liquid.
    E. decrease, if the liquid is sufficiently volatile.

69. Which of the following can be inferred from the heating curve shown?

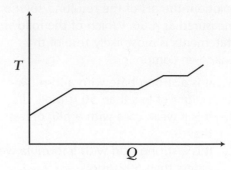

    A. The boiling point temperature is more than double the melting point temperature.
    B. The heat of vaporization is greater than the heat of fusion.
    C. The heat capacity in the gas phase is greater than that of the liquid phase.
    D. The heat capacity in the solid phase is greater than that of the liquid phase.
    E. The heat capacity in the liquid phase is greater than that of the solid phase.

70. Which of the following transformations could occur at the anode of an electrochemical cell?

    A. $Cr_2O_7^{2-}$ $\rightarrow$ CrO_4^{2-}
    B. Cr^{2+} $\rightarrow$ CrO_4^{2-}
    C. $Cr_2O_7^{2-}$ $\rightarrow$ Cr^{2+}
    D. CrO_4^{2-} $\rightarrow$ Cr^{3+}
    E. Cr^{3+} $\rightarrow$ Cr^{2+}

GO TO THE NEXT PAGE.

71. Which one of the following correctly matches the structure ~~Fischer~~ projection?

A. 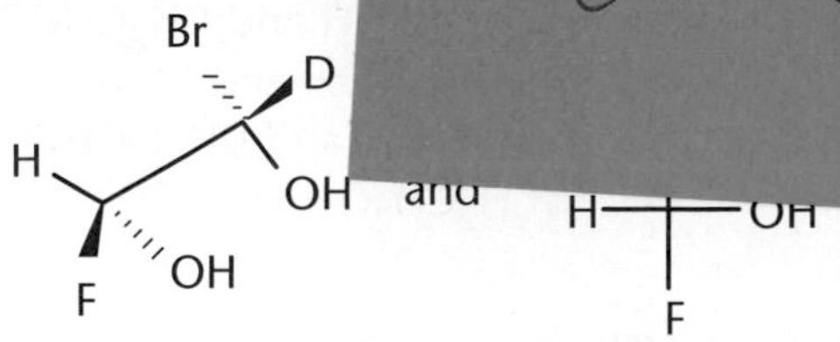 and

B. 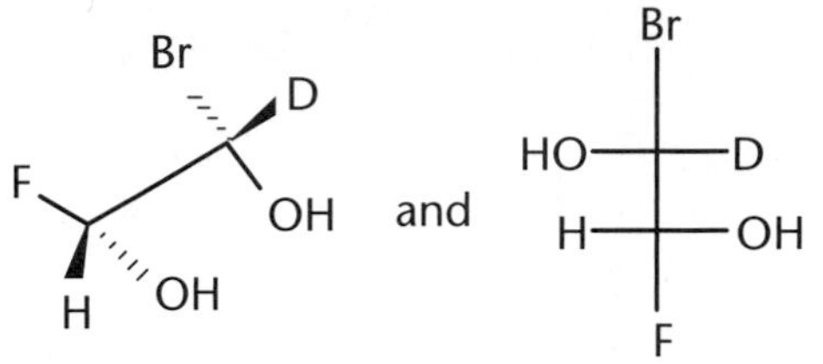 and

C. 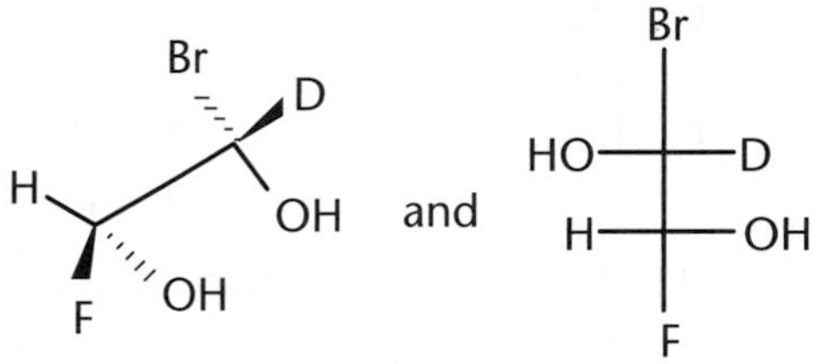 and

D. 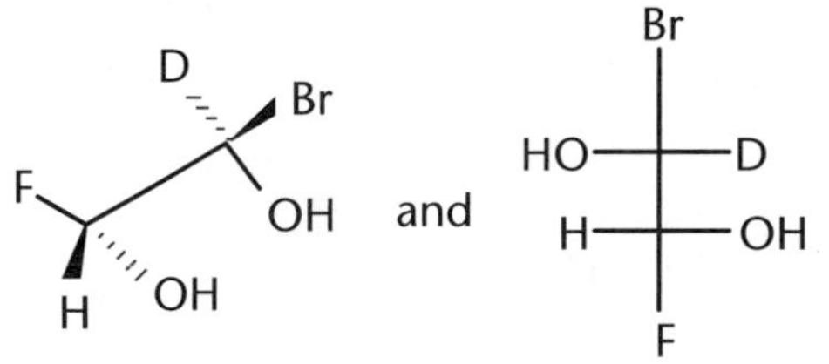 and

E. 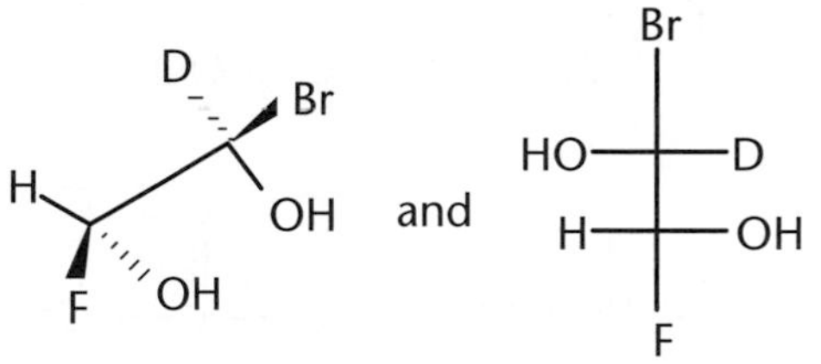 and

72. Which of the following alcohols is least soluble in water?

A. 1-Propanol
B. 2-Methyl-2-propanol
C. 2,3-Butanediol
D. 2-Butanol
E. 3-Pentanol

73. What is the correct IUPAC name of the compound pictured below?

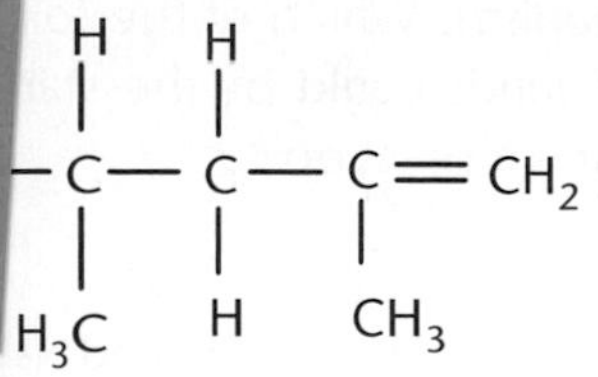

A. 2,4-Dimethyl-1-pentene
B. 2,4,4-Trimethyl-1-butene
C. 1,1,3-Trimethyl-3-butene
D. 2,4-Dimethyl-4-pentene
E. 2-Methyl-4-methylpentane

74. Which of the structures below has the least amount of nonbonded strain?

A.

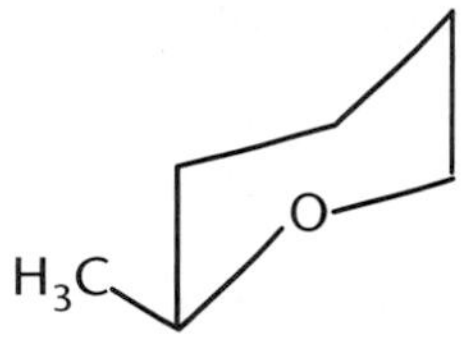

B.

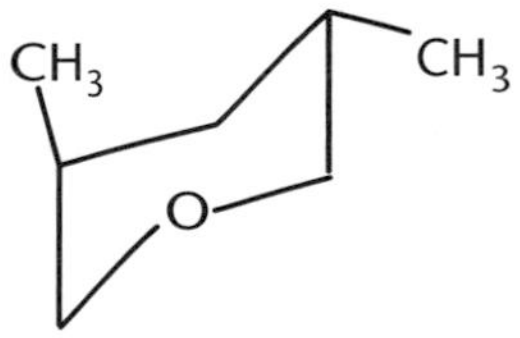

C.

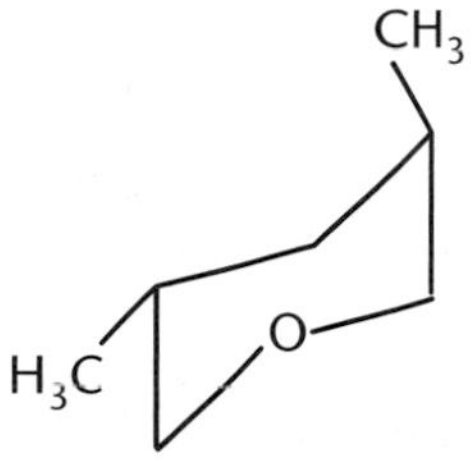

D.

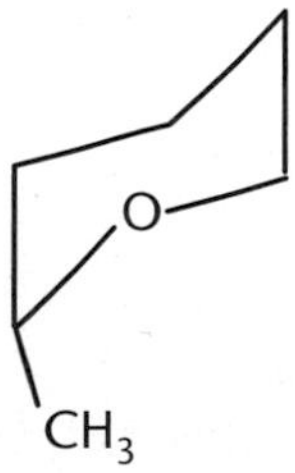

E.

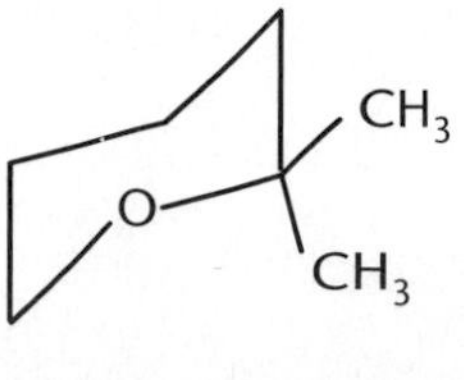

GO TO THE NEXT PAGE.

75. The Williamson ether synthesis is used to produce asymmetric ethers via an S_N2 mechanism. Which of the following pairs of compounds could be the starting materials for such a reaction?

A. $CH_3CH_2CH_2\overset{\overset{\displaystyle O}{\|}}{C}CH_2CH_3$ and $Na\overset{\overset{\displaystyle O}{\|}}{OC}CH_2CH_2CH_3$

B. $CH_3\overset{\overset{\displaystyle CH_3}{|}}{\underset{\underset{\displaystyle Cl}{|}}{C}}CH_2CH_2CH_3$ and $CH_3CH_2CH_2CH_2CH_2ONa$

C. (phenyl)ONa and (phenyl)CHO

D. CH_3CH_2ONa and $CH_3CH_2CH_2CH_2Cl$

E. $CH_3CH_2OCH_2CH_3$ and $CH_3CH_2CH_2CH_2CH_2ONa$

76. Which of the choices below best describes the two structures shown?

A. Enantiomers
B. Geometric isomers
C. Conformational isomers
D. Constitutional isomers
E. Diastereomers

77. Which of the following is a pair of structural isomers?

A. CH_3CH_2COOH and $CH_3CH_2CH_2OH$
B. CH_3CH_2COOH and $CH_2CHCOOH$
C. $CH_3CH_2CH_2OH$ and CH_3CH_2OH
D. CH_3CH_2CHO and CH_3OCHCH_2
E. $CH_3CH_2CH_2OH$ and $(CH_2CHCHO)_n$

78. Given the reaction

$$RY + NaCN \xrightarrow{DMSO} RCN + NaY$$

which of the following is the most likely identity of Y?

A. I
B. CH_3
C. SH
D. PH_2
E. OCH_3

79. Which one of the compounds pictured below is most capable of intramolecular hydrogen bonding?

A. $H_2C\!=\!\overset{\overset{\displaystyle }{}}{\underset{\underset{\displaystyle H}{|}}{C}}\!-\!\overset{\overset{\displaystyle O}{\|}}{C}\!-\!\overset{\overset{\displaystyle O}{\|}}{C}\!-\!CH_2CH_3$

B. $CH_3CH_2\overset{\overset{\displaystyle O}{\|}}{C}\!-\!CH_2COOH$

C. $H_2C\!=\!\overset{\overset{\displaystyle }{}}{\underset{\underset{\displaystyle H}{|}}{C}}\!-\!\overset{\overset{\displaystyle O}{\|}}{C}\!-\!\overset{\overset{\displaystyle O}{\|}}{C}\!-\!\overset{\overset{\displaystyle H}{|}}{C}\!=\!CH_2$

D. $H_2C\!=\!\overset{\overset{\displaystyle H}{|}}{\underset{\underset{\displaystyle }{}}{C}}\!-\!\overset{\overset{\displaystyle O}{\|}}{C}\!-\!\overset{\overset{\displaystyle O}{\|}}{C}\!-\!CH_3$

E. $CH_3CH_2\overset{\overset{\displaystyle O}{\|}}{C}\!-\!OCH_2CH_3$

GO TO THE NEXT PAGE.

80. What is the correct IUPAC name for the compound pictured below?

$$CH_3CHCH_2CHCH_2CH_3$$

with substituent $CH_2CH_2CH_3$ on the first CH and CH_2CH_3 on the lower position

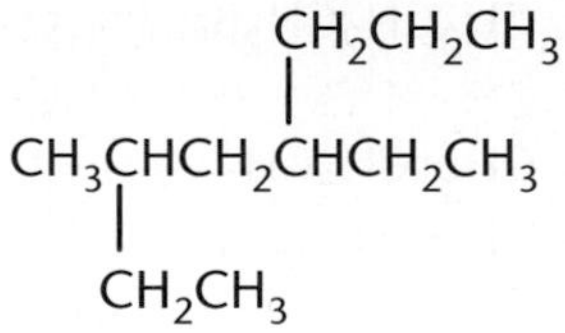

A. 2-Ethyl-4-propylhexane
B. 3-Propyl-5-ethylhexane
C. 5-Ethyl-3-propylhexane
D. 2,4-Diethylheptane
E. 5-Ethyl-3-methyloctane

81. Which of the following will be most reactive towards an S_N1 reaction?

A.

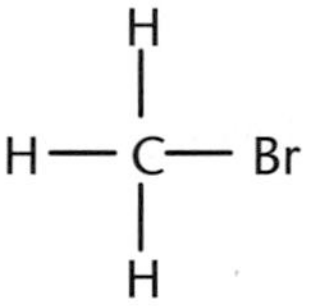

H—C—Br (with H, H, H attached)

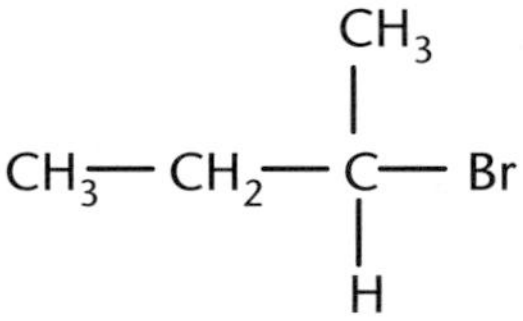

B.

CH_3—CH_2—C—Br (with CH_3 and H attached)

C.

CH_3—C—Br (with CH_3, CH_3, CH_3 attached)

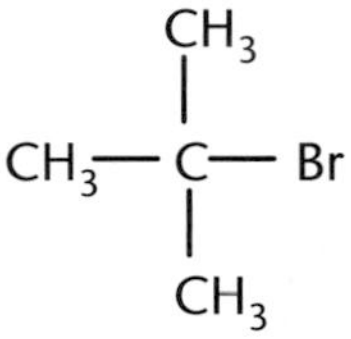

D.

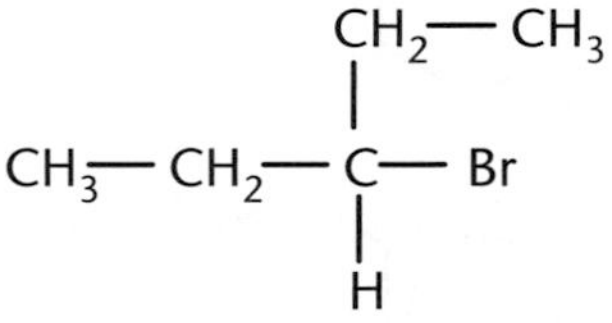

CH_3—CH_2—C—Br (with CH_2—CH_3 and H attached)

E.

CH_3—CH_2—C—Br (with H and H attached)

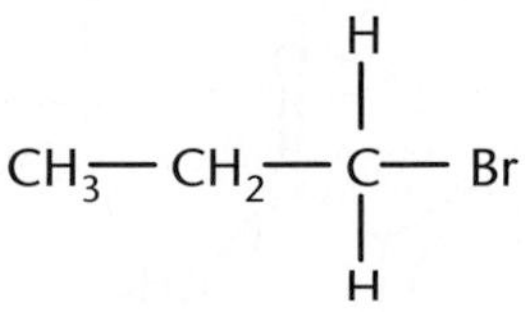

82. The compound pictured below

CHO
H——OH
H——OH
CHO

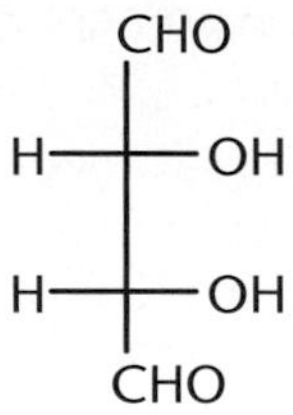

A. has two chiral carbons and is thus optically active.
B. is one of the four diastereomers possible for this compound.
C. has an internal plane of symmetry and thus rotates plane-polarized light.
D. has an axis of rotational symmetry and thus rotates plane-polarized light.
E. has two chiral carbons and is optically inactive.

83. Which of the compounds pictured below is aromatic?

A.

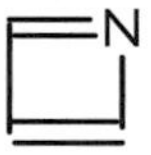

B.

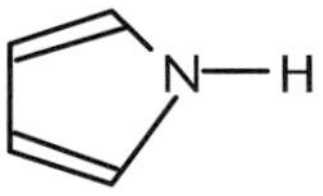

C.

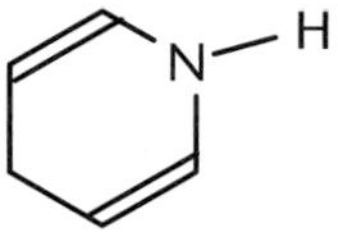

D.

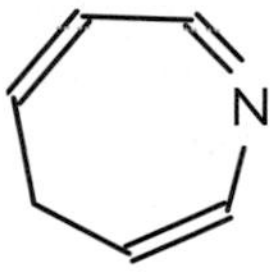

E.

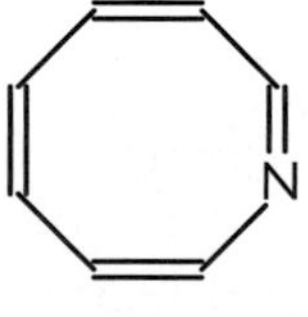

GO TO THE NEXT PAGE.

84. Which of the following structures properly represents an E isomer?

A.

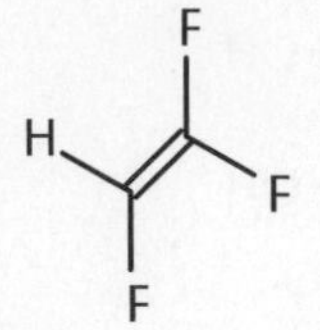

B.

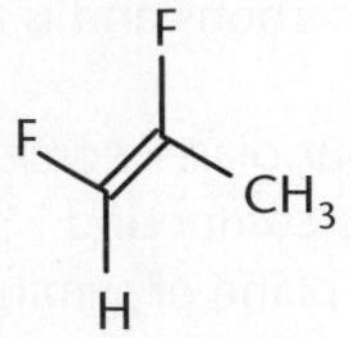

C.

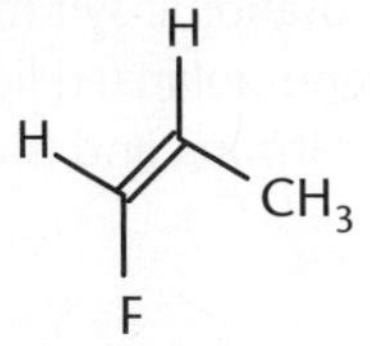

D.

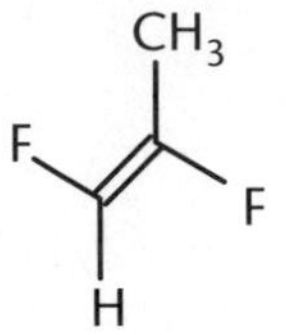

E.

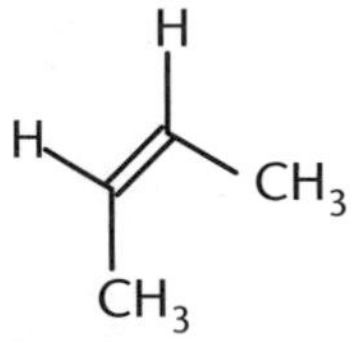

85. A portion of an organic molecule is pictured below, though not necessarily with accurate geometry. What are the approximate degree measures of angles *a*, *b*, and *c*, respectively?

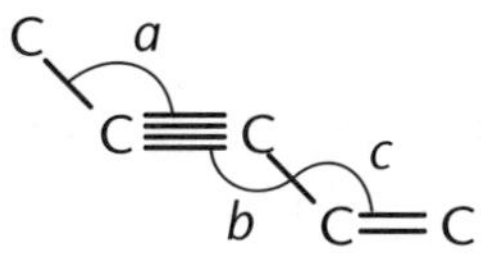

A. 109.5°, 109.5°, and 109.5°
B. 109.5°, 120°, and 109.5°
C. 120°, 120°, and 120°
D. 120°, 180°, and 120°
E. 180°, 180°, and 120°

86. Which of the following bromoalkanes is least likely to undergo an S_N2 reaction?

A. $CH_3CH_2CH_2CH_2Br$

B. $CH_3CHBrCH_2CH_3$

C.

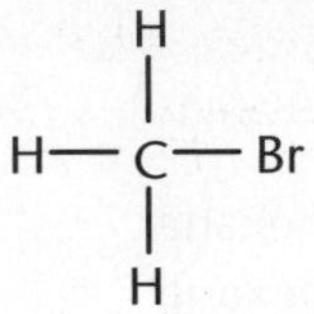

D.

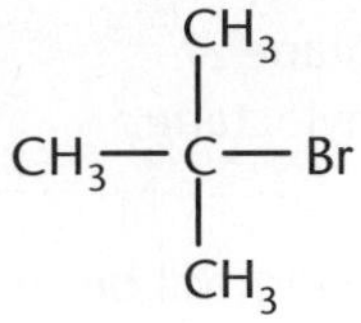

E. CH_3CH_2Br

87. Which of the following is most reactive toward CH_3NH_2?

A.

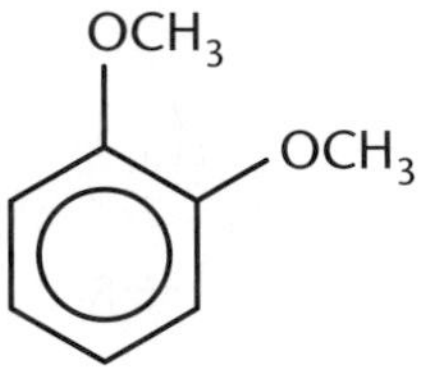

B.

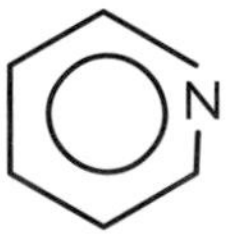

C.

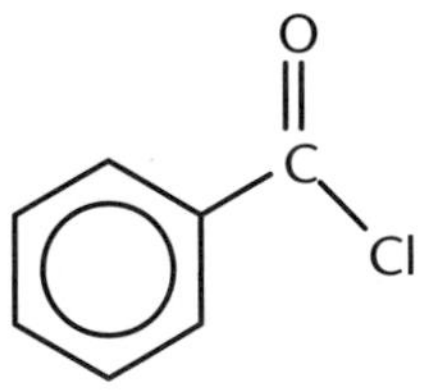

D.

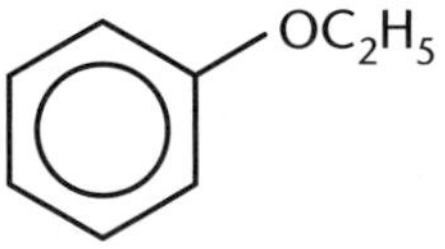

E.

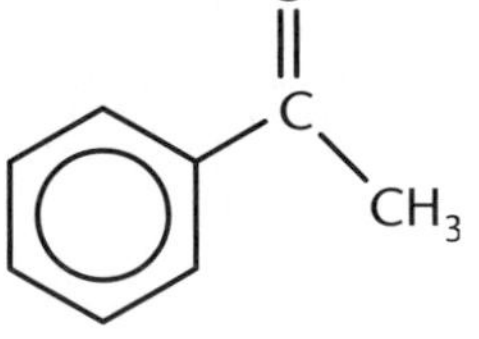

GO TO THE NEXT PAGE.

88. Which of the reagents below could be used to carry out the following conversion?

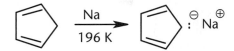

A. LiAlH$_4$/THF, followed by H$^+$/H$_2$O
B. aqueous Hg(CH3COO)$_2$, followed by NaBH$_4$ and KOH
C. KOH/C$_2$H$_5$OH
D. BH$_3$/THF, followed by H$_2$O$_2$ and KOH
E. CrO$_3$, H$_2$SO$_4$

89. 1,3-Cyclopentadiene reacts with sodium metal at low temperatures according to

What is the best explanation for this observation?

A. The reactant is more unstable at reduced temperatures.
B. The cation formed is stabilized by aromaticity.
C. Sodium metal is highly specific for cycloalkanes.
D. The rehybridization of the saturated carbon atom provides additional stability to the product.
E. The anion formed is stabilized by aromaticity.

90. What is the final product, Z, of the synthesis below?

A.
B.
C.
D.
E.

91. The compound pictured below

CH$_3$CH$_2$C—OCH$_2$CH$_3$

A. is optically active.
B. can be hydrolyzed to yield acetic acid and ethanol.
C. can be hydrolyzed to yield acetic acid and propanol.
D. is a *meso* compound.
E. can be hydrolyzed to yield propionic acid and ethanol.

GO TO THE NEXT PAGE.

92. Which of the following is an appropriate resonance form of the conjugate base of *p*-aminobenzoic acid?

A.

B.

C.

D.

E.

93. What is the major organic product of the reaction below?

A.

B.

C.

D.

E.

GO TO THE NEXT PAGE.

94. IR spectroscopy would be most useful in distinguishing between which of the following pairs of compounds?

A. CH$_3$CH$_2$CH$_2$COOH and CH$_3$CCH$_2$CH$_2$CH$_3$ (with =O)

B.
CH$_3$

CH$_3$CCH$_2$CH$_2$CH$_3$ and CH$_3$CH$_2$CH$_2$CH$_2$CH$_2$CH$_3$

C. (benzene ring with C=O–CH$_2$CH$_3$) and (benzene ring with C=O–CH$_3$)

D. CH$_3$CH$_2$OCH$_2$CH$_2$CH$_3$ and
CH$_2$CH$_2$CH$_2$CH$_2$OCH$_3$

E. CH$_3$CH$_2$CH$_2$CH$_2$OCH$_3$
CH$_3$CH$_2$CHOCHCH$_3$

95. Which of the following is a termination step in the free radical bromination of ethane?

A. CH$_3$CH$_2$• + Br• → CH$_3$CH$_2$Br
B. CH$_3$CH$_3$• + Br• → CH$_3$CH$_2$Br + H•
C. CH$_3$CH$_3$ + Br$_2$ → CH$_2$BrCH$_2$Br
D. CH$_3$CH$_2$• + Br• → CH$_3$CH$_2$Br + CH$_3$•
E. CH$_3$CH$_2$• + Br$_2$ → CH$_3$CH$_2$Br + Br•

96. What is the major product of the elimination reaction below?

$$\text{CH}_3-\underset{\underset{Cl}{|}}{\overset{\overset{H}{|}}{C}}-\underset{\underset{H}{|}}{\overset{\overset{H}{|}}{C}}-\underset{\underset{H}{|}}{\overset{\overset{H}{|}}{C}}-\text{CH}_3 \xrightarrow[\text{alcohol}]{\text{KOH}} \; ?$$

A.

B.

C.

D.

E.

GO TO THE NEXT PAGE.

97. Which of the following is a major organic product of the reaction below?

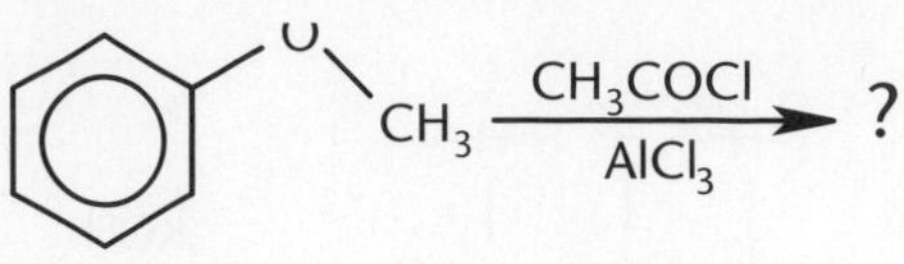

$$\text{(phenyl methyl ether)} \xrightarrow[\text{AlCl}_3]{\text{CH}_3\text{COCl}} ?$$

A.

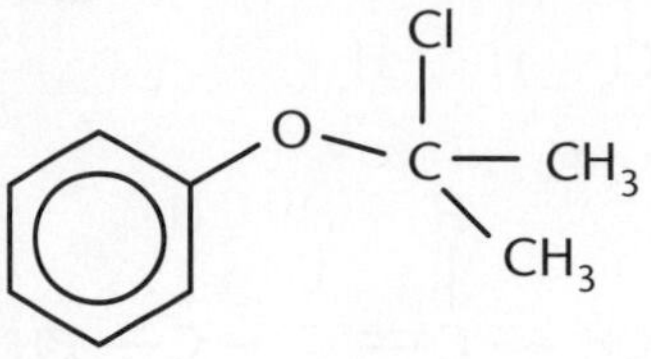

B.

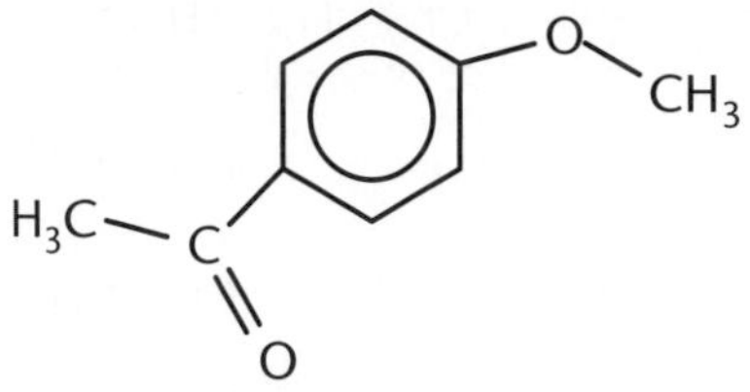

C.

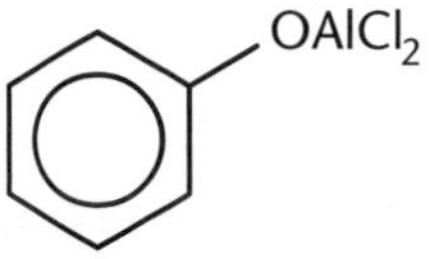

D.

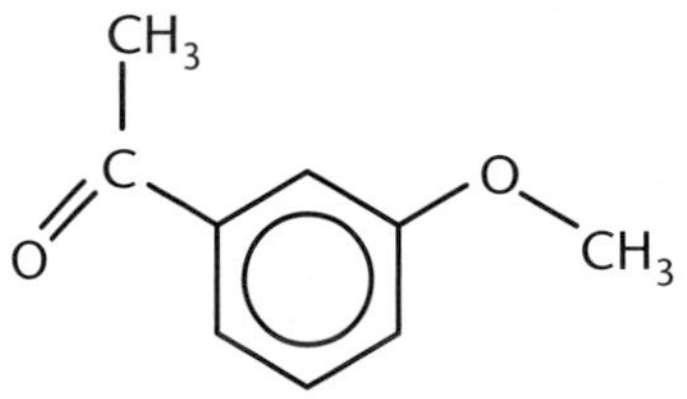

E.

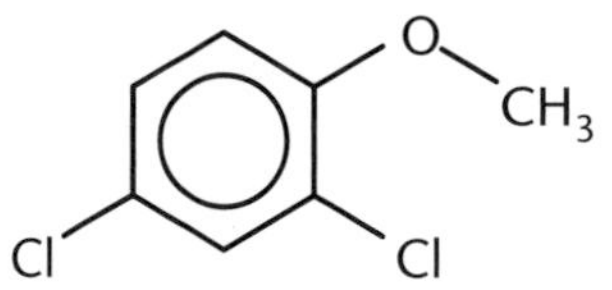

98. Which of the following is the conjugate acid of diethylamine?

A. $CH_3CH_2NH^-$
B. $(CH_3CH_2)_2NH$
C. $(CH_3CH_2)_2NH^+$
D. $(CH_3CH_2)_2NH2^+$
E. $(CH_3CH_2)_2N^-$

99. What are the major products of the reaction sequence shown below?

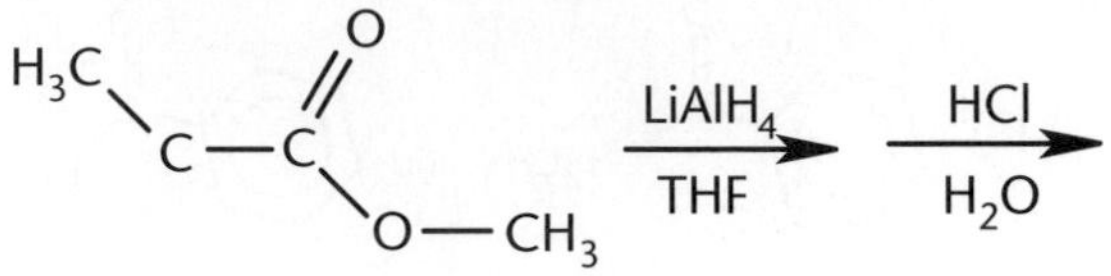

$$\xrightarrow[\text{THF}]{\text{LiAlH}_4} \xrightarrow[\text{H}_2\text{O}]{\text{HCl}}$$

A. CH_3CH_2COOH and $CH3OH$
B. CH_3CH_2COOH and $HCOOH$
C. $CH_3CH_2CH_2OH$ and CH_3OH
D. CH_3CH_2CHO and CH_3OH
E. $CH_3CH_2CH_2OH$ and CH_2O

GO TO THE NEXT PAGE.

100. Which of the following is a major organic product of the reaction sequence below?

A.

B.

C.

D.

E.

STOP. IF YOU FINISH BEFORE TIME HAS EXPIRED, CHECK YOUR WORK. YOU MAY GO BACK TO ANY QUESTION IN THIS PART ONLY.

Perceptual Ability Test
90 questions (6 parts)—60 minutes

PART 1

For questions 1 through 15:

For each question, a three-dimensional object is displayed at left. This figure is followed by outlines of five openings or apertures.

The assignment is the same for each question. Imagine how the object at left looks from all directions, not just the one shown. Choose one of the five openings presented that would allow the object to pass through if the proper side were inserted first. Mark the letter on your answer grid that corresponds to the selected aperture.

Basic Rules:

1. The irregular object at left may be rotated in any manner. It may be inserted through the aperture starting with a side not shown.
2. Once the irregular object has started through the aperture, it may not be rotated or turned in any way. The object must pass completely through the aperture. The aperture is always the exact shape of the external outline of the object.
3. Both the irregular object and openings are drawn to the same scale.
4. There are no irregularities in any hidden part of the object. If a figure has symmetric indentations, hidden portions are symmetric with visible parts.
5. There is only one correct answer choice for each object.

Try the following example:

___

Example:

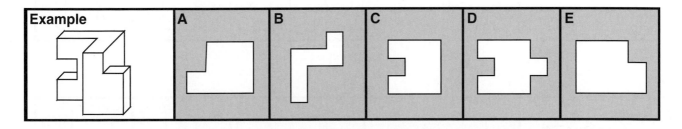

The correct answer is choice (B), since the object would pass through this aperture if the top were inserted first.

Proceed to Questions

GO TO THE NEXT PAGE.

1.

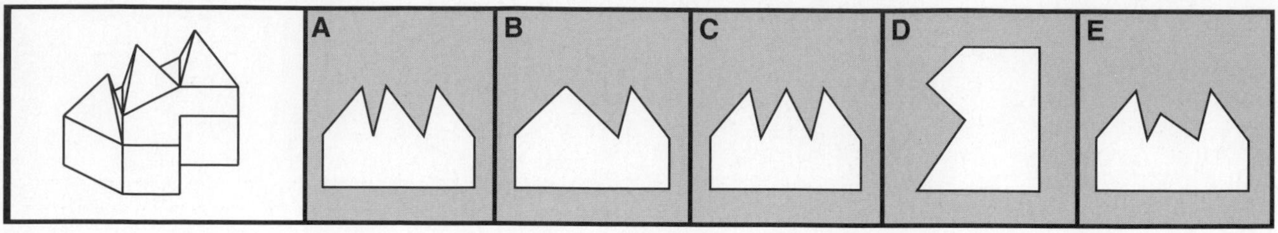

	A	B	C	D	E

2.

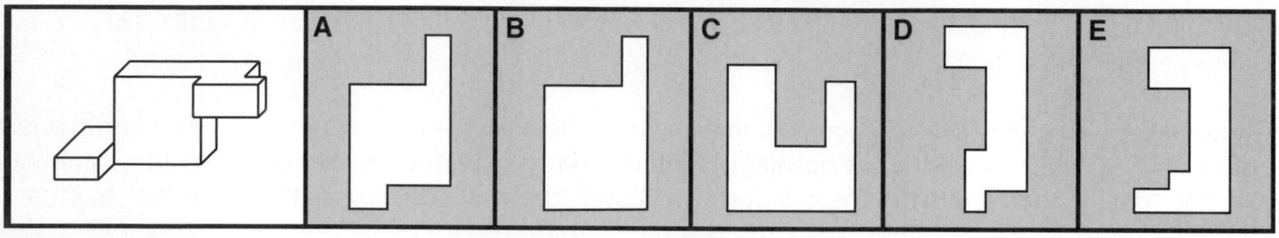

	A	B	C	D	E

3.

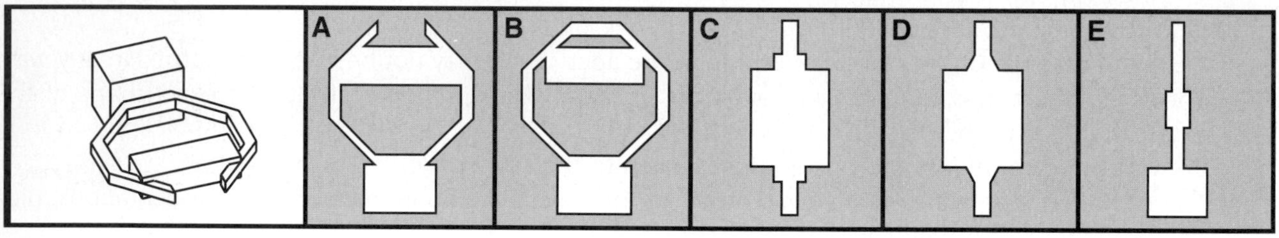

	A	B	C	D	E

4.

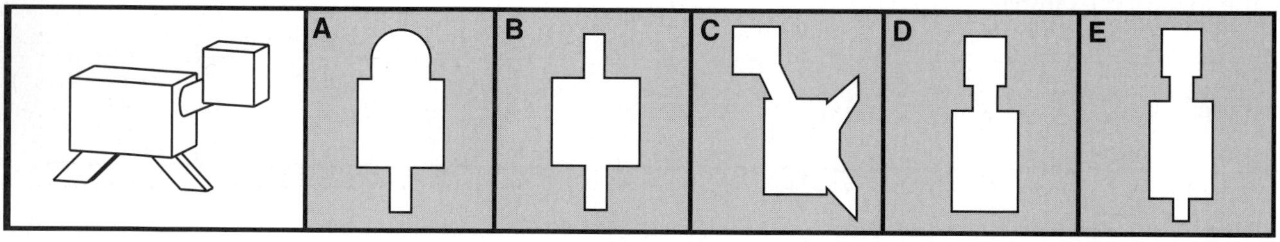

	A	B	C	D	E

5.

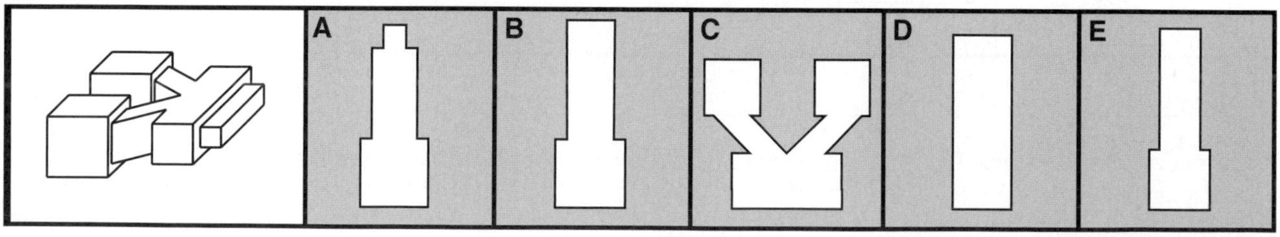

	A	B	C	D	E

GO TO THE NEXT PAGE.

6.

7.

8.

9.

10.

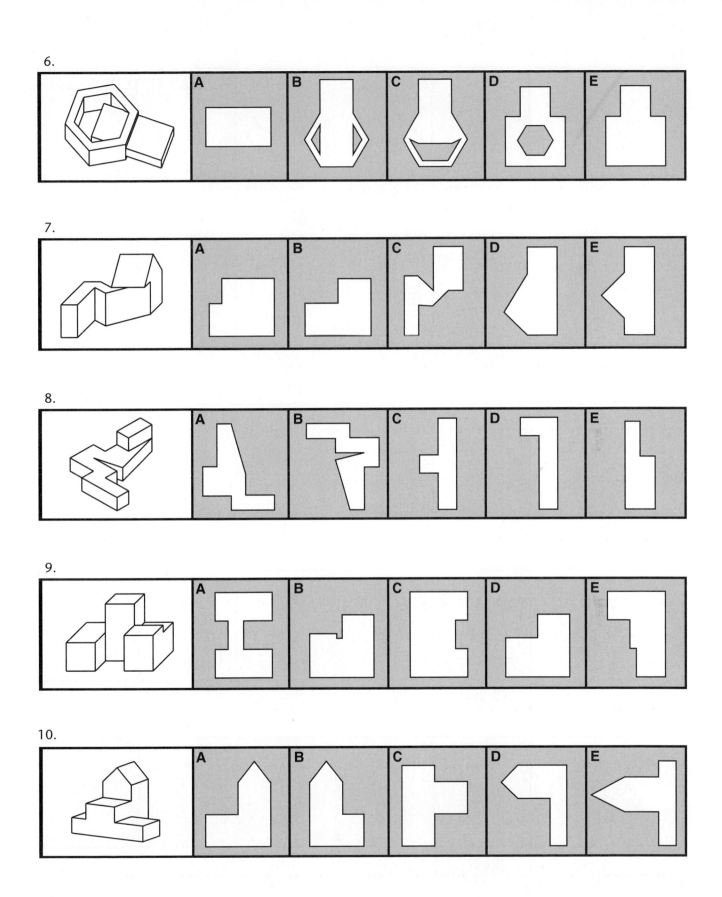

GO TO THE NEXT PAGE.

11.

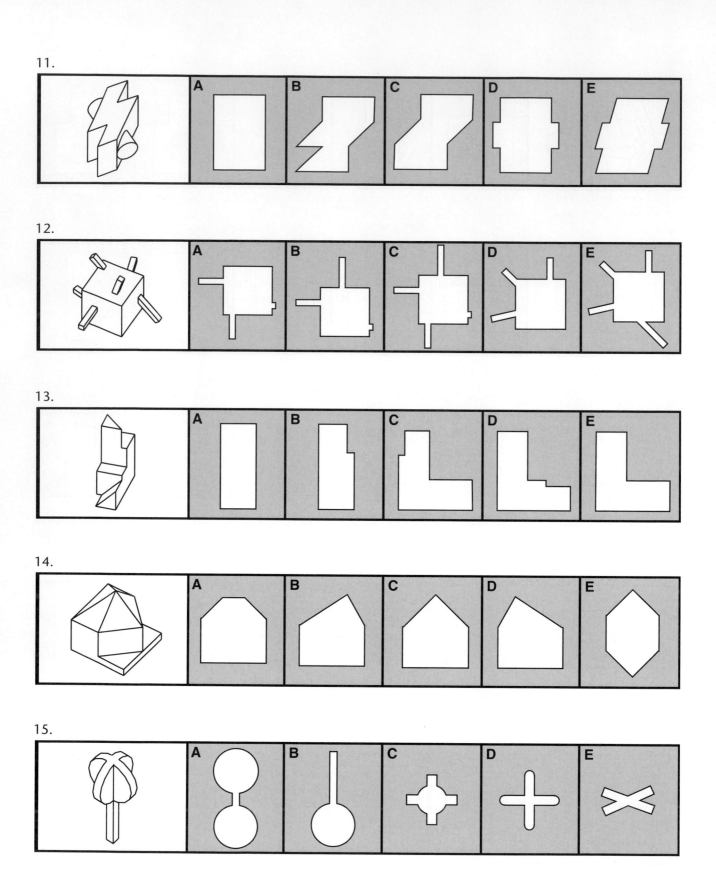

12.

13.

14.

15.

GO TO THE NEXT PAGE.

PART 2

For questions 16 through 30:

Presented are top, front, and end views of various solid objects. All views are presented without perspective. Points in the viewed surface are presented along parallel lines of sight.

The TOP VIEW image of the object presents the projection of looking down on the object. The FRONT VIEW image presents a view of the object from the front. The END VIEW illustrates a lateral view of the object from the right. These views are always in the same position.

Lines that cannot be seen in some perspectives are represented by DOTTED lines.

The problems that follow present two views of a particular object. Four alternatives are shown to complete the set. Select the correct alternative and mark the corresponding letter on the answer grid. Try the following example:

Example: Choose the correct **END VIEW**

TOP VIEW

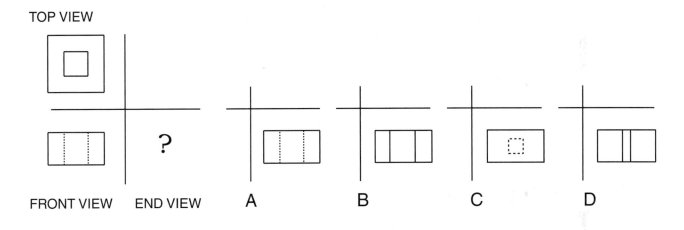

FRONT VIEW   END VIEW   A   B   C   D

The correct answer is choice (A). The following views are shown:

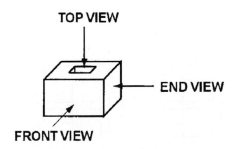

TOP VIEW

END VIEW

FRONT VIEW

Proceed to Questions

GO TO THE NEXT PAGE.

16. Choose the correct **END VIEW.**

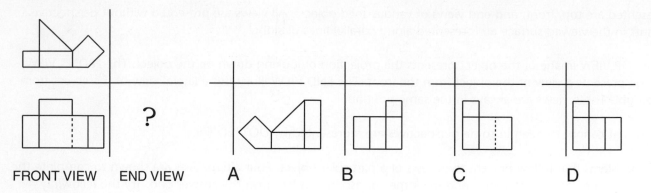

FRONT VIEW   END VIEW   A   B   C   D

17. Choose the correct **END VIEW.**

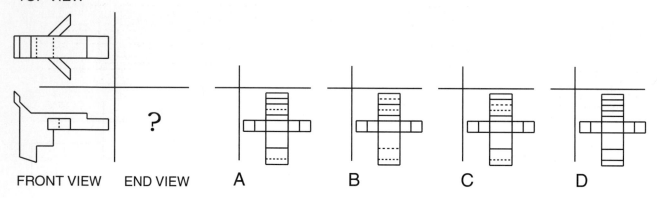

FRONT VIEW   END VIEW   A   B   C   D

18. Choose the correct **END VIEW.**

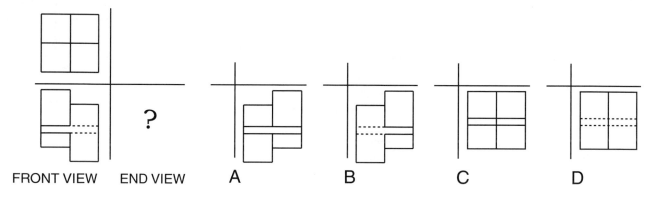

FRONT VIEW   END VIEW   A   B   C   D

GO TO THE NEXT PAGE.

19. Choose the correct **TOP VIEW.**

TOP VIEW

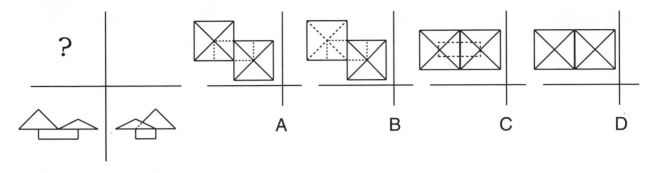

FRONT VIEW   END VIEW

20. Choose the correct **TOP VIEW.**

TOP VIEW

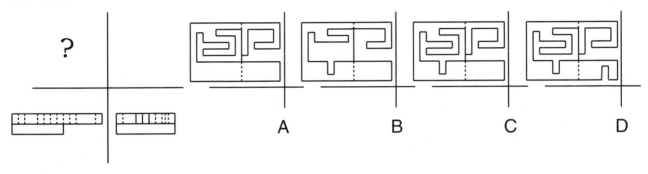

FRONT VIEW   END VIEW

21. Choose the correct **TOP VIEW.**

TOP VIEW

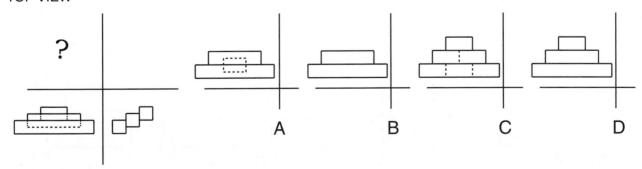

FRONT VIEW   END VIEW

GO TO THE NEXT PAGE.

22. Choose the correct **FRONT VIEW.**

TOP VIEW

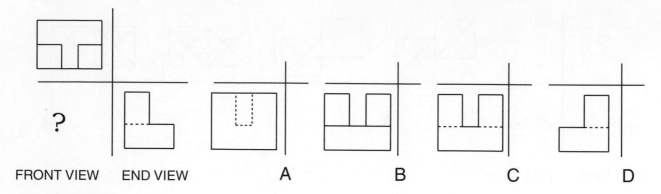

FRONT VIEW   END VIEW   A   B   C   D

23. Choose the correct **FRONT VIEW.**

TOP VIEW

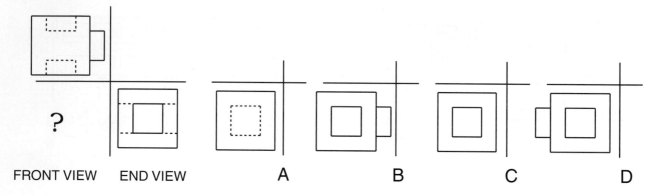

FRONT VIEW   END VIEW   A   B   C   D

24. Choose the correct **FRONT VIEW.**

TOP VIEW

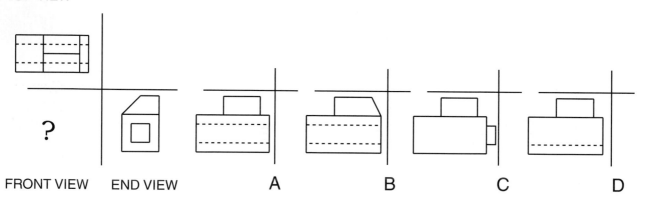

FRONT VIEW   END VIEW   A   B   C   D

GO TO THE NEXT PAGE.

25. Choose the correct **FRONT VIEW.**

TOP VIEW

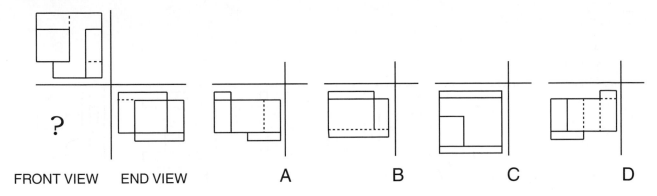

FRONT VIEW   END VIEW   A   B   C   D

26. Choose the correct **FRONT VIEW.**

TOP VIEW

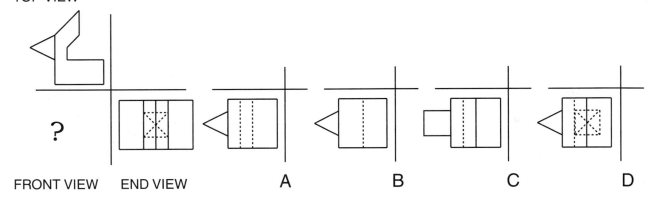

FRONT VIEW   END VIEW   A   B   C   D

27. Choose the correct **END VIEW.**

TOP VIEW

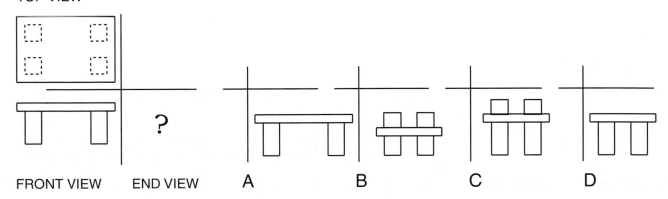

FRONT VIEW   END VIEW   A   B   C   D

GO TO THE NEXT PAGE.

28. Choose the correct **END VIEW.**

TOP VIEW

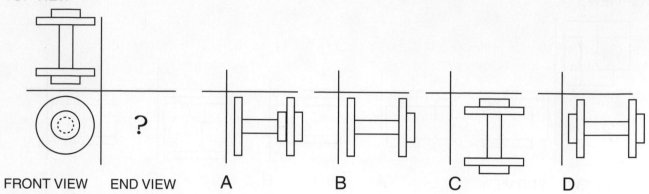

FRONT VIEW   END VIEW   A   B   C   D

29. Choose the correct **END VIEW.**

TOP VIEW

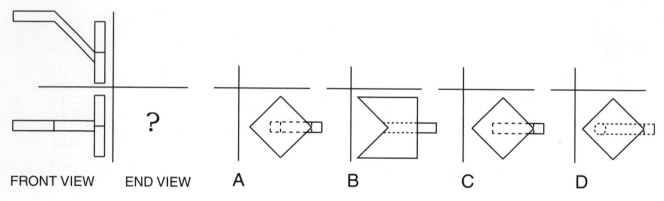

FRONT VIEW   END VIEW   A   B   C   D

30. Choose the correct **END VIEW.**

TOP VIEW

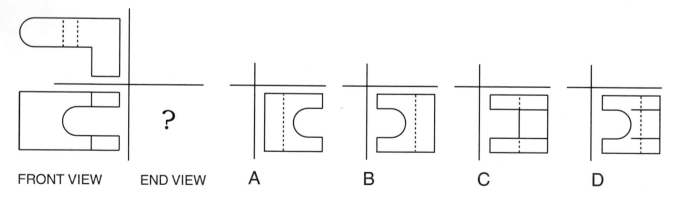

FRONT VIEW   END VIEW   A   B   C   D

GO TO THE NEXT PAGE.

PART 3

For questions 31 through 45:

Each question in this section presents four INTERIOR angles, labeled 1 through 4. Examine the four interior angles presented in each question.

Rank each question's angles in order from smallest to largest. Select the answer choice that represents the correct ranking and mark that answer choice on the answer grid. Try the following example problem:

Example:

1   2   3   4

(A) 4-1-2-3
(B) 2-1-4-3
(C) 1-4-2-3
(D) 3-2-1-4

The correct ranking of the angles from small to large is 4-1-2-3. Therefore, the correct answer is choice (A).

Proceed to Questions

GO TO THE NEXT PAGE.

31.

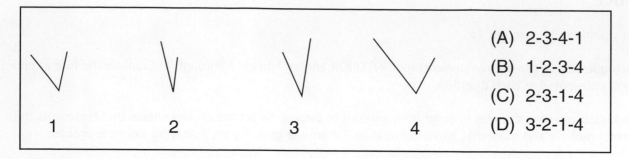

1 2 3 4

(A) 2-3-4-1
(B) 1-2-3-4
(C) 2-3-1-4
(D) 3-2-1-4

32.

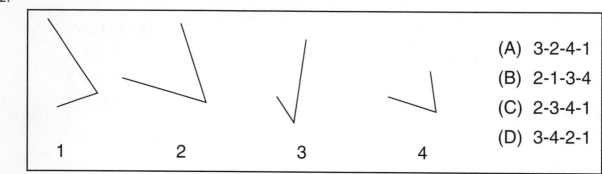

1 2 3 4

(A) 3-2-4-1
(B) 2-1-3-4
(C) 2-3-4-1
(D) 3-4-2-1

33.

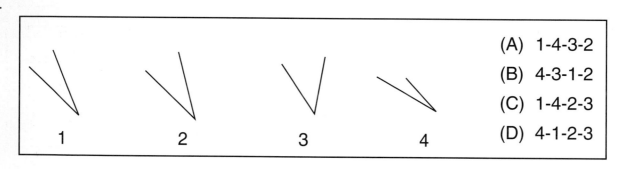

1 2 3 4

(A) 1-4-3-2
(B) 4-3-1-2
(C) 1-4-2-3
(D) 4-1-2-3

34.

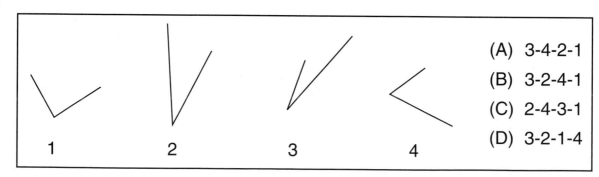

1 2 3 4

(A) 3-4-2-1
(B) 3-2-4-1
(C) 2-4-3-1
(D) 3-2-1-4

GO TO THE NEXT PAGE.

35.

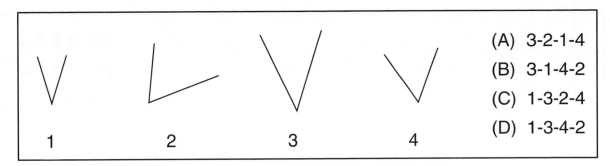

1   2   3   4

(A) 3-2-1-4
(B) 3-1-4-2
(C) 1-3-2-4
(D) 1-3-4-2

36.

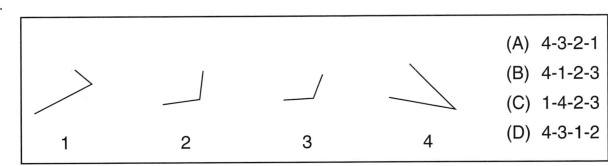

1   2   3   4

(A) 4-3-2-1
(B) 4-1-2-3
(C) 1-4-2-3
(D) 4-3-1-2

37.

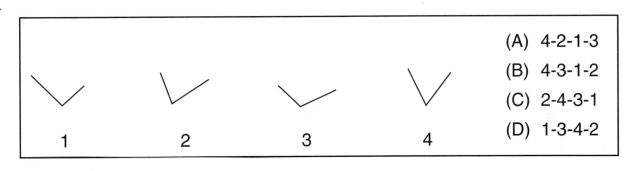

1   2   3   4

(A) 4-2-1-3
(B) 4-3-1-2
(C) 2-4-3-1
(D) 1-3-4-2

38.

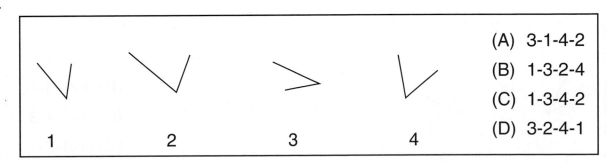

1   2   3   4

(A) 3-1-4-2
(B) 1-3-2-4
(C) 1-3-4-2
(D) 3-2-4-1

GO TO THE NEXT PAGE.

39.

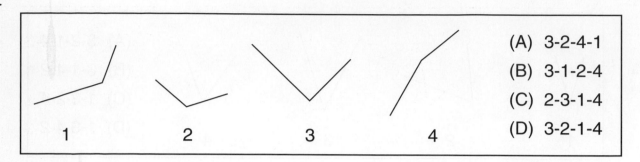

(A) 3-2-4-1

(B) 3-1-2-4

(C) 2-3-1-4

(D) 3-2-1-4

40.

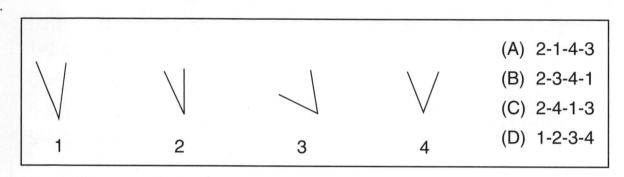

(A) 2-1-4-3

(B) 2-3-4-1

(C) 2-4-1-3

(D) 1-2-3-4

41.

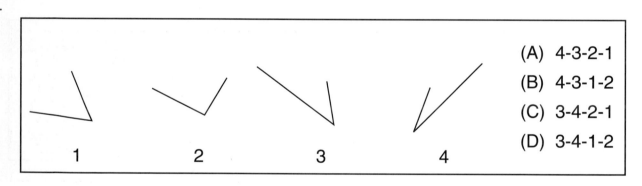

(A) 4-3-2-1

(B) 4-3-1-2

(C) 3-4-2-1

(D) 3-4-1-2

42.

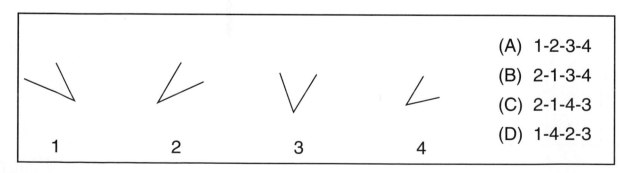

(A) 1-2-3-4

(B) 2-1-3-4

(C) 2-1-4-3

(D) 1-4-2-3

GO TO THE NEXT PAGE.

43.

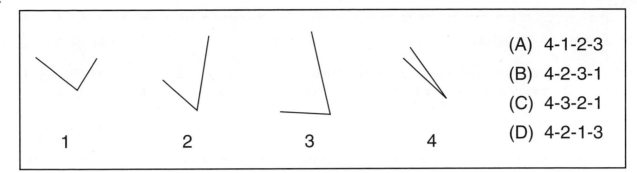

(A) 4-1-2-3

(B) 4-2-3-1

(C) 4-3-2-1

(D) 4-2-1-3

44.

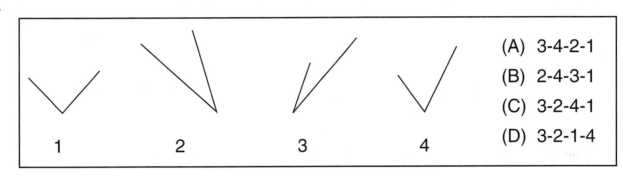

(A) 3-4-2-1

(B) 2-4-3-1

(C) 3-2-4-1

(D) 3-2-1-4

45.

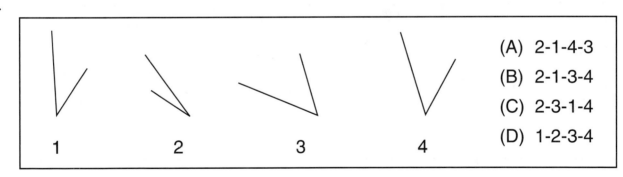

(A) 2-1-4-3

(B) 2-1-3-4

(C) 2-3-1-4

(D) 1-2-3-4

GO TO THE NEXT PAGE.

PART 4

For questions 46 through 60:

In these questions, a flat, square piece of paper is folded one or more times. Broken lines indicate the original position of the paper, and solid lines indicate the position of the folded paper. The folded paper remains within the boundaries of the original, flat sheet. The paper is not turned or twisted. There are one, two, or three folds per question.

Once the final fold is performed, a hole is punched in the paper. Once the hole is punched, mentally unfold the paper and ascertain the position(s) of the hole(s) on the original flat sheet.

Select the answer choice that represents the same pattern of dark circles that would reflect the position of holes on the unfolded sheet. There is only one correct pattern for each question. Try the following example:

Example:

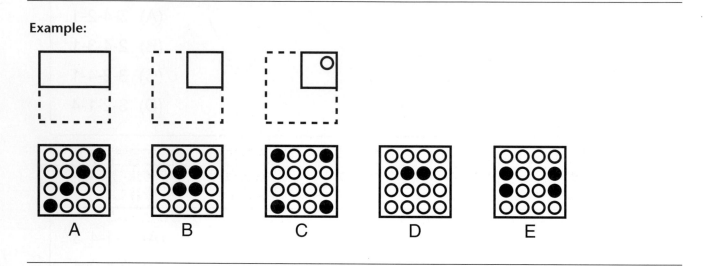

A   B   C   D   E

The correct answer is choice (C).

Proceed to Questions

GO TO THE NEXT PAGE.

46.

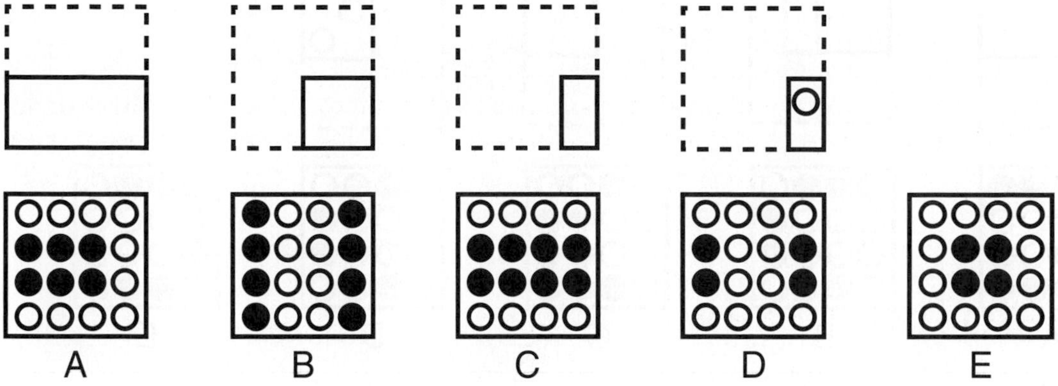

A   B   C   D   E

47.

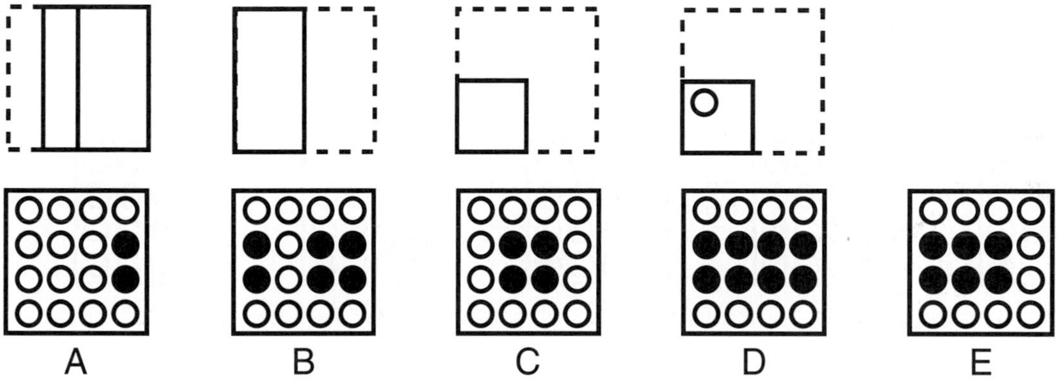

A   B   C   D   E

48.

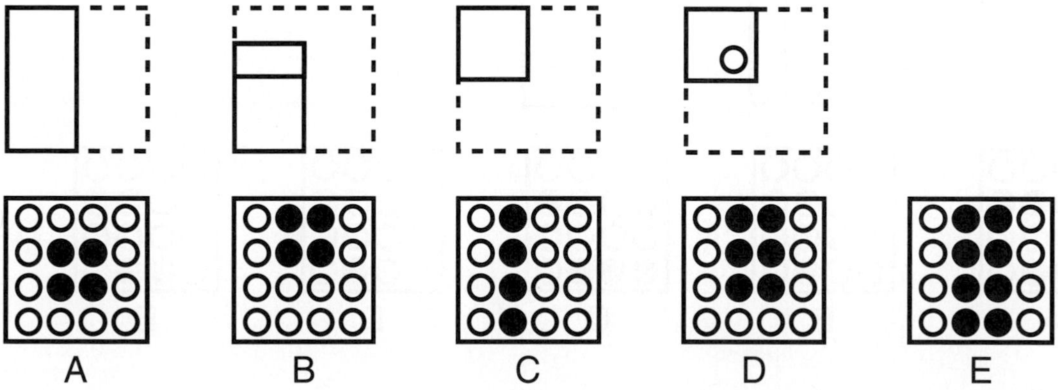

A   B   C   D   E

GO TO THE NEXT PAGE.

49.

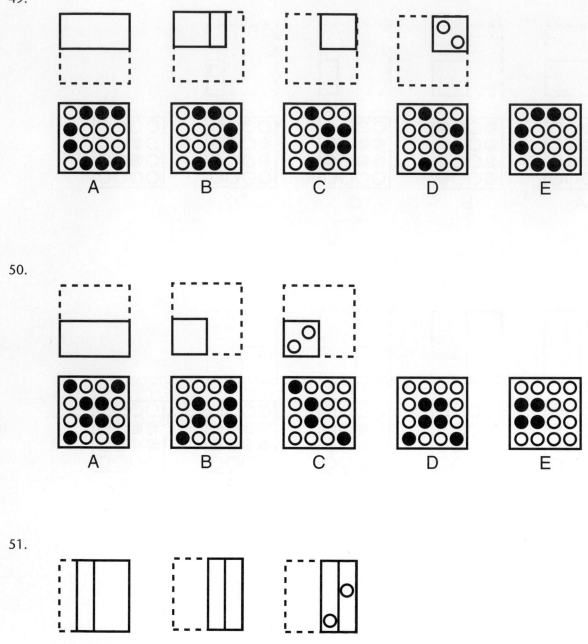

50.

51.

GO TO THE NEXT PAGE.

52.

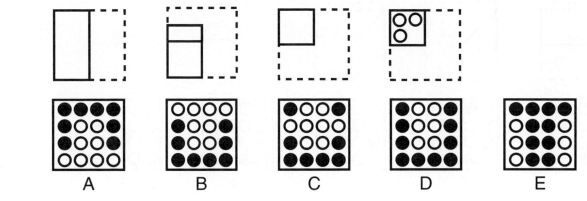

53.

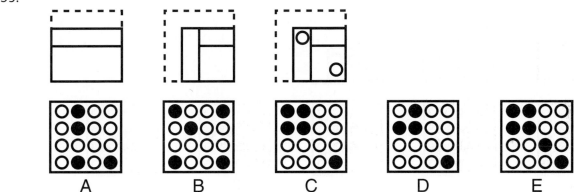

54.

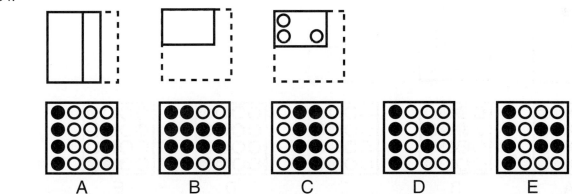

GO TO THE NEXT PAGE.

55.

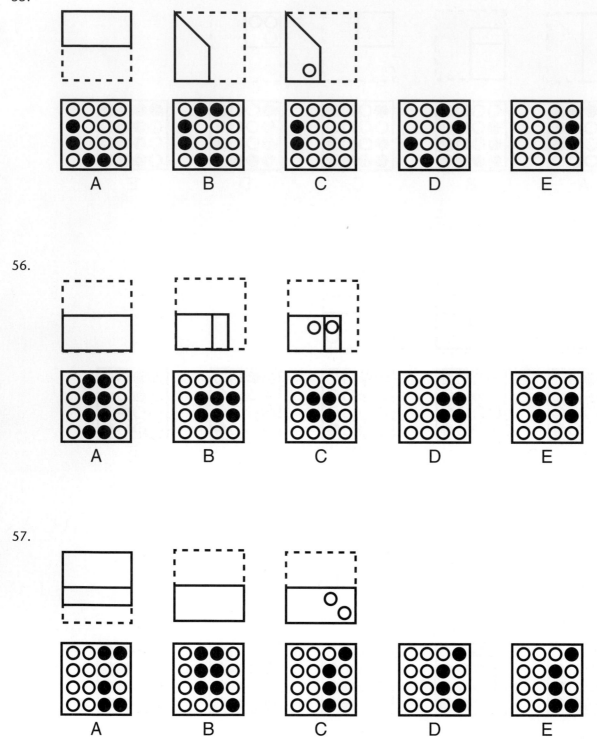

56.

57.

GO TO THE NEXT PAGE.

58.

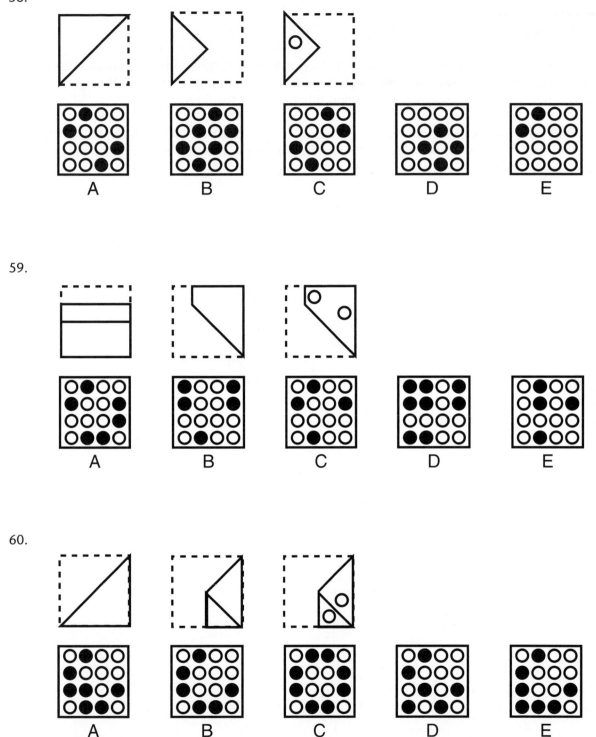

A   B   C   D   E

59.

A   B   C   D   E

60.

A   B   C   D   E

GO TO THE NEXT PAGE.

PART 5

For questions 61 through 75:

Each figure presented in this section has been constructed by cementing together identical cubes. After being cemented, each figure was varnished on all sides EXCEPT for the bottom (the side on which the figure rests). The only hidden cubes are the ones necessary to support other cubes in the figure.

Examine each figure carefully regarding the number of sides on each cube that have been varnished. The following questions ask for this information. Select the correct answer choice from the ones provided and darken the corresponding letter on your answer grid.

Note: Zero (0) is not the correct answer for any question.

Example:

In the Example Figure, how many cubes have two of their exposed sides painted?

Example Figure

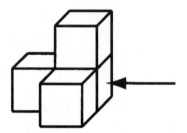

    A. 1 cube
    B. 2 cubes
    C. 3 cubes
    D. 4 cubes
    E. 5 cubes

The correct answer is choice (A). The cube is indicated with an arrow above.

Proceed to Questions

GO TO THE NEXT PAGE.

Problem A

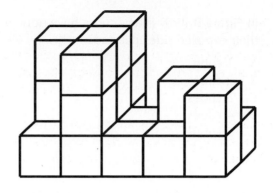

61. In Figure A, how many cubes have none of their exposed sides painted?

    A. 1 cube
    B. 2 cubes
    C. 3 cubes
    D. 4 cubes
    E. 5 cubes

62. In Figure A, how many cubes have one of their exposed sides painted?

    A. 1 cube
    B. 2 cubes
    C. 3 cubes
    D. 4 cubes
    E. 5 cubes

63. In Figure A, how many cubes have four of their exposed sides painted?

    A. 1 cube
    B. 2 cubes
    C. 3 cubes
    D. 4 cubes
    E. 5 cubes

64. In Figure A, how many cubes have five of their exposed sides painted?

    A. 1 cube
    B. 2 cubes
    C. 3 cubes
    D. 4 cubes
    E. 5 cubes

GO TO THE NEXT PAGE.

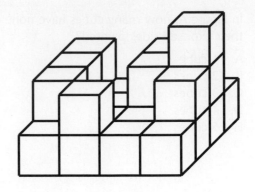

65. In Figure B, how many cubes have none of their exposed sides painted?

    A. 1 cube
    B. 2 cubes
    C. 3 cubes
    D. 4 cubes
    E. 5 cubes

66. In Figure B, how many cubes have two of their exposed sides painted?

    A. 1 cube
    B. 2 cubes
    C. 3 cubes
    D. 4 cubes
    E. 5 cubes

67. In Figure B, how many cubes have four of their exposed sides painted?

    A. 1 cube
    B. 2 cubes
    C. 3 cubes
    D. 4 cubes
    E. 5 cubes

68. In Figure B, how many cubes have five of their exposed sides painted?

    A. 1 cube
    B. 2 cubes
    C. 3 cubes
    D. 4 cubes
    E. 5 cubes

GO TO THE NEXT PAGE.

Figure C

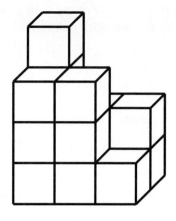

69. In Figure C, how many cubes have one of their exposed sides painted?

    A. 1 cube
    B. 2 cubes
    C. 3 cubes
    D. 4 cubes
    E. 5 cubes

70. In Figure C, how many cubes have three of their exposed sides painted?

    A. 1 cube
    B. 2 cubes
    C. 3 cubes
    D. 4 cubes
    E. 5 cubes

71. In Figure C, how many cubes have four of their exposed sides painted?

    A. 1 cube
    B. 2 cubes
    C. 3 cubes
    D. 4 cubes
    E. 5 cubes

72. In Figure C, how many cubes have five of their exposed sides painted?

    A. 1 cube
    B. 2 cubes
    C. 3 cubes
    D. 4 cubes
    E. 5 cubes

GO TO THE NEXT PAGE.

Problem D

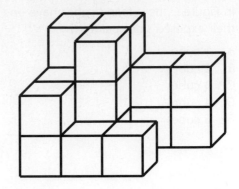

73. In Figure D, how many cubes have one of their exposed sides painted?

   A. 1 cube
   B. 2 cubes
   C. 3 cubes
   D. 4 cubes
   E. 5 cubes

74. In Figure D, how many cubes have three of their exposed sides painted?

   A. 1 cube
   B. 2 cubes
   C. 3 cubes
   D. 4 cubes
   E. 5 cubes

75. In Figure D, how many cubes have four of their exposed sides painted?

   A. 1 cube
   B. 2 cubes
   C. 3 cubes
   D. 4 cubes
   E. 5 cubes

GO TO THE NEXT PAGE.

PART 6

For questions 76 through 90:

In the following questions, a flat pattern is presented. This pattern will be folded into a three-dimensional figure, and the correct three-dimensional figure is one of the four answer choices illustrated at the right of the pattern. There is only one correct three-dimensional figure for each question. The pattern at the left represents the outside of the figure.

Select the three-dimensional figure that directly corresponds to the pattern at the left. Mark the appropriate answer choice on your answer grid that represents the correct figure. Try the following example:

Example:

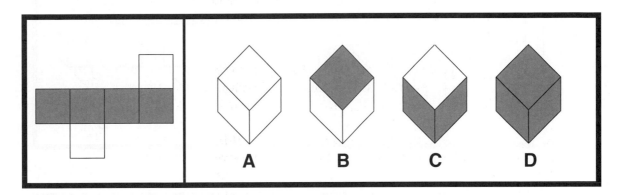

The correct answer is choice (C).

Proceed to Questions

GO TO THE NEXT PAGE.

76.

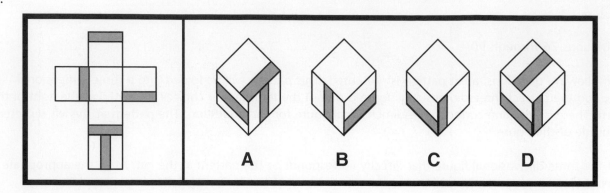

77.

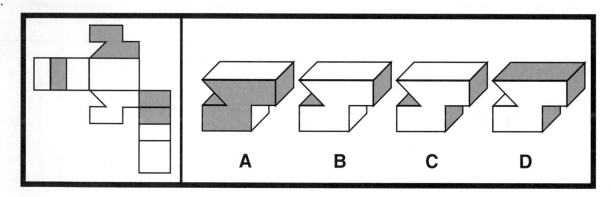

78.

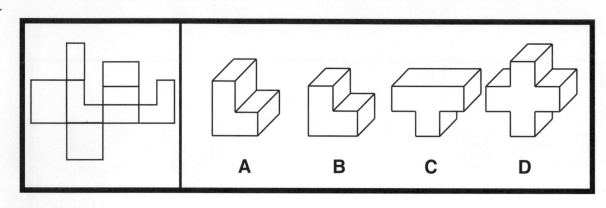

79.

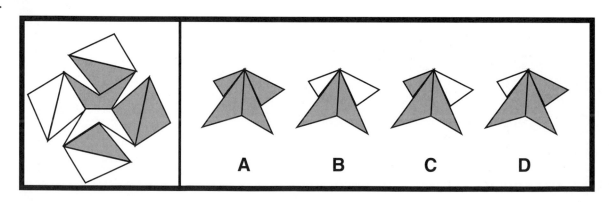

GO TO THE NEXT PAGE.

80.

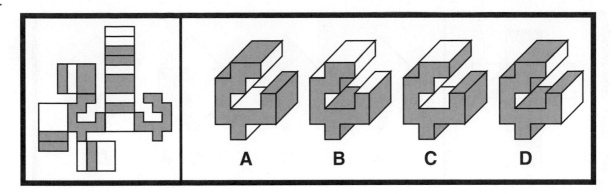

81.

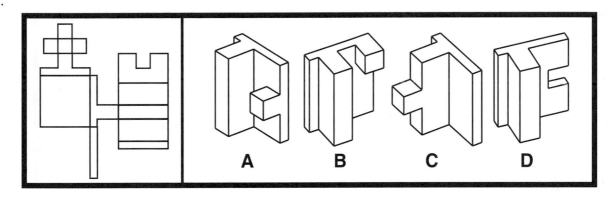

82.

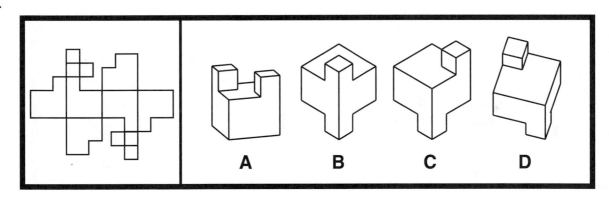

83.

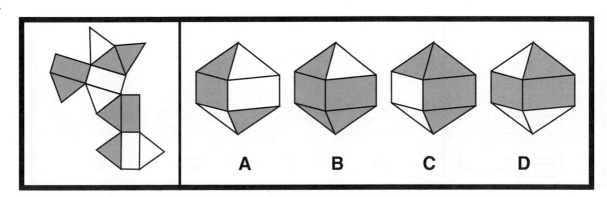

GO TO THE NEXT PAGE.

84.

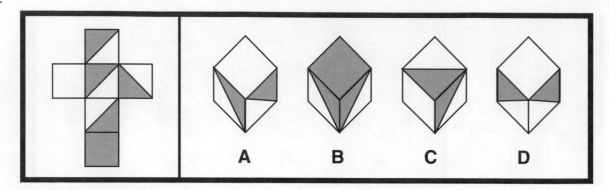

A   B   C   D

85.

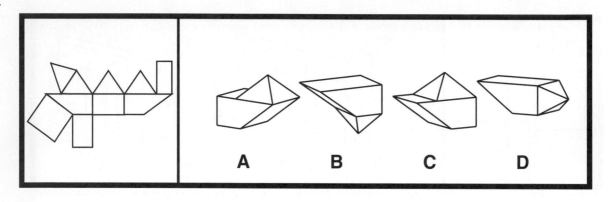

A   B   C   D

86.

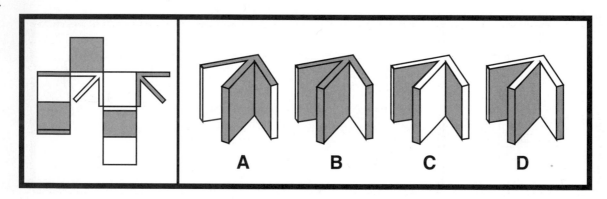

A   B   C   D

87.

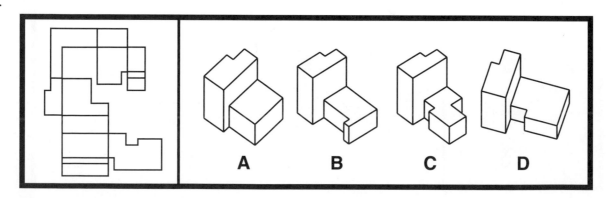

A   B   C   D

GO TO THE NEXT PAGE.

88.

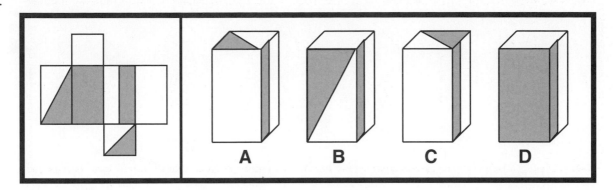

89.

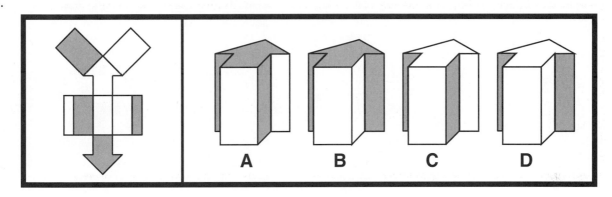

90.

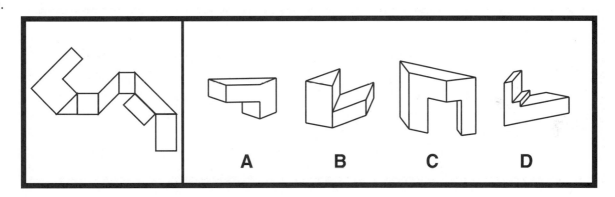

STOP. IF YOU FINISH BEFORE TIME HAS EXPIRED, CHECK YOUR WORK. YOU MAY GO BACK TO ANY QUESTION IN THIS PART ONLY.

Reading Comprehension
50 questions—50 minutes

DIRECTIONS: Read each passage carefully, and, when you believe you have sufficient comprehension of the passage, go on to the questions. Each question item consists of a question or an unfinished sentence followed by possible answers or completions. After reading a question, decide which choice is best and mark your answer.

When atoms on the surface of a solid interact with molecules of a gas or liquid, they may alter the structure of the molecules ever so slightly, thereby promoting unusual chemical reactions. Indeed, by investigating the interactions between molecules and the surfaces of solids, researchers have learned to synthesize a myriad of novel substances, develop chemical processes of unprecedented efficiency, and remove pollutants from the environment. Yet the study of chemistry on solid surfaces will have the most impact . . . on the technology of catalysts—substances that increase the rates of desirable chemical reactions at the expense of others. . . .

When applying the results of surface studies to commercial catalysis, investigators face a difficult problem. The tools of surface chemistry require vacuum conditions, whereas most practical catalysis must work in a high-pressure environment. . . . Researchers need to be careful about how they apply the findings of surface chemistry to high-pressure catalytic reactions. The great disparity in pressure means a vast difference in the number of gas molecules hitting a catalyst at any one time, and therefore the kinetics of the laboratory reaction may differ from the dynamics of the high-pressure reaction. . . . [Chemists have] learned to extrapolate the behavior of high-pressure catalytic reactions from idealized surface studies.

An elegant example of how the pressure gap can be bridged is the story of a set of surface chemistry experiments aimed at improving the technology of catalytic converters for automobiles. The primary function of the converters is to remove nitric oxide (NO) and carbon monoxide (CO) from automobile exhaust. Nitric oxide reacts rapidly with air to form nitrogen-oxygen compounds (NO_x), which are harmful to the environment, notably because they contribute to acid rain. Carbon monoxide is also extremely toxic to most forms of life. . . .

A typical catalytic converter consists of particles of platinum (Pt) and rhodium (Rh) deposited on a ceramic honeycomb. The platinum and rhodium particles catalyze the reactions that remove NO_x, CO, and uncombusted hydrocarbons from car exhaust. The ceramic honeycomb and small particle size serve the dual function of maximizing the exposure of the metals to the exhaust fumes and minimizing the quantity of platinum and rhodium—two very expensive metals.

In the mid-1980s researchers at General Motors and elsewhere set out to investigate how rhodium interacts with the nitric oxide and carbon monoxide from car exhausts. To do so, they studied reactions of NO and CO on single crystals of rhodium. Employing HREEL spectroscopy and other methods, the workers identified key steps in the breakdown of nitric oxide, and they determined how the arrangement of rhodium atoms on the surface influenced catalysis.

Yet it was not clear at first whether these results were applicable to the technology of catalytic converters: The experiments were conducted under vacuum conditions, whereas the rhodium particles used in catalytic converters are exposed to gases at high pressure. To demonstrate that practical information could be gained from the surface chemistry studies, the GM workers tested the rate of NO reduction on a rhodium surface in an environment that replicated the pressure conditions in a catalytic converter. By analyzing the action of rhodium in vacuum conditions and under high pressure, the researchers devised a mathematical model of the catalytic process. The model has allowed the results of the surface studies to be used in determining how new kinds of catalytic materials will operate under high pressures.

The GM group also found that the dissociation of NO was sensitive to the arrangement of atoms

GO TO THE NEXT PAGE.

on the rhodium surface. They arrived at this conclusion by using infrared spectroscopy. This technique is similar to HREEL spectroscopy, but it uses infrared radiation, instead of electrons, to cause molecular vibrations. Infrared spectroscopy has an advantage, however: It can be used both under vacuum conditions and at high pressures. Researchers at GM were therefore able to study, at high and low pressure, how nitric oxide interacts with irregular particles of rhodium and how it binds to a rhodium surface in which the atoms are arranged in a hexagonal pattern. Infrared spectroscopy identified differences in the vibrations of NO on the two types of surfaces, proving that surface structure influences bonding and ultimately the catalytic process. . . .

Surface chemistry has also helped researchers understand the catalytic process for removing sulfur from fossil fuels. Traces of sulfur in fossil fuels harm the environment in two ways. First, when fuel is burned in an engine, some sulfur reacts with air to form sulfur-oxygen compounds, which contribute to acid rain. Second, sulfur sticks to the platinum and rhodium in catalytic converters, thereby shutting down their activity and indirectly increasing the emission of NO and CO.

Sulfur is removed from petrochemicals at refineries as crude oil is transformed into such useful hydrocarbons as octane. Ideally, the desulfurization process should extract all the sulfur without destroying the valuable hydrocarbons. The process therefore requires a catalyst that encourages desulfurization but discourages the breakdown of pure hydrocarbons. [At the time of writing], the best catalyst for desulfurization is a mixture of molybdenum, cobalt, and sulfur itself. Because the material has a very complicated structure, chemists have had difficulty figuring out how petrochemicals interact with the catalyst. . . .

[A general model formulated by researchers at Harvard University] describes how thiols, a major class of sulfur-containing petrochemicals, interact with various molybdenum surfaces. Thiols consist of a hydrogen atom attached to a sulfur atom, which in turn is bonded to some combination of carbon and hydrogen. To study the interaction between thiols and molybdenum catalysts, [the researchers] used crystals of pure molybdenum so that the atoms on the surface would form a highly

ordered pattern. The regular structure limits the number of different kinds of sites available for bonding. By introducing various components to the molybdenum surface in a systematic way, the role of each component in desulfurization could be inferred.

Many years ago chemists made an astonishing discovery about molybdenum-induced desulfurization. The performance of pure molybdenum is actually enhanced when it is contaminated with sulfur, whereas most metals lose their ability to catalyze reactions when sulfur bonds to them. To study the role of surface sulfur, researchers compared how thiols react on clean molybdenum surfaces with how they perform on molybdenum covered with an ordered array of sulfur. Thiols interact with molybdenum catalysts to produce hydrocarbons, hydrogen gas, surface carbon, and sulfur. For example, ethanethiol (CH_3CH_2SH) is broken down into sulfur and one of two hydrocarbons: ethane (CH_3CH_3) and ethene (CH_2CH_2). Ideally, the catalyst should promote only the production of hydrocarbons and the removal of sulfur; it should discourage the synthesis of surface carbon and hydrogen gas, which have little value.

The molybdenum surface coated with sulfur removes sulfur from thiols more slowly than the clean surface can, but at the same time, the sulfur on the molybdenum surface decreases the rate of reactions that lead to undesirable products, thereby increasing the yield of useful hydrocarbons. Indeed, sulfur deposited on a molybdenum surface is beneficial for the desulfurization not only of thiols but also of other petrochemicals. . . .

[The Harvard researchers] used synchrotron, infrared, and other techniques to figure out what the stages of the desulfurization are and what steps are crucial in setting the overall rate of the reaction. The first step is the cleavage of the sulfur-hydrogen bond. . . . [T]his step occurs very rapidly and is favored because both sulfur and hydrogen form strong bonds to the molybdenum surface. In subsequent steps, the carbon-sulfur bond must break, and one carbon-hydrogen bond is either formed or broken to yield the hydrocarbon products from the thiol. . . . [The researchers] have found evidence that for any thiol molecule, the strength of the carbon-sulfur bond determines the overall rate of the desulfurization reaction.

GO TO THE NEXT PAGE.

By using [the] general model and information about the strength of the carbon-sulfur bond, [the Harvard researchers] have been able to predict the rates of reaction and the types of products formed during the desulfurization of thiols on molybdenum surfaces. Surface-bound carbon and gaseous hydrogen—the undesirable products—are formed at a rate that depends largely on whether a carbon-hydrogen bond can be broken before the breaking of the carbon-sulfur bond. According to fundamental principles of chemistry, therefore, the fraction of thiol intermediates that lead to useful hydrocarbons is proportional to the rate of carbon-sulfur bond breaking relative to the rate of carbon-hydrogen bond breaking. Thiols with low carbon-sulfur bond strengths—that is, high rates of bond breaking—would yield a large fraction of hydrocarbons. This conclusion has been borne out by experiments. . . .

Excerpt from "Catalysis on Surfaces," by Cynthia M. Friend, *Scientific American*, April 1993, © 1993 by *Scientific American*. Reprinted by permission. All rights reserved.

1.   It can be inferred from the passage that HREEL spectroscopy

   A.   can be used under a variety of conditions, including both high and low pressure.
   B.   uses infrared spectroscopy to cause molecular vibrations.
   C.   cannot be used at high pressures.
   D.   was developed by researchers at General Motors.
   E.   was developed by researchers at Harvard University.

2.   All of the following are reasons given for why it is difficult for scientists to apply the results of surface chemistry to commercial catalysts EXCEPT

   A.   There is a large difference in the number of gas molecules colliding with the catalyst.
   B.   The rate equations for the two conditions may be vastly different.
   C.   Most catalysis takes place at high pressure, whereas surface chemistry must be performed under vacuum conditions.
   D.   Commercial catalysts are difficult to access and, therefore, little experimentation is performed on them.
   E.   It is necessary to extrapolate the behavior of one to the other.

3.   The primary function of catalytic converters is

   A.   to prevent nitric oxide from reacting with water to generate nitrogen-oxygen compounds.
   B.   to maximize the exposure of Pt and Rh to exhaust fumes.
   C.   to regenerate Pt and Rh.
   D.   to remove nitric oxide and carbon monoxide from auto exhaust.
   E.   to clean the environment.

4.   All of the following were characteristics of the surface chemistry investigations carried out in the mid-1980s EXCEPT

   A.   HREEL spectroscopy was employed.
   B.   Vacuum conditions were applied.
   C.   There was uncertainty of the applicability of the results of these investigations to catalytic converters.
   D.   The effect of the arrangement of atoms on the rhodium surface on the dissociation of NO was studied.
   E.   The rate of NO oxidation on a rhodium surface was tested at high pressure.

GO TO THE NEXT PAGE.

5. It can be inferred from the passage that the performance of a molybdenum surface is best assessed in terms of

    A. the rate of reactions that produce undesirable products.
    B. the yield of useful hydrocarbons.
    C. the rate at which sulfur is removed from thiol.
    D. the rate of production of surface carbon and hydrogen gas.
    E. the rate at which sulfur is added to petrochemicals.

6. The first step in the desulfurization process is

    A. cleavage of the carbon-sulfur bond.
    B. formation of a carbon-hydrogen bond.
    C. the cleavage of one carbon-hydrogen bond.
    D. production of the hydrocarbon products from thiol.
    E. cleavage of the sulfur-hydrogen bond.

7. The rate at which surface-bound carbon and gaseous hydrogen are produced during desulfurization is principally determined by

    A. whether a C–H bond can be broken at all.
    B. whether a C–H bond can be broken prior to the cleavage of the C–S bond.
    C. the fraction of thiol intermediates present.
    D. the properties of the molybdenum surface.
    E. what technique is used to determine the stages of desulfurization.

8. Which of the following is a way in which traces of sulfur in fossil fuels harm the environment?

    A. Sulfur adheres to the platinum and rhodium in catalytic converters and enhances their activity.
    B. Sulfur produces toxic gases when released into the environment.
    C. Sulfur reacts with air to form sulfur-oxygen compounds, which contribute to acid rain.
    D. Sulfur in petrochemicals prevents useful hydrocarbons from being produced.
    E. Sulfur reacts with organic compounds in the soil, reducing the pH of the soil and disrupting the organisms.

9. When thiols with high carbon-sulfur bond strengths are subjected to the desulfurization reaction, the products would include

    A. a small fraction of useful hydrocarbons.
    B. a large fraction of useful hydrocarbons.
    C. a combination of hydrocarbons and carbon dioxide.
    D. a combination of hydrocarbons and sulfur dioxide.
    E. Cannot be determined

10. By investigating the interactions between molecules and the surfaces of solids, researchers have made progress in all of the following areas EXCEPT

    A. technology of catalysts.
    B. the study of gas phase decomposition mechanisms.
    C. the synthesis of novel substances.
    D. the development of efficient chemical processes.
    E. the removal of pollutants from the environment.

GO TO THE NEXT PAGE.

11. The best catalyst for desulfurization is a mixture of

   A. iron, oxygen, and hydrogen.
   B. carbon, nitrogen, and iron.
   C. sulfur and cobalt only.
   D. molybdenum, cobalt, and sulfur.
   E. sulfur, manganese, and cobalt.

12. Pt and Rh in catalytic converters function

   A. as coenzymes in the reactions that remove nitric acid and carbon monoxide from the car exhaust.
   B. to coat the ceramic honeycomb in order to minimize heat loss due to friction.
   C. to provide additional surface area for catalysis to take place.
   D. to maximize exposure to the exhaust fumes.
   E. to catalyze the reactions that remove nitrogen-oxygen compounds, carbon monoxide, and uncombusted hydrocarbons from car exhaust.

13. The goal of desulfurization is to

   A. break down the hydrocarbon products, as well as remove the sulfur.
   B. remove all the sulfur without destroying the hydrocarbons.
   C. convert sulfur from a solid form to a gaseous form.
   D. convert sulfur from a solid to a liquid form.
   E. remove the hydrocarbons.

14. A thiol consists of

   A. a hydrocarbon chain only.
   B. two hydrogen atoms, which are bonded to alternating carbons and phosphates.
   C. a sulfur and phosphate, which are bonded to a hydrocarbon chain.
   D. a hydrogen atom attached to a sulfur atom, which in turn is bonded to some combination of carbon and hydrogen.
   E. a nitrogen atom bonded to alternating sulfur and hydrogen atoms.

15. According to this passage, why is it necessary to minimize the quantity of platinum and rhodium used in a catalytic converter?

   A. They are very expensive metals.
   B. They are a limited resource.
   C. They can themselves pollute the environment if used in too great a quantity.
   D. If used in too great a quantity, they generate a large amount energy, which is difficult to dissipate.
   E. They have long half-lives.

16. According to the passage, all of the following are harmful to the environment and/or living organisms EXCEPT

   A. nitric oxide.
   B. carbon monoxide.
   C. sulfur-oxygen compounds.
   D. nitrogen-oxygen compounds.
   E. thiols.

GO TO THE NEXT PAGE.

The body reacts to tissue injury through a series of remarkable vascular and cellular changes designed to isolate and destroy the cause of injury. In a relatively simple animal, such as the hydra, cells cluster around and isolate the injurious agent, which is subsequently dissolved and destroyed. Essentially the same process occurs in humans—except that it involves the vascular system and more complex reactions.

In general, *inflammation* can be defined as the local, protective response of living tissues to injury. Acute inflammation is usually of sudden onset and is dominated by local vascular and exudative responses. Chronic inflammation is a slow, progressive process that may be either a continuation of the acute form or a prolonged low-grade form. Acute inflammation can be a reaction to a variety of noxious stimuli, including bacteria, trauma, and chemicals. Medical observers have long recognized it as a basic pathological process. Celcus, a Roman physician in the 1st century C.E., noted the four cardinal signs of inflammation as tumor, calor, rubor, and dolor (swelling, heat, redness, and pain).

The development of the microscope allowed scientists to observe the subtle vascular and cellular changes that are physiologically responsible for the outward signs of acute inflammation. In the 19th century, the German pathologist Julius Cohnheim described the changes in blood vessels during acute inflammation. Cohnheim's Russian contemporary Elie Metchnikoff added the insight that white blood cells (leukocytes) can play a key defensive role during inflammation by ingesting particulate matter, such as bacteria, in a process called phagocytosis.

Scientists now understand that inflammation develops as a series of interdependent but distinct cellular events and vascular changes, many of which affect the terminal vascular bed, a complex mesh where arterioles connect with venules via thin-wall bypass channels. The initial event, vasoconstriction, is typically a short-lived contraction of the arterioles in the immediate vicinity of the injurious agent and is rarely intense enough to result in complete ischemia (a local deficiency of blood). Vascular contraction is followed by vasodilation of the local blood vessels and a consequent increase in blood flow through the affected tissue. Blood flow initially increases through the most direct

routes leading to the veins. However, as the precapillary sphincters open, increasing amounts of blood are diverted into capillary side channels, resulting in hyperemia (a local excess of blood).

In close association with increased blood flow, the permeability of the capillaries and venules increases, and plasma escapes through the widened intercellular slits of the vessels' endothelial lining. Eventually, large quantities of fluids containing fibrinogen and other proteins leak from the blood vessels into interstitial spaces. A key event in inflammation is the walling off of the affected area due to the formation of fibrinogen clots in the interspaces of the tissue.

In addition to vascular changes, an inflamed area is invaded by leukocytes and other cells. A preliminary, limited line of cellular defense involves macrophages already present in the tissue. Such cells are active in the phagocytosis of infectious or toxic agents but are relatively few in number. Macrophages, however, can play a critical role later in the inflammatory process when monocytes migrate to the injured tissue, swell, mature, and develop into macrophages capable of phagocytosis.

Some of the most important defensive cells in the acute phase of the inflammatory reaction are polymorphonuclear leukocytes (also called granulocytes), which include polymorphonuclear neutrophils, polymorphonuclear basophils, and polymorphonuclear eosinophils. Neutrophils, the most numerous of the three types, are very motile and phagocytic. They constitute slightly more than 60 percent of circulating leukocytes (an adult human normally has about 7,000 white blood cells per cubic millimeter of blood, but the count can go as high as 30,000 cells/mm^3 during acute inflammation).

Within a few hours after its onset, acute inflammation is characterized by an increase in the number of neutrophils in the blood by as much as four- to fivefold in response to a combination of chemicals (collectively called leukocytosis-inducing factor) released from the inflamed tissue. This factor diffuses from the inflamed tissue to the blood and is carried to the bone marrow, where it mobilizes the neutrophils stored in the marrow tissue.

Enzymes, necrotic products, bacterial toxins, and chemicals released from the inflamed tissues can cause neutrophils and monocytes to move

GO TO THE NEXT PAGE.

from the circulatory system to the injured tissue. These products affect the permeability of the capillaries and small venules, allowing neutrophils and monocytes to actively squeeze through the pores of the blood vessels by diapedesis. The products also can damage the capillary walls and cause large amounts of neutrophils and monocytes to adhere to the capillaries' endothelial cells, a process called margination. Margination further facilitates rapid diapedesis of the white blood cells. Neutrophils and monocytes can be drawn towards the inflamed tissues by chemotaxis.

Ranging from 10 to 12 microns in diameter, neutrophils can phagocytize particles up to 5 or 6 microns in diameter. The neutrophil projects pseudopodia around the particle, creating a chamber containing the particle. The chamber invaginates and breaks from the outer cell membrane of the neutrophil to form a free-flowing vesicle in the cytoplasm. There the particle is digested by proteolytic enzymes released from lysosomes.

Eosinophils normally make up 2 to 3 percent of all blood leukocytes. While eosinophils are phagocytic and exhibit chemotaxis, they are not nearly as efficient as neutrophils in phagocytosis. These white blood cells, however, are particularly effective in defending against relatively large quantities of histamine, bradykinin, serotonin, and a number of lysosomal enzymes. Such chemical agents can cause local vascular and tissue reactions during the allergic response.

In summary, many of the cardinal signs of inflammation first described by Celsus can be explained by the vascular and cellular events now known to occur during inflammation. Calor (heat) and rubor (redness) are due to the dilation of the blood vessels and the resulting local excess of blood. Tumor (swelling) is caused by the accumulation of fluid leaking from blood vessels to the damaged tissue. Dolor (pain) probably results from swelling that stretches tissue over inflamed areas, as well as the chemical substances released in response to injurious agents.

17. The initial vascular event in inflammation is

   A. the contraction of local vessels.
   B. vasodilation.
   C. changes in the adhesiveness of capillary walls.
   D. an increase in circulating neutrophils.
   E. ischemia.

18. Inflammation can best be characterized as

   A. a pathological destruction of tissue.
   B. an injury to blood vessels.
   C. the formation of cell clusters around injurious agents.
   D. a protective, local response that follows tissue injury.
   E. a generalized response consisting of swelling, heat, and pain.

19. Scientists during the 19th century recognized for the first time

   A. the outward signs of inflammation.
   B. that leukocytes carry out pinocytosis.
   C. that inflammation is a pathological process.
   D. that a variety of injuries can lead to inflammation.
   E. how blood vessels change during inflammation.

20. A local deficiency of blood in tissues is called

   A. hyperemia.
   B. acute inflammation.
   C. leukocytes.
   D. ischemia.
   E. diapedesis.

21. The opening of precapillary sphincters leads directly to

   A. an expansion of arterioles.
   B. a closing of the direct routes to the veins.
   C. increased blood in capillary side channels.
   D. edema in inflamed tissues.
   E. invasion of inflamed area by leukocytes.

GO TO THE NEXT PAGE.

22. Which of the following statements is true about neutrophils?

    A. They can engulf particles twice their own size.
    B. They are the most effective leukocytes.
    C. They are the body's first cellular line of defense against infectious agents.
    D. They use enzymes to dissolve bacteria.
    E. Eosinophils are more efficient than neutrophils in phagocytosis.

23. During phagocytosis by a neutrophil, the particle is digested in

    A. the outer wall of the cell membrane.
    B. lysosomes.
    C. the pseudopodia.
    D. local capillaries.
    E. the cellular cytoplasm.

24. After the onset of inflammation, the number of neutrophils in the blood can reach as high as

    A. 7,000 cells/mm^3.
    B. 18,000 cells/mm^3.
    C. 30,000 cells/mm^3.
    D. 75,000 cells/mm^3.
    E. 8,000 cells/mm^3.

25. The body's isolation of an inflamed area is traceable to

    A. glucose and urea diffusing out of blood vessels.
    B. crystallization around the inflamed tissues.
    C. increased leakage of proteins into interstitial spaces.
    D. clotting in local blood vessels.
    E. increased concentration of K$^+$ ions intracellularly.

26. Enzymes, necrotic products, bacterial toxins, and chemicals cause all of the following EXCEPT

    A. change in the permeability of the capillaries.
    B. retention of neutrophils and monocytes within the circulatory system.
    C. neutrophils and monocytes to stick to the capillaries' endothelial cells.
    D. damage to the capillary walls.
    E. margination.

27. It is now known that "tumor" is most directly caused by

    A. invasion by eosinophils.
    B. certain chemical substances.
    C. dilation of blood vessels.
    D. extensive swelling that stretches tissue over inflamed areas.
    E. the buildup of fluid leaking from blood vessels to damaged tissue.

28. All of the following are characteristics of leukocytosis-inducing factor EXCEPT

    A. It causes an increase in the number of neutrophils.
    B. It is stored in the bone marrow.
    C. It activates neutrophils stored in marrow tissue.
    D. It is ultimately transported to the bone marrow.
    E. It is released initially from inflamed tissue.

29. Which of the following was NOT considered one of the cardinal signs of inflammation according to Celcus?

    A. Tumor
    B. Calor
    C. Cancer
    D. Rubor
    E. Dolor

GO TO THE NEXT PAGE.

30. One of the primary functions of eosinophils is

   A. to carry out chemotaxis on other foreign cells.
   B. to mark cells that contain foreign antigens so neutrophils can carry out phagocytosis on these cells at a later point.
   C. to lyse cells containing foreign antigens on their surface.
   D. to carry out phagocytosis on any foreign bacteria.
   E. to defend against chemical agents that cause vascular and tissue reactions during an allergic response.

31. The author of this passage would most likely agree with which of the following statements?

   A. The mechanism by which humans respond to tissue injury is unique to them.
   B. Little progress has been made in elucidating the mechanisms underlying the symptoms associated with inflammation.
   C. Most of the cardinal signs of inflammation as first described by Celsus are now better understood, since they can be explained by underlying vascular and cellular events.
   D. To understand completely the vascular and cellular events associated with inflammation, a large amount of further research is needed.
   E. Inflammation is maladaptive response that is widespread in the animal kingdom.

32. It can be inferred from the passage that macrophages

   A. develop from monocytes.
   B. are generated only when tissue is inflamed.
   C. include neutrophils, basophils, and eosinophils.
   D. are responsible for the process of margination.
   E. constitute about 30 percent of circulating leukocytes.

33. Which of the following is NOT a step in the process of phagocytosis by neutrophils?

   A. Release of proteolytic enzymes
   B. Projection of pseudopodia
   C. Formation of vesicle in cytoplasm
   D. Movement towards inflamed tissue via chemotaxis
   E. Invagination of particle-containing chamber

GO TO THE NEXT PAGE.

Lesch-Nyhan syndrome (LNS) was first described 32 years ago by Lesch and Nyhan. Lesch-Nyhan syndrome appears to be distributed evenly among different geographic locations and occurs in approximately 1 in every 380,000 births. The disease is characterized by hypoxanthine-guanine phosphoribosyltransferase (HPRT) deficiency. The syndrome is a neurologic disorder characterized by cerebral palsy manifested in the form of bilateral involuntary movements preceded by generalized hypotonia and delayed motor development, spasticity, and compulsive self-mutilation, mainly in the form of biting away lips and the ends of fingers. There has been some debate over whether these children are mentally retarded. Nyhan originally wrote that "a severe degree of mental retardation is one of the cardinal features of the disease." However, he and others since 1977 have observed that many patients with LNS appear more intelligent than test scores indicate. The severe disabilities combined with self-abusive tendencies and the need for physical restraints complicate the testing process. In a survey study done with 42 patients, Anderson et al. concluded that "most individuals with Lesch-Nyhan syndrome are not mentally retarded." In 1995, Matthews et al. performed the first systematic study to assess the cognitive functioning of Lesch-Nyhan patients. On the Stanford Binet Intelligence Scale, scores in each of the four domains assessed by this battery, as well as the general composite score, ranged from moderately mentally retarded to low average intelligence. Areas of weakness included attention, the manipulation of complex visual images, the understanding of complex or lengthy speech, mathematical ability, and multistep reasoning.

At birth, children with LNS appear normal. The first indication that something is wrong may be the passage of brown-red/orange "sand" in the diaper and extreme irritability of the infant. Until six to eight months of age, gross motor milestones may be reached appropriately. Between 8 and 24 months of age, however, choreoathetosis develops, and a loss of early milestones is seen. At first the infants are hypotonic, but later they develop hypertonia and hyperreflexia. Pyramidal symptoms consisting of increased deep tendon reflexes, a sustained ankle clonus, scissoring of the lower extremities, and extensor plantar responses are usually present by one year of age. By four years of age, many of the children are beginning

to exhibit the classic manifestation of LNS: self-mutilation. By eight to ten years of age, almost all children exhibit self-injurious behavior and demonstrate the neurologic manifestations of the disorder, including spasticity, choreoathetosis, opisthotonos, and facial dystonia. The development of communication is hindered by poor articulation due to pseudobulbar palsy and obstructed airflow. However, most affected children appear to comprehend quite well. The motor and physical development of affected children are grossly impaired with subnormal height and weight. Severely affected children are never able to walk. The life span of patients is usually less than 20 years. Patients usually die by the third decade from infection or renal failure secondary to crystal nephropathy due to decrease in lymphocyte and IgG levels.

A compulsive aggressiveness and self-mutilation, usually beginning by three years of age, are the most variable features of Lesch-Nyhan disease. These children are capable of feeling pain and would in most cases prefer to be restrained so they are unable to hurt themselves. Behavioral abnormalities can be highly variable.

In 1994, a study was performed on 40 male patients with Lesch-Nyhan, ranging in age from 2 to 32 years. Twenty-six different types of self-injury were reported by the parents. Biting some part of the body was the most common type of self-injury, followed by throwing an arm, leg, or head out as they were wheeled through a doorway. In addition, aggression against others, both physical and verbal, was as common as self-injury. There was considerable intra-individual fluctuation in the severity of the self-injurious behavior. All patients had episodes ranging from a few days to a few weeks when the self-injury was much worse than at other times. These periods of high self-injury were related to stressful physical and emotional events. When the patients were calm, enjoying themselves, and free from illness or pain, the tendency to self-injure was low. In addition, it was found that in general, the patient had control over self-injury and when/how restraints should be used. Most patients wanted to be restrained most of the time and were happiest when restrained in a way that made self-injury impossible. However, during certain activities or during low-stress periods, they requested that the restraints be removed. There was a correlation between the

GO TO THE NEXT PAGE.

severity of self-injury and the age when a physical problem was first noticed by the parents. The earlier the physical problem, the worse the self-injury eventually became.

Aggressive behavior against others is also included in the unusual behavior of these children. This can be in the form of hitting, spitting, or kicking. Verbal aggression is also present in some cases, with some children using a shocking vocabulary of profanity and other words that are socially unacceptable. Frequent projectile vomiting is also used by older children as one of their weapons, especially when they become upset. Although such bizarre behavior may be expected to alienate others, these children are actually very charming and responsive, being fully aware and sensitive to their environment. They have a good sense of humor and smile and laugh easily. In some cases, their personality attributes make them seem more intelligent than actually indicated by intelligence tests.

The disease is interesting in that an exact metabolic error leads to a complex set of clinical manifestations and, in addition, despite all the behavioral and neurologic abnormalities, autopsies on these patients have shown no anatomical abnormalities in the brain. However, a defect of neurotransmitter function has been found with a decrease of all functional aspects of dopamine-neuron terminals when compared to control values in the striatum. There is also a dopamine deficit in the mouse model.

Prior to 1996, the strongest support for a dopaminergic dysfunction was from the postmortem findings of a deficit in dopamine, homovanillic acid, and dopa decarboxylase in the basal ganglia of three patients with Lesch-Nyhan disease. However, in a later study by Ernst et al., the brain was able to be visualized and dopa decarboxylase activity was able to be measured, using the tracer 6-fluorodopa F 18, the precursor of dopamine, in conjunction with positron-emission tomography to measure presynaptic accumulation of fluorodopa F 18 tracer in the dopaminergic regions of the brain. The study population consisted of 15 healthy subjects and 12 male patents with Lesch-Nyhan disease. The fluorodopa F 18 ratio was significantly lower in the putamen (31 percent of control), caudate nucleus (39 percent), frontal cortex (44 percent), and ventral tegmental com-

plex (substancia nigra and ventral tegmentum, 57 percent) in the patients with Lesch-Nyhan disease than in the controls. Uptake of the tracer was abnormally low even in the youngest patients tested, with Lesch-Nyhan subjects having values 31 to 57 percent of those in normal subjects, and there was no overlap between the two groups. The conclusion was made that patients with Lesch-Nyhan disease have abnormally few dopaminergic nerve terminals and cell bodies. The abnormality involves all dopaminergic pathways and is not restricted to the basal ganglia. These dopaminergic deficits are pervasive and appear to be developmental in origin, which suggests that they may contribute to the characteristic neuropsychiatric manifestations of the disease.

Lesch-Nyhan is a rare X-linked recessive disorder of purine synthesis. The primary abnormality is found in a structural gene on the X chromosome coding for the synthesis of the enzyme hypoxanthine-guanine phosphoribosyltransferase (HPRT), which is virtually absent in this disorder. Patients show a striking degree of phenotypic and genotypic variation, with a prevalence of single DNA base substitutions.

The enzyme is composed of four identical subunits, each containing 217 amino acids, not counting the N-terminal methionine with a molecular mass of 24.47 kDa. The enzyme has several substrates: magnesium phosphoribosylpyrophosphate (PRPP), hypoxanthine, and guanine. HPRT is encoded by a single copy of an X-linked gene composed of nine exons spanning about 44 kb of DNA in position Xq26-27. Several mutations have been identified in the gene in patients with Lesch-Nyhan disease. These mutations result in virtually a complete loss of function of the enzyme HPRT, which normally catalyzes the conversion of hypoxanthine and guanine to their respective nucleotides, inosinic acid and guanylic acid. These purine nucleotides are the building blocks of DNA and RNA and are thus essential for the normal activity of the cell.

The enzyme HPRT is normally expressed in all cells of the body, with the highest activity found in cells of the basal ganglia and testes. If the basal ganglia is damaged, problems with movement can occur, and failure of sexual maturation and atrophic testes can result from problems in the

GO TO THE NEXT PAGE.

testes. In some patients, HPRT activity is absent in all cells, and in others, the HPRT activity in dialyzed erythrocyte lysates may range from less than 0.01 to 10 percent or 20 percent of the normal. In addition to the decrease in activity of HPRT in patients with a severe deficiency, there is also an increase in the activity of adenine phosphoribosyltransferase in erythrocytes but not fibroblasts, which convert adenine to its nucleotide. HPRT activity in fibroblasts of affected children is higher than is found in their erythrocytes, with values of around 1 to 3 percent of the activity found in normal fibroblasts. The amount of residual activity in fibroblasts correlates inversely with the severity of clinical symptoms.

HPRT and its companion, adenine phosphoribosyltransferase, reuse preformed purine bases that result from cell turnover and metabolism through a salvage pathway. If HPRT and this salvage pathway are missing, PRPP synthetase activity increases and PRPP accumulates within the cell, giving rise to accelerated purine production de novo, which results in overproduction of uric acid, which leads to increased blood concentrations of uric acid (hyperuricemia), increased amounts of uric acid in the urine (3–4 times that of normal individuals), tophaceous gouty arthritis, urinary tract calculi, and urate nephropathy (disease of the kidney).

There is currently no effective treatment available to correct many of the abnormalities which occur in this syndrome. Prenatal and carrier testing are available through both biochemical as well as molecular methods. In addition, preimplantation diagnosis is another alternative that might be discussed with at-risk couples.

34. Carrying out intelligence testing in individuals with Lesch-Nyhan syndrome is difficult because

A. these individuals frequently refuse to cooperate.
B. these individuals can act very charming and be very responsive to both others and their environment.
C. of their inability to speak.
D. of their tendency to self-injure and because of their disabilities.
E. of their tendency to be aggressive towards others.

35. In the 1994 study of patients with Lesch-Nyhan syndrome, it was found that

A. there was little variation in the type of self-mutilation behavior done by these individuals.
B. self-mutilation behavior fluctuated in severity over time.
C. environmental events had little influence on the severity of self-abusive behavior.
D. most patients resisted when restraints were applied.
E. these patients have an increased pain threshold.

36. All of the following were found to be areas of weakness in individuals with Lesch-Nyhan syndrome according to the Stanford Binet Intelligence Scale EXCEPT

A. ability to comprehend difficult language.
B. mathematical skills.
C. perceptual ability involving basic visual images.
D. attention span.
E. multistep reasoning.

GO TO THE NEXT PAGE.

37. Individuals with Lesch-Nyhan syndrome are often perceived as being more intelligent than they really are. According to the passage, what is the best explanation for this?

A. Individuals with Lesch-Nyhan syndrome are very creative.
B. Individuals with Lesch-Nyhan syndrome have the ability to devise intricate plans to self-mutilate themselves.
C. Individuals with Lesch-Nyhan syndrome can carry out planned acts of aggression towards others.
D. Individuals with Lesch-Nyhan syndrome have a relatively large vocabulary of profane and socially unacceptable words.
E. Individuals with Lesch-Nyhan syndrome have very likable personality traits.

38. In the Ernst et al. study, dopa decarboxylase activity was studied by

A. examining basal ganglia of deceased Lesch-Nyhan patients.
B. measuring the level of dopa decarboxylase in the synapses in the dopaminergic regions of the brain.
C. measuring the activity of 6-fluorodopa F 15 in dopaminergic regions of the brain.
D. measuring the presynaptic accumulation of fluorodopa F 18 tracer in dopaminergic regions of the brain.
E. measuring the postsynaptic buildup of fluorodopa F 18 in dopaminergic regions of the brain.

39. At birth, infants with Lesch-Nyhan syndrome typically display

A. hypertonia.
B. hyperreflexia.
C. hypotonia.
D. clinodactly.
E. hyperactivity.

40. Which of the following are examples of purine nucleotides?
    I. hypoxanthine
    II. guanine
    III. inosinic acid
    IV. guanylic acid

A. I and II only
B. III and IV only
C. All of the above
D. I and III only
E. II and IV only

41. In severely affected patients with Lesch-Nyhan syndrome, which of the following is true?

A. They have a decrease in activity of adenine phosphoribosyltransferase.
B. They have an increase in activity of HPRT.
C. They have an increase in activity of adenine phosphoribosyltransferase only in erythrocytes.
D. They have an increase in activity of adenine phosphoribosyltransferase only in fibroblasts.
E. Activity of HPRT is decreased uniformly in all cells.

42. Children with Lesch-Nyhan syndrome typically begin to engage in self-mutilating behavior

A. before the age of 2.
B. around the ages of 3 and 4.
C. around the ages of 4 and 5.
D. around the ages of 6 and 7.
E. between the ages of 8 and 10.

43. What type of inheritance pattern is found in Lesch-Nyhan syndrome?

A. Mitochondrial inheritance
B. Autosomal recessive
C. Autosomal dominant
D. X-linked dominant
E. X-linked recessive

GO TO THE NEXT PAGE.

44. All of the following were conclusions reached as a result of the Ernst et al. study EXCEPT

A. Dopaminergic deficits may contribute to the neuropsychiatric characteristics of Lesch-Nyhan disease.
B. Dopaminergic deficits appear to be developmental in origin.
C. Regions affected in this disorder include only the putamen and caudate nucleus.
D. Individuals with Lesch-Nyhan syndrome have only a small number of dopaminergic nerve terminals and cell bodies.
E. All dopaminergic pathways are involved in Lesch-Nyhan syndrome.

45. Children affected with Lesch-Nyhan syndrome typically display all of the following symptoms EXCEPT

A. poor communication skills.
B. poor ability to comprehend speech.
C. below average height and weight.
D. difficulty with walking.
E. shortened life span.

46. What is the most common type of mutation found in individuals with Lesch-Nyhan syndrome?

A. A single base substitution
B. A deletion
C. An insertion
D. A frameshift mutation
E. An inversion

47. Overproduction of uric acid in patients with Lesch-Nyhan syndrome results from

A. decreased de novo production of inosinic acid and guanylic acid.
B. the conversion of hypoxanthine and guanine into inosinic acid by HPRT.
C. accumulation of HPRT in the cells.
D. decreased activity of PRPP.
E. increased activity of magnesium phosphoribosylpyrophosphate synthetase.

48. Pyramidal symptoms include all of the following EXCEPT

A. scissoring of lower extremities.
B. extensor plantar responses.
C. increased deep tendon reflexes.
D. dysmorphic facial features.
E. sustained ankle clonus.

49. Which of the following is NOT mentioned as an example of aggressive behavior of children with LNS?

A. Projectile vomiting
B. Hitting
C. Verbal abuse
D. Lip biting
E. Kicking

50. The salvage pathway mentioned in the passage

A. increases PRPP synthetase activity.
B. allows preformed purine bases to be reused.
C. accelerates de novo purine production.
D. increases blood concentration of uric acid.
E. All of the above

STOP. IF YOU FINISH BEFORE TIME HAS EXPIRED, CHECK YOUR WORK. YOU MAY GO BACK TO ANY QUESTION IN THIS PART ONLY.

Quantitative Reasoning

40 questions—45 minutes

DIRECTIONS: Select the best answer for each question and mark your answer grid.

1. The ratio of boys to girls in a class is 5:3. If there are 120 students, how many girls are there?

   A. 75
   B. 72
   C. 45
   D. 48
   E. 200

2. What percent of $\sqrt{0.005}$ is $\sqrt{2}$?

   A. 0.05%
   B. 5%
   C. 20%
   D. 200%
   E. 2000%

3. An architect draws a blueprint so that $3\frac{1}{8}$ inches represents 125 feet. How many square inches are used to represent the area of a room 20 feet by 20 feet?

   A. $\frac{1}{4}$

   B. $\frac{5}{64}$

   C. $\frac{1}{2}$

   D. $\frac{2}{5}$

   E. $\frac{625}{64}$

4. The Jones's living room floor measures 10 ft. × 15 ft. If one carpeting firm charges $0.80 per square foot and another $7.50 per square yard, how much will the Joneses save by hiring the cheaper firm to do the job?

   A. $5
   B. $10
   C. $12
   D. $120
   E. $125

5. A car travels at the rate of 60 miles per hour. Find the car's rate in feet per second. (5,280 feet = 1 mile)

   A. 8
   B. 10
   C. 30
   D. 60
   E. 88

6. Given the information shown, find angle PQT.

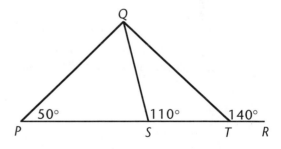

   A. 50°
   B. 80°
   C. 90°
   D. 110°
   E. 140°

GO TO THE NEXT PAGE.

7. What is the approximate length, in feet, of a ladder that is 45 feet from the foot of a building and reaches 24 feet up the wall of the building?

    A. 24
    B. 38
    C. 45
    D. 51
    E. 69

8. Given three externally tangent circles as shown, if the diameters of the circles are d, d_1, and d_2, respectively, what is the perimeter of the triangle formed by joining their centers?

    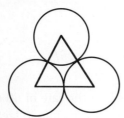

    A. $\frac{1}{2}(d + d_1 + d_2)$

    B. $\frac{1}{3}(d + d_1 + d_2)$

    C. $2(d + d_1 + d_2)$

    D. $d + d_1 + d_2$

    E. $3d$

9. Six people went shopping. Five spent $16 each, and the sixth spent $5 more than the average of all six. How much did the last person spend?

    A. $20
    B. $21
    C. $22
    D. $23
    E. $24

10. An express train leaves a station 3 hours after a freight train. The express train travels at 60 miles per hour and after 2 hours finds that it is still 20 miles behind the freight train. At what rate is the freight train traveling?

    A. 20 mph
    B. 24 mph
    C. 28 mph
    D. 30 mph
    E. 32 mph

11. A motorist travels 50 miles at 20 mph. He returns the same distance at 50 mph. What is his average rate for the entire trip?

    A. $24\frac{2}{7}$

    B. $28\frac{4}{7}$

    C. $29\frac{6}{7}$

    D. 30

    E. $32\frac{2}{7}$

12. Billy walks to school in 3 minutes. The school is 3 blocks from his house, and each block is 528 feet. What is Billy's average speed, in miles per hour? (5,280 feet = 1 mile)

    A. 0.3
    B. 0.6
    C. 3
    D. 5
    E. 6

GO TO THE NEXT PAGE.

13. A test consists of 60 problems to be done in 1 hour. A student does 30 problems in 20 minutes. How much time can he use for each of the remaining problems?

A. $\frac{1}{2}$ min

B. $\frac{3}{4}$ min

C. $1\frac{1}{4}$ min

D. $1\frac{1}{3}$ min

E. $1\frac{1}{2}$ min

14. A man bought 8 books at an average price of $6.00 and 10 books at an average price of $2.40. Find the average cost of the books.

A. $3.60
B. $4.00
C. $4.20
D. $6.00
E. $7.20

15. Fifteen movie theaters average 600 customers per day. If six are shut down but the same number of people still attend the movies, what is the new average attendance for the movies that remain open?

A. 66
B. 100
C. 500
D. 1,000
E. 1,500

16. Solve for x in the equation $\dfrac{32 - 10\sqrt{5x}}{3} = 4$.

A. $\frac{2\sqrt{5}}{5}$

B. $\frac{1}{5}$

C. $\frac{2}{5}$

D. $\frac{\sqrt{2}}{5}$

E. $\frac{4}{5}$

17. When the expression $\sqrt{1 + \dfrac{9}{16}}$ is simplified, which of the following is obtained?

A. $\sqrt{\dfrac{5}{8}}$

B. $\dfrac{\sqrt{17}}{4}$

C. $1\frac{3}{4}$

D. $1\frac{1}{4}$

E. $\dfrac{\sqrt{17}}{16}$

18. Put the following in increasing order:

I. $\dfrac{\sqrt{2}}{3}$ II. $\dfrac{\sqrt{3}}{4}$ III. $\dfrac{\sqrt{5}}{5}$

A. I, II, III
B. I, III, II
C. II, I, III
D. II, III, I
E. III, I, II

19. 15 is 6% of what number?

A. 250

B. $\dfrac{9}{10}$

C. 25

D. 90

E. 900

GO TO THE NEXT PAGE.

20. From the charts below, what percent of the world's coal is produced in Ohio?

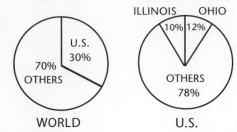

WORLD   U.S.

A. 0.3%
B. 1.2%
C. 3.6%
D. 4%
E. 36%

21. The circumference of a circle is increased by 20%. Find the percent of increase in the area.

A. 40%
B. 44%
C. 10%
D. 22%
E. 400%

22. If the diameter of a cylinder is increased by 20% and the height is decreased by $16\frac{2}{3}$%, by what percent is the volume changed?

A. −10%
B. +10%
C. +20%
D. +24%
E. $+83\frac{1}{3}$%

23. The numerator of a fraction is doubled, and the denominator is halved. The value of the fraction is

A. divided by 2.
B. divided by 4.
C. multiplied by 2.
D. multiplied by 4.
E. unchanged.

24. The length of a rectangle is twice the width. If the perimeter of a square equals the perimeter of the rectangle, what is the ratio of the area of the rectangle to the area of the square?

A. 1:1
B. 1:4
C. 4:1
D. 2:3
E. 8:9

25. A railroad must pay a tax of 6% on all revenue exceeding $50,000. How much tax must be paid on $150,000 of revenue?

A. $6,000
B. $9,000
C. $10,000
D. $12,000
E. $12,500

26. A picket fence is 60 feet long. Its pickets are $1\frac{1}{2}$ feet apart. If the fence is extended to 80 feet, without adding any pickets, what is the new distance, in feet, between pickets?

A. $1\frac{1}{8}$
B. 2
C. $\frac{8}{9}$
D. $2\frac{1}{8}$
E. 3

GO TO THE NEXT PAGE.

27. A rectangular swimming pool 24 feet × 16 feet is filled to a height of 1 foot. How high would the same amount of water reach in a pool 20 feet × 8 feet?

A. $\frac{5}{12}$ ft

B. $\frac{3}{5}$ ft

C. $\frac{5}{6}$ ft

D. $2\frac{2}{5}$ ft

E. $2\frac{3}{5}$ ft

28. $x + y + 3z = 7$; $3x + 6y + 6z = 8$. What is the numerical value of $(y - z)$?

A. $-\frac{13}{3}$

B. -6

C. 13

D. $\frac{29}{3}$

E. $-\frac{22}{3}$

29. A, B, and C have 24 marbles between them. A has more marbles than B, and B has more marbles than C. What is the largest number of marbles that B can have?

A. 8
B. 9
C. 10
D. 11
E. 12

30. Line ℓ is perpendicular to the line with the equation $y = -\frac{1}{5}x$, and the point $(3, -10)$ is on line ℓ. Which of the following is an equation of line ℓ ?

A. $y = -\frac{1}{5}x - \frac{47}{5}$

B. $y = 5x - 25$

C. $y = 5x$

D. $y = 5x - 5$

E. $y = \frac{1}{5}x - \frac{53}{5}$

31. Which of the following is equal to cos 59°?

A. sin 31°

B. cos 31°

C. sin 59°

D. $\cos \left(\frac{1}{59}\right)^{\circ}$

E. $\sin \left(\frac{1}{59}\right)^{\circ}$

32. Which of the following is true for all values of x such that $0 < x < \frac{\pi}{2}$?

A. $\sin x = \cos^2 + 1$

B. $\tan x = (\sin x)(\cos x)$

C. $\tan x = \frac{\cos x}{\sin x}$

D. $\sin^2 x = 1 - \cos^2 x$

E. $\sin x = \frac{1}{\cos x}$

33. Suppose that $-4 \le x \le 2$ and $3 \le y \le 5$. Which value for x and which value for y in their respective ranges will make $(x^2 - 6)(y + 7)$ its largest possible value?

A. $x = 2$ and $y = 5$
B. $x = 2$ and $y = 3$
C. $x = 1$ and $y = 4$
D. $x = -4$ and $y = 3$
E. $x = -4$ and $y = 5$

GO TO THE NEXT PAGE.

34. What is the length of side *AB* in equilateral triangle *ABC* if the length of altitude *AD* is 12?

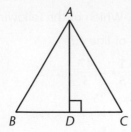

A. $8\sqrt{3}$
B. $10\sqrt{2}$
C. 18
D. $12\sqrt{3}$
E. 24

35. Evaluate the expression $\dfrac{6\times10^{-4}}{30\times10^{5}}$.

A. 2×10^{-1}
B. 5×10^{-10}
C. 2×10^{-10}
D. 5×10^{-9}
E. 2×10^{-9}

36. Five students taking an exam have to sit one behind the other. How many different ways can they arrange themselves?.

A. 5
B. 20
C. 50
D. 60
E. 120

37. There are five purple marbles and six yellow marbles in a bag. If two marble are drawn at random (one after the other without replacement), what is the probability of selecting two purple marbles?

A. $\dfrac{20}{121}$

B. $\dfrac{25}{121}$

C. $\dfrac{2}{11}$

D. $\dfrac{5}{11}$

E. $\dfrac{25}{36}$

38. Anne has a total of $34 in nickels, dimes, and quarters. If she has 3 times as many dimes as quarters and 2 times as many nickels as dimes, how many dimes does she have?

A. 12
B. 40
C. 51
D. 60
E. 120

39. What is the distance between $(-6, -9)$ and $(3, 3)$?

A. $3\sqrt{5}$
B. 15
C. 3
D. $\sqrt{21}$
E. 21

40. What is the average of 3, 5, 5, 11, and 13?

A. $7\dfrac{2}{5}$

B. 8

C. $6\dfrac{2}{5}$

D. $9\dfrac{1}{4}$

E. 5

STOP. IF YOU FINISH BEFORE TIME HAS EXPIRED, CHECK YOUR WORK. YOU MAY GO BACK TO ANY QUESTION IN THIS PART ONLY.

FULL-LENGTH PRACTICE DAT
ANSWER KEY

Survey of the Natural Sciences

#	Ans	#	Ans	#	Ans
1.	A	42.	D	86.	D
2.	C	43.	E	87.	C
3.	B	44.	D	88.	A
4.	C	45.	E	89.	E
5.	B	46.	E	90.	C
6.	A	47.	E	91.	E
7.	C	48.	B	92.	E
8.	E	49.	E	93.	C
9.	C	50.	D	94.	A
10.	D	51.	C	95.	A
11.	B	52.	D	96.	E
12.	E	53.	A	97.	B
13.	B	54.	A	98.	D
14.	A	55.	B	99.	C
15.	D	56.	D	100.	D
16.	A	57.	D		
17.	D	58.	C		
18.	C	59.	D		
19.	B	60.	D		
20.	C	61.	B		
21.	C	62.	C		
22.	B	63.	C		
23.	C	64.	B		
24.	C	65.	B		
25.	A	66.	A		
26.	A	67.	E		
27.	E	68.	D		
28.	A	69.	B		
29.	D	70.	B		
30.	E	71.	D		
31.	C	72.	E		
32.	D	73.	A		
33.	D	74.	A		
34.	D	75.	D		
35.	A	76.	D		
36.	B	77.	D		
37.	D	78.	A		
38.	E	79.	B		
39.	E	80.	E		
40.	D	81.	C		
41.	A	82.	E		
		83.	B		
		84.	D		
		85.	E		

Perceptual Ability

#	Ans	#	Ans
1.	A	46.	C
2.	D	47.	A
3.	C	48.	D
4.	E	49.	A
5.	A	50.	A
6.	E	51.	C
7.	B	52.	D
8.	B	53.	C
9.	D	54.	E
10.	C	55.	E
11.	A	56.	B
12.	E	57.	C
13.	B	58.	A
14.	C	59.	B
15.	B	60.	B
16.	D	61.	A
17.	A	62.	C
18.	B	63.	C
19.	A	64.	B
20.	C	65.	A
21.	D	66.	D
22.	C	67.	C
23.	B	68.	B
24.	A	69.	B
25.	D	70.	C
26.	A	71.	B
27.	D	72.	A
28.	D	73.	D
29.	A	74.	C
30.	C	75.	E
31.	C	76.	C
32.	A	77.	A
33.	D	78.	B
34.	B	79.	B
35.	D	80.	D
36.	B	81.	A
37.	A	82.	D
38.	A	83.	C
39.	D	84.	A
40.	A	85.	C
41.	B	86.	B
42.	C	87.	D
43.	B	88.	A
44.	C	89.	A
45.	A	90.	B

Reading Comprehension

#	Ans	#	Ans
1.	C	26.	B
2.	D	27.	E
3.	D	28.	B
4.	E	29.	C
5.	B	30.	E
6.	E	31.	C
7.	B	32.	A
8.	C	33.	D
9.	A	34.	D
10.	B	35.	B
11.	D	36.	D
12.	E	37.	E
13.	B	38.	D
14.	D	39.	C
15.	A	40.	B
16.	E	41.	C
17.	A	42.	B
18.	D	43.	E
19.	E	44.	C
20.	D	45.	B
21.	C	46.	A
22.	D	47.	E
23.	E	48.	D
24.	B	49.	D
25.	C	50.	B

Quantitative Reasoning

#	Ans	#	Ans
1.	C	21.	B
2.	E	22.	C
3.	A	23.	D
4.	A	24.	E
5.	E	25.	A
6.	C	26.	B
7.	D	27.	D
8.	D	28.	A
9.	C	29.	D
10.	C	30.	B
11.	B	31.	A
12.	E	32.	D
13.	D	33.	E
14.	B	34.	A
15.	D	35.	C
16.	E	36.	E
17.	D	37.	C
18.	D	38.	E
19.	A	39.	B
20.	C	40.	A

FULL–LENGTH PRACTICE DAT
Estimated Scaled Score Conversion Chart*

SCALED SCORE	Quantitative Reasoning	Reading Comp.	Biology	General Chemistry	Organic Chemistry	Science (Total Sci.)	PAT
30	40	–	–	–	30	100	90
29	39	50	40	–	–	99	89
28	–	49	–	30	29	98	88
27	–	48	–	–	–	97	–
26	38	47	39	–	–	96	87
25	37	46	–	29	28	95	85 to 86
24	36	45	38	–	–	94	84
23	35	44	–	28	27	92 to 93	81 to 83
22	33 to 34	42 to 43	37	–	–	89 to 91	78 to 80
21	31 to 32	40 to 41	35 to 36	27	26	86 to 88	74 to 77
20	29 to 30	38 to 39	34	26	25	81 to 85	70 to 73
19	27 to 28	35 to 37	32 to 33	24 to 25	23 to 24	76 to 80	65 to 69
18	24 to 26	31 to 34	30 to 31	22 to 23	21 to 22	70 to 75	59 to 64
17	22 to 23	27 to 30	27 to 29	20 to 21	19 to 20	63 to 69	52 to 58
16	19 to 21	24 to 26	24 to 26	18 to 19	17 to 18	56 to 62	46 to 51
15	16 to 18	21 to 23	21 to 23	16 to 17	15 to 16	48 to 55	39 to 45
14	14 to 15	18 to 20	18 to 20	13 to 15	13 to 14	41 to 47	32 to 38
13	11 to 13	15 to 17	15 to 17	11 to 12	11 to 12	33 to 40	26 to 31
12	9 to 10	13 to 14	12 to 14	9 to 10	8 to 10	27 to 32	21 to 25
11	7 to 8	10 to 12	10 to 11	7 to 8	7	21 to 26	17 to 20
10	6	8 to 9	8 to 9	6	5 to 6	17 to 20	13 to 16
9	5	6 to 7	6 to 7	4 to 5	4	13 to 16	10 to 12
8	4	5	5	3	3	10 to 12	7 to 9
7	3	4	4	–	–	7 to 9	6
6	2	3	3	2	2	5 to 6	4 to 5
5	–	2	2	–	–	4	3
4	–	–	–	1	1	3	2
3	1	1	1	–	–	2	–
2	0	0	–	–	–	–	–
1	–	–	0	0	0	0 to 1	0 to 1

*Conversion information estimated from released DAT material.

SURVEY OF THE NATURAL SCIENCES:
Answers and Explanations

ANSWER KEY

1. A	26. A	51. C	76. D
2. C	27. E	52. D	77. D
3. B	28. A	53. A	78. A
4. C	29. D	54. A	79. B
5. B	30. E	55. B	80. E
6. A	31. C	56. D	81. C
7. C	32. D	57. D	82. E
8. E	33. D	58. C	83. B
9. C	34. D	59. D	84. D
10. D	35. A	60. D	85. E
11. B	36. B	61. B	86. D
12. E	37. D	62. C	87. C
13. B	38. E	63. C	88. A
14. A	39. E	64. B	89. E
15. D	40. D	65. B	90. C
16. A	41. A	66. A	91. E
17. D	42. D	67. E	92. E
18. C	43. E	68. D	93. C
19. B	44. D	69. B	94. A
20. C	45. E	70. B	95. A
21. C	46. E	71. D	96. E
22. B	47. E	72. E	97. B
23. C	48. B	73. A	98. D
24. C	49. E	74. A	99. C
25. A	50. D	75. D	100. D

EXPLANATIONS

1. A The electron transport chain (ETC) is a complex carrier mechanism that generates ATP through oxidative phosphorylation, and it occurs in the inner mitochondrial membrane.

Choice (B) is incorrect because glycolysis is the oxidative breakdown of glucose into two molecules of pyruvate, and it occurs in the cytoplasm.

Choice (C) is incorrect because the Krebs cycle occurs in the mitochondrial matrix. The Krebs cycle begins when acetyl CoA combines with OAA to form citrate. Then a complicated series of reactions follows, which results in the release of 2 CO_2 and the regeneration of OAA.

Choice (D) is incorrect because fatty acid degradation occurs in microbodies called peroxisomes, which beak down fat into smaller molecules to use as fuel.

Choice (E) is incorrect because ATP synthesis occurs in the matrix (Krebs cycle), inner mitochondrial membrane (ETC), and cytoplasm (glycolysis).

2. C With each round of replication, the original DNA material gets halved. After four rounds of replication, the amount of original DNA will $= \left(\frac{1}{2}\right)^4 = \frac{1}{16} = 6.25\%.$

The original strand of DNA is comprised of two sister strands. After four rounds of replication, you would have 16 strands of DNA comprised of 32 sister strands. The two original sister strands are 6.25% of the 32 sister strands that you have at the end of the replication.

3. B The prokaryotic cell wall is composed of peptidoglycans, which are polysaccharides cross-linked by short peptide (protein) chains. The cell walls in plants, which are eukaryotes, are not composed of peptidoglycans.

Choice (A) is incorrect because photosynthetic granules (or grana) are components of the eukaryotic chloroplast. The granules are stacks of thylakoid membranes within the chloroplast.

Choice (C) is incorrect because mRNA is not unique to prokaryotes. mRNA (messenger RNA) is found in both prokaryotes and eukaryotes and transports genetic information from the DNA to the ribosome.

Choice (D) is incorrect because cell walls made of cellulose are found in plants, which are eukaryotes.

Choice (E) is incorrect because linear DNA, bundled on histones and packaged as chromosomes, is only found in eukaryotes. Prokaryotes have circular DNA.

4. C The statement in choice (C) is false: One molecule of glucose (6-carbon sugar) breaks down into two molecules of pyruvate (pyruvate is a 3-carbon molecule). Hence, this is the choice we are looking for.

Choice (A) is a true statement and therefore NOT the correct response: Glycolysis occurs in the cytoplasm.

Choice (B) is also true. Glycolysis is anaerobic and occurs in both eukaryotes and prokaryotes. In anaerobic conditions or in anaerobic bacteria, it is the first step in fermentation. In eukaryotes, pyruvate is reduced to lactic acid, and in prokaryotes, it is reduced to ethanol.

Choice (D) is an accurate statement. In glycolysis, one molecule of glucose is broken down and 4 ATP are formed. However, due to the initial investment of 2 ATP, the net production of ATP is 2. Also, two molecules of NAD^+ are reduced to NADH. These molecules will later enter the electron transport chain to produce ATP.

5. B Adenine and guanine are purines, while cytosine, uracil, and thymine are pyrimidines.

Choice (A) is an accurate statement. The basic unit of DNA is a nucleotide, which is made up of a phosphate group, a deoxyribose sugar, and a nucleic acid.

Choice (C) is also a true statement: The strands are antiparallel; that is, one strand has a $5' \rightarrow 3'$ polarity, and its complementary strand has a $3' \rightarrow 5'$ polarity.

Choice (D) is correct. Guanine always bonds with cytosine with three hydrogen bonds. Adenine will bond with either thymine or uracil with two hydrogen bonds.

Choice (E) is correct. The sugar molecule in DNA is deoxyribose, while in RNA it is ribose.

6. A Carbohydrates have a H:O ratio of 2:1, while fats have a H:O ratio much greater than 2:1, meaning that they have much more hydrogen than oxygen.

Choice (B) is incorrect because as implied above, the opposite is true.

Choice (C) is incorrect: Carbohydrates release 4 kcal/g, while fats release 9 kcal/g.

Choice (D) is incorrect because lipids do not form polymers. Carbohydrates form polymers known as polysaccharides, which are chains of repeating monosaccharide subunits.

Choice (E) is incorrect because neither carbohydrates nor lipids contain nitrogen. Proteins and amino acids contain nitrogen.

7. C Blastulation begins when the morula develops a fluid-filled cavity called the blastocoel, which, by the fourth day of human development, will become a hollow sphere of cells called the blastula.

Choice (A) is incorrect because the zygote is the diploid (2N) cell that results from the fusion of two haploid (N) gametes.

Choice (B) is incorrect: The morula is the solid ball of cells that results from the early stages of cleavage in an embryo.

Choices (D) and (E) are incorrect. The gastrula is the embryonic stage characterized by the presence of endoderm, ectoderm, the blastocoel, and the archenteron. The early gastrula is two layered; later a third layer, the mesoderm, develops.

8. E The lysosome is like the stomach of the cell and is characterized as a membrane-bound organelle that stores hydrolytic enzymes.

Choice (A) is incorrect because chloroplasts are found only in algae and plant cells. They contain chlorophyll and are the site of photosynthesis. Chloroplasts contain their own DNA and ribosomes and may have evolved by symbiosis.

Choice (B) is incorrect because microbodies are membrane-bound organelles specialized as containers for metabolic reactions.

Choice (C) is incorrect because phagosomes are vesicles that are involved in the transport and storage of materials, which are ingested by the cell through phagocytosis.

Choice (D) is incorrect. Vacuoles and vesicles are membrane-bound sacs involved in the transport and storage of materials that are ingested, secreted, processed, or digested by the cells. Vacuoles are larger than vesicles and are more likely to be found in plant cells.

9. C If the frequency of the dominant allele is three times that of the recessive allele, then $p = 3q$. According to Hardy–Weinberg equilibrium, $p + q = 1$, so $3q + q = 1$. Solving for q, we get $4q = 1$; $q = 0.25$ and $p = 0.75$. Again according to Hardy–Weinberg, the frequency of the heterozygotes is equal to $2pq$. Substituting in our values for p and q, we have the equation $2(0.75)(0.25)$, which equals 0.375 or 37.5%.

10. D The endoderm will develop into the epithelial linings of the digestive and respiratory tracts, parts of the liver, pancreas, thyroid, and the bladder lining.

Choice (A) is incorrect because the lens of the eyes will develop from the ectoderm.

Choice (B) is incorrect because the gonads are developed from the mesoderm.

Choice (C) is incorrect because the nervous system is developed from the ectoderm.

Choice (E) is incorrect because the connective tissue is developed from the mesoderm.

11. B The allantois is a saclike structure involved in respiration and excretion. It contains numerous blood vessels to transport O_2, CO_2, water, salt, and nitrogenous wastes. Later during development, the vessels enlarge and become the umbilical vessels, which will connect the fetus to the placenta.

Choice (A) is incorrect because the chorion lines the inside of the shell and is a moist membrane that permits gas exchange.

Choice (C) is incorrect because the amnion is the membrane that encloses the amniotic fluid. Amniotic fluid provides an aqueous environment that protects the developing embryo from shock.

Choice (D) is incorrect because the yolk sac encloses the yolk. Blood vessels in the yolk sac transfer food to the developing embryo.

Choice (E) is incorrect because the placenta and the umbilical cord are outgrowths of the four previous membranes. This system delivers oxygen and nutrients to the fetus while removing carbon dioxide and metabolic wastes.

12. E Platelets are cell fragments that lack nuclei and are involved in clot formation.

Choice (A): Erythrocytes are the oxygen-carrying components of the blood. They contain hemoglobin, which can bind up to four molecules of oxygen.

Choice (B): Macrophages carry out phagocytosis of foreign particles and bacteria, digest them, and present the fragments on their cell surface.

Choice (C): T cells lyse virally infected cells or secrete proteins that stimulate the development of B or other types of T cells.

Choice (D): B cells mature into memory cells or antibody-producing cells during immune responses.

13. B In ten turns of the Calvin cycle, 20 PGAL are formed from 6 carbon dioxide and 6 RBP molecules.

14. A Sulfur is sometimes found in proteins but never in nucleic acids. The famous Hershey–Chase experiment took advantage of this to determine whether proteins or nucleic acids carried the genetic information of the cell.

The other choices are incorrect. Nucleic acids contain the elements C, H, O, N, and P. They are polymers of subunits called nucleotides, and they code all the information needed by an organism to produce proteins and replicate.

15. D In plants, spores are haploid and produce the haploid gametophyte generation. Therefore, since they have 18 chromosomes, that would be the haploid number. The diploid number would be 36.

16. A Any male born from that mating will receive an X chromosome from his mother and a Y from his father. The X he receives will either carry fragile X syndrome or color blindness, so he has a 50% chance of having fragile X syndrome and a 50% chance of being color-blind, neither of which are phenotypically normal.

17. D The cell walls of bacteria are made of peptidoglycans, whereas the cell walls of plants and fungi are made up of cellulose.

All the other choices are true of the cytoskeleton: The cytoskeleton is composed of microtubules and microfilaments and gives the cell mechanical support, maintains its shape, and functions in cell motility.

18. C At approximately 50°C, heat alters the shape of the active site of the enzyme molecule and deactivates it, leading to a rapid drop in rate.

Choice (A) is incorrect: Up to approximately 40°C, the rate of enzyme action increases; after that, the protein will denature.

Choice (B) is incorrect because the optimum temperature for most enzymes is 37°C, physiological temperature. Some enzymes can work at higher temperature, but those will be in specialized organisms, such as the bacteria that thrive in hot springs.

Choice (D) is incorrect because an increase in energy in the system will increase effective collisions until the temperature becomes so high as to denature the enzyme.

19. B Plant cells are rigid and cannot form a cleavage furrow. They divide by the formation of a cell place, an expanding partition that grows outward from the interior of the cell until it reaches the cell membrane.

Choice (A) is incorrect because plant cells lack centrioles. The spindle apparatus is synthesized by microtubule organizing centers, which are not visible.

Choice (C) is incorrect: Cytokinesis in animal cells proceeds through formation of cleavage furrow.

Choice (D) is incorrect because animal cells have centrioles from which the spindle apparatus arises.

Choice (E) is incorrect because most cell divisions have equal cytokinesis, except for cells such as yeast that bud.

20. C 32 ATP are produced by the electron transport chain and oxidative phosphorylation. Ultimately, 1 molecule of glucose will be catalyzed to produce 36 ATP (32 from oxidative phosphorylation, 2 from the citric acid cycle, and 2 from glycolysis).

21. C Before considering the Punnett square for the offspring, we will determine the phenotype of the parents. A red-eyed fly with red-eyed and sepia-eyed parents must be heterozygous, because its sepia-eyed parent can only contribute the recessive sepia allele. If this heterozygous fly is crossed with a homozygous recessive (sepia-eyed) fly, 1/2 the offspring will be red eyed because they will receive the red, dominant allele from the heterozygous fly. The Punnett square will look like this:

red-eyed parent	R	r
sepia-eyed parent		
r	Rr (red)	rr (sepia)
r	Rr (red)	rr (sepia)

22. B The retina develops from the ectoderm. The ectoderm develops into the nervous system, the epidermis, the lens of the eye, and the inner ear. The endoderm develops into the lining of the digestive tract, lungs, liver, and pancreas. The mesoderm develops into the muscles, skeleton, circulatory system, gonads, and kidneys.

23. C Osmosis is a special type of diffusion involving water and is a form of passive transport. Hypertonic means high solute and low solvent. Hypotonic means high solvent and low solute. Solvent always flows spontaneously from an area of high solvent concentration to an area of low solvent concentration. Therefore, water will flow from a hypotonic environment to a hypertonic environment.

24. C Disruptive selection occurs when selection acts to eliminate the intermediate type and favor the extremes. A stabilizing selection eliminates both extremes and increases the occurrence of the intermediate type. A directional selection eliminates one of the extremes and increases the occurrence of the other extreme. Genetic drift is a random change in the gene pool that occurs over time. Genetic drift is felt strongly in small populations where random changes have significant effects on the gene pool. Gene flow occurs when groups migrate from place to place, carrying new alleles to a previously isolated population.

25. A The snake is a secondary consumer because it eats the mouse, a primary consumer. Primary consumers feed directly on plants, which are the primary producers in the ecosystem. An aphid is a primary consumer because it feeds directly on wheat. The fungus in choice (C) is a "detrivore" or decomposer that feeds on dead matter. It can also be viewed as a primary consumer that feeds directly on the green plant. Photosynthetic bacteria are primary producers. The hawk in choice (E) is a tertiary consumer.

26. A The medulla controls many vital functions, including breathing, heart rate, and gastrointestinal activity.

Choice (B) is wrong because the hypothalamus controls such things as hunger, thirst, sex drive, water balance, blood pressure, and temperature regulation. It also plays an integral role in controlling the endocrine system.

Choice (C) is wrong because the cerebrum (usually referred to as the cerebral cortex) processes and integrates sensory input and motor responses and is important for memory and creative thought.

Choice (D) is wrong because the cerebellum is important in coordinating muscles. It aids in balance (it receives input from the inner ear), hand-eye coordination, and the timing of rapid movements.

Choice (E) is wrong because the pituitary gland, along with the hypothalamus, plays an integral role in controlling the endocrine system.

27. E Once a virus has injected its genetic material into the cytoplasm of a host cell, it can enter either the lytic cycle or the lysogenic cycle. In the lysogenic cycle, the viral DNA integrates into the host genome (if it is an RNA virus, the RNA is first transcribed into DNA using reverse transcriptase) and lies dormant. At this stage, the virus is referred to as a provirus, so choice (C) is correct. The viral DNA can remain dormant indefinitely, making choice (B) correct, as it replicates along with the host, making choice (A) correct. At some later time, the viral DNA can be activated, and the bacteria will enter the lytic cycle in which the bacteria takes control of the host's genetic machinery and makes numerous progeny. In the last stage, the virus produces an enzyme that causes the cell to burst, releasing all the new viruses.

28. A The posterior pituitary releases two hormones, the oxytocin hormone and the antidiuretic hormone (ADH, also called vasopressin). choice (B), FSH, is released by the anterior pituitary. Choice (C), glucagon, is released by the alpha cell of the islets of Langerhans in the pancreas. Choice (D), estrogen, is released by the graafian follicle within the ovary during the menstrual cycle. Choice (E), calcitonin, is released by the thyroid gland.

29. D When a symbiotic relationship between two organisms benefits both species involved, it is referred to as mutualism.

Parasitism, choice (A), is the symbiotic relationship wherein one species benefits at the expense of the other. An example is heartworm in dogs. The worm parasites nourish themselves on the blood of the dog host, which can be potentially fatal to the dog.

Commensalism, choice (B), is when one organism is benefited by the association and the other is not affected. An example is barnacles and whales. Barnacles attach themselves to whales, thereby obtaining more feeding opportunities, while the whale is unaffected by the barnacles' presence.

Predation, Choice (C), is free-living organisms feeding on other living organisms. Unlike the other relationships above, predation is not a symbiotic relationship.

30. E In the modern system of classification, all organisms are named as follows: kingdom, phylum, subphylum, class, order, family, genus, species. In the Linnaen classification system, all organisms are assigned a scientific name consisting of only the genus and species name of that organism. This scheme was originated by the biologist Carl Linn. Therefore *Homo* refers to the genus, and *sapiens* refers to the species.

31. C Luteinizing hormone (LH) is first released as a surge midway through the menstrual cycle. This surge causes the mature follicle to burst, releasing the ovum from the ovary. Following ovulation, LH induces the ruptured follicle to develop into the corpus luteum (hence the name), which then secretes estrogen and progesterone.

Choice (A) is incorrect because progesterone and estrogen inhibit GnRH release (thereby inhibiting FSH and LH release, thus preventing additional follicles from maturing).

Choice (B) is incorrect because LH is secreted by the anterior pituitary. The ovary secretes estrogen and progesterone.

Choice (D) is describing the function of progesterone, not LH.

Choice (E) is describing the function of prolactin, not LH.

32. D If a piece of cardiac muscle were placed in a petri dish and nourished properly, it would contract at intrinsic beat. Cardiac muscle, unlike any other muscle type, is capable of depolarizing spontaneously, which causes a contraction. Other muscle types require some type of stimulation to cause depolarization and contraction (usually a neurotransmitter).

Choice (A) is incorrect because cardiac muscle is innervated by the autonomic nervous system. The somatic motor system controls voluntary actions—walking, running, etc.

Cardiac muscle is striated, eliminating choice (B), and it has only one or two centrally located nuclei, eliminating choice (C).

Choice (E) is incorrect because cardiac muscle, like skeletal muscle and smooth muscle, requires Ca^{2+} for contraction.

33. D Fixed action patterns are complex, coordinated, innate behavioral responses to specific patterns of stimulation in the environment. These responses are controlled from all levels of the central nervous system. The characteristic movement of heard animals is an example of a fixed action pattern.

The startle response, Choice (A), is an example of a complex reflex pattern. These responses are controlled from the brainstem or cerebrum.

Choice (B) is an example of a simple reflex. These responses are controlled at the spinal cord.

Circadian rhythms, Choice (C), are an example of a behavior cycle. These behaviors are a response to both internal and external stimuli, and they control such behaviors as sleep and wakefulness and eating and satiation.

34. D The stamen is the male organ of a flower and consists of the stalklike filament, on top of which is the anther. The anther produces monoploid spores, which develop into pollen grains.

The female organ of the flower consists of the stigma (E), the site of pollen deposition; the style (A), a tubelike structure that connects the stigma to the ovary; and the ovary, which contains ovules and is the site of fertilization and seed development.

The petal, Choice (B), is a specialized leaf that serves to protect the female organs of the plant and to attract insects to aid in fertilization.

35. A Pioneer organisms are the first species that inhabit an area that was previously devoid of life. Typically, these organisms have to be able to survive in harsh conditions, such as living on rocky surfaces. Lichens, which are a symbiotic relationship between alga and fungi, are capable of living on rocky surfaces. The acid produced by lichens aids in soil formation, which allows other organisms to colonize the area. Mosses (B) usually follow lichens in colonization but cannot serve as a pioneer organism. Grasses are typically the next succeeding organism, followed by ferns, then birches.

36. B The area in the kidney with the lowest solute concentration is the cortex. Filtrate that enters the nephron travels through the proximal convoluted tubule, then through the loop of Henle, followed by the distal convoluted tubule, collecting duct, and renal pelvis, and then out of the kidney to the bladder. The convoluted tubules are within the cortex, and the collecting duct and pelvis are in the medulla. As filtrate travels from the cortex to the medulla, it constantly experiences an increasing concentration gradient, the purpose of which is to reabsorb water so that the urine is concentrated.

Choice (A) is incorrect because the solute concentration within the nephron varies according to the region of the kidney through which filtrate is traveling.

Choice (C) is incorrect because the medulla has a very high concentration gradient, which is necessary in order for an organism to produce concentrated urine.

Choice (D) is incorrect because the pelvis, which is in the medulla, has a very high concentration gradient so that water can be reabsorbed.

Choice (E) is incorrect because epithelia does not refer to a region within the kidney.

37. D A niche defines the functional role of an organism it its ecosystem. A niche describes what the organism eats, where and how it obtains its food, the nature of its parasites and predators, how it reproduces, etc. Organisms occupying the same niche compete for the same limited resources, such as food, water, light, oxygen, and space. This competition will either cause one species to be driven to extinction, eliminating Choice (A), or cause the species to evolve in divergent directions, changing the niches they occupy and eliminating competition.

Choice (B) is wrong because the two species involved may or may not be nocturnal (since they occupy the same niche, they are either both nocturnal or not).

Choice (C) is wrong because the species will evolve so that they are more distinct from each other (divergent), not more similar (convergent).

Choice (E) is incorrect because two species may indeed occupy two niches, and it is the ensuing competition that drives evolution.

38. E The resting membrane potential across a nerve cell membrane depends on the physiology of two ions: Na^+ and K^+. The Na^+/K^+ pump is an active transport protein that maintains an electrochemical gradient across the membrane by pumping 3 Na^+ out and 2 K^+ in. This makes the cell negative on the inside relative to the outside and creates a high concentration of Na^+ outside the cell relative to the inside and a high concentration of K^+ inside relative to the outside. The membrane is more permeable to K^+ than Na^+, and it is the balance between the pump and the "leaky" membrane that determines the cell's resting potential.

39. E As discussed in question 26, the cerebellum is involved in balance, hand-eye coordination, and the timing of rapid movements. If a tumor were located in the cerebellum, you would expect loss of hand-eye coordination.

Choices (A) and (D) are incorrect because the hypothalamus is responsible for temperature regulation and hunger and thirst drives.

Choice (B) is incorrect because the medulla is responsible for controlling heart rate.

Choice (C) is incorrect because the cerebrum is responsible for processing sensory input, such as vision, smell, and taste.

40. D Chlorophyll, the green pigment that participates in the light reactions of photosynthesis, has a magnesium atom in its center. Zinc, copper, and manganese are involved in a variety of cellular functions, none of which need to be memorized. Iron is found in hemoglobin and provides the ability to bind and release oxygen.

41. A With the exception of the noble gases, which occupy the last column of the periodic table, the electronegativity of elements increases as one goes towards the upper right-hand corner. The five elements listed in Choice (A) are in the same column (or group) but occupy positions that are farther and farther down. The electronegativity thus decreases, and this is what we are looking for.

Choice (B) is incorrect because it contains elements in the same row (or period) in the order of increasing atomic number (moving to the right). The electronegativity increases.

Choice (C) is incorrect because the elements move towards the upper-right hand corner (i.e., in the direction of increasing electronegativity).

Choice (D) is incorrect because the elements are moving up a group, and hence electronegativity is increasing.

Choice (E) is incorrect because the elements are all noble (or inert) gases and all have very low electronegativity.

42. D The second ionization energy is the energy needed to remove a second electron from an already positively charged ion. In other words, for the process

$$X^+ \rightarrow X^{2+} + e^- \qquad \Delta E = ?$$

ΔE is the second ionization energy of the element X. An element with a high second ionization energy, then, would have a cation with a very stable electron configuration. In particular, if X^+ has an electronic configuration similar to that of a noble gas, then X will have a high second ionization energy. Choices (D) and (E), Rb and Cs, are both in the first column of the periodic table. A first ionization would form Rb^+ and Cs^+, both of which will a noble gas configuration. (Rb^+ will have the configuration of Kr, while Cs^+ will have the configuration of Xe.) Kr has a higher ionization energy than Xe, since its valence orbital has a lower principal quantum number. Rb^+, therefore, has a higher ionization energy than Cs^+, which in turn means that Rb has a higher second ionization energy than Cs.

Choices (A), (B), and (C) are incorrect because they are Group II elements. A first ionization would cause each of them to be isoelectronic to a Group I element, which has a low ionization energy, since another ionization would bring them to a stable octet of a noble gas configuration.

43. E Phosphorus has five valence electrons. It thus needs three more to complete its octet. It can do this by forming three covalent bonds: two to hydrogen and one to chlorine. The Lewis structure is as follows:

$$H-\overset{\displaystyle :\ddot{C}l:}{\underset{\displaystyle ..}{P}}-H$$

The Lewis structure, however, does not necessarily give an accurate representation of the three-dimensional appearance of the molecule. For that, we have to use VSEPR theory. There are four regions of electron density around the central P atom—three bonding electron pairs and one non-bonding pair. These will want to be as far apart as possible, resulting in a tetrahedral electronic geometry. In describing the actual molecular geometry, however, we ignore the nonbonding pair and would thus describe the molecule as trigonal pyramidal. It is similar to the structure of NH_3:

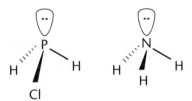

44. D Virtually no calculation is needed for this question. The pressure has slightly less than doubled on going from 1.00 atm to 1.80 atm. Since temperature and volume are not changing, the number of moles of gas needs to increase proportionally (i.e., it needs to increase to slightly less than the double, 6.00 moles). The only choice that fits this requirement is (D): An extra 2.4 moles would bring the total number of moles of gas to 5.4 moles.

For completeness, the setup is as follows. Rearrange the ideal gas law:

$$\frac{P_1}{n_1} = \frac{P_2}{n_2} = \frac{RT}{V} = \text{constant}$$

$$n_2 = \frac{n_1}{P_1} \times P_2 = \frac{3.00}{1.00} \times 1.80 = 5.40 \text{ moles}$$

The extra number of moles needed is therefore 5.4 – 3.0 = 2.4.

(A sidenote: Be careful when applying this approach to questions dealing with changes in temperature. Make sure you are using absolute temperature, in Kelvin. An increase from 20°C to 40°C is NOT a doubling of temperature!)

45. E First we must determine the order of the reaction. On going from experiment 1 to experiment 2, the concentration of B has increased, but the rate of reaction remains the same. The reaction therefore appears to be independent on the concentration of B, or in other words, it is zero order with respect to B. Comparing experiments 1 and 3, we see that the concentration of A has tripled, while the rate of reaction has increased by about a factor of 9. The reaction is second order in A. We can therefore write:

$$\text{rate} = k[A]^2$$

To determine the rate constant, we need only to arrange the above equation and substitute in values for [A] and the rate for any one experiment:

$$k = \frac{\text{rate}}{[A]^2} = \frac{1.87}{(0.181)^2}$$

Note that the rate constant will have units (of $M^{-1}s^{-1}$ for second-order reactions), but we are ignoring that in this particular question.

46. E The spontaneity of a reaction is determined by the free energy change, ΔG. A reaction goes from being spontaneous to nonspontaneous (or vice versa) when the value of ΔG crosses the value of 0. Since $\Delta G = \Delta H - T\Delta S$, and we are told to assume that the values of ΔH and ΔS are not sensitive to changes in temperature, we can solve for the temperature at which the value of ΔG becomes zero. The tricky part is that ΔH and ΔS are

reported in different units, and we must be careful to be consistent. We change the value of ΔH from 131 kJ/mol to 131,000 J/mol:

$$0 = 131,000 - T(134)$$

$$T = \frac{131,000}{134}$$

This is slightly less than 1,000 K. (Remember: We always use the absolute temperature in cases like this!) To convert from Kelvin to degrees Celsius, we need to subtract about 300. This brings the value to about 700, which is Choice (E).

The ΔH and ΔS values are reported in different energy units not just to trap you. The magnitude of the enthalpy change is usually much greater than the magnitude of the entropy change for a given reaction, so expressing one with kJ and the other with J (or kcal and cal) is a common practice.

Choice (C) may have been tempting if you had forgotten to convert from K to °C.

47. E A mole of ideal gas, regardless of the species, occupies 22.4 L at STP, which corresponds to 1 atm pressure and 0°C (or 273 K). The conditions specified in the question stem are thus STP conditions. The mixture occupies a volume of 44.8 L, which means there are 2 moles of gas present. If the mixture contains 1.5 moles of argon, then there must be 2 – 1.5 = 0.5 mol Ne present.

48. B Halogens are Group VII elements, occupying the second to last column on the periodic table. It includes F, Cl, Br I, and At. Alkaline earth metals are the Group II elements, the ones in the second column. It includes Be, Mg, Ca, etc. Transition metals are the block of elements in the middle columns of the periodic table, from Sc to Hg. Cr, in Group VIB, is a transition metal.

Choice (A)—Cl, Na, Sr—is incorrect because it lists a halogen, an alkali metal (a Group I element), and an alkaline earth metal.

Choice (C) is incorrect because Se is not a halogen and Sn is not a transition metal.

Choices (D) and (E) are incorrect because Rd is an alkali metal, not a halogen or an alkaline earth metal.

49. E The percentage of oxygen by mass is the mass of oxygen divided by the total mass of the compound, multiplied by 100%. Even though we are told that the sample weighs 200 g, we actually don't need this to get the answer. Any sample of $CuSO_4 \bullet 5H_2O$, regardless of its weight, will have the same percentage of O by mass, since this is dictated by the stoichiometric relationships in the chemical formula. We can work with the convenient quantity of 1 mole. The weight of a 1-mole sample is just the molecular weight of the compound: $63.55 + 32.06 + 4 \times 16 + 5 \times (2 \times 1 + 16) = 63.55 + 32.06 + 64 + 90 \approx 250$ g. The mass of oxygen in this 1-mole sample is $4 \times 16 \times 5 \times 16 = 144$, where the first four come from the sulfate and the other five come from the five water molecules hydrated to the compound. The percentage by mass of oxygen is therefore

$$\frac{144}{250} \times 100\%$$

Since 144 is more than half of 250, the percentage is more than 50%, making (E) the correct choice.

Failure to realize that there are five water molecules (each of which contains an oxygen atom) may have led you to choice (C).

Note, again, that nowhere did we use the fact that the sample weighs 200 g.

50. D Nonmetallic elements are found in the right of the periodic table and, if neutral, will always have valence electrons in the p subshell, which can hold a maximum of six electrons. (If it is not neutral, there is a possibility that electrons have been added or removed so that there are only s valence electrons.) The requirement that it be in its ground state means that the orbitals are filled in accordance with the Aufbau principle. Only choice (D) satisfies these criteria.

Choice (A) is incorrect because its valence electrons are in the s subshell. If it is a neutral species, this would be Mg, which is a metal. If it is a nonmetal, it must have had electrons removed or added, making it not neutral (e.g., Al^+.)

Choice (B) is incorrect because it has three electrons in an s subshell, which can accommodate a maximum of only two electrons (since it contains only one orbital).

Choice (C) is incorrect because the $4s$ orbital should not have filled before the $3p$ orbitals: It does not represent a ground-state species.

Choice (E) is incorrect because the p subshell, with three orbitals, can only have a maximum of six electrons.

51. C Nitrogen is in the second period, and hence its valence shell does not have a d subshell. It cannot expand its octet and can form no more than four bonds. Choice (C) is the only structure in which neither nitrogen forms more than four bonds.

All the other choices contain at least one nitrogen forming five bonds.

52. D For a molecule to be polar, it must contain polar bonds (bonds formed between elements of different electronegativity, in which electron density is not shared equally), and the dipole moments carried by these polar bonds must not cancel vectorially. Choices (A), (B), and (C) are incorrect because even though they all contain polar bonds, these bonds are arranged spatially so that they cancel one another:

BF_3 has a trigonal planar geometry, and the dipole moments of the polar B–F bonds, when added together vectorially, yield no net dipole moment. The same goes for the tetrahedral CF_4 and CBr_4.

Choice (D) is correct because the two polar C–Cl bonds do not completely cancel each other. Compared to choice (E), a C–Cl bond is more polar than a C–Br bond, since Cl is more electronegative than Br. The C–Cl bonds thus have a greater dipole moment.

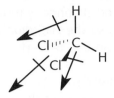

net dipole moment

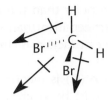

net dipole moment

53. A This question tests our knowledge of both stoichiometry and gas laws. First, we need to determine how many moles of hydrogen gas are generated from the reaction, then calculate the volume of the gas under the conditions described. For the first part, the dimensional setup is as follows:

number of moles of H_2 produced =

$$5.05 \text{ g Zn} \times \frac{1 \text{ mol Zn}}{65.4 \text{ g}} \times \frac{1 \text{ mol hydrogen}}{1 \text{ mol Zn}} = \frac{5.05}{65.4}$$

where the atomic weight of Zn of 65.4 g/mol is read off the periodic table and the stoichiometric relationship between Zn and H_2 is read from the balanced equation given in the question stem. For the second part of calculating the volume, we need to use the ideal gas law. We need to be careful about units, because we are using the value of R as given in the question stem to determine the volume in liters, but that means that we need our temperature to be in Kelvin and our pressure to be in atmospheres. We know 40°C = 313 K, and since 1 atm = 760 torr, 763 torr = 763/760 atm.

$$PV = nRT$$

$$V = \frac{nRT}{P} = \text{number of moles of}$$

$$H_2 \times \frac{(0.0821 \text{ L} \bullet \text{atm/mol} \bullet \text{K})(313 \text{ K})}{763/760 \text{ atm}}$$

$$= \text{number of moles of } H_2 \times \frac{760}{763} \times 0.0821 \times 313$$

$$= \frac{5.05}{65.4} \times \frac{760}{763} \times 0.0821 \times 313$$

which is Choice (A).

54. A Isotopes of an element have the same atomic number but different mass numbers. The atomic number is the same as the number of protons, and the mass number is the sum of protons and neutrons. The isotope given in the question

has a mass number of 208 and an atomic number of 82; it therefore has 82 protons and 208 − 82 = 126 neutrons. Another isotope of the same element must therefore also have 82 neutrons (an atomic number of 82) but a different number of neutrons. Choice (A) is correct.

Choices (B) and (C) are incorrect because each would imply that the two isotopes are the same.

Choices (D) and (E) are incorrect because isotopes of the same element must have the same atomic number (same number of protons)—in this case, 82.

55. B The empirical formula gives the simplest whole number ratio of the different elements in a compound. Since in this question, the number of moles of each element in the compound has been given to us already, all we need to do is to find the simplest whole number ratio among them. We know 1.074 is twice the value of 0.537, so N:H:Cl = 0.537:1.074:0.537 = 1:2:1. The empirical formula is thus NH_2Cl.

(Note that in most questions involving empirical formulas, we would probably just be given the mass of each element in the sample, and we would first have to determine the number of moles of each by dividing by the atomic mass of the elements.)

56. D Hess's Law tells us that the standard change in enthalpy of a reaction, $\Delta H°$, is equal to the sum of the standard enthalpies of formation of the products minus the sum of the standard enthalpies of formation of the reactants. Therefore, for the first reaction in the table, we can write:

$\Delta H° = 729.8 \text{ kcal} = 6 \times \Delta H°_f (CO_2) +$
$3 \times \Delta H°_f (H_2O) - \Delta H°_f (C_6H_5OH) - 7 \times \Delta H°_f (O_2)$

O_2 is already in its standard state, so its enthalpy of formation is zero. The last term in the equation thus vanishes. The enthalpy of formation of carbon dioxide is the enthalpy change of the second reaction in the table (i.e., 94.4 kcal/mol). The enthalpy of formation of one mole of H_2O is *one-half* the enthalpy change of the third reaction (i.e., 68.4 kcal/mol). (The reaction leads to the formation of *two* moles of H_2O.) We can now substitute in these values and solve for the unknown, the enthalpy of formation of C_6H_5OH:

$$729.8 = 6 \times 94.4 + 3 \times 136.8 - \Delta H^\circ_f\ (C_6H_5OH)$$

$$\Delta H^\circ_f\ (C_6H_5OH) = 6 \times 94.4 + 3 \times 68.4 - 729.8 \approx 600 + 210 - 730$$

With this approximation, we can see that only Choice (D) is close enough to be correct.

57. D The percent yield is the actual yield divided by the theoretical yield, multiplied by 100 percent. The theoretical yield is the amount of product expected based purely on stoichiometry. In this question, the theoretical yield is determined as follows:

amount of $C_6H_5NO_2$ expected =

$$\frac{78g\ C_6H_6}{78\ g/mol\ C_6H_6} \times \frac{1\ mol\ C_6H_6}{mol\ C_6H_5NO_2} \times$$
$$123\ g/mol\ C_6H_5NO_2 = 123\ g\ C_6H_5NO_2$$

The actual yield is 82 g. The percent yield is therefore $\frac{82}{123} \times 100$ percent. Without actually performing the division, we note that 82 is certainly more than half of 123, so the percentage is greater than 50 percent.

Choice (D) is the only possible response.

58. C Hydrogen bonds are a specific type of dipole-dipole interaction. When hydrogen is bound to a highly electronegative atom, such as oxygen or fluorine, the hydrogen atom carries little of the electron density of the covalent bond. This partially positively charged hydrogen atom interacts with the partial negative charge located on the electronegative atoms of nearby molecules. Water is a liquid at room temperature because each molecule can form two hydrogen bonds with neighboring molecules. Hydrogen fluoride can form only one intermolecular hydrogen bond.

Choice (A) is incorrect because H2O and HF differ by only 2 amu; this difference is insignificant relative to boiling point determination.

Choice (B) is incorrect because the H–F bond is more polar than the H–O bond (fluorine is more electronegative than oxygen), so the H–F dipole-dipole attraction is stronger than that of O–H.

Choice (D) is incorrect because dispersion forces only exist between nonpolar atoms or molecules. So the dispersion forces between H–F and H–O are insignificant.

Choice (E) is incorrect because intermolecular forces are measured with pure samples only.

59. D The easiest way to answer this question is to eliminate wrong answer choices.

Choices (A) and (B) can be eliminated because the unknown compound resulted in an acidic solution, so it cannot be a base.

We can eliminate choice (C) as follows: We are given a pH of 4.56. Since pH = $-\log[H^+]$, then the $[H^+] = 1 \times 10^{-pH}$. The $[H^+]$ must then be between 1×10^{-5} M and 1×10^{-4} M. Since the volume is 1L, then there are between 1×10^{-5} M and 1×10^{-4} mol H^+. Looking at choice (C), if the acid had a formula weight of $50\ \frac{g}{mol}$ and 100 g was added to the water, then 2 mol of H^+ would form if it were a strong acid. From the previous calculation, we know that is impossible. The unknown must be a weak acid.

Choice (E) is incorrect because there is no acid (weak or strong) that has a formula weight of less than $10\ \frac{g}{mol}$.

We can confirm choice (D) as the correct answer as follows: The formula for $K_a = \frac{[H^+][A^-]}{[HA]}$. Since the unknown compound must be a weak acid, there will be more undissociated acid in solution than dissociated, making the $[HA] > [H^+][A^-]$, so then $K_a < 1$. If $K_a < 1$, then $pK_a > 1$.

60. D The molarity of the acid solution can be calculated using the neutralization formula: $M_A V_A = M_B V_B$. Since we are given that both the acid and base are monoprotic, the normalities equal the molarities. Solving for the acid molarity and plugging in, we get $M_A = \dfrac{M_B V_B}{V_A} = \dfrac{(0.1)(35)}{50}$, choice (D).

61. B Freezing point depression is a colligative property—one that depends only on the amount of the substance present. Since the compound in the question is ionic, the formula for the freezing point depression has to be multiplied by the number of particles formed upon dissolving. The formula for freezing point depression is $\Delta T_f = k_f m \bullet x$; where x is the number of particles formed.

$\Delta T_f = \dfrac{\text{mass/MW}}{\text{kg}} = \dfrac{22.2/111}{1} \approx (2)(0.2) = 0.4°C.$

The observed freezing point is $-1.12°C$, which is 3 times as much as the calculated value. The unknown ionic compound must therefore dissociate into 3 particles, making (B) the correct choice.

62. C

A. $\begin{array}{cc} 2 + x = 0 & x - 2 - 2 = 0 \\ \uparrow\ \ \uparrow & \uparrow\ \ \uparrow\ \ \uparrow \\ +1\ \ \ x & x\ \ -2\ \ -1 \\ H_2S & SOCl_2 \\ S = -2 & S = +4 \end{array}$

B. $\begin{array}{cc} 2 + x - 8 = 0 & x - 2 - 2 = 0 \\ \uparrow\ \ \uparrow\ \ \uparrow & \uparrow\ \ \uparrow\ \ \uparrow \\ +1\ \ \ x\ \ -2 & x\ \ -2\ \ -1 \\ H_2SO_4 & SOCl_2 \\ S = +6 & S = +4 \end{array}$

C. $\begin{array}{cc} 2 + x - 6 = 0 & x - 2 - 2 = 0 \\ \uparrow\ \ \uparrow\ \ \uparrow & \uparrow\ \ \uparrow\ \ \uparrow \\ +1\ \ \ x\ \ -2 & x\ \ -2\ \ -1 \\ H_2SO_3 & SOCl_2 \\ S = +4 & S = +4 \end{array}$

D. $\begin{array}{cc} 2 + x = 0 & 2 + x - 8 = 0 \\ \uparrow\ \ \uparrow & \uparrow\ \ \uparrow\ \ \uparrow \\ +1\ \ \ x & +1\ \ \ x\ \ -2 \\ H_2S & H_2SO_4 \\ S = -2 & S = +6 \end{array}$

E. $\begin{array}{cc} 2 + x - 6 = 0 & 2 + x - 8 = 0 \\ \uparrow\ \ \uparrow\ \ \uparrow & \uparrow\ \ \uparrow\ \ \uparrow \\ +1\ \ \ x\ \ -2 & +1\ \ \ x\ \ -2 \\ H_2SO_3 & H_2SO_4 \\ S = +4 & S = +6 \end{array}$

63. C In beta decay, a neutron decays into a proton and an electron: $_0^1 n \rightarrow\ _1^1 p +\ _{-1}^0 e$. The generic for beta decay is $_Z^A X \rightarrow\ _{Z+1}^A Y +\ _{-1}^0 e$. In this example, the formula is $_6^{14}C \rightarrow X +\ _{-1}^0 e$. X must be $_7^{14}N$.

64. B The best oxidizing agent is the species getting reduced. The nitrogen goes from +5 in NO_3^- to -3 in NH_3, getting reduced and serving as an oxidizing agent.

Choice (A) is wrong because aluminum goes from 0 in Al_s to +3 in $Al(OH)_4^-$.

Choices (C) and (D) are wrong because they represent products of the reaction.

Choice (E) is wrong because neither the oxygen nor hydrogen in OH^- are changed in the reaction.

65. B This question requires no calculation. Since we are dealing with a base, choices (C), (D), and (E) can all be eliminated. Choice (A) is impossible because the pH can never exceed 14. That leaves only (B) as a possibility.

66. A The point on the pressure temperature curve where all three phases exist together in equilibrium is the triple point. The triple point is at point D, answer choice (A).

67. E Condensation, the conversion of a gas to a liquid, occurs along the gas-liquid boundary, which includes point Z and point D, the triple point.

68. D Vapor pressure is the amount of pressure the gas phase of a substance exerts over the liquid phase. The vapor pressure of a liquid is effected by temperature and pressure, as viewed on the diagram in questions 66–67, as well as by the amount of any solute dissolved in the liquid, as determined by Raoult's Law. In this question, the only thing that is changing is the amount of liquid in the container; this will have no effect on the ability of liquid molecules to become gas molecules. Therefore, the vapor pressure will remain the same.

69. B The heat of vaporization is the amount of energy required to turn a liquid into a gas and is represented by the top plateau on the graph. The heat of fusion is the amount of energy required to turn a solid into a liquid and is represented by the bottom plateau on the graph. Since vaporization requires a greater Q than that of fusion, choice (B) is correct. Stated simply, it requires less energy to allow particles to move past one another (solid → liquid) than it does to separate them from one another completely (gas → liquid).

Heat capacity is the amount of heat required to raise the temperature of an object by 1 K (or 1°C). The heat capacity of the different phases can be compared by examining the slope of the T vs. Q curve. The steeper the slope, the less heat (Q) was required to increase the temperature; therefore, the lower the heat capacity. The slope for each of the phases is too close to draw any accurate conclusions of their relative values.

Choice (A) is incorrect because the graph does not give absolute values for the boiling point and melting point, so you cannot tell if one is more than double the other.

70. B Oxidation occurs at the anode and reduction at the cathode (mnemonic: An Ox—Red Cat). Only in the reaction shown in choice (B) is chromium being oxidized.

A. $2x - 14 = -2$ $\qquad\qquad$ $x - 8 = -2$

$\uparrow \quad \uparrow$ $\qquad\qquad\qquad\qquad$ $\uparrow \quad \uparrow$

$x \quad -2$ $\qquad\qquad\qquad\qquad\;$ $x \quad -2$

$Cr_2O_7^{2-}$ $\longrightarrow$ $\qquad\qquad$ CrO_4^{2-}

$Cr = +6$ $\qquad\qquad\qquad\qquad$ $Cr = +6$

B. $\qquad\qquad\qquad\qquad\qquad\qquad$ $x - 8 = -2$

$\qquad\qquad\qquad\qquad\qquad\qquad$ $\uparrow \quad \uparrow$

$\qquad\qquad\qquad\qquad\qquad\qquad$ $x \quad -2$

Cr^{2+} $\longrightarrow$ $\qquad\qquad\;\;$ CrO_4^{2-}

$\qquad\qquad\qquad\qquad\qquad\qquad$ $Cr = +6$

C. $2x - 14 = -2$

$\uparrow \quad \uparrow$

$x \quad -2$

$Cr_2O_7^{2-}$ $\longrightarrow$ $\qquad\qquad$ Cr^{2+}

$Cr = +6$

D. $x - 8 = -2$

$\uparrow \quad \uparrow$

$x \quad -2$

CrO_4^{2-} $\longrightarrow$ $\qquad\qquad$ Cr^{3+}

$Cr = +6$

E. Cr^{3+} $\longrightarrow$ Cr^{2+}

71. D Recall that the convention of Fischer projections is that horizontal lines are bonds projecting towards the front, while vertical lines are bonds towards the back. The Fischer projection given in choice (D) is thus equivalent to this:

$$
\begin{array}{c}
Br \\
HO - C - D \\
H - C - OH \\
F
\end{array}
$$

If we then mentally rotate about the C–C single bond (the vertical solid line above), we can verify that indeed it is similar to the first structure shown in choice (D).

A correct Fischer projection that should be drawn for each of the other choices is shown below:

72. **E** Since the –OH group is polar and is capable of hydrogen bonding, alcohols whose alkyl portions are not too big will dissolve in water. (Alkyl groups are nonpolar and thus do not dissolve readily in polar solvents: "Like dissolves like!") Among the answer choices, 3-pentanol has the longest alkyl chain and thus will be the least soluble in water.

73. **A** The longest carbon chain containing the double bond (the principal functional group in this case) is made up of five carbon atoms. We can therefore eliminate all choices except (A) and (D). We want the position of the double bond to be designated by as low a number as possible, so we number the carbon atoms from right to left. The alkene functionality thus occurs at carbon number 1, and there are methyl groups attached to carbons #2 and #4, making the molecule 2,4-dimethyl-1-pentene.

74. **A** The oxacyclohexane with the least amount of nonbonded strain will have the least steric hindrance by virtue of equatorial positioning of the ring substituents. Methyl groups (or other relatively bulky substituents) in the axial position

will experience repulsion from the electron clouds of other substituents (H atoms) occupying axial positions. For example, there are repulsive interactions between the methyl group and each of the pictured H atoms below:

Choice (A) does not have a methyl group in the axial position, so it has the least nonbonded strain.

75. **D** Ethers have the generic formula ROR', and asymmetric ethers are ones where R ≠ R'. However, we do not even need to know this to answer the question correctly. As indicated in the question, the Williamson ether synthesis is an S_N2 reaction, so we want first of all to identify compounds that will participate in an S_N2 reaction. Choice (D) contains the only pair that satisfies the criteria: The alkoxide ion $CH_3CH_2O^-$ in CH_3CH_2ONa is a strong base, and $CH_3CH_2CH_2CH_2Cl$ possesses a good leaving group (the chloride ion) and is not sterically hindered (it is a primary alkyl halide). The two will therefore readily react via the S_N2 mechanism. The product is an asymmetric ether (R = butyl group, R' = ethyl group).

Choice (A) is incorrect because $CH_3CH_2CH_2$ COONa is the salt of a carboxylic acid and is thus not a particularly strong base. The ketone on the left also does not have a good leaving group.

Choice (B) is incorrect because even though we have a strong base in $CH_3CH_2CH_2CH_2CH_2O^-$, the alkyl halide is tertiary and thus will not react readily via S_N2.

Choice (C) is incorrect because the phenoxide ion ($C_6H_5O^-$) is not as strong a base as an alkoxide ion and benzaldehyde (C_6H_5CHO) does not have a good leaving group.

Choice (E) is incorrect because the substrate is already an ether, which does not have a good leaving group.

76. D The connectivity of the atoms is different between the two compounds. Note that the compound on the left has a vinylic hydrogen (attached directly to an sp^2 hybridized carbon) but the compound on the right does not: Both carbon atoms of the double bond are substituted. They are thus constitutional or structural isomers.

77. D Structural isomers have the same molecular formula: the same number of each kind of atoms. Only choice (D) satisfies this requirement. Their molecular formula is both C_3H_6O. (Each has three carbon atoms, six hydrogen atoms, and one oxygen atom.) The connections between the atoms, however, are different:

$$CH_3CH_2\overset{\overset{\textstyle O}{\|}}{CH} \qquad \overset{\textstyle H_3CO}{\underset{\textstyle H}{}}C{=}CH_2$$

The other choices are incorrect because they do not have the same molecular formula. They are not isomers of any kind.

78. A The reaction is an SN2 reaction: DMSO is a polar aprotic solvent; CN^- is a strong nucleophile; and the leaving group is Y^-, which acts as the counter-ion to Na^+ in the product. We thus expect Y^- to be a reasonable leaving group. If Y were I, this would indeed be the case: I^- is a weak base and is a good leaving group.

The other choices are incorrect because CH_3^-, SH^-, PH_2^-, and OCH_3^- are not good leaving groups.

79. B Hydrogen bonding can occur when there is a hydrogen atom bonded to a highly electronegative atom. In such a case, the hydrogen atom may interact with the electronegative atom

from another molecule (i.e., other than the one to which it is covalently bonded). This question asks about *intra*molecular hydrogen bonding, which is a more unusual phenomenon. Even if we were not familiar with intramolecular hydrogen bonding, we can still pick the correct answer as choice (B) because it is the only structure where we have a hydrogen atom bonded to an oxygen atom (in the carboxylic acid functional group). The intramolecular part comes in because the hydrogen can also interact with the carbonyl oxygen on the ketone group:

hydrogen bond

80. E The longest carbon chain contains eight carbon atoms: Do not be misled by the way the structure is drawn!

The molecule is thus an octane. This alone is enough for us to pick choice (E) as the correct answer. To verify, we notice that a methyl group and an ethyl group fall outside the octane chain. If we started numbering the carbon from the bottom up, we would get 5-ethyl-3-methyl; if we numbered the carbon starting from the top, we would get 4-ethyl-6-methyl. As usual, we go for the option with the lowest number (in this case the lowest sum). $5 + 3 < 4 + 6$, so the name of the compound is 5-ethyl-3-methyloctane.

81. C The first (and rate-determining) step in an S_N1 reaction is the departure of the leaving group, leaving behind a carbocation intermediate.

The more stable the carbocation intermediate, the more rapidly this step, and the reaction overall, proceeds. Carbocations are stabilized by the presence of electron-donating alkyl groups, so the more substituted the carbon bearing the positive charge, the more stable the carbocation. Among the answer choices, choice (C), being a tertiary halide, is the most substituted and will form the most stable tertiary carbocation.

Choice (A) is a methyl halide, which, having no alkyl group attached to the carbon atom, will not react via an S_N1 reaction.

Choices (B) and (D) are both secondary alkyl halides. They will undergo S_N1 reactions but not as readily as a tertiary alkyl halide.

Choice (E) is a primary alkyl halide, and the carbocation it forms is not stable.

82. E The structure shown is a *meso* compound. It possesses two chiral carbon atoms (indicated by an asterisk in the figure below), but it also has an internal plane of symmetry and thus is achiral (optically inactive).

$$
\begin{array}{c}
\text{CHO} \\
\text{H} - \!\!\!\!\overset{*}{\vert}\!\!\!\!- \text{OH} \\
\text{- - - - - - - - - - - - - -} \quad \text{plane of} \\
\text{H} - \!\!\!\!\overset{*}{\vert}\!\!\!\!- \text{OH} \quad \text{symmetry} \\
\text{CHO}
\end{array}
$$

83. B Aromatic compounds are cyclic, planar, and contain $(4n + 2)$ π electrons that can be delocalized. All the choices contain a nitrogen atom in the ring, making these all heterocyclic compounds. (Nitrogen, as a "noncarbon," is known as a heteroatom.) The nitrogen atom contains a lone pair of electrons, which may or may not be part of the π system, depending on the orientation of the orbital holding these nonbonding electrons. For the nonbonding electrons to be part of the π system (and thus be counted among the $4n + 2$), the orbital must be perpendicular to the plane of the ring, parallel to the π orbitals of the double bond. Choice (B) satisfies all the criteria for aromaticity. All the carbon atoms in the ring are sp^2 hybridized,

forming a delocalized π system with their 4 π electrons. The nitrogen atom in the ring forms three bonds that are in a plane. It is thus also sp^2 hybridized, and the nonbonding electrons are in an unhybridized *p*-orbital that is perpendicular to the plane. These nonbonding electrons can thus be conjugated with the π electrons of the double bond, giving a total of 6 (= 4 × 1 + 2) π electrons.

orbital holding nonbonding
electrons of nitrogen

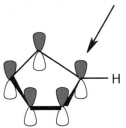

Choice (A) is incorrect because the nonbonding electrons of nitrogen are in an orbital lying in the plane of the ring. They thus do not form part of the π system, and the compound only has the 4 π electrons, one from each atom in the ring. It does not satisfy Hückel's rule.

nonbonding electrons

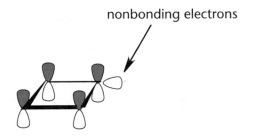

Choice (C) is not aromatic because the carbon opposite to the nitrogen is a saturated sp^3 hybridized carbon. Because the C–C–C bond angle is 109.5° for saturated carbons, the molecule is actually not planar.

Choice (D) is not correct for the same reason as Choice (C).

Choice (E) is not aromatic because it has 8 π electrons and thus does not satisfy Hückel's rule.

84. D An E isomer is one in which the higher-priority group on each end of the double bond faces opposite sides (E = "<u>e</u>pposite"). Priority is assigned based on atomic weight. In choice (D), the higher-priority group is F on both ends, and these two F atoms are on opposite sides. It is thus an E isomer.

Choice (A) is incorrect because the molecule does not have geometric isomers: The carbon atom on one end of the double bond is bonded to the same group (F).

Choice (B) is a Z isomer because the higher priority groups (again, F's on each end) are on the same side.

Choice (C) is incorrect because the higher-priority group on one end is F, while it is a methyl group on the other. These two are on the same side, making this also a Z isomer. In fact, since the lower priority group is H on both ends, we can forego the Z/E designation and refer to the compound as the *cis* isomer.

Choice (E) is incorrect because the higher-priority methyl groups are on the same side. Again, we can refer to it as the *cis* isomer (*cis*-2-butene).

85. E Numbering the carbon atoms from left to right, we notice that carbon 2 and carbon 3 form a triple bond and a single bond each. They are thus both *sp* hybridized, and the bond angles *a* and *b* must be 180° (i.e., carbons 1–4 are linear). Carbon 4 forms a double bond and a single bond (with presumably another single bond, not shown, to a hydrogen atom or something else). It is thus sp^2 hybridized with a bond angle of 120°. A more accurate representation of the structure of the molecule may be as follows:

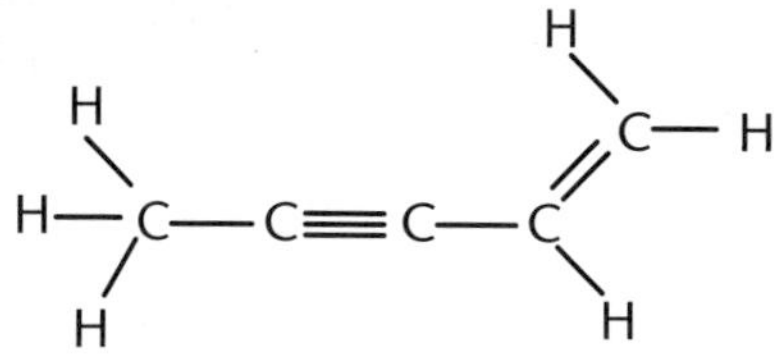

86. D A more substituted alkyl halide is less likely to undergo an S_N2 reaction, because the incoming nucleophile is sterically hindered from approaching the substrate. Choice (D) is a tertiary alkyl halide and is thus the most sterically hindered.

87. C The compound in choice (C) is an alkyl halide, which is a very reactive species formed from a carboxylic acid and a chlorinating group, such as PCl_3 or $SOCl_2$. Acyl chlorides react with amines to form amides (carboxylic acids and amines can also form amides, but the acyl chloride form is much more reactive).

Answer choices (A) and (D) are ethers, which are very stable and do not react with amines.

Answer choice (B) is pyridine, which is even more stable than benzene. Considering that benzene will not react with amines, pyridine certainly will not.

Answer choice (E) is a ketone. It resembles the acyl chloride of choice (C), but here instead of Cl^- as the leaving group, a primary cabanion (CH_3^-), would have to serve as the leaving group, a very unstable compound. Therefore the amine will not react with choice (E).

88. A In this reaction, a carboxylic acid is being reduced to an alcohol. The correct answer must therefore be a strong reducing agent. $LiAlH_4$ is a strong reducing agent (THF is just a solvent—reactions involving $LiAlH_4$ must be anhydrous) that can donate H^- to bring the acid down to the alcohol.

Choice (B) is incorrect because organomercury compounds are unreactive and cannot be used to yield the given product.

The reactants in choice (C) would produce an ester.

The reactants in choice (D) are used to convert an alkene to an alcohol. They will not convert a carboxylic acid to an alcohol.

The reactants in choice (E) promote oxidation, not reduction.

89. E When 1,3-cyclopentadiene reacts with sodium, it goes from a nonaromatic to an aromatic compound. A cyclic compound is aromatic if it satisfies Hückel's rule; that is, it has $4n+2$ π electrons, where *n* is any integer. The product of the reaction has 6 π electrons, so it is therefore aromatic. An aromatic compound is very stable because the π electrons are delocalized throughout ring. In this reaction, the products are much more stable, so the reaction will have a very negative ΔH, so the reaction will still be spontaneous $(-\Delta G)$, even under low temperatures (as determined by the formula $\Delta G = \Delta H - T\Delta S$).

90. C The reactants used to produce compound X, an alkyl halide and Lewis acid, promote Friedel–Crafts alkylation. The alkyl group attached to the chlorine will add to the benzene ring, and the product will be isopropyl benzene.

In the next step, the reactants promote halogenation of the benzene ring. The chlorine will add *para* to the isopropyl group of product X (R groups are *o/p* directing). Notice this eliminates choices (A) and (B).

In the final step, a free radical halogenation reaction, bromine will add to the most substituted carbon atom (since it is the most stable free radical intermediate). The most substituted carbon is the tertiary carbon attaching the isopropyl group to the ring. This leaves only choice (C) as the correct answer.

91. E The compound pictured is ethyl propionate—the ester formed from the dehydration reaction of ethanol and propionic acid. If water is added to an ester, the parent acid and alcohol are formed.

Choice (A) and (D) are incorrect because there are no chiral carbons in the molecule.

Choices (B) and (C) are incorrect because propionic acid would be formed, not acetic acid.

92. E When *p*-aminobenzioc acid dissociates, it assumes a −1 charge. Any resonance structure that can be drawn must have the same charge. This eliminates choice (A) as a possible answer.

Answer choices (B) and (D) are not even benzene derivative; rather they are a pyridine derivative.

Choice (C) can be eliminated because the carbonyl carbon has only three bonds and no formal charge. This leaves only choice (E) as the correct answer.

93. C This question is nearly the same as the final reaction in question 90. The halide in free radical halogenation reactions always adds to the most substituted carbon. The most substituted carbon is the tertiary carbon connecting the isopropyl group to the benzene ring, making choice (C) the only possibility.

Choices (A), (B), and (D) are incorrect because the free radical reaction will not involve the benzene ring (don't confuse this with a halogenation reaction, which requires a Lewis acid catalyst).

Choice (E) is incorrect because the bromination will not cause the benzene ring to open up.

94. A IR spectroscopy is useful in distinguishing different functional groups of a molecule. Only in choice (A) do the two molecules pictured have different functional groups.

95. A There are three steps in a radical reaction: initiation, propagation, and termination. Termination is when two radicals combine, forming a compound with an even number of electrons. Since termination reactions decrease the number of free radicals, terminations decrease the reaction rate and eventually cause the reaction to stop. Only choice (A) depicts two free radicals combining to form a compound with an even number of electrons.

Choices (B) and (D) depict propagation steps. Choice (C) is not a radical reaction, and choice (E) does not even occur during the course of a radical reaction.

96. E Elimination reactions involve the removal of inorganic acid (hydrogen and a halide) from an alkane to form an alkene. This bit of information eliminates all the incorrect answer choices: Choices (A), (C), and (D) still have the chlorine attached, and choice (B) is an alkyne. This leaves only choice (E).

97. B We can recognize this reaction as a Friedel–Crafts acylation—we are reacting a benzene ring with an acyl halide and a Lewis acid. The $CH_3C=O$ will add to the ring with the aid of the $AlCl_3$ Lewis acid catalyst, either *ortho* or *para* to the alkoxide group, because O–R groups are activating *o/p* directors. Choice (B) is the only answer that assigns the correct placement of the $CH_3C=O$ group.

Choices (A) and (C) are incorrect because the ether functional group will not react with the acyl halide.

Choice (D) is incorrect because the acyl group is *meta* to the alkoxide group. It must be either *ortho* or *para*, since that is where O–R groups direct addition reactions.

Choice (E) would be formed if Cl_2 and $FeCl_3$ were being added.

98. D When diethylamine, $(CH_3CH2)_2NH$, acts as a Brønstead–Lowry base and binds an H^+, it forms the conjugate acid $(CH_3CH2)_2NH_2^+$, answer choice (D).

99. C When an ester is reduced, the alcohol function of the ester is first liberated, then the carboxylic acid is converted into a primary alcohol. The reduction of methyl propanoate would thus yield methanol and propanol.

$$R-C(=O)-O-R' \xrightarrow[\text{THF}]{\text{LiAlH}_4} RCH_2OH + R'OH$$

$$H_3C-CH_2-C(=O)-O-CH_3 \xrightarrow[\text{THF}]{\text{LiAlH}_4} CH_3CH_2CH_2OH + CH_3OH$$

The addition of acid to the alcohol mixture will have no effect, so the correct answer is (C).

100. D The first step of the reaction will lead to the addition of a nitro group to the ring through a diazonium intermediate. The nitro group will add either *ortho* or *para*, as R groups are *o/p* directors. This leaves only choices (D) and (E) as possibilities. In the second step of the reaction, the potassium permanganate will oxidize the toluene to benzoic acid. Therefore the answer must be (D).

PERCEPTUAL ABILITY TEST
Answers and Explanations

ANSWER KEY

1. A	13. B	25. D	37. A	49. A	61. A	73. D	85. C
2. D	14. C	26. A	38. A	50. A	62. C	74. C	86. B
3. C	15. B	27. D	39. D	51. C	63. C	75. E	87. D
4. E	16. D	28. D	40. A	52. D	64. B	76. C	88. A
5. A	17. A	29. A	41. B	53. C	65. A	77. A	89. A
6. E	18. B	30. C	42. C	54. E	66. D	78. B	90. B
7. B	19. A	31. C	43. B	55. E	67. C	79. B	
8. B	20. C	32. A	44. C	56. B	68. B	80. D	
9. D	21. D	33. D	45. A	57. C	69. B	81. A	
10. C	22. C	34. B	46. C	58. A	70. C	82. D	
11. A	23. B	35. D	47. A	59. B	71. B	83. C	
12. E	24. A	36. B	48. D	60. B	72. A	84. A	

EXPLANATIONS

1.   A

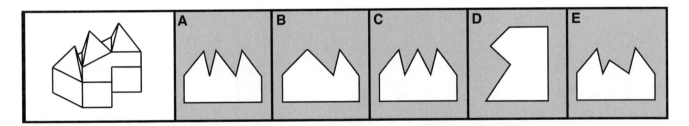

Projections

BOTTOM (Top)

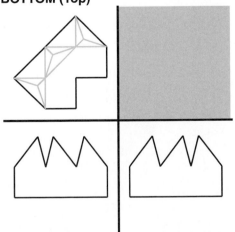

BACK (Front)   **RIGHT (End)**

2. D

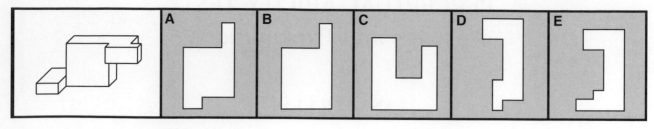

Projections

BOTTOM (Top)

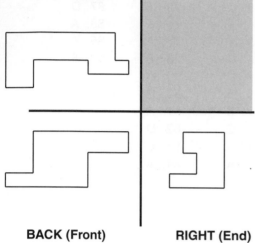

BACK (Front)   **RIGHT (End)**

3. C

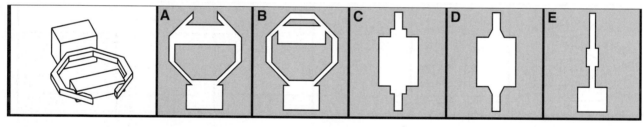

Projections

BOTTOM (Top)

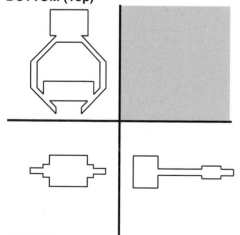

BACK (Front)   **RIGHT (End)**

4.   E

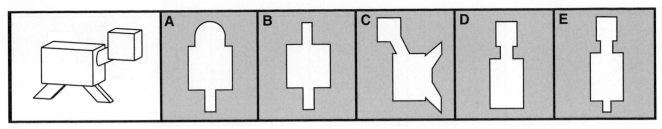

Projections

BOTTOM (Top)

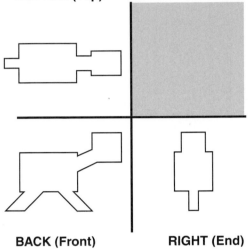

BACK (Front)   **RIGHT (End)**

5.   A

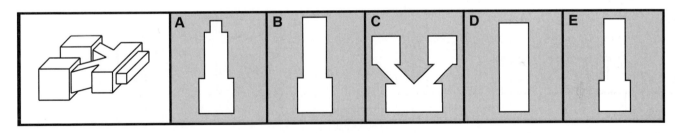

Projections

BOTTOM (Top)

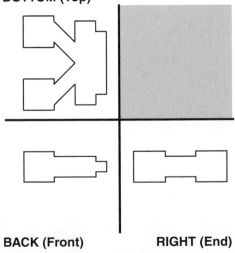

BACK (Front)   **RIGHT (End)**

6. E

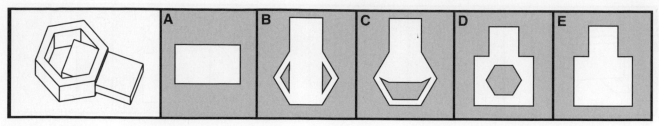

Projections

BOTTOM (Top)

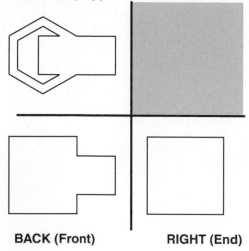

BACK (Front)   **RIGHT (End)**

7. B

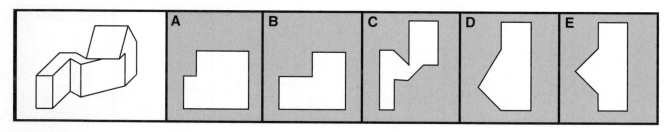

Projections

BOTTOM (Top)

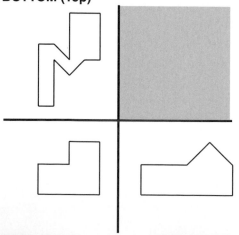

BACK (Front)   **RIGHT (End)**

8. B

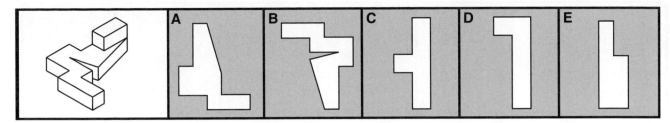

Projections

BOTTOM (Top)

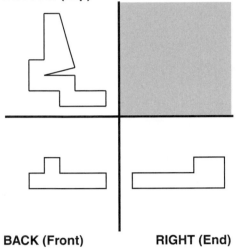

BACK (Front)   **RIGHT (End)**

9. D

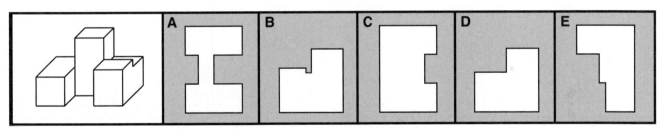

Projections

BOTTOM (Top)

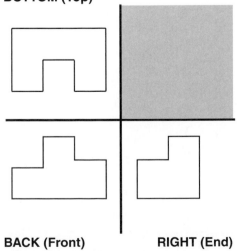

BACK (Front)   **RIGHT (End)**

10. C

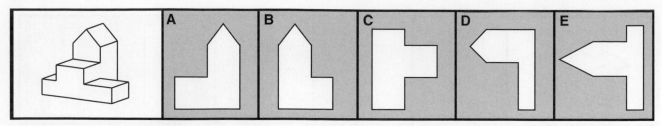

Projections

BOTTOM (Top)

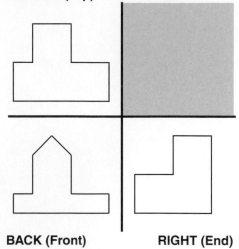

BACK (Front)   **RIGHT (End)**

11. A

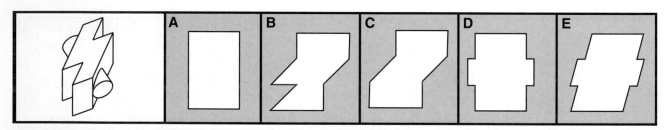

Projections

BOTTOM (Top)

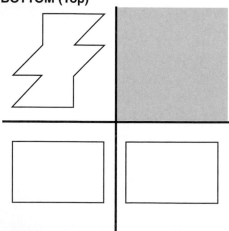

BACK (Front)   **RIGHT (End)**

12. E

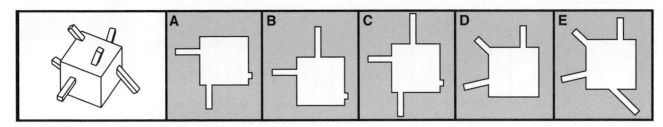

Projections

BOTTOM (Top)

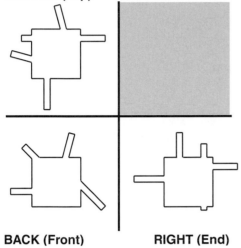

BACK (Front)   **RIGHT (End)**

13. B

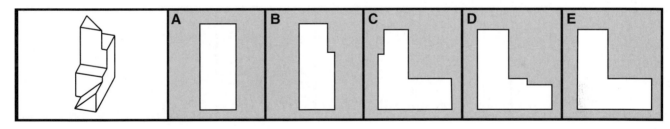

Projections

BOTTOM (Top)

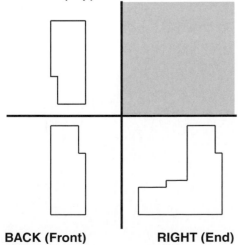

BACK (Front)   **RIGHT (End)**

14. C

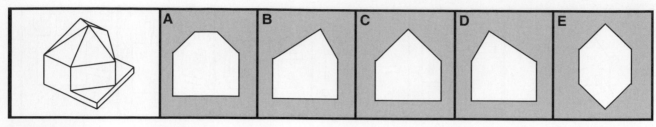

Projections

BOTTOM (Top)

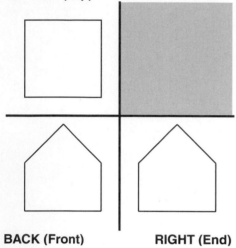

BACK (Front)   **RIGHT (End)**

15. B

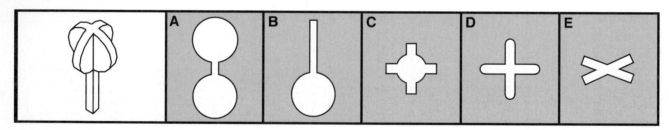

Projections

BOTTOM (Top)

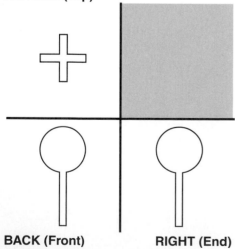

BACK (Front)   **RIGHT (End)**

750

16.   D

TOP VIEW

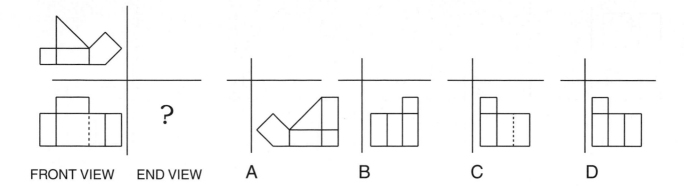

FRONT VIEW   END VIEW   A   B   C   D

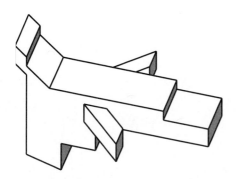

17.   A

TOP VIEW

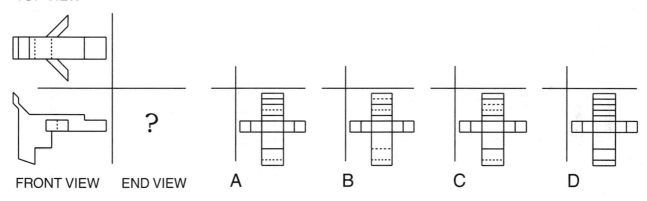

FRONT VIEW   END VIEW   A   B   C   D

18. B

TOP VIEW

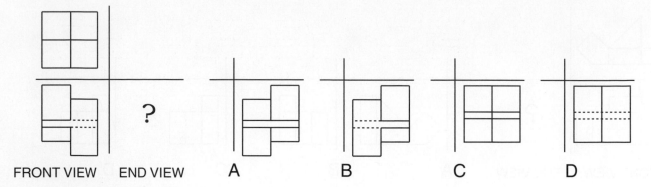

FRONT VIEW   END VIEW   A   B   C   D

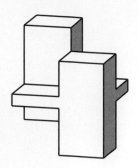

19. A

TOP VIEW

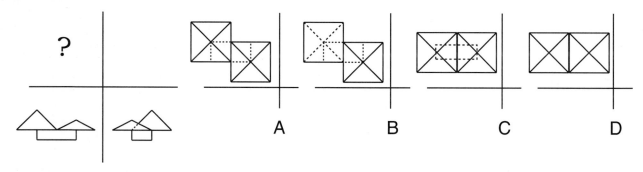

FRONT VIEW   END VIEW

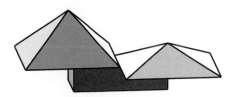

20. C

TOP VIEW

?

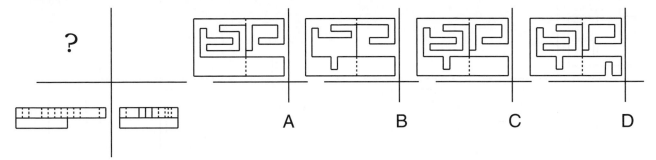

A   B   C   D

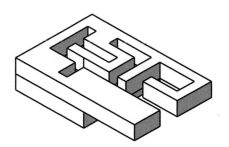

FRONT VIEW   END VIEW

21. D

TOP VIEW

?

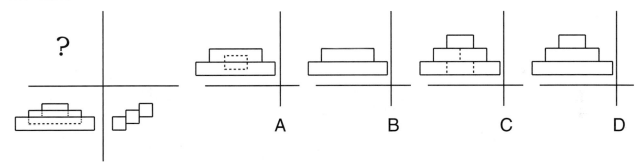

A   B   C   D

FRONT VIEW   END VIEW

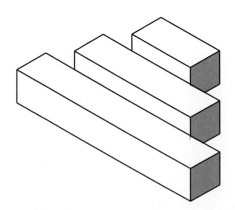

22. C

TOP VIEW

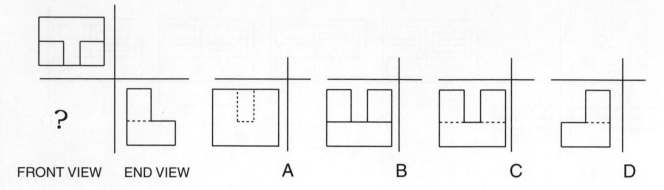

?

FRONT VIEW   END VIEW   A   B   C   D

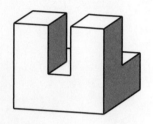

23. B

TOP VIEW

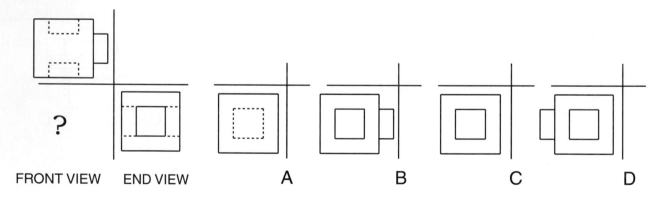

?

FRONT VIEW   END VIEW   A   B   C   D

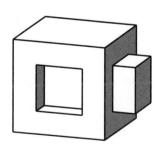

24. A

TOP VIEW

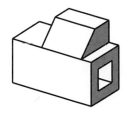

?

FRONT VIEW   END VIEW   A   B   C   D

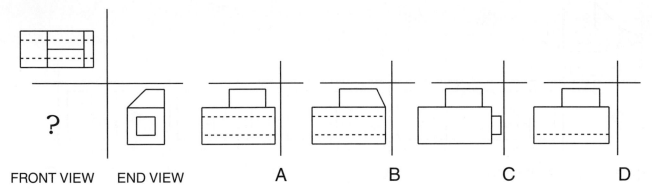

25. D

TOP VIEW

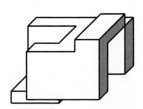

?

FRONT VIEW   END VIEW   A   B   C   D

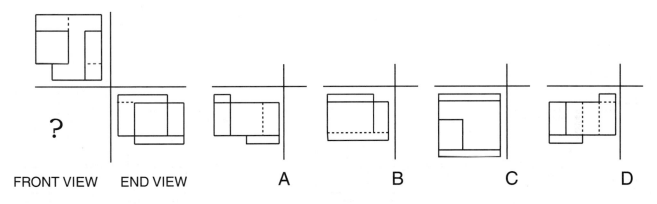

26. A

TOP VIEW

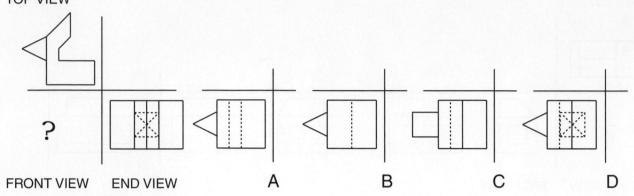

?

FRONT VIEW   END VIEW   A   B   C   D

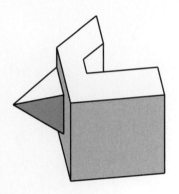

27. D

TOP VIEW

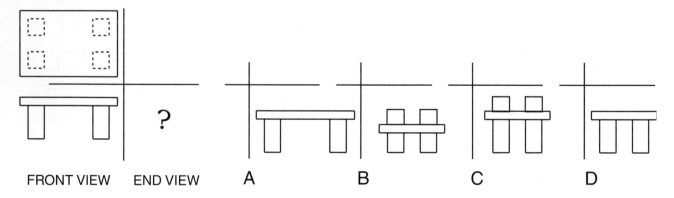

FRONT VIEW   END VIEW   A   B   C   D

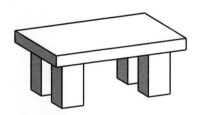

28. D

TOP VIEW

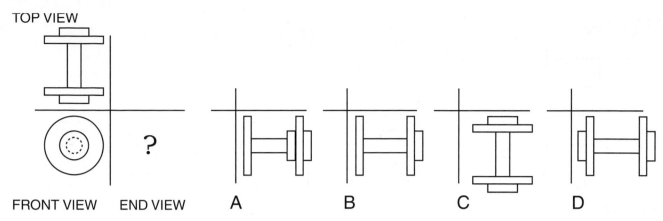

FRONT VIEW   END VIEW   A   B   C   D

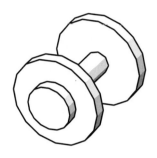

29. A

TOP VIEW

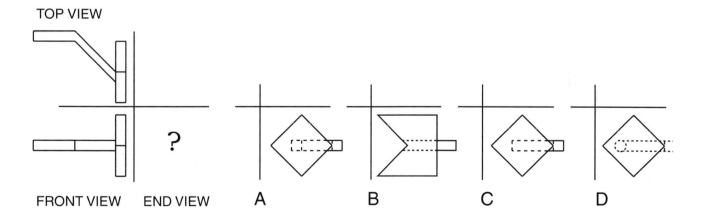

FRONT VIEW   END VIEW   A   B   C   D

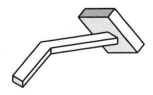

30. C

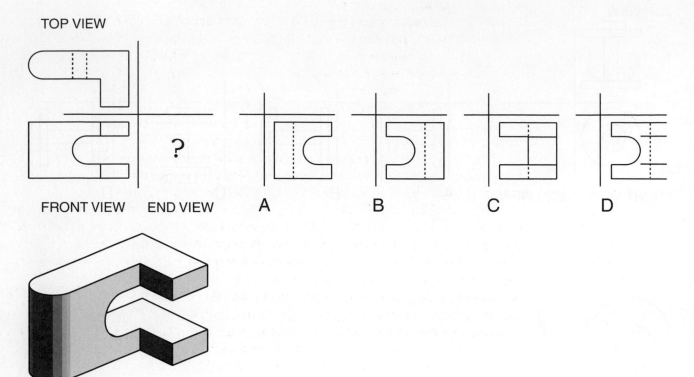

TOP VIEW

FRONT VIEW   END VIEW   A   B   C   D

?

31. C

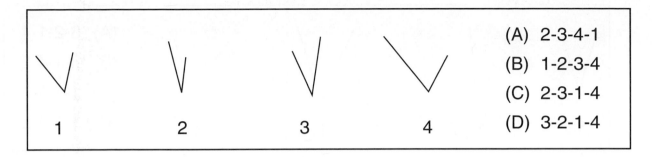

(A) 2-3-4-1
(B) 1-2-3-4
(C) 2-3-1-4
(D) 3-2-1-4

32. A

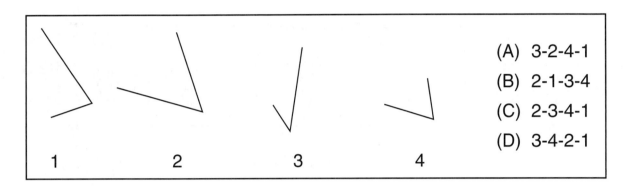

(A) 3-2-4-1
(B) 2-1-3-4
(C) 2-3-4-1
(D) 3-4-2-1

33. D

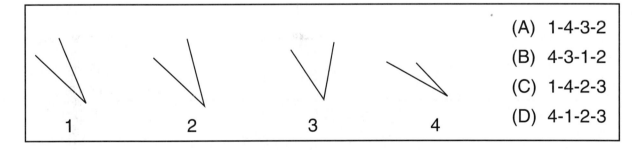

(A) 1-4-3-2
(B) 4-3-1-2
(C) 1-4-2-3
(D) 4-1-2-3

34. B

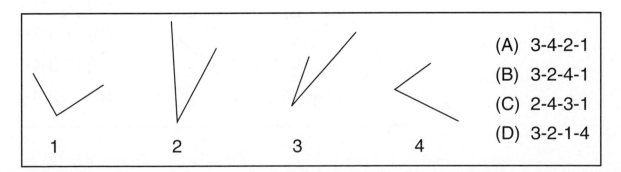

(A) 3-4-2-1
(B) 3-2-4-1
(C) 2-4-3-1
(D) 3-2-1-4

35. D

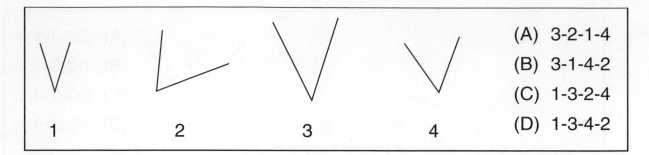

(A) 3-2-1-4
(B) 3-1-4-2
(C) 1-3-2-4
(D) 1-3-4-2

36. B

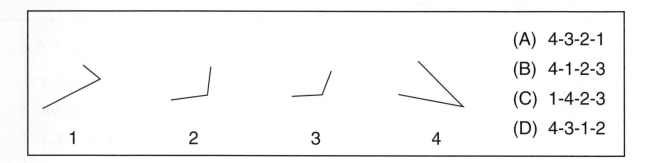

(A) 4-3-2-1
(B) 4-1-2-3
(C) 1-4-2-3
(D) 4-3-1-2

37. A

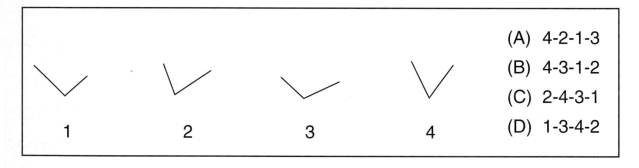

(A) 4-2-1-3
(B) 4-3-1-2
(C) 2-4-3-1
(D) 1-3-4-2

38. A

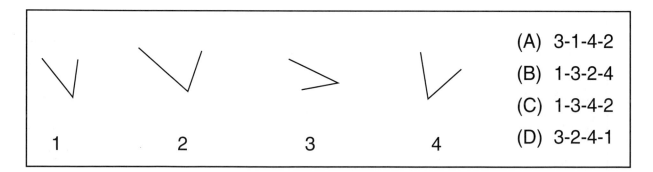

(A) 3-1-4-2
(B) 1-3-2-4
(C) 1-3-4-2
(D) 3-2-4-1

39. D

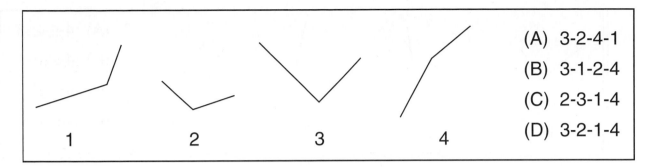

1   2   3   4

(A) 3-2-4-1
(B) 3-1-2-4
(C) 2-3-1-4
(D) 3-2-1-4

40. A

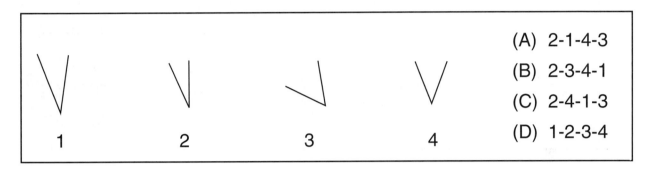

1   2   3   4

(A) 2-1-4-3
(B) 2-3-4-1
(C) 2-4-1-3
(D) 1-2-3-4

41. B

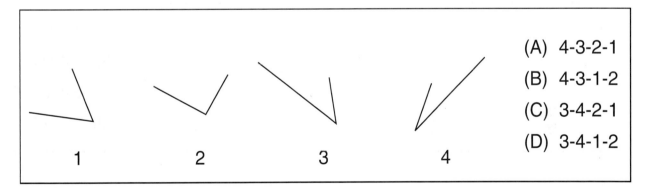

1   2   3   4

(A) 4-3-2-1
(B) 4-3-1-2
(C) 3-4-2-1
(D) 3-4-1-2

42. C

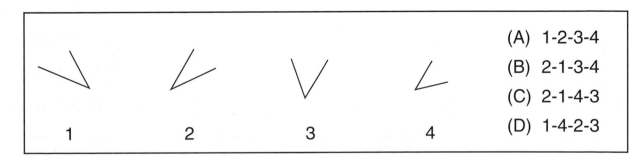

1   2   3   4

(A) 1-2-3-4
(B) 2-1-3-4
(C) 2-1-4-3
(D) 1-4-2-3

43. B

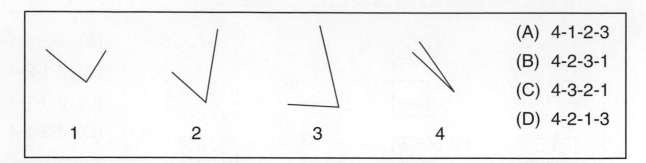

(A) 4-1-2-3

(B) 4-2-3-1

(C) 4-3-2-1

(D) 4-2-1-3

44. C

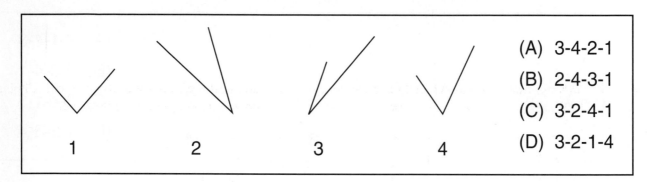

(A) 3-4-2-1

(B) 2-4-3-1

(C) 3-2-4-1

(D) 3-2-1-4

45. A

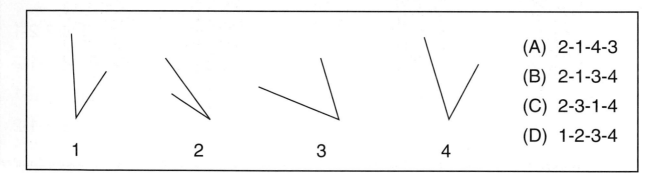

(A) 2-1-4-3

(B) 2-1-3-4

(C) 2-3-1-4

(D) 1-2-3-4

46. C Always make sure to eliminate answer choices by looking at the symmetry of the first fold. In this problem, we cannot eliminate any answer choices because all of the answers are symmetrical across the first fold.

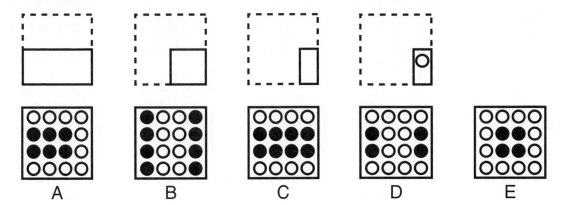

47. A Always make sure to eliminate answer choices by looking at the symmetry of the first fold. Eliminate (B) and (C) because they are not symmetrical about the line generated by the first fold.

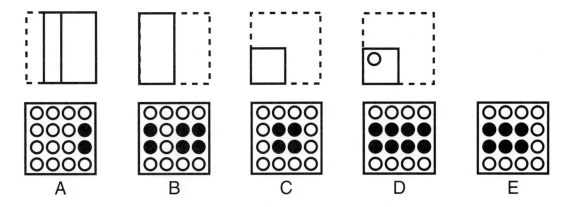

48. D Always make sure to eliminate answer choices by looking at the symmetry of the first fold. Eliminate choice (C).

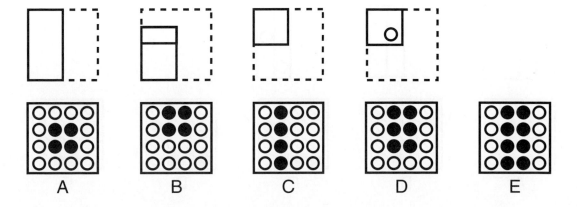

49. A Always make sure to eliminate answer choices by looking at the symmetry of the first fold. It is not possible to eliminate any answer choices in this problem because they are all symmetrical about the line generated by the first fold.

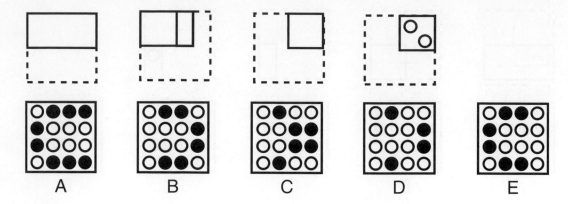

50. A Always make sure to eliminate answer choices by looking at the symmetry of the first fold. Eliminate choices (B), (C), and (D).

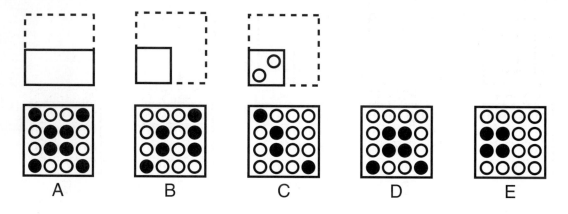

51. C Always make sure to eliminate answer choices by looking at the symmetry of the first fold. Eliminate (B), (D), and (E).

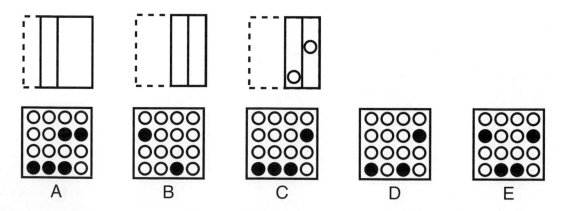

52. **D** Always make sure to eliminate answer choices by looking at the symmetry of the fold. Eliminate choices (A), (B), (C), and (E).

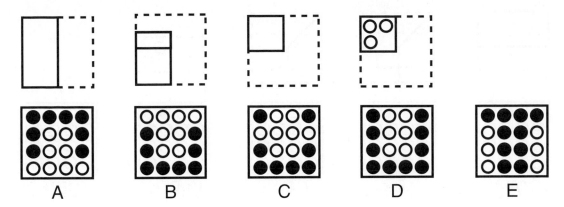

53. **C** Always make sure to eliminate answer choices by looking at the symmetry of the first fold. Eliminate (A), (B), and (D) because they are not symmetrical about the line generated by the first fold!

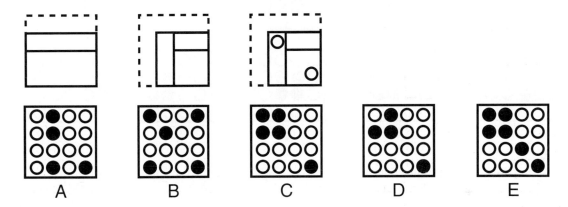

54. **E** Always make sure to eliminate answer choices by looking at the symmetry of the first fold. Eliminate (A), (C), and (D).

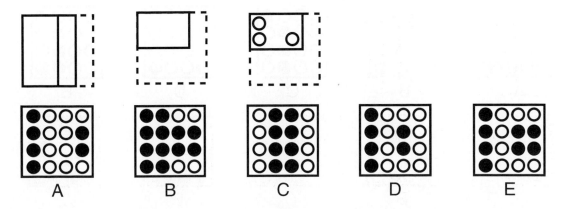

55. **E**   Always make sure to eliminate answer choices by looking at the symmetry of the first fold. Eliminate (A) and (D).

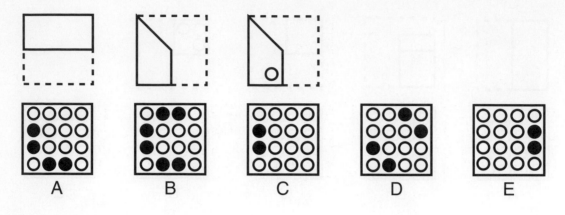

56. **B**

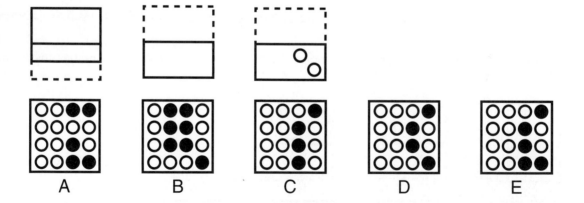

57. **C**   Always make sure to eliminate answer choices by looking at the symmetry of the first fold. Eliminate (A), (B), (D), and (E).

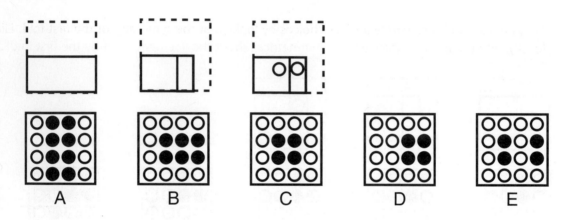

58. **A** Always make sure to eliminate answer choices by looking at the symmetry of the first fold. Eliminate (D) and (E).

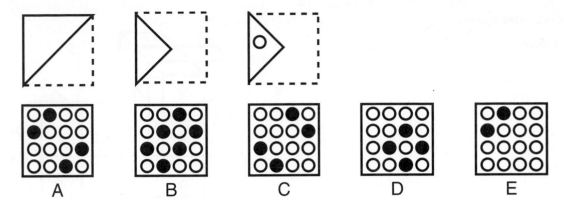

59. **B** Always make sure to eliminate answer choices by looking at the symmetry of the first fold. Eliminate (A), (C), and (E).

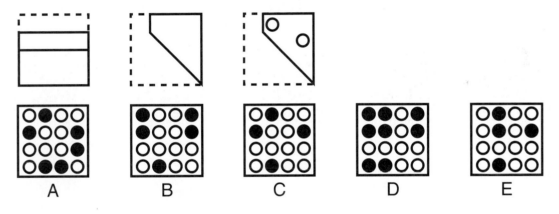

60. **B** Always make sure to eliminate answer choices by looking at the symmetry of the first fold. Eliminate (C).

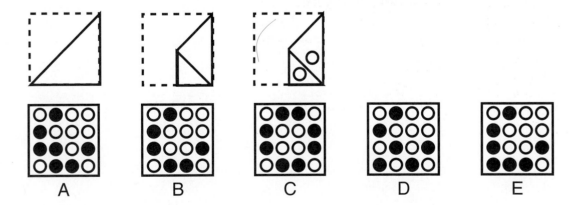

Problem A

61. In Figure A, how many cubes have none of their
    exposed sides painted?

    A. 1 cube
    B. 2 cubes
    C. 3 cubes
    D. 4 cubes
    E. 5 cubes

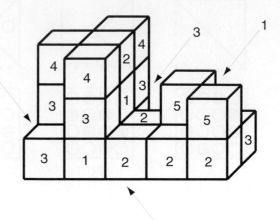

62. In Figure A, how many cubes have one of their
    exposed sides painted?

    A. 1 cube
    B. 2 cubes
    C. 3 cubes
    D. 4 cubes
    E. 5 cubes

63. In Figure A, how many cubes have four of their
    exposed sides painted?

    A. 1 cube
    B. 2 cubes
    C. 3 cubes
    D. 4 cubes
    E. 5 cubes

64. In Figure A, how many cubes have five of their
    exposed sides painted?

    A. 1 cube
    B. 2 cubes
    C. 3 cubes
    D. 4 cubes
    E. 5 cubes

Figure B

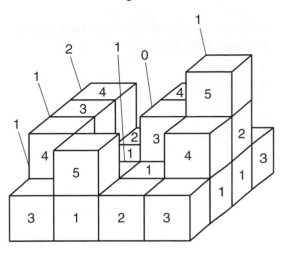

65. In Figure B, how many cubes have none of their exposed sides painted?

   A. 1 cube
   B. 2 cubes
   C. 3 cubes
   D. 4 cubes
   E. 5 cubes

66. In Figure B, how many cubes have two of their exposed sides painted?

   A. 1 cube
   B. 2 cubes
   C. 3 cubes
   D. 4 cubes
   E. 5 cubes

67. In Figure B, how many cubes have four of their exposed sides painted?

   A. 1 cube
   B. 2 cubes
   C. 3 cubes
   D. 4 cubes
   E. 5 cubes

68. In Figure B, how many cubes have five of their exposed sides painted?

   A. 1 cube
   B. 2 cubes
   C. 3 cubes
   D. 4 cubes
   E. 5 cubes

Problem C

69. In Figure C, how many cubes have one of their exposed sides painted?

    A. 1 cube
    B. 2 cubes
    C. 3 cubes
    D. 4 cubes
    E. 5 cubes

70. In Figure C, how many cubes have three of their exposed sides painted?

    A. 1 cube
    B. 2 cubes
    C. 3 cubes
    D. 4 cubes
    E. 5 cubes

71. In Figure C, how many cubes have four of their exposed sides painted?

    A. 1 cube
    B. 2 cubes
    C. 3 cubes
    D. 4 cubes
    E. 5 cubes

72. In Figure C, how many cubes have five of their exposed sides painted?

    A. 1 cube
    B. 2 cubes
    C. 3 cubes
    D. 4 cubes
    E. 5 cubes

Figure C

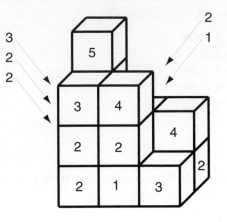

770

Problem D

73. In Figure D, how many cubes have one of their exposed sides painted?

    A. 1 cube
    B. 2 cubes
    C. 3 cubes
    D. 4 cubes
    E. 5 cubes

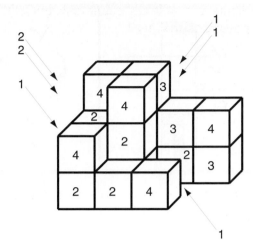

74. In Figure D, how many cubes have three of their exposed sides painted?

    A. 1 cube
    B. 2 cubes
    C. 3 cubes
    D. 4 cubes
    E. 5 cubes

75. In Figure D, how many cubes have four of their exposed sides painted?

    A. 1 cube
    B. 2 cubes
    C. 3 cubes
    D. 4 cubes
    E. 5 cubes

76. C

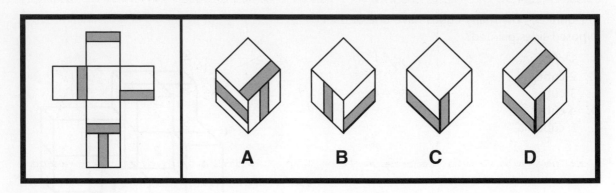

77. A

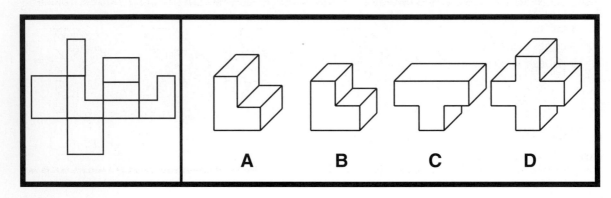

78. B

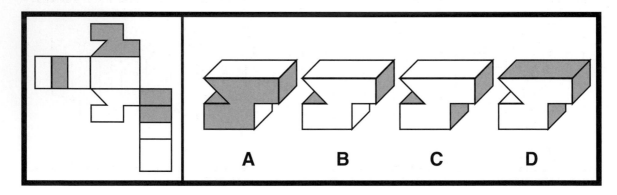

79. B

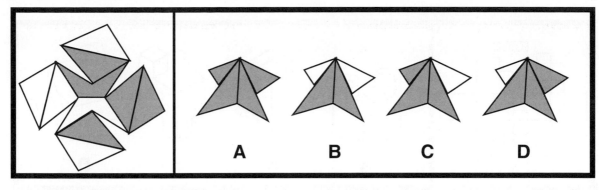

80. D

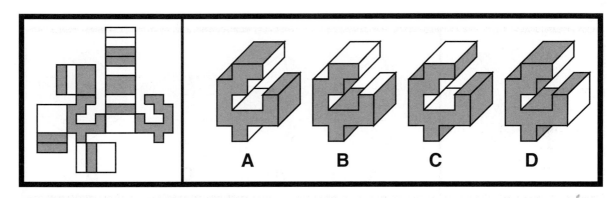

81. A

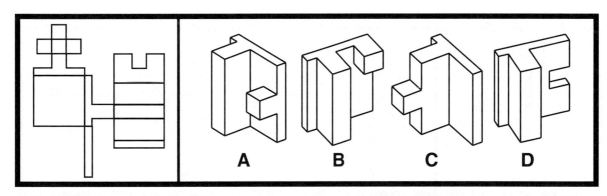

82. D

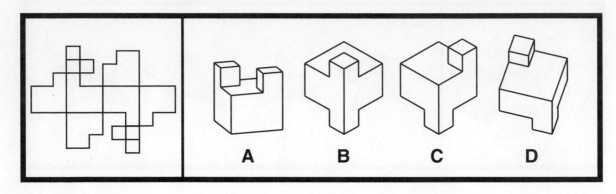

83. C

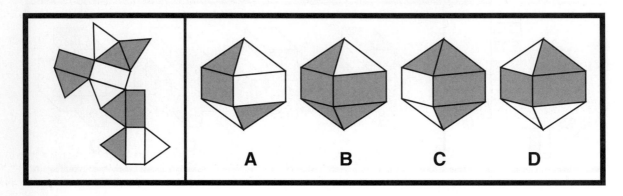

84. A

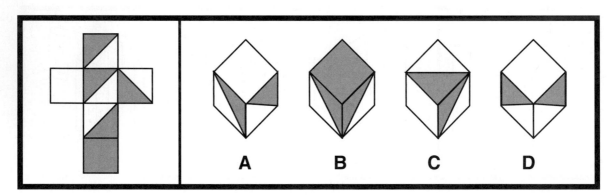

85. C

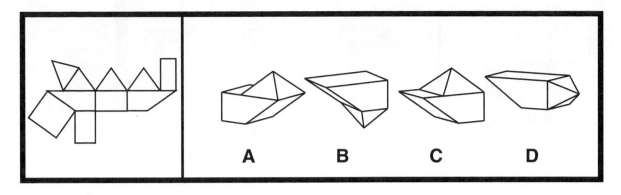

86. B

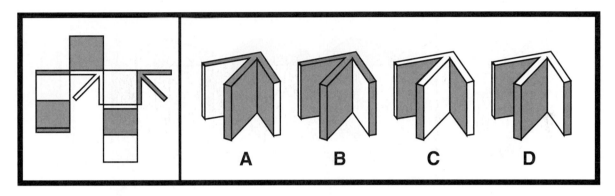

87. D

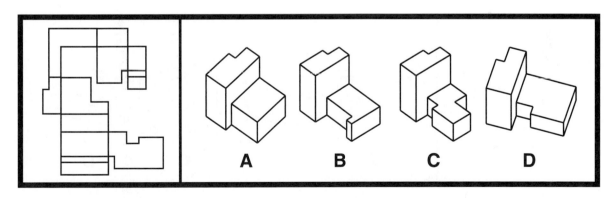

88. A

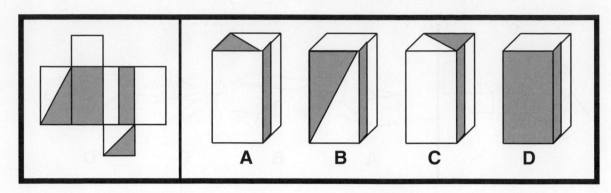

89. A

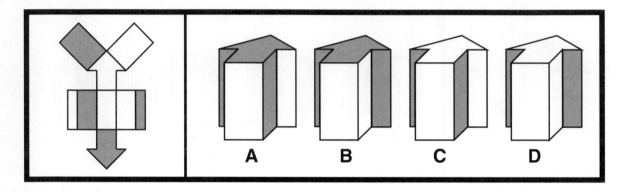

90. B

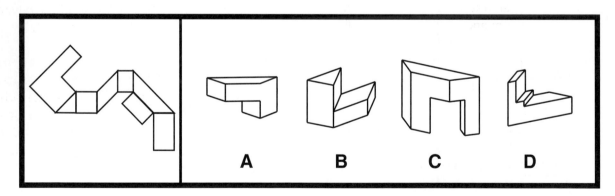

READING COMPREHENSION:
Answers and Explanations

ANSWER KEY

1. C	14. D	27. E	40. B
2. D	15. A	28. B	41. C
3. D	16. E	29. C	42. B
4. E	17. A	30. E	43. E
5. B	18. D	31. C	44. C
6. E	19. E	32. A	45. B
7. B	20. D	33. D	46. A
8. C	21. C	34. D	47. E
9. A	22. D	35. B	48. D
10. B	23. E	36. D	49. D
11. D	24. B	37. E	50. B
12. E	25. C	38. D	
13. B	26. B	39. C	

EXPLANATIONS

1. C The different types of spectroscopy are discussed in paragraphs five, six, and seven. Paragraphs five and six tell us that HREEL was used under vacuum conditions. Midway through paragraph seven, the author states that IR spectroscopy has an advantage over HREEL because it can be used under both vacuum and high-pressure conditions. We can infer from this that HREEL cannot be used under high-pressure conditions, making answer choice (C) correct.

Choice (A) is wrong, given the above discussion. Choice (B) is wrong based on further information provided in paragraph seven—that is, HREEL uses electrons to cause vibrations. The context of choices (D) and (E) are out of the scope of the passage and can be eliminated.

2. D The difficulties applying the results of surface chemistry to commercial catalysts are discussed in paragraph two. Choice (C) is a valid reason, and it is the reason why choices (A) and (B) are also valid reasons. The surface chemistry experiments were done under vacuum (no pressure) conditions, while commercial catalysts operate

under high pressure, resulting in more molecules impacting the surface. This alters the kinetics of the reaction. Choice (E) is also valid and is derived from the last line in the second paragraph.

Choice (D), the availability of catalysts, was never discussed in the passage and so is the correct answer.

3. D The correct answer to this question can be found in paragraph three, specifically from the sentence that begins with "The primary function of the converters . . ."

Choice (A) is incorrect because nitric oxide reacts with air, not water.

Choice (B) does not describe the function of catalytic converters but rather why they have a certain shape (honeycomb).

Choice (C) is fundamentally incorrect—catalysts need not be regenerated.

Choice (E) is incorrect because catalytic converters serve to minimize further pollution of the environment; they do not clean the environment.

4. E The experiments conducted in the mid-1980s are discussed in paragraphs five, six, and seven. Midway through paragraph six, the author states that the GM workers studied the reduction of NO. Choice (E) states that oxidation of NO was studied, which is incorrect, making (E) the correct answer choice.

5. B The question stem is referencing the second sentence of paragraph 11. At the end of the same paragraph, we are told that catalysts should promote the production of useful hydrocarbons, remove sulfur, and not promote the production of carbon and hydrogen. We can then measure the performance based any of these three measures. Choices (A), (C), (D), and (E) address the rate of the reactions, while choice (B) addresses yield.

The measure of performance is determine by the amount produced (or not produced), not how fast it does so. Therefore, (B) is the correct choice.

6. E The desulfurization process is discussed in paragraph 13. The second sentence reads, "The first step is the cleavage of the sulfur-hydrogen bond." This leaves only choice (E) as the correct choice.

7. B The rate of formation of carbon and hydrogen is addressed in the last paragraph. Carbon and hydrogen will be formed if a C–H bond is broken before a C–S bond. This is stated accurately in choice (B).

8. C The effects sulfur has on the environment are briefly addressed in paragraph eight. The author states that sulfur-oxygen compounds contribute to acid rain, as also stated in choice (C).

Choices (A) and (D) do not involve the environment and so are incorrect. Choice (B) could be applied to carbon emissions (CO is toxic), not sulfur emissions. Choice (E) is a true statement but is never addressed by the author, so it is also incorrect.

9. A This question addresses the same concepts as in question 7. At the end of the last paragraph, we are told that thiols with low carbon-sulfur bond strengths will yield a large fraction of hydrocarbons. So if a compound has high bond strengths, it would yield a small fraction of hydrocarbons—choice (A).

10. B The correct statements in this question are taken directly from the first paragraph. The technology (A), synthesis (C), and development (D) of catalysts are all stated, as well as the removal of pollutants (E). The study of decomposition mechanisms is never mentioned, making (B) the correct answer choice.

11. D The answer to this question can be found in paragraph nine. The question stem is lifted directly from the passage, and the correct answer merely fills in the blank, "[At the time of writing], the best catalyst for desulfurization is ...."

12. E The role of Pt and Rh in catalytic converters is discussed in paragraph four. The metals function to remove NO, CO, and uncombusted hydrocarbons, choice (E).

Choice (A) is incorrect because the metals are catalysts, not coenzymes. The metals do not serve any role in heat and friction, making choice (B) incorrect. Choices (C) and (D) are incorrect because it is the ceramic honeycomb surface to which the metals are deposited that influences the surface area, not the metals themselves.

13. B The correct answer to this question can be found in paragraph nine. The desulfurization process encourages sulfur removal without breaking down pure hydrocarbons. Choice (B) is the only one that properly addresses this.

14. D The nature of thiols is described in paragraph ten. The passage states that thiols are hydrocarbons that have attached a sulfur atom to some combination of carbon and hydrogen, as described in choice (D).

15. A The construction of a catalytic converter is delivered in paragraph four. The amount of metals used in a catalyst is minimized because they are very expensive. None of the other choices are mentioned. (Again, don't be tempted by a true statement if it is not addressed in the passage, such as choice [B].)

16. E The environmental dangers of nitric oxide, nitrogen-oxygen compounds, and carbon monoxide are addressed in paragraph three. The danger of sulfur-oxygen compounds is addressed in paragraph eight. The dangers of thiols are never addressed. The passage states that sulfur compounds have to be burned before they become harmful, but it never addresses the dangers of thiols released directly into the atmosphere.

17. A The series of events involved in an inflammation reaction is described in paragraph four. The initial event in inflammation is vasoconstriction of the arterioles near the area of injury. Choice (E) is tempting, but it can be eliminated based on the fact that ischemia develops as a result of vasoconstriction and so cannot occur first.

18. D The definition of *inflammation* is provided in the first sentence of the second paragraph. Choices (A) and (B) are incorrect because they describe events that would incite an inflammatory response. Choice (C) is too specific—it describes only one part of the inflammatory response. Choice (E) is incorrect because inflammation is a local response, not a generalized one, as described in the first sentence of the second paragraph.

19. E The findings of 19th-century scientists, specifically those of Cohnheim and Metchnikoff, are discussed midway through the third paragraph. The advent of the microscope allowed scientists to learn about the vascular and cellular changes that are responsible for the signs of inflammation. Choice (A) is incorrect because the outward signs of inflammation were described as early as the 1st century C.E. (paragraph two). Choice (B) misrepresents the work of Metchnikoff. It was not pinocytosis that was studied but rather the process of phagocytosis. Choice (C) is an incorrect statement for reasons addressed in the previous question. Choice (D), although a correct statement, was not described in relation to 19th-century studies and was understood well before that.

20. D "A local deficiency of blood in tissues" is the definition of *ischemia*. The definition is provided in the fourth paragraph.

21. C The opening of precapillary sphincters is one of the vascular events that occurs during inflammation, as discussed in paragraph four. Going to the passage to prephrase our answer before looking at the choices, we know that the answer must involve hyperemia, described as a local excess of blood. Only choice (C) involves hyperemia.

22. D Neutrophils are discussed in paragraph ten. We can eliminate choice (A), as neutrophils can engulf particles up to half their size, not twice their size. Choice (B) can be eliminated: The relative effectiveness of leukocytes is never addressed. Choice (C) is also incorrect. Paragraph six informs us that macrophages are the first line of cellular defense. Choice (E) can also be eliminated— paragraph 11 states that eosinophils are not nearly as efficient as neutrophils in phagocytosis. Only choice (D) is correct.

23. E We can go back to paragraph ten to answer this question. Phagocytosed particles are digested in free-flowing vesicles in the cytoplasm. Since *vesicle* is not an answer choice, choice (E), the cytoplasm, must be the correct answer. The only other tempting choice is (B), lysosomes. We can eliminate this by looking at the last sentence of the paragraph—lysosomes are the source of the digestive enzymes but are not where digestion occurs.

24. B To get this question correct, we have to combine two pieces of information provided for us in paragraph seven. We are told that neutrophils constitute about 60 percent of circulating leukocytes and that the number of leukocytes can reach a high of 30,000 cells/mm^3. So the number of neutrophils can reach a high of $0.60 \times 30,000$ or 18,000 cells/mm^3.

25. C At the end of paragraph five, we are told that a key event in inflammation is the walling off of the affected area by fibrin clots. The fibrin was able to enter the area from the blood because of the increased permeability of the blood vessels. This makes choice (C) the only possibility.

26. B The effects of enzymes, toxins, etc. are described in paragraph nine. The effects include stimulating inflammatory cells to migrate to the area, marginate, and then pass through the vessel wall. The cells can pass through because the products also increase the permeability of the capillaries and damage their walls. Answer choice (B) is the opposite of what happens—cells are induced to leave the circulatory system, not stay within.

27. E In the last paragraph of the passage, the author attaches modern definitions to the first-century terms used to describe inflammation. Tumor is caused by the accumulation of fluid leaking from blood vessels to the damaged tissue.

28. B Leukocytosis-activating factor is discussed in paragraph eight. The chemical is released from inflamed tissue and travels in the blood to the bone marrow, where it activates neutrophils. The factor is not stored in the bone marrow, making choice (B) the correct response to this EXCEPT question.

29. C The four cardinal signs of inflammation are tumor, calor, rubor, and dolor (see paragraph two).

30. E Eosinophils are discussed in paragraph 11. The author states that eosinophils are particularly effective in defending against chemical agents, such as histamine. Choice (A) is incorrect because chemotaxis and margination were only discussed with respect to neutrophils and monocytes (paragraph nine).

31. C The author would agree with the statement in choice (C), as it correlates well with the discussion in the last paragraph. Choice (A) is wrong because the author describes how hydra respond to injury in the opening paragraph. The author cited several examples of the progress that has been made in understanding the mechanisms behind inflammation (paragraph three) and so would disagree with choice (B). Given the extent of the discussion of the events involved in inflammation, the process is very well understood, so the author would disagree with choice (D). Additionally, the author never mentions how much further research may be needed. The author would certainly disagree with choice (E), as inflammation is a remarkable response that protects living tissues and is definitely not maladaptive.

32. A At the end of paragraph six, we are told that monocytes migrate into injured tissues and mature into macrophages, making choice (A) correct. Choice (B) is incorrect because macrophages are already present in tissues. Choice (C) is describing granulocytes, not macrophages. Choice (D) is incorrect because margination is only discussed in relation to neutrophils and monocytes. Choice (E) is incorrect because we are never given the percent composition of macrophages in the blood.

33. D The process of phagocytosis is addressed in paragraph ten. Choice (D) describes margination and is the correct answer choice.

34. D The middle of the first paragraph describes the difficulties in testing patients with Lesch-Nyhan syndrome (LNS). The testing is complicated by the patients' severe disabilities, combined with their self-abusive tendencies and the need for physical restraints. Their behavior towards others is not mentioned, so we can eliminate choices (A), (B), and (E). Choice (C) is incorrect because LNS patients are able to speak.

35. B The 1994 study of LNS patients is described in paragraph four. Lines 9–11 state that there was considerable fluctuation in the severity of the self-injurious behavior. This makes choice (B) the correct statement and negates choice (A) as a possible answer. The author also states that the periods of high self-injury were related to stressful physical and emotional events, which negates Choice (C). Choice (D) is incorrect because patients were happy when restraints were used to prevent self-injury. Choice (E) is incorrect, because the level of pain threshold in LNS patients was never addressed.

36. D The areas of weakness in LNS patients are described at the end of the first paragraph. Attention span, choice (D), is not among the weaknesses listed.

37. E The answer to this question can be found at the end of paragraph five. The author writes that the personality attributes of LNS patients (good sense of humor, smile and laugh easily) make them seem more intelligent than tests indicate.

38. D The Ernst et al. study is described in paragraph seven. Choice (D) is taken directly from the passage—the presynaptic accumulation of a labeled dopamine precursor was measured. Choice (A) describes studies performed prior to the Ernst study. Choices (B) and (E) are stated incorrectly: The level of dopamine in the presynaptic cells was measured, not the levels in the synapse or postsynaptic cell. Choice (C) attempts to trick you on detail—the compound used is 6-fluorodopa F 18, not F 15.

39. C As stated in paragraph two, LNS infants are at first hypotonic.

40. B The classification of the purine nucleotides is addressed at the end of paragraph nine. Inosinic acid and guanylic acid are purine nucleotides.

41. C The role that the enzyme HPRT and its substrate PRPP play in LNS is discussed in paragraphs 10 and 11. We can eliminate choice (A) because there is an increase, not a decrease, in APRT (adenine phosphoribosyl-transferase) activity. Choice (B) can be eliminated because there is a decrease, not an increase, in HPRT activity. Choice (C) is correct—whenever two answer choices are in direct opposition to one another, as with choices (A) and (C), one of the two is usually correct. Choice (D) is incorrect because the increase in APRT activity is seen in erythrocytes, not fibroblasts. Choice (E) can be eliminated because paragraph 10 states that the HPRT activity in erythrocytes is affected differently.

42. B Paragraph two states that by four years of age, many children with LNS begin to exhibit the classic sign of self-mutilation. Later, in paragraph three, the author states that the self-mutilation usually begins at age three. Therefore, choice (B) is correct.

43. E The first line of paragraph eight states that LNS is a rare X-linked recessive disorder.

44. C The Ernst et al. study is described in paragraph seven. The study showed that several regions of the brain are affected, including the putamen, the caudate nucleus, frontal cortex, and ventral tegmental complex. Choice (C) is therefore an exception and the correct answer to the question.

45. B The physical and mental manifestations of LNS are addressed in paragraphs one and two. LNS patients' communication skills are impaired due to palsy and impaired airflow. They have subnormal weight and height, are spastic, and have a life span of less than 20 years. However, affected children can comprehend quite well, so choice (B) must be the answer.

46. A At the end of paragraph eight, the author writes that there is a prevalence of single DNA base substitutions.

47. E The cause of uric acid production is described in paragraph 11. Prephrasing our answer by going back to the relevant section in the passage, we expect the correct answer to involve in whole or in part the absence of the HPRT salvage pathway, resulting in increased PRPP synthetase activity and PRPP accumulation. This results in accelerated purine production. Looking at the answer choices, only (E) is satisfactory.

48. D The description of pyramidal symptoms begins at line ten in paragraph two. All but choice (D), dysmorphic features, are described as pyramidal symptoms.

49. D Examples of aggressive behavior can be found in the beginning of paragraph five. Choice (D) is not an example of aggressive behavior; rather, it is a form of self-mutilation.

50. B The salvage pathway is discussed in paragraph 11. The pathway allows preformed purine bases to be recycled, as stated in choice (B). Choices (A), (C), and (D) are incorrect because they each result from the absence of the salvage pathway.

QUANTITATIVE REASONING:
Answers and Explanations

ANSWER KEY

1. C	11. B	21. B	31. A
2. E	12. E	22. C	32. D
3. A	13. D	23. D	33. E
4. A	14. B	24. E	34. A
5. E	15. D	25. A	35. C
6. C	16. E	26. B	36. E
7. D	17. D	27. D	37. C
8. D	18. D	28. A	38. E
9. C	19. A	29. D	39. B
10. C	20. C	30. B	40. A

EXPLANATIONS

1. C The question stem states that the ratio of boys to girls is $\frac{5}{3}$, so for every 8 students, there are 3 girls. We can express this as the fraction

$$\frac{3 \text{ girls}}{8 \text{ students}}.$$

If there are 120 students, then the number of girls = 120 students $\times \dfrac{3 \text{ girls}}{8 \text{ students}}$ = 45 girls.

2. E To solve verbal math problems, you have to change the words into math:

What percent of $\sqrt{0.005}$ is $\sqrt{2}$?
$\downarrow$ $\downarrow$ $\downarrow$ $=$ $\downarrow$
$y\%$ $\times$ $\sqrt{0.005}$ $=$ $\sqrt{2}$?

$$y = \frac{\sqrt{2}}{\sqrt{0.005}} \times 100\%$$

When we divide two radicals, we can divide the numbers under one radical sign.

$$x = \sqrt{\frac{2}{0.005}} \times 100\% = \sqrt{\frac{2,000}{5}} \times 100\% =$$
$$\sqrt{400} \times 100\% = 20 \times 100\%.$$

$y = 2{,}000\%$, choice (E).

3. A We can solve for the length of the side of the room in inches as it would appear on the blueprint by using the conversion given in the question stem:

$$\frac{3\frac{1}{8} \text{ blueprint in.}}{125 \text{ feet}} = \frac{\frac{25}{8} \text{ in.}}{125 \text{ feet}} = \frac{\frac{1}{8}}{5} = \frac{1 \text{ in.}}{40 \text{ feet}}.$$

Converting the length of the room, we get

$$20 \text{ ft} \times \frac{1 \text{ in.}}{40 \text{ feet}} = \frac{1}{2} \text{ in.}$$

The area is then $\frac{1}{2} \times \frac{1}{2} = \frac{1}{4}$ in^2.

4. A Since the dimensions of the floor are given in feet, we'll change all the costs to dollars per square foot. The area of the floor = $10 \times 15 = 150$ ft^2.

One firm: Cost = 150 ft$^2 \times \$0.80/ft^2 = 150 \times \dfrac{4}{5} = 30 \times 4 = \$120$.

Another firm: Cost = $\dfrac{\$7.50}{\text{yd}^2} \times \dfrac{1 \text{ yd}^2}{9 \text{ ft}^2} \times 150 \text{ ft}^2 = \dfrac{7.50}{3} \times 50 = 2.50 \times 50 = \$125$.

The possible savings is $\$125 - \$120$ or $\$5$.

5. E We can solve this question using dimensional analysis. We take the expression we are given and multiply it by conversion fractions to cancel out units until we are left with the units we are looking for:

$$\frac{60 \text{ miles}}{\text{hour}} \times \frac{5{,}280 \text{ feet}}{1 \text{ mile}} \times \frac{1 \text{ hour}}{60 \text{ min}} \times \frac{1 \text{ min}}{60 \text{ sec}} =$$
$$\frac{(60)(5{,}280)}{3{,}600} = \frac{88 \text{ ft}}{\text{sec}}.$$

6. C We can use the internal triangles of the figure to solve for angles 1 and 2, then add them to find the answer. Remember that the sum of the angles of a triangle equals 180°.

Angle 1: $\angle a = 180° - 110° = 70°$. Therefore, $50° + 70° + \angle 1 = 180°$; $\angle 1 = 60°$.

Angle 2: $\angle b = 180° - 140° = 40°$. Therefore, $110° + 40° + \angle 2 = 180$; $\angle 2 = 30°$.

Therefore, angle $PQT = 60 + 30 = 90°$.

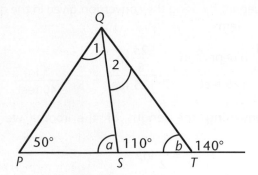

7. D The wall and ground make a right triangle, as shown in the diagram. Notice this is the Pythagorean triple 8:15:17, with each leg multiplied by 3. The length of the hypotenuse (ladder) is then $17 \times 3 = 51$ ft.

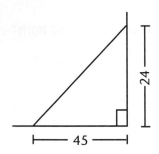

8. D The important concept here is that the line connecting the centers of tangent circles goes through the point of tangency. The lines connecting the centers of the circles in the diagram form a triangle because the circles are tangent to one another. OA and OB are radii of circle O. Therefore, $OA + OB = d$. Similarly, $PA + PC = d_1$ and $QC + QB = d_2$. The sum of all these radii is the perimeter of the triangle. Therefore the perimeter $= d + d_1 + d_2$.

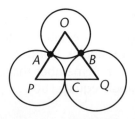

9. C Let $x =$ the amount the sixth woman spent. We are told that she spent \$5 more than the average of all six. Therefore,

$$x = \frac{5(16) + x}{6} + 5; \ 6x = 80 + x + 30; \ 5x = 110; \ x = \$22.$$

10. C The freight train travels 3 hours longer than the express train. Also, it has traveled 20 miles more than the express. Arrange this information in boxes:

	rate	$\times$	time	$=$	distance
Freight	?	$\times$	$3 + 2$	$=$	$120 + 20$
Express	60	$\times$	2	$=$	120

The freight train traveled 140 miles in 5 hours. Its rate is therefore $\frac{140}{5}$ or 28 mph, choice (C).

11. B Average rate $= \dfrac{\text{total distance}}{\text{total time}}$.

The trip going takes $2\frac{1}{2}$ hours. The trip returning takes 1 hour. Total time $= 3\frac{1}{2}$ hrs $= \frac{7}{2}$ hrs.

Average rate $= \dfrac{50 + 50}{\frac{7}{2}} = \dfrac{200}{7} = 28\frac{4}{7}$ mph.

12. E Billy walks 3 blocks in 3 minutes, which is the same as 1 block per minute.

528 feet per minute $= \dfrac{1}{10}$ mile per $\dfrac{1}{60}$ hour $= \dfrac{1}{10} \times \dfrac{60}{1} = 6$ mph.

13. D Total problems: 60; total time: 60 minutes.

Problems done: 30; time taken: 20 minutes.
Problems remaining: $60 - 30 = 30$; time remaining: $60 - 20 = 40$ minutes.

Average time remaining per problem $= \dfrac{40}{30} = 1\frac{1}{3}$ min.

14. B Average cost per book $= \dfrac{\text{total cost}}{\text{total books}} =$

$\dfrac{8(\$6.00) + 10(\$2.40)}{8 + 10} = \dfrac{\$48 + \$24}{18} = \dfrac{\$72}{18} = \$4.$

8($6.00) = $48 is the total cost of the $6.00 books. 10($2.40) is the total cost of the $2.40 books. The sum, $72, is the total cost of all the books.

15. D Total customers per day = 15(600). (Don't multiply out any product at first!) If six theaters shut down, then nine remain open. If we let x be the average number of customers per day for each of the nine theaters, 15(600) = 9x, because we are told that the number of customers remains the same.

$$15(600) = 9x; \ 9,000 = 9x; \ x = 1,000.$$

16. E $\dfrac{32 - 10\sqrt{5x}}{3} = 4$

Cross multiply: $32 - 10\sqrt{5x} = 12$

Transpose: $20 = 10\sqrt{5x}$

Divide by 10: $2 = \sqrt{5x}$

Square both sides: $4 = 5x$

Solve for x: $x = \dfrac{4}{5}$

17. D

$$1 + \frac{9}{16} = \frac{16}{16} + \frac{9}{16} = \frac{25}{16}; \ \sqrt{1 + \frac{9}{16}} = \sqrt{\frac{25}{16}} = \frac{5}{4} = 1\frac{1}{4}.$$

18. D Square all the terms to get rid of the radicals.

$$I^2 = \frac{2}{9} = \frac{1}{4.5}$$
$$II^2 = \frac{3}{16} = \frac{1}{5.3}$$
$$III^2 = \frac{5}{25} = \frac{1}{5}$$

If numerators are equal, the smallest fraction is the one with the largest denominator. Thus, the values in increasing order are $\dfrac{3}{16}, \dfrac{1}{5}, \dfrac{2}{9}$ or (D): II, III, I.

19. A 15 is 6% of what number? Here, the % term is 6%; the part term is 15. We need to find the whole. % × whole = part. 6% of x = 15; $x = 15 \div 6\% = 1,500 \div 6 = 250$.

20. C Thirty percent of the world's coal is produced in the United States. Twelve percent of U.S. coal is produced in Ohio. Therefore, 12% of 30%, or 3.6%, of the world's coal is produced in Ohio.

21. B Since the circumference and the radius of a circle are directly proportional ($C = 2\pi r$), the percent increase will be the same for both. If the circumference increases by 20%, then the radius increases by 20%. If we let the radius of the original circle be 5, the radius of the new circle is 5 + (20% of 5) = 5 + 1 = 6.

The area of a circle is proportional to the square of the radius ($A = \pi r^2$). The area of the original circle = $\pi 5^2 = 25\pi$. The area of the new circle = $\pi 6^2 = 36\pi$.

Therefore, the % increase = $\dfrac{\text{amount of increase}}{\text{original amount}} \times$

$100\% = \dfrac{36\pi - 25\pi}{25\pi} \times 100\% = \dfrac{11}{25} \times 100\% = 44\%.$

22. C Pick numbers since you are given percents and asked for percents.

Volume of cylinder = Area of base × Height.

Let radius of the first cylinder = 5.

It is increased by 20%: New radius = $5 + \dfrac{1}{5}(5) = 6$.

Let the height of the first cylinder = 6.

It is decreased by $16\dfrac{2}{3}$%: New height = $6 - \dfrac{1}{6}(6) = 5$.

A cylinder has a circular base.

Therefore, volume of first cylinder = $\pi(5)^2 \times 6 = 25\pi \times 6 = 150\pi$.

Volume of new cylinder = $\pi(6)^2 \times 5 = 36\pi \times 5 = 180\pi$.

% increase in volume = $\dfrac{\text{increase in volume}}{\text{original volume}} =$

$\dfrac{30\pi}{150\pi} = \dfrac{1}{5} = 20\%.$

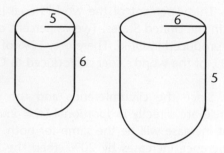

23. D When the numerator is doubled, the value of the fraction is doubled. When the denominator is halved, the value of the fraction is again doubled. The net result is quadrupling (multiplying by 4), choice (D).

24. E Let the width be 10 (for the rectangle). Therefore, the length is 20, and the perimeter is $2(10 + 20) = 60$. The perimeter of the square is also 60, which gives a side of 15. The area of the rectangle is $(10)(20) = 200$. The area of the square is $(15)(15) = 225$. The ratio $= 200:225 = 40:45 = 8:9$.

25. A No tax is paid on the first \$50,000. A tax of 6% is paid on the remaining \$100,000. The amount of tax $= 6\% \times \$100,000 = \$6,000$, choice (A).

26. B In a 60-foot fence, there are forty $1\frac{1}{2}$-foot sections (distance between pickets). Forty sections are made by 41 pickets. If the fence is extended to 80 feet without adding any pickets, there are still 41 pickets and 40 sections formed. Each section is $\frac{80}{40}$ or 2 ft.

27. D No matter the shape of the pool, a given amount of water will take up the same volume. The volume of a swimming pool in the shape of a rectangular solid equals length × width × height.

Let h = the height the water would reach in the second pool.

(24 feet)(16 feet)(1 foot) = (20 feet)(8 feet)(h feet).

Cancel like factors: $12 \text{ feet}^2 = 5h \text{ feet}^2$; $h = 2\frac{2}{5}$ feet.

28. A $x + y + 3z = 7$; $3x + 6y + 6z = 8$.

We want to solve for $(y - z)$, so we first have to eliminate x. Multiply the first equation by 3 and subtract it from the second equation.

$$3x + 6y + 6z = 8$$
$$- [\, 3x + 3y + 9z = 21\,]$$
$$\overline{ 3y - 3z = -13}$$
$$3(y - z) = -13$$
$$y - z = -\frac{13}{3}$$

29. D B will have his maximum number of marbles when the others (A and C) have their minimum number according to the constraints. Since C has less than both A and B, his minimum is 0. Therefore, A and B have 24 together. If A is to have more than B and B is to have a maximum, A will have 13, and B will have 11.

30. B The graph of a line has to satisfy the equation $y = mx + b$, where m is the slope and b is the y-intercept. If two lines are perpendicular to each other, then the slope of one line is the negative inverse of the other. We are told that line ℓ is perpendicular to the line $y = -\frac{1}{5}x$, so the slope of ℓ must equal 5. In the $y = mx + b$, we know that m must equal 5. To find b, we substitute the point $(3, -10)$ into the equation. We are given that the point $(3, -10)$ is on the line, so $x = 3$ and $y = -10$ must satisfy the equation $y = 5x + b$. By substituting $x = 3$ and $y = -10$, we get

$$y = mx + b$$
$$y = 5x + b$$
$$-10 = 5\,(3) + b$$
$$-10 = 15 + b$$
$$-10 - 15 = b$$
$$-25 = b$$

Now we know that $m = 5$ and $b = -25$, so our equation is $y = 5x - 25$, which is choice (B).

31. A Using a simple mnemonic and some common sense, this question can be answered quickly. Recalling the mnemonic SOH CAH TOA, $\sin\theta = \dfrac{\text{opposite}}{\text{hypotenuse}}$ and $\cos\theta = \dfrac{\text{adjacent}}{\text{hypotenuse}}$. From this, it is easy to see that the functions sine and cosine are not inversely related. The true relationship is $\cos\theta = \sin(90 - \theta)$. Therefore, the $\cos 59° = \sin 31°$.

If you were not sure of the relationship between the sine and cosine functions, you can still get this question correct by eliminating answer choices. Answer choices (B) and (D) can easily be eliminated—the only cosine function that can equal the $\cos 59°$ is the $\cos 59°$. Answer choice (C) can also be eliminated—since the functions of sine and cosine are different, the cosine of an angle cannot equal the sine of the same angle.

32. D Choice (D) happens to be a rearrangement of the trigonometric identity:

$$\sin^2 x + \cos^2 x = 1$$

This is true for all values of x. If you didn't know this identity—and you aren't required to memorize identities for the DAT—you could easily solve this problem by picking values for x, plugging them in, and seeing which choice works. We'll pick a value between 0 and $\dfrac{\pi}{2}$. How about $\dfrac{\pi}{4}$? Remember that $\dfrac{\pi}{4} = 45°$.

(A)
$$\sin\frac{\pi}{4} = \cos^2\frac{\pi}{4} + 1$$
$$\frac{\sqrt{2}}{2} = \left(\frac{\sqrt{2}}{2}\right)^2 + 1$$
$$\frac{\sqrt{2}}{2} = \frac{2}{4} + 1$$
$$\frac{\sqrt{2}}{2} = 1.5 \qquad \text{No.}$$

(B)
$$\tan\frac{\pi}{4} = (\sin\frac{\pi}{4})(\cos\frac{\pi}{4})$$
$$1 = \left(\frac{\sqrt{2}}{2}\right)\left(\frac{\sqrt{2}}{2}\right)$$
$$1 = \frac{2}{4}$$
$$1 = 0.5 \qquad \text{No.}$$

(C)
$$\tan\frac{\pi}{4} = \frac{\cos\frac{\pi}{4}}{\sin\frac{\pi}{4}}$$
$$1 = \frac{\frac{\sqrt{2}}{2}}{\frac{\sqrt{2}}{2}}$$
$$1 = 1 \qquad \text{Possible . . .}$$

(D)
$$\sin^2\frac{\pi}{4} = 1 - \cos^2\frac{\pi}{4}$$
$$\left(\frac{\sqrt{2}}{2}\right)^2 = 1 - \left(\frac{\sqrt{2}}{2}\right)^2$$
$$\frac{2}{4} = 1 - \frac{2}{4}$$
$$0.5 = 0.5 \qquad \text{Possible . . .}$$

(E)
$$\sin\frac{\pi}{4} = \frac{1}{\cos\frac{\pi}{4}}$$
$$\frac{\sqrt{2}}{2} = \frac{1}{\frac{\sqrt{2}}{2}}$$
$$\frac{\sqrt{2}}{2} = \frac{2}{\sqrt{2}} \qquad \text{No.}$$

So now let's check (C) and (D) with another value. We'll use $\dfrac{\pi}{6}$ or 30°.

(C)
$$\tan\frac{\pi}{6} = \frac{\cos\frac{\pi}{6}}{\sin\frac{\pi}{6}}$$
$$\frac{1}{\sqrt{3}} = \frac{\frac{\sqrt{3}}{2}}{\frac{1}{2}}$$
$$\frac{1}{\sqrt{3}} = \sqrt{3} \qquad \text{No.}$$

Therefore, (D) must be the correct answer.

33. E Let's look at each term of the expression $(x^2 - 6)(y + 7)$ separately. In evaluating the term $x^2 - 6$, notice that x is being squared, so the term is largest when the absolute value for x is largest. Since x ranges from -4 to 2, the largest value will be when $x = -4$. In evaluating the value for y, the term $y + 7$ will be greatest when y is greatest. Since y ranges from 3 to 5, the largest value will be when $y = 5$.

34. A We are given that $\triangle ABC$ is equilateral, which means that each leg of the triangle is equal. The altitude of an equilateral triangle bisects the base, so $BD = CD = \frac{1}{2}AB$. Labeling the legs as shown, we can use the Pythagorean theorem to solve for the length of AB.

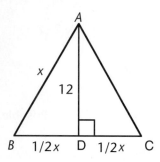

$$\left(\frac{1}{2}x\right)^2 + 12^2 = x^2$$

$$\frac{1}{4}x^2 + 144 = x^2$$

$$x^2 - \frac{1}{4}x^2 = 144$$

$$\frac{3}{4}x^2 = 144$$

$$x^2 = 144 \times \frac{4}{3}$$

$$x^2 = 48 \times 4$$

$$x = \sqrt{192} = 8\sqrt{3}$$

35. C This is a simple arithmetic problem, as long as you remember the rules for handling exponents and scientific notation.

$$\frac{6 \times 10^{-4}}{30 \times 10^5} = \frac{6}{30} \times 10^{-9}$$

$$= \frac{1}{5} \times 10^{-9}$$

$$= 0.2 \times 10^{-9}$$

$$= 2 \times 10^{-10}$$

36. E The number of different ways to arrange x number of objects, given no repeats, is $x!$, the factorial of x. The number of ways to arrange 5 students equals $5! = 5 \times 4 \times 3 \times 2 \times 1 = 120$.

37. C The probability of two independent events occurring together is the product of their individual probabilities. The probability of selecting the first marble is $\frac{5}{11}$, and the probability of selecting the second marble is $\frac{4}{10}$ (don't forget to subtract 1 since you are not putting the second one back!). The probability of drawing two purple marbles is then $\frac{5}{11} \times \frac{4}{10} = \frac{20}{110} = \frac{2}{11}$.

38. E To solve verbal math problems, you have to convert words into equations:

1. "$34 in nickels, dimes, and quarters" is expressed as $\$34 = (n)\left(\frac{1}{20}\right) + (d)\left(\frac{1}{10}\right) + (q)\left(\frac{1}{4}\right)$,

where
     n = # of nickels, which is one-twentieth of a dollar
     d = # of dimes, which is one-tenth of a dollar
     q = # of quarters, which is one-fourth of a dollar

2. "3 times as many dimes as quarters" is expressed as $3q = d$.

3. "2 times as many nickels as dimes" is expressed as $n = 2d$.

Substituting the equations for q and n (from steps 2 and 3 above) into the equation from step, and then solving for d, we get

$$\$34 = (n)\left(\frac{1}{20}\right) + (d)\left(\frac{1}{10}\right) + (q)\left(\frac{1}{4}\right)$$

$$\$34 = (2d)\left(\frac{1}{20}\right) + (d)\left(\frac{1}{10}\right) + \left(\frac{d}{3}\right)\left(\frac{1}{4}\right)$$

$$= \frac{d}{10} + \frac{d}{10} + \frac{d}{12}$$

$$= \frac{2d}{10} + \frac{d}{12}$$

$$= \frac{24d}{120} + \frac{10d}{120}$$

$$34 = \frac{34d}{120}$$

$$d = 120$$

39. B To find the distance between two points on the coordinate plane, plot the points and construct a right triangle. The distance between the points is measured by the hypotenuse of the right triangle (see figure). The lengths of legs are measured using the graph, and the hypotenuse is calculated using the Pythagorean is theorem ($a^2 + b^2 = c^2$). Plugging in the lengths of the legs of the triangle in this example yields $9^2 + 12^2 = c^2$. Notice that these values are the triple 3, 4, 5 multiplied by 3, so the hypotenuse = 15.

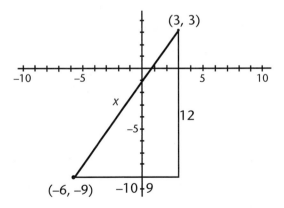

40. A The average of a set of numbers equals $\frac{\text{sum of the numbers}}{\text{number of items}}$. The average of the given set of numbers = $\frac{3 + 5 + 5 + 11 + 13}{5} = \frac{37}{5} = 7\frac{2}{5}$.

INDEX

A

A band, 112
AB blood type, 82
abiotic environment, 141
ABO blood type, 51, 81–82
absolute configuration, 328–329
absolute refractory period, 115
absolute values (DAT quantitative reasoning), 601–602, 631–632
absorbed (digestion), 117, 165
absorption, 11, 121
absorption spectra, 186
acetal formation, 385
acetic acid, 11
acetoacetic ester condensation, 411
acetylcholine, 97, 101, 114
acetylcholinesterase, 97, 98
acetylide ion, 359
achiral object, 327
acid anhydrides, 403
acid dissociation constant (K_a), 281
acidic amino acids, 459–460
acidic side chains (amino acid), 457
acidity (pH), 143, 394–396
acids, 277–288, 401
acromegaly, 86
ACTH (adrenocorticotrophic hormone), 83, 86
actin molecules, 112
actinide series, 193
action potentials, 94, 95, 112
activated complex, 230
activation energy (E_a), 230, 246
active immunity, 80
active site, 20
active transport, 94, 127
actual yield, 223
acylation, 367, 407
acyl halide, 399, 401, 414

adaptation, 121, 176
adaptive advantage, 169
adaptive radiation, 176, 177
adaptive responses, 133
adenine (A), 55
adenosine triphosphate (ATP), 413
ADH (antidiuretic hormone), 87, 88, 129
adiabatic process, 239
adipose tissue, 465
adol condensation, 388–389
adrenal cortex, 83
adrenal glands, 83–85
adrenal hormones, 85
adrenal medulla, 83, 84–85
adsorbant, 428
aerobic respiration, 12, 24, 125
afferent neurons, 98
agarose gel electrophoresis, 433
agglutinate, 80
agonistic displays, 138
airways, 107
alarm defensive substances (behavior), 139
alcohol, 319, 369–376, 383
alcohol fermentation, 24
aldehydes, 320–321, 381–391
aldonic acids, 449
aldosterone, 84, 91
algae, 164
algebra (DAT quantitative reasoning), 591–602
alimentation, 165
aliphatic compounds, 363–364
alkali metals, 197
alkaline earths, 195, 197
alkanes, 313–316, 318–322, 343–350
alkanoyl halides, 401
alkenes, 316–318, 351–358, 383
alkyl (R), 364, 409
alkyl alkanoates, 409

alkyation of ammonia, 417–419
alkyl halides, 346–349
alkynes, 318, 358–362
alkoxyalkanes, 376
allantois, 71, 72
allergic reactions, 81
alleles, 45, 50, 174
all-or-none response, 95, 114
alpha decay, 304
  helix, 463
  state, 438
altitude and terrestrial biome, 158–160
alveoli, 107
American Dental Association, 3
amides, 401, 402–403, 406, 407–408, 410, 414, 415
amines, 322, 415–420
amino acids, 57, 79, 453–460, 466
aminoacyl-tRNA synthetase, 60
aminopeptidases, 122
amino-terminal residue, 461
ammonia, 28, 125, 386–387
amnion, 71, 72
amoeba, 117
amorphous (solid), 260
amphibians, 71, 167
amphioxus, 167
amphiprotic species, 284
amphoteric species, 284–285, 454
amylase, 123
anaerobic respiratory processes, 12, 24
analogous structures, 170
anaphase, 32, 35
anatomy, comparative, 170
androgens, 84
angle ranking (PAT), 472, 509–514
angular quantum number, 187
anhydrides, 401, 403–407, 414

animal behavior, 131–139
animalia, 163, 164–168
animals, sexual reproduction in, 37–38
animals, vascular systems in, 75–82
annelids, 76, 104, 106, 110, 118–119, 125, 166
anode, 292
anomers, 448
antagonistic displays, 138
anterior pituitary gland, 85, 86, 88
antiaromatic compound, 363
antibodies, 80
antibonding orbital, 212, 338
anticholinesterases, 98
anticodon, 60
anticonformation, 333–334
antigens, 80, 81
anus, 118
aorta, 76
aortic loops, 76
aphotic zone, 143, 159
appendicular skeleton, 111
appendix, 171
aquatic biomes, 158–160
aqueous humor, 102
aqueous solution, 267, 268
arachnids, 166
arbitrary stimulus, 134
arenas, 364
arithmetic (DAT quantitative reasoning), 577–589
aromatic compounds, 363–368
Arrhenius acids, nomenclature of, 278
Arrhenius definition, 277
arteries, 76, 77
arterioles, 76
arthropods, 75, 104, 106, 110, 119, 126, 166
aryl compounds (Ar), 364

Tear-Out, Quick Reference Study Sheets for Biology, General Chemistry and Organic Chemistry

The following DAT Study Sheets are your one-stop resource for the key diagrams, charts, equations, and formulas that you are sure to see on the exam. This color-coded guide is separated into three DAT subtopics: Biology, General Chemistry, and Organic Chemistry. Each topic features the most important highlights you will want to review in-between study sessions and before your test day. Carefully tear out the pages to create a light and portable on-the-go resource that you can use to study anytime, anywhere.

DAT STUDY SHEET – BIOLOGY

THE CELL

FLUID MOSAIC MODEL AND MEMBRANE TRAFFIC
- Phospholipid bilayer with cholesterol and embedded proteins
- Exterior hydrophilic phosphoric acid region
- Interior hydrophobic fatty acid region

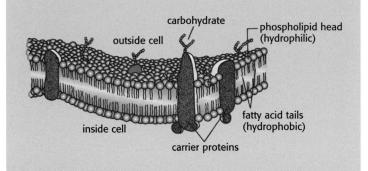

carbohydrate

outside cell

phospholipid head (hydrophilic)

fatty acid tails (hydrophobic)

inside cell

carrier proteins

HOMEOSTASIS

HORMONAL REGULATION
Aldosterone
- stimulates Na^+ reabsorption and K^+ secretion, increasing water reabsorption, blood volume and blood pressure
- secreted from adrenal cortex
- is regulated by renin-angiotensin system

ADH
- increases collecting duct's permeability to water to increase water reabsorption
- is secreted from posterior pituitary with high [solute] in the blood

THE LIVER'S ROLES IN HOMEOSTASIS
1. gluconeogenesis
2. processing of nitrogenous wastes (urea)
3. detoxification of wastes/chemicals/drugs
4. storage of iron and vitamin B12
5. synthesis of bile and blood proteins
6. beta-oxidation of fatty acids to ketones
7. interconversion of carbs, fat, and amino acids

ENZYMES

REGULATION
- **Allosteric**: binding of an affector molecule at allosteric site.
- **Feedback inhibition**: end product inhibits an initial enzyme pathway
- **Reversible inhibition**: competitive inhibitors bind to active site; noncompetitive inhibitors to the allosteric site

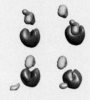

GLUCOSE CATABOLISM
Glycolysis occurs in the cell cytoplasm: $C_6H_{12}O_6 + 2ADP + 2P_i + 2NAD^+ \rightarrow 2Pyruvate + 2ATP + 2NADH + 2H^+ + 2H_2O$.

Fermentation occurs in anaerobic conditions. Pyruvate is converted into lactic acid (in muscle) or ethanol (in yeast).

Respiration occurs in aerobic conditions.
- **Pyruvate decarboxylation**: Pyruvate converted to acetyl CoA in the mitochondrial matrix.
- **Citric acid cycle**: Acetyl CoA enters, coenzymes exit.
- **Electron transport chain**: Coenzymes are oxidized, and energy is released as electrons are transferred from carrier to carrier.
- **Oxidative phosphorylation**: Electrochemical gradient caused by NADH and FADH² oxidation provides energy for ATP synthase to phosphorylate ADP into ATP.

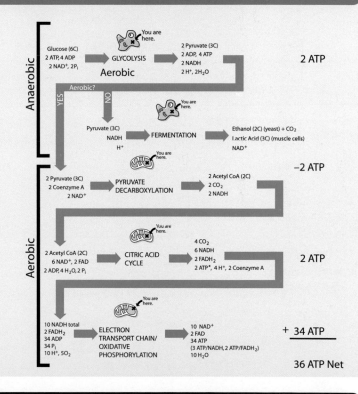

MUSCULOSKELETAL SYSTEM

Sarcomere
- contractile unit of the fibers in skeletal muscle
- contains thin actin and thick myosin filaments

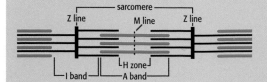

CONTRACTION
Initiation:
- Depolarization of a neuron leads to action potential.

BONE FORMATION AND REMODELLING
- Osteoblasts: builds bone
- Osteoclasts: breaks down bone
- Reformation: inorganic ions are absorbed from the blood for use in bone
- Degradation (Resorption): inorganic ions are released into the blood

ENDOCRINE SYSTEM

Direct hormones directly stimulate organs, tropic hormones stimulate other glands.
Mechanisms of hormone action: **Peptides** act via secondary messengers and **steroids** act via a hormone/receptor binding to DNA. Amino acid derivatives may do either.

Hormone	Source	Action
Follicle-stimulating (FSH)		Stimulates follicle maturation; spermatogenesis
Luteinizing (LH)		Stimulates ovulation; testosterone synthesis
Adrenocorticotropic (ACTH)		Stimulates adrenal cortex to make and secrete glucocorticoids
Thyroid-stimulating (TSH)	Anterior pituitary	Stimulates the thyroid to produce thyroid hormones
Prolactin		Stimulates milk production and secretion
Endorphins		Inhibit the perception of pain in the brain
Growth hormone		Stimulates bone and muscle growth/lipolysis
Oxytocin	Hypothalamus; stored in posterior pituitary	Stimulates uterine conteractions during labor, milk secretion during lactation
Vasopressin (ADH)		Stimulates water reabsorption in kidneys
Thyroid hormones (T_4, T_3)	Thyroid	Stimulate metabolic activity
Calcitonin		Decreases (tones down) blood calcium level
Parathyroid hormone	Parathyroid	Increases the blood calcium level
Glucocorticoids	Adrenal cortex	Increase blood glucose level and decrease protein synthesis
Mineralocorticoids		Increase water reabsorption in kidneys
Epinephrine, Norepinephrine	Adrenal medulla	Increases blood glucose level and heart rate
Glucagon		Stimulates conversion of glycogen to glucose in the liver, increases blood glucose
Insulin	Pancreas	Lowers blood glucose, increases glycogen stores
Somatostatin		Supresses secretion of glucagon and insulin
Testosterone	Testes	Maintains male secondary sexual characteristics
Estrogen	Ovary/Placenta	Maintains female secondary sexual characteristics
Progesterone		Promotes growth/maintenance of endometrium
Melatonin	Pineal	Unclear in humans
Atrial natriuretic peptide	Heart	Involved in osmoregulation and vasodilation
Thymosin	Thymus	Stimulates T lymphocyte development

REPRODUCTION

CELL DIVISION

- G_1: cell doubles its organelles and cytoplasm
- S: DNA replication
- G_2: same as G_1
- M: the cell divides in two
- Mitosis = PMAT
- Meiosis = PMAT × 2

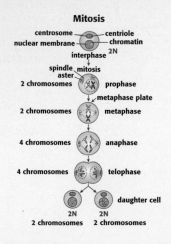

SEXUAL REPRODUCTION

Meiosis I:
- Two pairs of sister chromatids form tetrads during prophase I.
- Crossing over leads to genetic recombination in prophase I.

Meiosis II:
- Identical to mitosis, but no replication.
- Meiosis occurs in **spermatogenesis** (sperm formation) and **oogenesis** (egg formation).

FOUR STAGES OF EARLY DEVELOPMENT

cleavage: mitotic divisions
implantation: embryo implants during blastulation
gastrulation: ectoderm, endoderm, and mesoderm form
neurulation: germ layers develop a nervous system

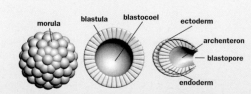

| Ectoderm "Attract-o-derm" | Nervous system, epidermis, lens of eye, inner ear | Endoderm "Endernal" organs | Lining of digestive tract, lungs, liver and pancreas | Mesoderm "Means-o-derm" | Muscles, skeleton, circulatory system, gonads, kidney |

DIGESTION

CARBOHYDRATE DIGESTION

Enzyme	Site of Production	Site of Function	Hydrolysis Reaction
Salivary amylase (ptyalin)	Salivary glands	Mouth	Starch → maltose
Pancreatic amylase	Pancreas	Small Intestine	Starch → maltose
Maltase	Intestinal glands	Small Intestine	Maltose → 2 glucoses
Sucrase	Intestinal glands	Small Intestine	Sucrose → glucose, fructose
Lactase	Intestinal glands	Small Intestine	Lactose → glucose, galactose

PROTEIN DIGESTION

Enzyme	Production Site	Function Site	Function
Pepsin	Gastric glands (chief cells)	Stomach	Hydrolyzes specific peptide bonds
Trypsin	Pancreas	Small Intestine	Hydrolyzes specific peptide bonds / Converts chymotrypsinogen to chymotrypsin
Chymotrypsin	Pancreas	Small Intestine	Hydrolyzes specific peptide bonds
Carboxypeptidase	Pancreas	Small Intestine	Hydrolyzes terminal peptide bond at carboxyl
Aminopeptidase	Intestinal glands	Small Intestine	Hydrolyzes terminal peptide bond at amino
Dipeptidases	Intestinal glands	Small Intestine	Hydrolyzes pairs of amino acids
Enterokinase	Intestinal glands	Small Intestine	Converts trypsinogen to trypsin

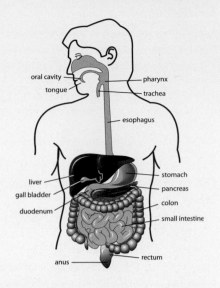

oral cavity, tongue, pharynx, trachea, esophagus, liver, gall bladder, duodenum, stomach, pancreas, colon, small intestine, anus, rectum

IMMUNE SYSTEM

- The body distinguishes between "self" and "nonself" (antigens)

HUMORAL IMMUNITY (specific defense)

B lymphocytes

memory cells ← → **plasma cells**

memory cells: remember antigen, speed up secondary response

plasma cells: make and release antibodies (**IgG, IgA, IgM, IgD, IgE**), which induce antigen phagocytosis

- **Active immunity**: antibodies are produced during an immune response.

- **Passive immunity**: antibodies produced by one organism are transferred to another organism.

CELL-MEDIATED IMMUNITY

T lymphocytes

cytotoxic T cells ← → **suppressor cells**

cytotoxic T cells: destroy cells directly

suppressor cells: regulate B and T cells to decrease anti-antigen activity

helper T cells: activate B and T cells and macrophages by secreting lymphokines

↓ **memory cells**

NONSPECIFIC IMMUNE RESPONSE

Includes skin, passages lined with cilia, macrophages, inflammatory response, and interferons (proteins that help prevent the spread of a virus).

LYMPHATIC SYSTEM

- lymph vessels meet at the thoracic duct in the upper chest and neck, draining into the veins of the cardiovascular system.

- vessels carry **lymph** (excess interstitial fluid), and capillaries (**lacteals**) collect fats by absorbing chylomicrons in the small intestine.

- **lymph nodes** are swellings along the vessels with phagocytic cells (leukocytes) that remove foreign particles from lymph.

CIRCULATION

BLOOD TYPING

Antigens are located on the surface of red blood cells

Blood type	RBC antigen	Antibodies	Donates to:	Receives From:
A	A	Anti-B	A, AB	A, O
B	B	Anti-A	B, AB	B, O
AB	A, B	None	AB only	All
O	None	Anti-A, B	All	O

Blood cells with Rh factor are Rh$^+$ and produce no antibody. Rh$^-$ lack antigen and produce an antibody.

MOLECULAR GENETICS

NUCLEIC ACID

- Basic unit: nucleotide (sugar, nitrogenous base, phosphate)
- DNA's sugar: deoxyribose. RNA's sugar: ribose.
- 2 types of bases: double-ringed purines (adenine, guanine) and single-ringed pyrimidines (cytosine, thymine, uracil).
- DNA double helix: antiparallel strands joined by base pairs (AT, GC).
- RNA is usually single-stranded: A pairs with U, not T.

TRANSCRIPTION REGULATION, PROKARYOTES

Regulated by the **operon**:

- structural genes: have DNA that codes for protein
- operator gene: repressor binding site
- promoter gene: RNA polyermase's 1st binding site
- Inducible systems need an inducer for transcription to occur. Repressible systems need a corepressor to inhibit transcription.

MUTATIONS

- **Point**: one nucleotide is substituted by another; they are silent if the sequence doesn't change.
- **Frameshift**: insertions or deletions shift reading frame. Protein doesn't form, or is nonfunctional.

VIRUSES

- acellular structures of double or single-stranded DNA or RNA in a protein coat.
- Lytic cycle: virus kills the host.
- Lysogenic cycle: virus enters host genome.

DNA REPLICATION

- **Semiconservative**: each new helix has an intact strand from the parent helix and a newly synthesized strand.

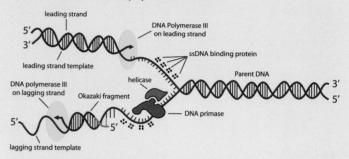

EUKARYOTIC PROTEIN SYNTHESIS

- **Transcription**: RNA polymerase synthesizes hnRNA using a DNA, "antisense strand" as a template.
- **Post-transcriptional processing**: introns are cut out of hnRNA, exons spliced to form mRNA.
- **Translation**: occurs on ribosomes in the cytoplasm.

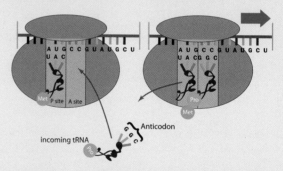

- **Post-translational modifications**: (i.e., disulfide bonds) made before the polypeptide becomes a functional protein.

EVOLUTION

- When frequencies are stable, the population is in Hardy-Weinberg equilibrium: no mutations, large population, random mating, no net migration, and equal reproductive success.

$$p + q = 1; p^2 + 2pq + q^2 = 1$$

p = freq. of dom. allele q = freq. of rec. allele

p^2 = freq of dom homozygotes

$2pq$ = freq of heterozygotes

q^2 = freq of recessive homozygotes

CLASSICAL GENETICS

- If both parents are Rr, the alleles separate to give a genotypic ratio of 1:2:1 and a phenotypic ratio of 3:1.

Law of independent assortment: Alleles of unlinked genes assort independently in meiosis.

- For two traits: AbBb parents will produce AB, Ab, aB, and ab gametes.
- The phenotypic ratio for this cross is 9:3:3:1.

STATISTICAL CALCULATIONS

- The probability of producing a genotype that requires multiple events to occur equals the *product* of the probability of each event.
- The probability of producing a genotype that can be the result of multiple events equals the *sum* of each probability.

GENETIC MAPPING

- Crossing over during meiosis I can unlink genes (Prophase I).
- Genes are most likely unlinked when far apart.
- One map unit is 1% recombinant frequency.

Given Recombination frequencies

X and Y: 8%

X and Z: 12%

Y and Z: 4%

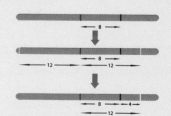

INHERITED DISORDERS in PEDIGREES

- Autosomal recessive: skips generations
- Autosomal dominant: appears in every generation
- X-linked (sex-linked): no male-to-male transmission, and more males are affected.

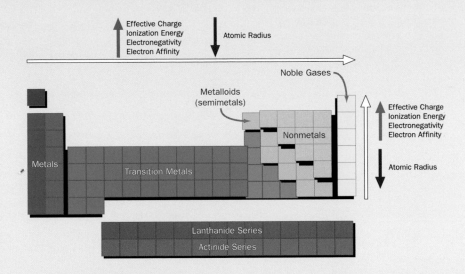

ATOMIC STRUCTURE

Atomic weight: the weight in grams of one mole (mol) of a given element and is expressed in terms of g/mol.

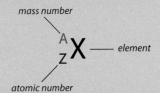

mass number

$$_Z^A X \quad \longleftarrow element$$

atomic number

A **mole** is a unit used to count particles and is represented by **Avogadro's number**, 6.022×10^{23} particles.

$$Moles = \frac{grams}{atomic\ or\ molecular\ weight}$$

Isotopes: For a given element, multiple species of atoms with the same number of protons (same atomic number) but different numbers of neutrons (different mass numbers).

Planck's quantum theory: Energy emitted as electromagnetic radiation from matter exists in discrete bundles called quanta.

Bohr's Model of the Hydrogen Atom

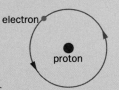

electron

proton

Angular momentum $= \dfrac{nh}{2\eta}$

Energy of electron $= E = \dfrac{-RH}{n^2}$

Electromagnetic energy of photons $= E = \dfrac{hc}{\lambda}$

The group of hydrogen emission lines corresponding to transitions from upper levels $n > 2$ to $n = 2$ is known as the **Balmer series**, while the group corresponding to transitions between upper levels $n > 1$ to $n = 1$ is known as the **Lyman series.**

Absorption spectrum: Characteristic energy bands where electrons absorb energy.

Quantum Mechanical Model of Atoms

Heisenberg uncertainty principle: It is impossible to determine with perfect accuracy the momentum and the position of an electron simultaneously.

Quantum Numbers:

#	Character	Symbol	Value
1st	Shell	n	n
2nd	Subshell	l	From zero to n−1
3rd	Orbital	m_ℓ	Between l and −l
4th	Spin	m_s	½ or −½

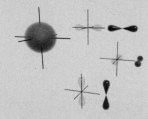

Principal Quantum Number (n): The larger the integer value of n, the higher the energy level and radius of the electron's orbit. The maximum number of electrons in energy level n is $2n^2$.

Azimuthal Quantum Number (l): Refers to subshells, or sublevels. The four subshells corresponding to $l = 0, 1, 2,$ and 3 are known as s, p, d and f, respectively. The maximum number of electrons that can exist within a subshell is given by the equation $4l+2$.

Magnetic Quantum Number (m_ℓ): This specifies the particular orbital within a subshell where an electron is highly likely to be found at a given point in time.

Spin Quantum Number (m_s): The spin of a particle is its intrinsic angular momentum and is a characteristic of a particle, like its charge.

Electron Configuration

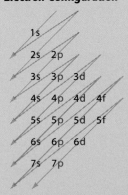

1s

2s 2p

3s 3p 3d

4s 4p 4d 4f

5s 5p 5d 5f

6s 6p 6d

7s 7p

Hund's rule: Within a given subshell, orbitals are filled such that there are a maximum number of half-filled orbitals with parallel spins.

Valence electrons: Electrons of an atom that are in its outer energy shell or that are available for bonding.

Experimental Determination of Rate Law: The values of k, x, and y in the rate law equation (rate = k [A]^x [B]^y) must be determined experimentally for a given reaction at a given temperature. The rate is usually measured as a function of the initial concentrations of the reactants, A and B.

Efficiency of Reactions

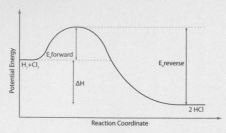

Factors affecting reaction rates: Reactant Concentrations, Temperature, Medium, Catalysts

Catalysts are unique substances that increase reaction rate without being consumed; they do this by lowering the activation energy.

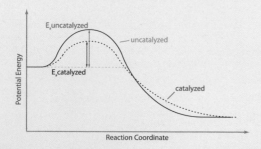

Law of Mass Action

$$a A + b B \rightleftharpoons c C + d D$$

$$K_c = \frac{[C]^c[D]^d}{[A]^a[B]^b}$$

K_c is the equilibrium constant. (c stands for concentration.)

Properties of The Equilibrium Constant

Pure solids/liquids don't appear in expression.

- K_{eq} is characteristic of a given system at a given temperature.
- If $K_{eq} \gg 1$, an equilibrium mixture of reactants and products will contain very little of the reactants compared to the products.
- If $K_{eq} \ll 1$, an equilibrium mixture of reactants and products will contain very little of the products compared to the reactants.
- If K_{eq} is close to 1, an equilibrium mixture of products and reactants will contain approximately equal amounts of the two.

A + B ⇌ C + heat	
Will shift to **RIGHT**	Will shift to **LEFT**
1. if more A or B added	1. if more C added
2. if C taken away	2. if A or B taken away
3. if pressure applied or volume reduced (assuming A, B, and C are gases)	3 if pressure reduced or volume increased (assuming A, B, and C are gases)
4. if temperature reduced	4. if temperature increased

Formal Charges

Formal charge = Valence electrons $- \frac{1}{2} N_{bonding} - N_{nonbonding}$

Intermolecular Forces

1. Dipole-Dipole Interactions: Polar molecules orient themselves such that the positive region of one molecule is close to the negative region of another molecule.

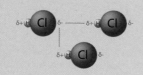

2. Hydrogen Bonding: The partial positive charge of the hydrogen atom interacts with the partial negative charge located on the electronegative atoms (F, O, N) of nearby molecules.

3. Dispersion Forces: The bonding electrons in covalent bonds may appear to be equally shared between two atoms, but at any particular point in time they will be located randomly throughout the orbital. This permits unequal sharing of electrons, causing rapid polarization and counter-polarization of the electron clouds of neighboring molecules, inducing the formation of more dipoles.

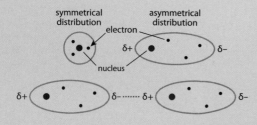

A **compound** is a pure substance that is composed of two or more elements in a fixed proportion.

A **mole** is the amount of a substance that contains the same number of particles that are found in a 12.000 g sample of carbon-12.

Combination Reactions: two or more reactants form one product.

$$S (s) + O_2 (g) \rightarrow SO_2 (g)$$

Decomposition Reactions: a compound breaks down into two or more substances, usually as a result of heating or electrolysis.

$$2HgO (s) \rightarrow 2Hg (l) + O_2 (g)$$

Single Displacement Reactions: an atom (or ion) of one compound is replaced by an atom of another element.

$$Zn (s) + CuSO_4 (aq) \rightarrow Cu (s) + ZnSO_4 (aq)$$

Double Displacement Reactions: also called metathesis reactions, elements from two different compounds displace each other to form two new compounds.

$$CaCl_2 (aq) + 2 AgNO_3 (aq) \rightarrow Ca(NO_3)_2 (aq) + 2 AgCl (s)$$

Net Ionic Equations: These types of equations are written showing only the species that actually participate in the reaction. So in the following equation,

$$Zn (s) + Cu^{2+} (aq) + SO_4^{2-} (aq) \rightarrow Cu (s) + Zn^{2+} (aq) + SO_4^{2-} (aq)$$

the spectator ion (SO_4^{2-}) does not take part in the overall reaction, but simply remains in solution throughout. The net ionic equation would be:

$$Zn (s) + Cu^{2+} (aq) \rightarrow Cu (s) + Zn^{2+} (aq)$$

Neutralization Reactions: These are a specific type of double displacements which occur when an acid reacts with a base to produce a solution of a salt and water:

$$HCl (aq) + NaOH (aq) \rightarrow NaCl (aq) + H_2O (l)$$

ACIDS AND BASES

Arrhenius Definition: An acid is a species that produces H+ (a proton) in an aqueous solution, and a base is a species that produces OH⁻ (a hydroxide ion).

Bronsted-Lowry Definition: An acid is a species that donates protons, while a base is a species that accepts protons.

Lewis Definition: An acid is an electron-pair acceptor, and a base is an electron-pair donor.

Properties of Acids and Bases

$$pH = -\log[H^+] = \log\left(\frac{1}{[H^+]}\right)$$

$$pH = -\log[OH^-] = \log\left(\frac{1}{[OH^-]}\right)$$

$$H_2O(l) \rightleftharpoons H^+(aq) + OH^-(aq)$$

$$K_w = [H^+][OH^-] = 10^{-14}$$

$$pH + pOH = 14$$

Weak Acids and Bases

$$HA(aq) + H_2O(l) \rightleftharpoons H_3O^+(aq) + A^-(aq)$$

$$K_a = \frac{[H_3O^+][A^-]}{[HA]}$$

$$K_b = \frac{[B^+][OH^-]}{[BOH]}$$

Salt Formation: Acids and bases may react with each other, forming a salt and (often, but not always) water in a neutralization reaction.

$$HA + BOH \rightarrow BA + H_2O$$

Titration and Buffers

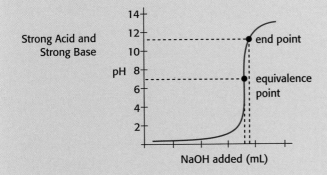

Strong Acid and Strong Base

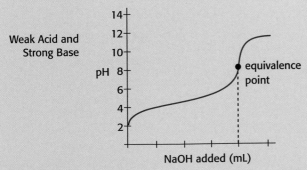

Weak Acid and Strong Base

Titration is a procedure used to determine the molarity of an acid or base by reacting a known volume of a solution of unknown concentration with a known volume of a solution of known concentration.

ACIDS AND BASES (cont.)

Henderson-Hasselbalch equation is used to estimate the pH of a solution in the buffer region where the concentrations of the species and its conjugate are present in approximately equal concentrations.

$$pH = pK_a + \log\frac{[conjugate\ base]}{[weak\ acid]}$$

$$pOH = pK_b + \log\frac{[conjugate\ acid]}{[weak\ base]}$$

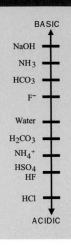

THE GAS PHASE

1 atm = 760 mm Hg = 760 torr

Do not confuse STP with standard conditions—the two standards involve different temperatures and are used for different purposes. STP (0°C or 273 K) is generally used for gas law calculations; standard conditions (25°C or 298 K) is used when measuring standard enthalpy, entropy, Gibbs free energy, and voltage.

Boyle's Law

$$PV = k \text{ or } P_1V_1 = P_2V_2$$

Law of Charles and Gay-Lussac

$$\frac{V}{T} = k \text{ or } \frac{V_1}{T_1} = \frac{V_2}{T_2}$$

Avagadro's Principle

$$\frac{n}{V} = k \text{ or } \frac{n_1}{V_1} = \frac{n_2}{V_2}$$

Ideal Gas Law

$$PV = nRT$$

Deviations due to Pressure: As the pressure of a gas increases, the particles are pushed closer and closer together. At moderately high pressure a gas' volume is less than would be predicted by the ideal gas law, due to intermolecular attraction.

Deviations due to Temperature: As the temperature of a gas decreases, the average velocity of the gas molecules decreases, and the attractive intermolecular forces become increasingly significant. As the temperature of a gas is reduced, intermolecular attraction causes the gas to have a smaller volume than would be predicted.

SOLUTIONS

Units of Concentration

$$\textbf{Percent Composition by Mass: } = \frac{\text{Mass of solute}}{\text{Mass of solution}} \times 100\ (\%)$$

$$\textbf{Mole Fraction: } \frac{\text{\# of mol of compound}}{\text{total \# of moles in system}}$$

$$\textbf{Molarity: } \frac{\text{\# of mol of solute}}{\text{liter of solution}}$$

$$\textbf{Molality: } \frac{\text{\# of mol of solute}}{\text{kg of solvent}}$$

$$\textbf{Normality: } \frac{\text{\# of gram equivalent weights of solute}}{\text{liter of solution}}$$

PHASES & PHASE CHANGES

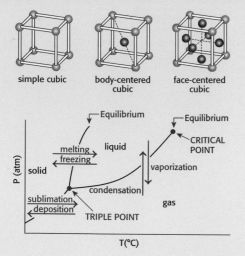

simple cubic   body-centered cubic   face-centered cubic

Colligative Properties: These are physical properties derived solely from the number of particles present, not the nature of those particles. These properties are usually associated with dilute solutions.

Freezing Point Depression

$$\Delta T_f = K_f m$$

Boiling Point Elevation

$$\Delta T_b = K_b m$$

Osmotic Pressure

$$\Pi = MRT$$

Vapor-pressure Lowering (Raoult's Law)

$$P_A = X_A P^\circ_A; \; P_B = X_B P^\circ_B$$

Solutions that obey Raoult's Law are called ideal solutions.

Graham's Law of Diffusion and Effusion

Diffusion: occurs when gas molecules diffuse through a mixture.

Effusion: is the flow of gas particles under pressure from one compartment to another through a small opening.

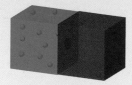

Effusion

Both diffusion and effusion have the same formula:

$$\frac{r_1}{r_2} = \left(\frac{MM_2}{MM_1}\right)^{\frac{1}{2}}$$

REDOX REACTIONS & ELECTROCHEMISTRY

Oxidation: loss of electrons

Reduction: gain of electrons

Oxidizing agent: causes another atom to undergo oxidation, and is itself reduced.

Reducing agent: causes another atom to be reduced, and is itself oxidized.

THERMOCHEMISTRY

Constant-volume and constant-pressure calorimetry: used to indicate conditions under which the heat changes are measured.

$q = mc\Delta T$, where q is the heat absorbed or released in a given process, m is the mass, c is the specific heat, and ΔT is the change in temperature.

States and State Functions: are described by the macroscopic properties of the system. These are properties whose magnitude depends only on the initial and final states of the system, and not on the path of the change.

Enthalpy (H): is used to express heat changes at constant pressure.

Standard Heat of Formation (ΔH°_f): the enthalpy change that would occur if one mole of a compound were formed directly from its elements in their standard states.

Standard Heat of Reaction (ΔH°_{rxn}): the hypothetical enthalpy change that would occur if the reaction were carried out under standard conditions.

$$\Delta H^\circ_{rxn} = (\text{sum of } \Delta H^\circ_{rxn} \text{ of products}) - (\text{sum of } \Delta H^\circ_{rxn} \text{ of reactants})$$

Hess's Law: states that enthalpies of reactions are additive.

The reverse of any reaction has an enthalpy of the same magnitude as that of the forward reaction, but its sign is opposite.

Bond Dissociation Energy: an average of the energy required to break a particular type of bond in one mole of gaseous molecules:

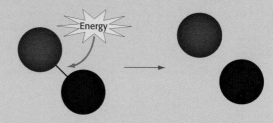

Entropy (S) the measure of the disorder, or randomness, of a system.

$$\Delta S_{universe} = \Delta S_{system} + \Delta S_{surroundings}$$

Gibbs Free Energy (G): combines the two factors which affect the spontaneity of a reaction—changes in enthalpy, ΔH, and changes in entropy, ΔS.

$$\Delta G = \Delta H - T\Delta S$$

if ΔG is negative, the rxn is spontaneous

if ΔG is positive, the rxn is not spontaneous

if ΔG is zero, the system is in a state of equilibrium; thus, $\Delta G = 0$ and $\Delta H = T\Delta S$

ΔH	ΔS	Outcome
−	+	Spontaneous at all temps.
+	−	Nonspontaneous at all temps.
+	+	Spontaneous only at high temps.
−	−	Spontaneous only at low temps.

Reaction Quotient (Q): Once a reaction commences, the standard state conditions no longer hold. For the reaction,

$$a A + b B \rightleftharpoons c C + d D$$

$$Q = \frac{[C]^c[D]^d}{[A]^a[B]^b}$$

DAT STUDY SHEET – ORGANIC CHEMISTRY

NOMENCLATURE

1. Find the longest carbon chain containing the principle functional group (highest priority groups are generally more oxidized).
2. Number the carbon chain so that the principle functional group gets lowest number (1).
3. Proceed to number the chain so that the lowest set of numbers is obtained for the substituents.
4. Name the substituents and assign each a number.
5. Complete the name by listing substituents in alphabetical order, place commas between numbers and dashes between numbers and words.

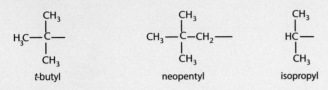

Functional Group	Suffix	Functional Group	Suffix
Carboxylic Acid	-oic acid	Ketone	-one
Ester	-oate	Thiol	-thiol
Acyl halide	-oyl halide	Alcohol	-ol
Amide	-amide	Amine	-amine
Nitrile/Cyanide	-nitrile	Imine	-imine
Aldehyde	-al	Ether	-ether

ISOMERS

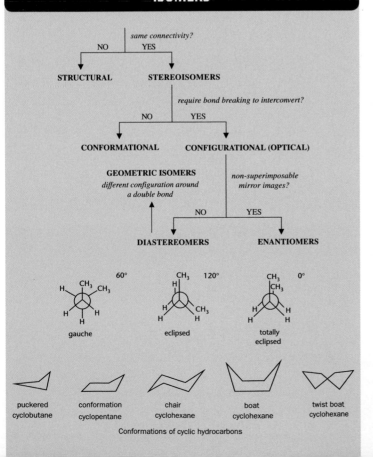

Conformations of cyclic hydrocarbons

BONDING

Bond order	single	double	triple
Bond type	sigma	sigma	sigma
		pi	2 pi
Hybridization	sp^3	sp^2	sp
Angles	109.5°	120°	180°
Example	C–C	C=C	C≡C

ALKANES

Free radical halogenation

- Initiation
- Propagation
- Termination

Combustion

$$C_3H_8 + 5O_2 \rightarrow 3CO_2 + 4H_2O + heat$$

Nucleophilicity and Basicity

$$RO^- > HO^- > RCO_2^- > ROH > H_2O$$

Nucleophilicity, size, and polarity

$$CN^- > I^- > RO^- > HO^- > Br > Cl^- > F^- > H_2O$$

Leaving groups (weak bases best)

$$I^- > Br^- > Cl^- > F^-$$

S_N1	S_N2
2 steps	1 step
Favored in polar protic solvents	Favored in polar aprotic solvents
3° > 2° > 1° > methyl	Methyl > 1° > 2° > 3°
Rate = k[RX]	Rate = k[Nu][RX]
Racemic products	Optically active and inverted products
Strong nucleophile not required	Favored with strong nucleophile

AMINO ACIDS, PEPTIDES, & PROTEINS

Amino acids have four substituents: amine group, carboxyl group, hydrogen, and R group. Amino acids are **amphoteric**—they can act as either acids or bases and often take the form of **zwitterions** (dipolar ions).

Structure

Primary: sequence of amino acids
Secondary: α-helix, β-pleated sheet
Tertiary: disulfide bridges, hydrophobic/hydrophilic interactions
Quaternary: arrangement of polypeptides

Henderson–Hasselbalch Equation

$$pH = pK_a + \log [conj.\ base]/[conj.\ acid]$$

ALKYNES

Alkynes have a terminal hydrogen that is appreciably more acidic than hydrogens on alkanes and alkenes.

Synthesis via double elimination of geminal or vicinal dihalide

Oxidation with $KMnO_4$, O_3

Reduction with Lindlar's Catalyst or liquid ammonia

Free radical addition

Electrophilic addition (anti orientation)

Hydroboration (cis alkene formed)

ALKENES

Cis isomers have higher boiling points than trans isomers due to their net dipole moment. Trans isomers have higher melting points than cis isomers due to more effective arrangement, more efficient packing.

Catalytic Reduction

Electrophilic Addition of HX

Electrophilic Addition of X_2

Electrophilic Addition of H_2O

Free Radical Addition (anti-Markovnikov)

Hydroboration (anti-Markovnikov, syn orientation)

Oxidation with $KMnO_4$

Oxidation with O_3

ALDEHYDES

The dipole moment of aldehydes causes an elevation of boiling point, but not as high as alcohols since there is no hydrogen bonding.

Synthesis

- Oxidation of primary alcohols
- Ozonolysis of alkenes
- Friedel–Crafts acylation

Reactions

Reactions of Enols (Michael additions)

Nucleophilic addition to a carbonyl

Aldol condensation

An aldehyde acts both as nucleophile (enol form) and target (keto form)

CARBOXYLIC ACIDS

Carboxylic acids have pKa's of around 4.5 due to resonance stabilization of the conjugate base. Electronegative atoms increase acidity with inductive effects. Boiling point is higher than alcohols because of the ability to form two hydrogen bonds.

Synthesis

Oxidation of primary alcohols with KMnO$_4$

Organometallic reagents with CO$_2$ (Grignard)

Hydrolysis of Nitriles

$$CH_3Cl \longrightarrow CH_3CN \longrightarrow CH_3COH + NH_4^+$$

Reactions

Formation of soap by reacting carboxylic acids with NaOH; arrange in micelles

nonpolar tail   polar head

Nucleophilic acyl substitution

Ester formation

Acyl halide formation

Reduction to alcohols

carboxylic acid

aldehyde

alcohol

ALCOHOLS

- Higher boiling points than alkanes
- Weakly acidic hydroxyl hydrogen

Synthesis

- Addition of water to double bonds
- S$_N$1 and S$_N$2 reactions
- Reduction of carboxylic acids, aldehydes, ketones and esters
  - aldehydes and ketones with NaBH$_4$
  - esters and carboxylic acids with LiAlH$_4$

Reactions

E1 dehydration reactions in strongly acidic solutions

minor
Hoffman product

major
Zaitsev product

Substitution reactions after protonation or leaving group conversion

tosyl chloride

Oxidation

- PCC takes a primary alcohol to an aldehyde

- Jones's reagent, KMnO$_4$, and alkali dichromate salts will convert secondary alcohols to ketones and primary alcohols to carboxylic acids

- Tertiary alcohols cannot be oxidized without breaking a carbon to carbon bond

Oxidation and reduction

Wittig Reaction

$$(C_6H_5)_3P + CH_3Br \longrightarrow (C_6H_5)_3\overset{+}{P}CH_3 + Br^-$$

phosphonium salt   ylide

CARBOXLIC ACID DERIVATIVES

Acyl halides

Nucleophilic acyl substitution

Friedel–Crafts acylation

Reduction

Anhydrides

Synthesis via reaction of carboxylic acid with an acid chloride

Hydrolysis
Conversion into esters and carboxylic acids
Addition of ammonia to form amides

Friedel–Crafts acylation

Amines & Nitrogen Containing Compounds

Amide   Carbamate   Imine   Enamine

Azide   Nitrile   Isocyanate

Direct alkylation of ammonia

$$CH_3Br + NH_3 \longrightarrow CH_3\overset{+}{N}H_3Br^- \xrightarrow{NaOH} CH_3NH_2 + NaBr + H_2O$$

Reduction from nitro compounds, nitriles, imines, and amides

$$CH_3CH_2C\equiv N \xrightarrow{LAH} CH_3CH_2CH_2NH_2$$

Exhaustive methylation (Hoffman elimination)

Gabriel Synthesis

Amides

Synthesis via reaction of acid chlorides with amines or acid anhydrides with ammonia
Hydrolysis
Hoffman rearrangement converts amides to primary amines

nitrene   isocyanate

Reduction with LAH

Esters

Synthesis via condensation of carboxylic acids and alcohols

Hydrolysis in acid or base
Conversion to amides

Transesterification
Grignard addition
Claisen Condensation

Reduction